Handbuch der experimentellen Pharmakologie

Vol. 44 Heffter-Heubner New Series

Handbook of Experimental Pharmacology

Heme and Hemoproteins

Contributors

K. W. Bock · F. De Matteis · G. H. Elder · L. G. Israels
G. S. Marks · J. D. Maxwell · U. A. Meyer · H. L. Rayner
H. Remmer · S. Sassa · B. A. Schacter · G. H. Tait
T. R. Tephly · D. P. Tschudy

Editors

Francesco De Matteis
W. Norman Aldridge

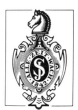

Springer-Verlag Berlin Heidelberg New York 1978

Dr. Francesco De Matteis
Dr. W. Norman Aldridge

Medical Research Council Labs., MRC Toxicology Unit, Woodmansterne Road, Carshalton, Surrey SM5 4EF, Great Britain

With 60 Figures

ISBN 3-540-08460-6 Springer-Verlag Berlin Heidelberg New York
ISBN 0-387-08460-6 Springer-Verlag New York Heidelberg Berlin

Library of Congress Cataloging in Publication Data. Main entry under title: Heme and hemoproteins. (Handbuch der experimentellen Pharmakologie: New series; v. 44). Bibliography: p. Includes index. 1. Porphyria—Etiology. 2. Heme. 3. Hemoproteins. 4. Drugs—Toxicology. I. Bock, Karl Walter. II. De Matteis, Francesco, 1932–. III. Aldridge, W. N. IV. Series. QP905.H3 vol. 44 [RC632.P6] 615′.1′08s 77-13134 [615′.39]

Typesetting, printing, and bookbinding: Universitätsdruckerei H. Stürtz AG, Würzburg
2122/3130-543210

Preface

The study of the biological effects of foreign chemicals (whether therapeutic drugs or chemicals present at work or in the environment) interests the biologist from a number of different and complementary viewpoints. Apart from the more obvious pharmacological and toxicological interest, the experimentalist often uses foreign chemicals to produce in experimental animals disease states similar to naturally occurring diseases, so that their pathogenetic mechanisms and therapy can be studied under controlled conditions. In addition — as Claude Bernard pointed out over a century ago — foreign chemicals can be employed as instruments to analyze the most delicate vital processes; much can be learned about the physiological processes themselves by a careful study of the mechanisms by which these are altered by chemicals.

The field of heme and hemoproteins offers an example of the interplay of these different approaches. Their metabolism can be altered by therapeutic drugs and other foreign chemicals and this results in a variety of biological responses that transcend the boundaries of pharmacology into the confines of clinical medicine, genetics, toxicology, biochemistry and physiology.

In this book a multidisciplinary approach to the study of heme metabolism is presented including the effect of chemicals on heme metabolism in patients, the results of experimental work in the whole animal, as well as in vitro studies. The major emphasis throughout is intended to be on the mechanisms by which drugs and foreign chemicals disturb heme metabolism, considering whenever possible the molecular events which are involved in the light of the information obtained from different approaches. Our intention has been to provide a critical assessment of the present state of knowledge (rather than a complete coverage of the literature) according to the various authors' current work and experience; to indicate areas of uncertainty where further work is required and to put forward interpretation and hypothesis which will stimulate further experiments.

Carshalton, Surrey

F. DE MATTEIS
W. N. ALDRIDGE

Table of Contents

CHAPTER 1

The Biosynthesis and Degradation of Heme. George H. Tait. With 6 Figures

A. Introduction 1
B. Structures of Porphyrins and Hemes 2
C. Function and Turnover of Hemoproteins 3
D. Enzymes of Heme Biosynthesis and Degradation 6
    I. Outline of Pathway 6
    II. Aminolevulinate Synthetase (E.C. 2.3.1.37) 8
    III. Aminolevulinate Dehydratase (E.C. 4.2.1.24) 12
    IV. Porphobilinogen Deaminase (E.C. 4.3.1.8) and Uroporphyrinogen III
        Cosynthetase 14
    V. Uroporphyrinogen Decarboxylase (E.C. 4.1.1.37) 18
    VI. Coproporphyrinogen Oxidase (E.C. 1.3.3.3) 19
    VII. Protoporphyrinogen Oxidase 21
    VIII. Heme Synthetase (E.C. 4.99.1.1) 21
    IX. Heme Oxygenase (E.C. 1.14.99.3) 23
    X. Biliverdin Reductase (E.C. 1.3.1.24) 25
E. Conjugation of Bilirubin 26
F. Control of Heme and Hemoprotein Biosynthesis 28
    I. Introduction 28
    II. Control in Erythropoietic Cells 29
    III. Control in Liver 31
Abbreviations 35
References 35

CHAPTER 2

Induction of Hepatic Hemoproteins. K.W. Bock and H. Remmer. With 6 Figures

A. Introduction 49
B. Use of the Term Induction in Studies on Mammalian Tissues 50
C. Tryptophan Pyrrolase (Dioxygenase) 52
D. Cytochromes of the Endoplasmic Reticulum 53
    I. Cytochrome(s) P-450 53
        1. Cytochrome P-450-Dependent Monooxygenase(s) 53
        2. Chemical Inducers 55
        3. Cytochrome P-450, One Hemoprotein or Many? 58

4. Studies on the Induction Mechanism of Cytochrome P-450 . . . 59
5. Factors Influencing the Induction of Cytochrome P-450 61
    a) Species Differences, Genetic Factors 61
    b) Developmental Factors 62
    c) Hormonal Factors 62
    d) Nutritional Factors 62
6. Connection Between the Induction of Cytochrome P-450 Dependent Monooxygenase(s) and Other Effects of Inducing Agents . 63
    a) Induction of Microsomal Enzymes and the Proliferation of
       Endoplasmic Reticulum Membranes 63
    b) General Cell Changes Induced by Treatment with Pheno-
       burbital 64
    c) Liver Growth 65
7. Reversibility of Induction Phenomena 65
    II. Cytochrome b_5 66
E. Catalase 67
F. Mitochondrial Cytochromes 68
G. Summary of Conclusions 69

Recommended Reviews 70

References 70

CHAPTER 3

Inhibition of Liver Hemoprotein Synthesis. THOMAS R. TEPHLY. With 2 Figures

A. Introduction 81
B. Agents Inhibiting Heme Biosynthesis and Hepatic Hemoprotein Synthesis 82
    I. 3-Amino-1, 2, 4-triazole 82
    II. The Effect of Metals on Heme Biosynthesis 84
       1. The Inhibition of Liver Heme Synthesis by Cobalt 84
       2. Effect of Manganese and Cadmium 88
    III. Role of Agents Which Affect the Availability of Glycine 89
    IV. Effect of Acetate on Heme Biosynthesis 90
C. Conclusions 91
Abbreviations 91
References 92

CHAPTER 4

Loss of Liver Cytochrome P-450 Caused by Chemicals. Damage to the Apoprotein and Degradation of the Heme Moiety. F. DE MATTEIS. With 7 Figures

A. Introduction 95
B. Loss of Liver Cytochrome P-450 Caused by Chemicals Which Require
   Metabolic Conversion to Reactive Derivatives 96

    I. 2-Allyl-2-isopropylacetamide and Related Drugs   97
       1. Loss of Pre-existing Cytochrome P-450   97
       2. Conversion of Heme into Unidentified "Green Pigments". . . .   98
       3. Importance of the Allyl Group and Role of the Drug-Metabolizing
          Activity of the Liver 102
       4. Possible Mechanisms Underlying the Loss of Heme 104
   II. Carbon Disulphide and Other Sulphur-Containing Chemicals . . . 104
       1. Oxidative Desulphuration of CS_2 105
       2. Loss of Cytochrome P-450 During Oxidative Desulphuration of
          Parathion and of Other Sulphur-Containing Chemicals. Liver
          Toxicity of Phosphorothionates 107
       3. Possible Mechanisms Underlying the Loss of Cytochrome P-450
          Caused by Sulphur-Containing Chemicals. Nature of the Primary
          Target Within the Hemoprotein 108
  III. Loss of Cytochrome P-450 Heme Caused by Carbon Tetrachloride
       in Rat Liver 109
 C. Increased Breakdown of the Heme of Liver Cytochrome P-450 Associated
    with Lipid Peroxidation 110
    I. Lipid Peroxidation in vitro 110
   II. Lipid Peroxidation in vivo 111
  III. Mechanisms Underlying the Production and Decomposition of Lipid
       Peroxides and the Associated Destruction of Heme 112
 D. Loss of Liver Cytochrome P-450 Caused by the Administration of Various
    Metals 115
    I. Increased Rate of Liver Heme Turnover and Stimulation of Heme
       Oxygenase 115
   II. Other Experimental Conditions Where Stimulation of Heme Oxygen-
       ase is Seen in Association with Decreased Levels of Cytochrome
       P-450 117
  III. Possible Mechanisms by Which Loss of Cytochrome P-450 and Stimu-
       lation of Heme Oxygenase may be Related 117
       1. The Heme of Cytochrome P-450 as an Inducer for Heme
          Oxygenase 118
       2. The Heme of Cytochrome P-450 as a Substrate for Heme
          Oxygenase 121
Abbreviations 121
References 121

CHAPTER 5

Hepatic Porphyrias Caused by 2-Allyl-2-isopropylacetamide, 3,5-Diethoxycarbonyl-1,4-dihydrocollidine, Griseofulvin and Related Compounds. F. DE MATTEIS. With 7 Figures

A. Introduction 129
   I. The Concept of Porphyria 129
  II. Drugs and Liver Porphyrin Metabolism: Two Types of Interaction . 129
 III. The Induction of Porphyria by Drugs in the Normal Liver 130

B. The Mechanism of Induction of Porphyria by Drugs 132
   I. Stimulation of 5-Aminoevulinate Synthetase (ALA-S). 132
      1. Interference by Drugs with the Regulation of the Pathway
         Through Loss of Liver Heme. The "Specific" Effect 133
         a) Increased Destruction of Liver Heme Caused by Allyl-Con-
            taining Acetamides and Barbiturates 134
         b) Inhibition of Liver Heme Synthesis Caused by DDC and
            Griseofulvin 135
         c) Requirement for Specific Chemical Structures 138
         d) Heme Pools Depleted in Porphyria. Importance of Heme with
            Rapid Turnover 140
      2. The Action Related to the Property of Lipid Solubility of Drugs.
         The Nonspecific Effect in the Stimulation of ALA-S. 143
         a) Drug Interactions in Experimental Porphyria 143
         b) Possible Mechanisms Underlying the Nonspecific Effect. . . 145
      3. Possible Role of Drug Metabolism and of Protein Synthesis in
         the Stimulation of ALA-S Caused by Drugs 146
Abbreviations 150
References 150

CHAPTER 6

Porphyria Caused by Hexachlorobenzene and Other Polyhalogenated Aromatic Hydrocarbons. G.H. ELDER. With 5 Figures

A. Introduction 157
B. Properties and Metabolism of Porphyrogenic Polyhalogenated Aromatic
   Hydrocarbons 159
   I. Chemistry and Nomenclature 159
   II. Absorption, Distribution in the Body, Metabolism and Excretion . 160
      1. Hexachlorobenzene 160
         a) Absorption and Distribution 160
         b) Metabolism and Excretion 161
      2. Other Porphyrogenic Polychlorinated Aromatic Hydrocarbons . 161
C. Porphyria Caused by Hexachlorobenzene and Other Halogenated Aromatic
   Hydrocarbons 162
   I. Hexachlorobenzene 162
      1. HCB Porphyria in Man 162
         a) Clinical Features 163
         b) Biochemical Features 164
         c) Porphyria due to Occupational Exposure to HCB 167
      2. HCB Porphyria in the Rat 167
         a) General Features 167
         b) Porphyrins in Urine, Faeces and Tissues 169
         c) Factors Influencing the Porphyrogenic Action of HCB in Rats 170

      3. HCB Porphyria in Other Species 171
        a) Mammals 171
        b) Birds 171
    II. Other Polyhalogenated Aromatic Hydrocarbons 172
      1. Polyhalogenated Biphenyls 172
      2. Porphyria Associated with the Manufacture of Chlorinated
        Phenols: TCDD 173
        a) Porphyria in Herbicide Factories 173
        b) TCDD 174
      3. Other Halogenated Aromatic Compounds 175
  III. Conclusion 176
D. The Effect of Polyhalogenated Aromatic Hydrocarbons on Heme
Metabolism in the Liver 176
    I. Effect on Hemoproteins in the Liver 177
      1. Microsomal Hemoproteins 177
      2. Other Hemoproteins 179
    II. Effect on Enzymes of the Heme Biosynthetic Pathway 180
      1. 5-Aminolaevulinate Synthetase (ALA-S) 180
      2. Uroporphyrinogen Decarboxylase (UROG-D) 181
      3. Coproporphyrinogen Oxidase (CPG-OX) 184
      4. Other Enzymes 185
      5. Conclusion 185
E. The Mechanism of the Porphyrogenic Action of Polyhalogenated Aromatic
Hydrocarbons 186
    I. The Mechanism of the Delayed Response to the Porphyrogenic
    Action of Polyhalogenated Aromatic Hydrocarbons 187
    II. The Relationship Between Porphyria and Morphological Changes
    in the Liver 187
   III. Inhibition of UROG-D by Porphyrogenic Compounds or Their Meta-
    bolites 189
   IV. The Role of Iron in the Production of Porphyria 190
F. General Conclusions 192
Abbreviations 193
References 193

CHAPTER 7

The Effect of Chemicals on Hepatic Heme Biosynthesis. Differences in Response to Porphyrin-Inducing Chemicals Between Chick Embryo Liver Cells, the 17-Day-Old Chick Embryo and Other Species. GERALD S. MARKS. With 15 Figures

A. Introduction 201
B. Porphyrin Induction in Chick Embryo Liver Cells 201
    1. Structure-Activity Relationships 201
    2. Pattern of Porphyrin Accumulation 209
    3. Mechanism of Action of Porphyrin-Inducing Drugs 212

C. Porphyrin Induction in 17-Day-Old Chick Embryos 217
D. Porphyrin Induction in Chickens and Japanese Quail 222
E. Differences in Response to Porphyrin-Inducing Drugs in Different Species
and Model Test Systems 222
    1. Comparison of Response in Chick Embryo and Rat Liver Cells
       in Culture 222
    2. Comparison of Response in Chick Embryo Liver Cells in Culture
       with the Response of the 17-Day-Old Chick Embryo 223
    3. Comparison of Responsiveness of 17-Day-Old Chick Embryo and
       the Chicken 223
    4. Comparison of Responsiveness of Avian and Mammalian Species 223
    5. Extrapolation of Results from Animal and Model Test Systems
       to Man 229
Abbreviations 233
References 233

CHAPTER 8

Pharmacogenetics in the Field of Heme Metabolism: Drug Sensitivity in Hereditary Hepatic Porphyria. J. DOUGLAS MAXWELL and URS A. MEYER. With 7 Figures

A. Hereditary Hepatic Porphyrias 239
   I. Enzyme Defects in the Hepatic Porphyrias 240
    1. Intermittent Acute Porphyria (IAP) 241
    2. Hereditary Coproporphyria (HCP) 241
    3. Variegate Porphyria (VP) 242
    4. Porphyria Cutanea Tarda (PCT) 242
   II. Biochemical Basis for Clinical Features in the Hepatic Porphyrias . 242
B. Precipitation of Hereditary Hepatic Porphyria by Drugs 243
C. Experimental Models for the Exacerbation of Hereditary Hepatic Porphyria
by Drugs 245
D. Common Basis for Induction of Hepatic ALA-Synthetase in Clinical and
Experimental Porphyria 249
References 252

CHAPTER 9

The Influence of Hormonal and Nutritional Factors on the Regulation of Liver Heme Biosynthesis. DONALD P. TSCHUDY

A. Introduction 255
B. The Influence of Nutritional Factors 255
   I. Carbohydrates and Protein 255
    1. The "Glucose Effect" in Experimental Porphyria 255

      2. The "Glucose Effect" in Human Hepatic Porphyria 256
      3. Possible Mechanisms Underlying the "Glucose Effect" 257
    II. Other Dietary Factors 263
C. The Influence of Hormonal Factors 264
References 267

CHAPTER 10

Effects of Drugs on Bilirubin Metabolism. H.L. RAYNER, B.A. SCHACTER, and L.G. ISRAELS

Definition of Certain Abnormalities of Bilirubin Metabolism 273
A. Introduction 273
B. Normal Bilirubin Metabolism 274
    I. Sources of Bilirubin 274
    II. Enzymatic Degradation of Heme 275
    III. Albumin Binding of Bilirubin 276
    IV. Hepatocellular Uptake 277
    V. Intracellular Binding 277
    VI. Conjugation of Bilirubin 278
    VII. Excretion to Bile 279
    VIII. Intestinal Fate of Bilirubin 280
C. Drug-Mediated Alterations in Bilirubin Metabolism 280
    I. Increased Bilirubin Production Due to Erythrocyte Destruction . . 280
      1. Hemolysis Related to Impaired Erythrocyte Metabolism . . . 281
      2. Hemolysis and Unstable Hemoglobins 282
      3. Drug-Induced Immune Hemolysis 282
    II. Effect of Drugs on Hepatic Hemoprotein Turnover 283
      1. Drugs and Bilirubin Production 284
      2. Drugs and Heme Oxygenase 286
      3. Heme Catabolism in Drug-Induced Porphyria 287
    III. Drugs and Protein Binding of Bilirubin 288
      Binding Capacity of Neonatal Albumin 290
    IV. Drugs and the Hepatocellular Uptake and Storage of Bilirubin . . 291
      1. Interference with Transport of Bilirubin Across Membranes . . 291
      2. Interference with Cytoplasmic Binding of Bilirubin 292
      3. Drug-Mediated Increases in Bilirubin Uptake and Storage . . . 293
    V. Drugs and the Glucuronyl Transferases 293
      1. Glucuronyl Transferase Assay Techniques 294
      2. Glucuronyl Transferase Induction 295
        a) Phenobarbital 295
        b) Glutethimide 297
        c) Antipyrine 297
        d) Dicophane (DDT) 298
        e) Clofibrate 298
        f) Other Agents 298
        g) GT Induction in Animals 299

3. Glucuronyl Transferase Inhibition. 299
   a) Novobiocin 300
   b) Vitamin K 300
   c) Other Agents 300
   d) GT Inhibition in Intact Cells 301
4. Alterations in UDP-Glucuronic Acid Availability 301
VI. Drugs and the Biliary Excretion of Bilirubin. 302
1. Drugs Increasing Bilirubin Excretion 303
2. Drugs Decreasing Bilirubin Excretion 303
3. Cholestasis Due to Drugs 303
4. Phenobarbital Therapy of Cholestasis 305
VII. Drugs and Bilirubin in the Intestine 305
VIII. Alternate Paths of Bilirubin Excretion 306
IX. Bilirubin Photodegradation 306
Abbreviations 309
References 309

CHAPTER 11

Toxic Effects of Lead, with Particular Reference to Porphyrin and Heme Metabolism. SHIGERU SASSA. With 5 Figures

A. Biosynthesis of Heme 333
I. Conversion of ALA to Porphobilinogen (PBG) 333
II. Conversion of PBG to Uroporphyrinogen III 334
III. Formation of Protoporphyrin IX. 335
IV. Formation of Heme 335
B. Effect of Lead on the Heme Biosynthetic Pathway. 336
I. Inhibition of ALA-Dehydratase (ALA-D) Activity 336
1. Assay of ALA-D Activity 338
2. Inhibition Kinetics 339
3. Genetic Factors Which Affect ALA-D Levels. 340
4. Erythrocyte GSH Concentration in Lead Poisoning 340
II. Inhibition of Ferrochelatase 341
1. Assay of Erythrocyte Proporphyrin 342
2. Increased Protoporphyrin is Chelated with Zinc. 344
III. Effects of Lead on ALA-Synthetase 345
IV. Effects on Other Enzymes of the Heme Biosynthetic Pathway . . . 345
V. Effect of Lead on Heme Degradation 346
C. Toxic Effects of Exposure to Lead 346
I. Effect on the Red Blood Cells 346
1. Distribution of Lead Between Red Cells and Plasma. 346
2. Effect of Lead on Globin Synthesis 347
3. Fast Hemoglobin 347
4. Basophilic Stippling of Erythrocytes in Lead Poisoning 348
5. Effects of Lead on Mitochondria 348
6. Anemia in Lead Poisoning 349

   II. Lead Effect on the Immune System 351
  III. Drug Metabolizing System 351
   IV. Lead Neuropathy 352
       1. Encephalopathy 352
       2. Neuropathy in Lead Poisoning and in Acute Intermittent Porphy-
          ria 353
    V. Lead Effects on the Kidney 354
   VI. Tumorigenic and Teratogenic Effects of Lead 355
D. Biological Defense Mechanisms Against Lead 356
E. Factors Affecting the Toxic Effects of Lead 356
    I. Alcohol 356
   II. Sickle Cell Anemia 357
  III. Diet 357
   IV. Iron Deficiency 358
F. Diagnosis of Lead Poisoning 358
G. Summary 360
Abbreviations 361
References 361

Author Index 373
Subject Index 425

B. Structures of Porphyrins and Hemes

Porphyrins are cyclic tetrapyrroles in which the pyrrole rings are linked through their α-carbon atoms by methene bridges. As shown in Figure 1 for the compound porphin, the pyrrole rings are conventionally designated as A, B, C, and D, their β-carbon atoms are numbered 1–8, and the methene bridge carbon atoms are labeled α, β, γ, and δ (FALK, 1964; GAJDOS and GAJDOS-TÖRÖK, 1969a). The porphyrins which occur in nature all have side chains on the β-carbon atoms of the pyrrole rings. Uroporphyrin has an acetic acid (carboxymethyl) and a propionic acid (2-carboxyethyl) side chain on each ring (Fig. 2), and coproporphyrin has a methyl and a propionic acid side chain on each ring. Thus, there are four isomers of each of these porphyrins. In isomer I, the side chains are arranged symmetrically around the ring; in isomer II, the substituents on rings B and D are reversed with respect to those on ring A; in isomer III, the substituents on ring D are reversed; and in isomer IV, the substituents on rings B and C are reversed. Only the I and III isomers of uroporphyrin (Fig. 2) and coproporphyrin occur in nature, and hemes, chlorophylls, and the corrin ring of vitamin B_{12} all have the III isomer structure. Protoporphyrin IX (Fig. 3), the other important porphyrin in nature, has both methyl and vinyl groups on rings A and B, and both methyl and pro-

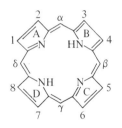

Fig. 1. Structure of porphin

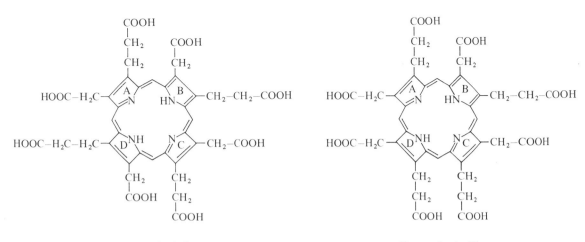

Uroporphyrin I   Uroporphyrin III

Fig. 2. Structures of uroporphyrin I and uroporphyrin III

pionic acid side chains on rings C and D. It is the only one of the 15 isomers to occur naturally.

Porphyrins are aromatic molecules and they have characteristic, strong absorption bands in the near ultraviolet and visible regions of the spectrum, and they also exhibit bright red fluorescence when exposed to ultraviolet light (FALK, 1964; GRANICK and MAUZERALL, 1961). These properties make it easy to detect trace amounts of porphyrins in biological samples, to follow their extraction and purification, and to identify them. Porphyrins can be reduced to the colorless, nonfluorescent hexahydroporphyrins (porphyrinogens). The most useful reducing agents are sodium amalgam (MAUZERALL and GRANICK, 1958) and sodium borohydride (see TAIT, 1972). Porphyrinogens are unstable and are very readily reoxidised to porphyrins by oxygen or light. Uroporphyrinogen III, coproporphyrinogen III and protoporphyrinogen IX, and not uroporphyrin and coproporphyrin, are the biosynthetic intermediates in the enzymic formation of protoporphyrin, while protoporphyrin is utilized in the synthesis of heme (MAUZERALL and GRANICK, 1958).

Free porphyrins normally occur in nature in only small amounts, instead, most of the porphyrin occurs as metal complexes. In animals the most important complex is between iron and protoporphyrin. The ferrous and ferric complexes are usually called protoheme and protohemin respectively; in a biological context, this is usually abbreviated to heme and hemin. Protohem(in) plays its functions as the prosthetic group of proteins to which it can be attached in one of two ways. In most of the hemoproteins—hemoglobin, myoglobin, catalase, peroxidase, tryptophan pyrrolase, cytochrome P-450, and cytochromes b, the protoheme is attached to the protein noncovalently by coordination between its iron atom and nitrogen atoms of the amino acid side chains. In cytochromes c, however, it is attached to the protein covalently by thioether bonds formed between the two vinyl groups of the heme and two cysteinyl residues in the protein. In cytochromes a, the noncovalently bound prosthetic group is heme a, a heme biosynthesized from protoheme (KIESE et al., 1958), which contains a formyl instead of a methyl group at position 8, and in which the vinyl group at position 2 in protohem is alkylated with a farnesyl residue (GRASSL et al., 1963 a, b). (For a further discussion of the nomenclature of porphyrins and hemoproteins see MARKS, 1969).

C. Function and Turnover of Hemoproteins

Although the exact mechanisms of intracellular protein breakdown are not yet known (GOLDBERG et al., 1974), it is clear that most proteins are continuously turning over at rapid, though different, rates (SCHIMKE, 1973). The methods which can be used to determine the half-lives of individual proteins have been discussed in recent reviews by SCHIMKE and DOYLE (1970), and SCHIMKE (1973). The loss of enzyme activity, or of protein reacting with specific antibody, can be measured at various times after giving animals inhibitors of protein synthesis. Methods based on loss of enzyme activity, which are the only ones that can be applied to proteins that cannot yet be purified, assume that this loss parallels destruction of the enzyme. This assumption is not valid for all enzymes, some of whose activities increase or decrease markedly for other reasons (HOLZER, 1969). These methods also assume that inhibition of synthesis of a protein does not affect its rate of destruction, an assumption which also does not hold for all proteins (SCHIMKE, 1973; KANAI et al., 1974). A more reliable measure of half-life can be obtained by injecting a radioactive amino acid into animals, killing them at various times thereafter, and measuring the rate of loss of radioactivity from the purified protein. For this method to give a true measure of the half-life, the radioactive amino acid once released from the protein molecule must not be reincorporated into protein. [^{14}C]-Leucine, which has been used in a number of studies, has been shown by POOLE (1971) to be extensively reused, thus giving falsely high half-lives for some proteins. Arginine labeled in the guanido group gives more reliable values since, in liver at least, the guanido group is rapidly converted to urea (IP et al., 1974). These workers have also used [^{14}C]-carbonate and measured the radioactivity in the arginyl residues of the purified protein.

The half-lives of hemoproteins or, more accurately, of their heme groups, can be measured using radioactive aminolevulinic acid (ALA) which is incorporated specifically into the heme moieties (DALY et al., 1967; DRUYAN et al., 1969); when the hemoprotein is degraded, the heme is not reutilized. By using tritiated aminolevulinic acid and [^{14}C]-amino acid in the same experiment, the half-lives of the heme and the protein moieties can be measured (see DRUYAN et al., 1969).

A detailed discussion of the functions of hemoproteins is outside the scope of this review. Hemoproteins can be classified into five groups (see GRANICK and GILDER, 1947); those which transport oxygen—hemoglobin and myoglobin; those which transport electrons—mitochondrial cytochromes; those which activate oxygen—cytochrome oxidase, tryptophan pyrrolase, cytochrome P-450; those which activate hydrogen peroxide—peroxidases; and those which decompose hydrogen peroxide—catalases. Except for hemoglobin, which is present only in erythrocytes and their precursors, and myoglobin, which is confined to muscle, the other hemoproteins are present in most mammalian cells. The cytochromes of the inner mitochondrial membrane function as part of the electron transport chain transferring reducing equivalents from NADH and succinate to oxygen, and producing energy in the process. Cytochromes b$_5$ and P-450 are components of microsomal electron transport chains. In liver, cytochrome b$_5$ seems to be involved in NADH-dependent desaturation of fatty acids. Cytochrome P-450 functions in a separate pathway, which may also include cytochrome b$_5$, to catalyze the NADPH-dependent hydroxylation of steroids, drugs, and other foreign compounds (LU et al., 1974). There seem to be at least three species of cytochrome P-450 in liver microsomes which differ in their molecular weights, their substrate specificities, and their inducibility by different compounds (COMAI and GAYLOR, 1973; WELTON and AUST, 1974). In some tissues, but not in liver, cytochrome P-450 is also present in mitochondria; i.e. bovine adrenal cortex (HARDING et al., 1964), rat ovary (COOPER and THOMAS, 1970), human placenta (MEIGS and RYAN, 1968) and chick kidney (GHAZARIAN et al., 1974). Catalase, which occurs in the peroxisomes (see LAZAROW and DE DUVE, 1973a), is also present in most tissues, with erythrocytes and liver having the highest activites (HARTZ et al., 1973). It decomposes hydrogen peroxide which is generated during mitochondrial aerobic metabolism (BOVERIS and CHANCE, 1973).

Hemoglobin and myoglobin are the two major hemoproteins in mammals; in normal man (70 kg body weight) there is about $500-700$ g of the former and $35-200$ g of the latter (see BERK et al., 1974a). Hemoglobin, unlike most other cellular proteins, is stable and, once synthesized, remains in the erythrocyte for the whole of its life of 120 days in man, sheep, and dog (LONDON, 1961), and about 60 days in the rat (ÅKESON et al., 1960). Myoglobin appears to turn over very slowly (DALY et al., 1967). The other hemoproteins—cytochromes, catalase, tryptophan pyrrolase—contain only a small percentage of the total heme in the body, but they turn over rapidly. Values reported in the literature for the concentrations and half-lives of hemoproteins of rat liver have been tabulated by MEYER and MARVER (1971a), MARVER and SCHMID (1972) and NICHOLLS and ELLIOTT (1974). In rat liver, the total content of heme is 70 nmoles/g wet weight, of which 43% is in mitochondrial cytochromes, 32% in cytochrome P-450, 17% in cytochrome b_5, and 7% in catalase (MEYER and MARVER, 1971a). The half-lives of rat liver hemoproteins are, $5.5-6$ days for mitochondrial cytochromes b, c and a; 4.4 days for mitochondrial cytochrome b_5; and 2.3 days for microsomal cytochrome b_5 (DRUYAN et al., 1969; ASCHENBRENNER et al., 1970; IP et al., 1974). The heme and protein moieties of the individual hemoproteins turn over at the same rate. Liver cytochrome P-450 shows a biphasic decay curve. The larger fraction turns over with a half-life of $7-10$ h and the smaller fraction with a half-life of $24-48$ h (LEVIN and KUNTZMAN, 1969; MEYER and MARVER, 1971b). Catalase has a half-life of 67.2 h (KANAI et al., 1974), and tryptophan pyrrolase one of 2.3 h (FEIGELSON et al., 1959). From the known concentrations and half-lives, MEYER and MARVER (1971a) and MARVER and SCHMID (1972) have calculated that rat liver has to make about 20 nmol of aminolevulinic acid (ALA)/h/g wet weight, and that 70% of this is required for incorporation into the heme of cytochrome P-450.

LONDON et al. (1950) and GRAY et al. (1950) gave ^{15}N-glycine to humans, and followed incorporation of label into fecal stercobilin. They found a peak of label, accounting for about 70% of the total, appearing at 120 days, and in addition a smaller peak, accounting for $15-20\%$ of the total, in the first week after giving ^{15}N-glycine. The major peak was clearly from the breakdown of erythrocyte hemoglobin, but the origin of the early peak was not known. Later $[^{14}C]$-glycine and $[^{14}C]$-ALA (which does not get incorporated into hemoglobin) were used and the radioactivity in serum or biliary bilirubin was measured (see YAMAMOTO et al., 1965; LEVITT et al., 1968). With $[^{14}C]$-glycine, there were two peaks of radioactivity, one at $12-24$ h and the other at $3-5$ days. With $[^{14}C]$-ALA there was only one peak of radioactivity at $1-6$ h. These results suggested that the radioactive bilirubin formed in the first 24 h was from breakdown of hepatic heme. This very early peak of labeled bilirubin also appeared to consist of two components; the first, which became radioactive within minutes of giving the radioactive precursor, from the breakdown of "free" hepatic heme, and the second from turnover of hepatic hemoproteins. Normally, all or almost all the heme in the body is converted by enzymes to equimolar amounts of bilirubin and carbon monoxide (LANDAW et al., 1970; BERK et al., 1974b). However, compounds such as allylisopropylacetamide cause the conversion of hepatic heme to unknown green pigments (LANDAW et al., 1970).

The early work, referred to above, had indicated that about 15−20% of the bilirubin formed per day was derived from hepatic heme. Direct measurement on patients with acute intermittent porphyria showed that of the 5−8 μmol total bilirubin formed/day/kg body weight, 0.7−1.7 μmol, or 13−21%, was produced by the liver (JONES et al., 1971). In normal individuals, the values are probably the same (see BERK et al., 1974b). From these results it can be calculated that the liver (weight 1.5 kg) of normal man (weight 70 kg) makes 1.5−3 nmol heme or 12−24 nmol ALA/h/g liver.

D. Enzymes of Heme Biosynthesis and Degradation

I. Outline of Pathway

The steps in the pathway are outlined in Figure 3.

Condensation of glycine and succinyl CoA to form aminolevulinic acid (ALA) is catalyzed by ALA synthetase, a mitochondrial enzyme that requires pyridoxal phosphate. ALA then passes into the cytoplasm where ALA dehydratase catalyzes the condensation of two molecules of ALA to form the pyrrole porphobilinogen (PBG). Two cytoplasmic proteins, PBG deaminase and uroporphyrinogen III cosynthetase, acting in unison, convert four molecules of PBG to uroporphyrinogen III. In this isomer, one of the PBG molecules, conventionally ring D, is inserted into the macrocycle the wrong way round. PBG deaminase acting on its own converts PBG to the symmetrical isomer uroporphyrinogen I. Another cytoplasmic enzyme, uroporphyrinogen decarboxylase, converts the four acetic acid side chains to methyl groups to give coproporphyrinogen III. The remaining steps in heme biosynthesis occur in the mitochondrion. Coproporphyrinogen oxidase oxidatively decarboxylates the two propionic acid side chains on rings A and B to vinyl groups, giving protoporphyrinogen IX, from which six hydrogen atoms are removed enzymically to yield protoporphyrin IX. Fe^{2+} is then inserted by heme synthetase, forming protoheme. Heme is incorporated into the hemoproteins of the cell. When these hemoproteins are degraded and the heme is released, it is cleaved at the α-methene bridge carbon atom by microsomal heme oxygenase to biliverdin IXα and carbon monoxide. The biliverdin is then reduced to bilirubin IXα by the cytoplasmic biliverdin reductase. Most cells in the body can perform all these enzymic reactions; however, as far as we know the liver is the major, if not the only, site of bilirubin metabolism. Bilirubin is transported from its sites of formation to the liver where the carboxyl groups on the propionic acid side chains are conjugated with glucuronic acid, glucose, xylose, etc. The conjugated compounds are then excreted in the bile, and then into the gut where additional modifications, which need not concern us here, are performed by gut bacteria.

The activities of the enzymes of heme biosynthesis and degradation are expressed by different authors in a number of ways, making comparison difficult. Rat liver, which has been used in many of the studies, contains, per gram wet weight, about 200 mg of total protein, 30 mg of nuclear protein, 50 mg each of mitochondrial and microsomal protein, and 70 mg of soluble protein (KRISHNAKANTHA and KURUP, 1972; SCHNEIDER, 1963; FLEISCHMANN et al., 1975).

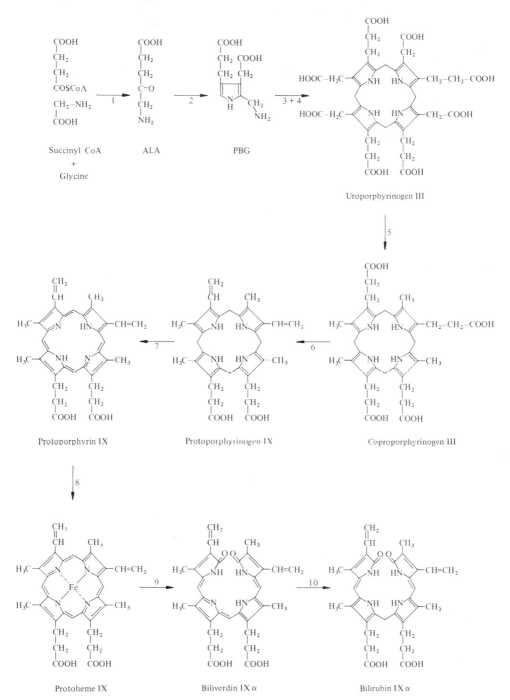

Fig. 3. Biosynthesis and degradation of heme. Enzymes catalyzing the interconversions are: 1. ALA synthetase. 2. ALA dehydratase. 3. PBG deaminase. 4. Uroporphyrinogen III cosynthetase. 5. Uroporphyrinogen decarboxylase. 6. Coproporphyrinogen oxidase. 7. Protoporphyrinogen oxidase. 8. Heme synthetase. 9. Heme oxygenase. 10. Biliverdin reductase

II. Aminolevulinate Synthetase (E.C. 2.3.1.37)

All the evidence to date is consistent with the formation of ALA from succinyl CoA and glycine, catalyzed by ALA synthetase, being the rate-limiting step in heme biosynthesis in mammalian and avian cells (GRANICK and SASSA, 1971), and much work has been done to try to establish how the activity, or the amount, of this enzyme in cells is regulated. In spite of the importance of this enzyme, we still know relatively little about its molecular properties, mainly because the enzyme from all sources is unstable to extraction and purification procedures, and in addition the mammalian and avian mitochondrial enzyme is difficult to solubilise. Recently, these difficulties have been overcome, and pure ALA synthetase has been obtained from a number of sources.

The general outline of the mechanism of this reaction has been known for a number of years (see NEUBERGER, 1961; JORDAN and SHEMIN, 1972). Glycine reacts with enzyme-bound pyridoxal phosphate to form a stable carbanion, with loss of a proton from the methylene carbon atom of glycine; the carbanion then reacts with the electrophilic carbonyl carbon atom of succinyl CoA to form α-amino-β-ketoadipic acid with loss of CoA. It was not known then whether α-amino-β-keto-adipic acid was decarboxylated to ALA before or after being released from the enzyme. Recent experiments with ALA synthetase purified from *Rhodopseudomonas spheroides* have given more detailed information on the sequence of the intermediate steps. FANICA-GAIGNIER and CLEMENT-METRAL (1973a, b) obtained spectral evidence that pyridoxal phosphate initially reacts with two groups on the enzyme, one an amino group and the other possibly an SH group, to form an aldamine. ZAMAN et al. (1973) showed that the hydrogen atom on the methylene carbon atom of glycine with R-configuration is specifically lost and that only the one with S-configuration is incorporated into ALA (Fig. 4). This evidence confirms that the carbanion is formed between pyridoxal phosphate and glycine with loss of a proton, and not with loss of the carboxyl group. ABBOUD et al. (1974) subsequently found that the H(S) of glycine occupies the S-configuration on carbon atom 5 of ALA (Fig. 4). The finding of a chiral center on this carbon atom means that the decarboxylation of α-amino-β-ketoadipic acid to ALA must occur on the enzyme surface, and not after α-amino-β-ketoadipic acid is released into solution. ALA is an inhibitor of ALA synthetase of *R. spheroides* (KIKUCHI et al., 1958; FANICA-GAIGNIER and CLEMENT-METRAL, 1973b), suggesting that the ALA formed during the enzymic reaction is bound to the enzyme, and subsequently released. Working with the partially purified cytoplasmic ALA synthetase from rat liver, SCHOLNICK et al. (1972a, b) came to similar conclusions about the mechanism. They found that this enzyme also requires SH groups for activity and that inhibition by SH reagents is blocked by pyridoxal phosphate. They proposed that pyridoxal phosphate initially

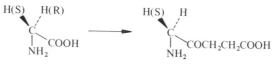

Fig. 4. Stereospecificity of incorporation of glycine into ALA

forms a thiohemiacetal with the enzyme. Metal ions stimulate activity, and it is suggested that they facilitate one or more of the steps in the overall reaction. ALA is not an inhibitor of this enzyme, and on this basis they think that decarboxylation of α-amino-β-ketoadipic acid and release of ALA occur simultaneously.

In mammalian and avian cells, ALA synthetase is normally found exclusively in mitochondria. The low activities found in other subcellular fractions, such as cytoplasm, are probably due to enzyme released from mitochondria which have been damaged or disrupted during tissue fractionation (cf. PATTON and BEATTIE, 1973). By comparing the distribution of ALA synthetase in sub-mitochondrial fractions from liver, with that of marker enzymes, it appears that ALA synthetase is free in the matrix, or loosely bound to the inner mitochondrial membrane (PATTON and BEATTIE, 1973; McKAY et al., 1969; BARNES et al., 1971; ZUYDERHOUDT et al., 1969). However in the livers, and kidneys, of animals treated with porphyrinogenic drugs, where ALA synthetase activity is much higher than normal, a significant proportion of the total activity is present in the cytoplasm (HAYASHI et al., 1969; BARNES et al., 1971), much more than can be accounted for by mitochondrial damage. The molecular weight of the rat liver cytoplasmic enzyme is higher than that of the mitochondrial enzyme (WHITING and ELLIOTT, 1972; HAYASHI et al., 1970), but in mouse liver they appear to be about the same size (GAYATHRI et al., 1973). Both mitochondrial and cytoplasmic enzymes are known to be synthesized on cytoplasmic ribosomes (GRANICK, 1966; HAYASHI et al., 1969; STEIN et al., 1970), and to account for the difference between them it is proposed that the enzyme undergoes modification on being incorporated into mitochondria (WHITING and ELLIOTT, 1972).

After treating animals, or cell cultures, with inhibitors of protein or nucleic acid synthesis, ALA synthetase activity falls rapidly, strongly suggesting that the enzyme has a short half-life. More reliable methods for measuring the rate of turnover (see Sect. C) have not yet been applied. In adult rat liver, the mitochondrial enzyme and its messenger RNA both have half-lives of about 70 min (TSCHUDY et al., 1965a; MARVER et al., 1966a; STEIN et al., 1970), while in fetal rat liver, the half-life of the enzyme is 34 min (WOODS, 1974). Adult rat liver cytoplasmic enzyme has a half-life of 20 min in the absence of hemin, and 120 min in its presence (HAYASHI et al., 1972). By contrast, both cytoplasmic and mitochondrial ALA synthetases of mouse liver appear to have half-lives of about 3 h (GAYATHRI et al., 1973). In chick embryo liver cells, the half-lives of ALA synthetase and its mRNA are 3 h and 5 h respectively (SASSA and GRANICK, 1970).

Molecular weights found for mammalian ALA synthetases, using partially purified preparations, vary over a wide range, and it seems likely that the different results are due to the ease with which the enzyme forms aggregates with other proteins (WHITING and ELLIOTT, 1972; KAPLAN, 1971). WHITING and ELLIOTT (1972) obtained values of 77,000 and 178,000 for rat liver mitochondrial and cytoplasmic enzymes, respectively, when precautions were taken to avoid aggregation. Higher values are given by SCHOLNICK et al. (1972a) and HAYASHI et al. (1970). Very recently, WHITING and GRANICK (1975) have purified the enzyme from chick embryo liver mitochondria to homogeneity. It has a molecular weight of 87,000, and consists of two polypeptide chains of molecular weight 49,000. The specific activity of the preparation, 30,000 nmol ALA/h/mg protein, is about a hundred times higher than the ALA synthetase (M.W. 200,000) purified, apparently to homogeneity, from rabbit reticulocytes by AOKI et al. (1971). This means either that the rabbit reticulocyte enzyme has a much lower specific activity, or that the preparation is still far from pure. The ALA synthetase from fetal rat liver mitochondria has a molecular weight of 47,000 (WOODS and MURTHY, 1975). It differs from the adult enzyme in having a shorter half-life and in not being inhibited by hemin. It is tempting to speculate that these differences in properties may be due to the fetal enzyme being a monomer, and the adult enzyme being a dimer. The ALA synthetases purified from *R. spheroides* (WARNICK and BURNHAM, 1971) and *M. denitrificans* (TAIT, 1973a) are both monomeric proteins; they have molecular weights of 57,000 and 68,000, and specific activities of 130,000 and 37,000 nmol ALA formed/h/mg protein respectively.

The activity of ALA synthetase in most mammalian and avian cells is normally very low, and thus sensitive assay techniques must be used. Tissue homogenates, or individual subcellular fractions, are incubated aerobically with suitable substrates, and the ALA formed is measured colorimetrically (GRANICK and URATA, 1963; MARVER et al., 1966b; HAYASHI et al., 1969). Alternatively, after incubating with radioactive succinate, α-ketoglutarate or citrate, or with 2-[^{14}C]-glycine, the amount of radioactivity incorporated into ALA is measured (IRVING and ELLIOTT, 1969; EBERT et al., 1970; STRAND et al., 1972a; FRESHNEY and PAUL, 1970). These methods, modified slightly by individual workers, are the ones most widely used. They all require that the ALA formed be purified before its amount is determined, and this is usually done by column chromatography or paper electrophoresis, either before or after converting ALA to a pyrrole by boiling with acetylacetone. In colorimetric assays, it is necessary to separate ALA from aminoacetone, which is formed from glycine and acetyl CoA by mitochondrial aminoacetone synthetase (URATA and GRANICK, 1963). EDTA is usually added to assays, since not only does it markedly reduce the amount of aminoacetone formed, but it also prevents conversion of ALA to PBG by inhibiting ALA dehydratase. In incubations with a radioactive substrate, the ALA formed has to be separated from unused substrate and from radioactive products formed during the incubation. In order to reduce the amounts of these products formed, metabolic inhibitors are added (see IRVING and ELLIOTT, 1969). During formation of ALA, the carboxyl carbon atom of glycine is lost as CO_2. Thus in assays with 1-[^{14}C]-glycine the [^{14}C]CO_2 can be trapped and counted directly (LEWIS et al., 1967). As long as the enzyme preparation does not contain any other enzymes which decarboxylate glycine, this would seem to be a rapid, sensitive assay method for ALA synthetase. It has been used with partially purified preparations of mammalian ALA synthetase (SCHOLNICK et al., 1972a; WOODS and MURTHY, 1975) and with bacterial extracts (see JORDAN and SHEMIN, 1972).

Where more than one of the above methods have been done with the same tissue extract, very similar activities have been found (cf. BOCK et al., 1971). However, it should be noted that optimum assay conditions with respect to the substrates and metabolic inhibitors added may be different with extracts from different tissues (EBERT et al., 1970).

When whole liver homogenates are used, there is no need to add succinate or a source of succinyl CoA since enough is made by the mitochondria themselves

(MARVER et al., 1966b). However, only mitochondrial ALA synthetase activity will be measured. To measure total tissue activity, an exogenous source of succinyl CoA has to be added. In assays with damaged mitochondria, or with other sub-cellular fractions, activity is very low unless succinyl CoA or a succinyl CoA-generating system (succinate, CoA, ATP and succinic thiokinase) is added (cf. GROSS and HUTTON, 1971). The succinic thiokinase used can be partially purified from a number of bacteria (cf. TAIT, 1973a), or an extract of a mutant of R. spheroides lacking ALA synthetase (LASCELLES and ALTSHULER, 1969) can be added.

ALA synthetase activity in liver and other tissues increases markedly when animals are treated in a variety of ways. In most of the work, ALA synthetase activity has been measured in tissue homogenates where the mitochondria are more or less intact. Changes in activity have been equated with changes in the amount of enzyme protein present, on the assumption that the specific activity of the enzyme does not change. Recently PATTON and BEATTIE (1973) have devised a very sensitive assay method which uses much lower concentrations of protein than previous methods. They found that with [^{14}C]-succinate as substrate, sonicated mitochondria from normal rat liver had about 10-times the activity of unsonicated mitochondria. Sonication of mitochondria caused a four-fold stimulation of activity in assays with [^{14}C]-citrate, but had no effect in assays with [^{14}C]-α-ketoglutarate. Interestingly, with [^{14}C]-succinate as substrate, sonicated liver mitochondria from normal and porphyric rats had the same high activity, while with unsonicated mitochondria the activity of the porphyric was about 10 times that of normal. AOKI et al. (1974) found that the total activity of ALA synthetase in human erythro-blast hemolysates increased by a factor of about 5 on sonication, and by a further factor of 3−4 on treating the sonicate with deoxycholate. These results indicate that when crude tissue extracts are assayed, the enzyme may not be optimally active, perhaps because its mode of binding to mitochondria does not allow free access of substrates, or because the active site may be partly blocked (KAPLAN, 1971), or because the enzyme is partially inhibited by hemin or some other inhibitor. An endogenous inhibitor of ALA synthetase has been detected in liver mito-chondria (IRVING and ELLIOTT, 1969; JONES and JONES, 1970), although its physi-ological importance is not known. Heme synthetase is bound to the inside of the inner mitochondrial membrane, and it is possible that the amount of heme present could affect the ALA synthetase activity of intact mitochondria (cf. MCKAY et al., 1969). Sonication of mitochondria, or treatment with detergents, may alter the conformation of the enzyme or separate it from inhibitors. It seems possible that the increase in ALA synthetase activity which occurs on making animals porphyric may be due, in part at least, to an increase in the specific activity of the enzyme, rather than to synthesis of new enzyme. In R. spheroides it has been clearly shown that ALA synthetase occurs in both a low and a high activity form, and that the former can be readily converted to the latter in vitro (DAVIES et al., 1973; HAYASAKA and TUBOI, 1974). The form in which the enzyme occurs in the whole bacterium is governed by the conditions of growth.

ALA synthetase activity has been measured in rat liver by many research workers, and values of between 10 and 100 nmol ALA formed/h/g liver have been reported, most values being towards the lower end of this range (see references below). Human liver (TSCHUDY et al., 1965b; SWEENEY et al., 1970; STRAND et al., 1970; see also review by Moore and Goldberg, 1974) and chick embryo liver (Korinek and Moses, 1973) have activities similar to that of rat liver. The activity of mouse liver (De Matteis et al., 1973) is about twice, and the activity of rabbit and guinea pig liver (Woods and Dixon, 1972) is about one-fifth to one-tenth that of rat liver. The activity in the livers of starved mice (Gross and Hutton, 1971) and rats (Bock et al., 1971) is about twice that of fed animals. In rats, activity decreases in the order spleen, liver, kidney, heart (Sardesai et al., 1972). Rabbit brain has high activity (90 nmol ALA/h/g tissue; Muzyka, 1972), as have human and guinea pig erythroblasts (Aoki et al., 1974; Tanaka and Bottomley, 1974). In rats and mice, the tissue with highest activity is the Harderian gland. In rats, its activity is about 100 times higher than that of liver (Wetterberg et al., 1971; Strand et al., 1972a), and in mice the activity, which varies with the strain, can be up to 10 times that of liver (Margolis, 1971). In the livers of fetal rabbits, rats, guinea pigs and mice, ALA synthetase activity is much higher than in adult animals (Woods and Dixon, 1972; Freshney and Paul, 1971). The activities start to fall before birth, and reach the adult values at birth or soon after. While the high activity in fetal liver may be due to the presence of erythropoietic cells, the proportion of these cells in the liver at different stages of development does not appear to correlate with the ALA synthetase activity, at least in the rabbit (Woods and Dixon, 1972). Alternatively these authors suggest that high activity is due to lack of repression of synthesis of the fetal liver enzyme by hemin (Woods and Murthy, 1975; Murthy and Woods, 1974). ALA synthetase activities in a variety of tissues have also been reported by Marver et al. (1966b) and Strand et al. (1972a).

Rat liver ALA synthetase is specific for succinyl CoA and glycine, and does not act on other acyl CoA esters or on other amino acids (Scholnick et al., 1972a). Mammalian enzymes have K_M values for glycine, succinyl CoA and pyridoxal phosphate of $5-19$ mM, $60-200$ µM and $1-10$ µM respectively (Muzyka, 1972; Woods and Murthy, 1975; Scholnick et al., 1972a; Kaplan, 1971; Whiting and Elliott, 1972; Aoki et al., 1971). The low affinity of the enzyme for glycine is worthy of note.

Like most bacterial ALA synthetases, most mammalian ones are markedly inhibited by hemin (see Jordan and Shemin, 1972; Whiting and Elliott, 1972; Kaplan, 1971); partially purified preparations are inhibited by about 50% by 50 µM hemin. The fetal liver enzyme, however, is not inhibited by hemin, but rather is slightly activated (Woods and Murthy, 1975).

III. Aminolevulinate Dehydratase (E.C. 4.2.1.24)

The properties of this enzyme, which has been purified from a number of bacterial, plant, avian, and mammalian sources, have been comprehensively reviewed by Shemin (1972). ALA dehydratase is a cytoplasmic enzyme which catalyzes the condensation of two molecules of ALA to form the pyrrole porphobilinogen (PBG) with the loss of two molecules of water (Fig. 3). One of the ALA molecules forms a Schiff's base through its keto group with an amino group on the enzyme, as shown by formation of a stable enzyme-substrate complex after reduction with sodium borohydride (Shemin, 1968, 1972; Gurba et al., 1972); this ALA molecule is the one which contributes the acetic acid side chain of PBG. The other molecule of ALA is probably also bound to the enzyme, but exactly how is not known.

ALA dehydratases purified to homogeneity from different mammalian tissues have very similar properties (SHEMIN, 1972). They have pH optima between 6.3 and 7, K_M values for ALA of between about 0.1 and 0.4 mM and, with the possible exception of the mouse liver enzyme (COLEMAN, 1966), they are all strongly inhibited by EDTA. They are SH enzymes. Although maximum activity is sometimes obtained with crude cell extracts in the absence of added thiol compounds (GIBSON and GOLDBERG, 1970; NARISAWA and KIKUCHI, 1966), the activity of partially purified preparations is generally very low, and optimum activity is only obtained after preincubation with glutathione or cysteine (GIBSON et al., 1955). More recently dithiothreitol has been found to be more effective (WILSON et al., 1972); its action is so rapid that preincubation is not required (GRANICK et al., 1973). Pb^{2+} and other heavy metal ions inhibit the enzyme (GIBSON et al., 1955; GIBSON and GOLDBERG, 1970). The inhibition by Pb^{2+} is reversed by thiol compounds and is noncompetitive with ALA (WILSON et al., 1972; GRANICK et al., 1973), suggesting that the thiol groups on the enzyme are not at the active site, but are involved in maintaining the correct enzyme conformation. The rat liver enzyme is markedly inhibited by Fe^{3+} (STEIN et al., 1970). Hemin, protoporphyrin and coproporphyrinogen III strongly inhibit the enzymes from liver, red blood cells, and spleen of rat and mouse (SATYANARAYANA RAO et al., 1970); coproporphyrinogen at 50 µM inhibits by 60–90%. The physiological significance of this "feedback" inhibition remains to be determined. Hemin appears to be a competitive inhibitor of the mouse liver enzyme (DOYLE and SCHIMKE, 1969) but a noncompetitive inhibitor of the enzymes from guinea pig liver and red cells (WEISSBERG and VOYTEK, 1974).

It is clear that ALA dehydratase is a multisubunit enzyme, but controversy remains regarding the exact number of subunits (see SHEMIN, 1972). For the beef liver enzyme, WILSON et al. (1972) report a molecular weight of 260,000 with 14 subunits; CHEH and NEILANDS (1973), a molecular weight of 280,000 with 7–8 subunits; and WU et al. (1974) a molecular weight of 282–289,000 with 8 identical subunits. WU et al. (1974) also present electron micrographic evidence which is consistent with there being 8 subunits. GURBA et al. (1972) conclude that bovine and rat liver enzymes have 6–7 subunits, each of which forms a Schiff's base with ALA, and DOYLE (1971) concludes that mouse liver enzyme has 6 identical subunits. Difficulties in measuring accurately the molecular weights of the intact enzyme and of the subunits probably account for these differences, and at the moment no final decision on the subunit structure of the enzyme can be made.

The marked inhibition by EDTA, first noted by GIBSON et al. (1955), suggested that mammalian ALA dehydratases were metalloenzymes. However, purified preparations were found to contain only small amounts of metal (see GURBA et al., 1972). CHEH and NEILANDS (1973) have now shown that activity is very low when purified bovine enzyme is assayed in solutions free of metal ion contamination, and that it increases to a maximum on adding 5–6 g atoms of Zn^{2+}/mol of enzyme. The enzyme can also be reactivated by Cd^{2+}. They conclude that ALA dehydratase is a metalloenzyme from which the metal is removed during purification, and that full activity is restored when four out of the eight subunits rebind Zn^{2+}. FINELLI et al. (1974) present evidence that zinc may also be required during the synthesis of the enzyme in rats.

In most mammalian tissues, the specific activity of ALA dehydratase is much higher than that of ALA synthetase. In liver, for example, it is 50–100 times higher. GIBSON et al. (1955) found activities of 0.70, 0.24, and 0.15 μmol PBG formed/h/g wet weight for rat liver, kidney, and Harderian gland respectively. In rabbit, liver (1.0 μmol PBG/h/g wet weight) also had highest activity, with lower activities in kidney (0.3), bone marrow (0.24), spleen (0.10), lung (0.07), brain (0.06), heart muscle (0.04), and skeletal muscle (0.01). Activities close to those of rat and rabbit liver have been reported for livers of man (TSCHUDY et al., 1965b), cow (BATLLE et al., 1967), guinea pig (WEISSBERG and VOYTEK, 1974), and mouse (HUTTON and GROSS, 1970). Red blood cells of different species also have high activity (WEISSBERG and VOYTEK, 1974; CALISSANO et al., 1966).

The activity of ALA dehydratase varies by a factor of 3–4 in the liver, kidney, and spleen of different strains of mice (COLEMAN, 1966; DOYLE and SCHIMKE, 1969); activity is under the genetic control of two alleles at the levulinate (LV) locus. The differences in activity are due to differences in the rates of synthesis of ALA dehydratase, since the hepatic enzymes from all strains of mice have the same half-life of 5−6 days, and the purified enzymes all have the same specific activity (COLEMAN, 1966; DOYLE and SCHIMKE, 1969).

In the liver of fetal mice (DOYLE and SCHIMKE, 1969; FRESHNEY and PAUL, 1971), and in the liver and red blood cells of fetal guinea pigs (WEISSBERG and VOYTEK, 1974) the activities of ALA dehydratase are higher than in the corresponding adult tissues. In both animals, the activities start to fall about 5 days before birth, and reach minimum values at, or soon after, birth. In mouse liver (DOYLE and SCHIMKE, 1969), and in the liver, but not in red blood cells, of the guinea pig (WEISSBERG and VOYTEK, 1974), the activities subsequently increase again to the adult level, which is about one-third to one-half the fetal level. In mouse liver, the loss of activity just before birth correlates with the rapid fall in the proportion of hematopoietic cells in the liver (DOYLE and SCHIMKE, 1969).

Since the activity of ALA dehydratase in tissues is much higher than that of ALA synthetase, it has been thought that it plays little part in regulating the overall rate of heme synthesis. However, the requirement for highly reducing conditions to obtain maximum activity in vitro suggests that the oxidation-reduction potential in intact cells may determine the rate at which this reaction occurs in vivo. There is some tentative evidence that the conversion of ALA to PBG may be the rate-limiting step in porphyrin and heme synthesis under some circumstances. SHARMA (1973) has shown that rats with iron-deficiency anaemia excrete more ALA but less PBG than control rats, and that the ALA dehydratase activities in their bone marrow and liver are markedly lower than the normal values. He suggests that the decrease in ALA dehydratase activity contributes to the reduction of porphyrin syntheses in iron deficiency. MURTY et al. (1970) have shown that rats with a deficiency of vitamin E have a low level of hepatic hemoproteins, and that the incorporations of injected [^{14}C] ALA and [^{14}C] PBG into their liver microsomal hemoproteins are 7% and 50% respectively of the incorporations obtained using normal animals.

IV. Porphobilinogen Deaminase (E.C. 4.3.1.8) and Uroporphyrinogen III Cosynthetase

Porphobilinogen deaminase catalyzes the condensation of four molecules of PBG to form the symmetrical cyclic tetrapyrrole uroporphyrinogen I, and four molecules of ammonia (BOGORAD, 1958a). With the enzyme isolated from most sources, the loss of PBG parallels the formation of uroporphyrinogen I, and intermediates such as di-, tri- and linear tetrapyrroles are not detected (see DAVIES and NEU-BERGER, 1973). This finding suggests that the four condensation steps take place sequentially on the enzyme surface, and that intermediates are firmly bound to the enzyme. The formation of uroporphyrinogen III from PBG, where one of the PBG units is inserted into the ring the wrong way round, occurs under the combined action of PBG deaminase and a second protein uroporphyrinogen III cosynthetase (BOGORAD, 1958b). On its own, uroporphyrinogen III cosynthetase does not react with PBG or with uroporphyrinogen I. It can be considered to be a "specifier protein" which in some way alters the mechanism of the reaction catalyzed by PBG deaminase (FRYDMAN and FEINSTEIN, 1974).

Human erythrocytes (STEVENS et al., 1968) and all mouse tissues tested (LEVIN, 1968a) have a much higher activity of uroporphyrinogen III cosynthetase than of PBG deaminase. This excess probably ensures that in vivo only the biologically useful III isomer is formed. Humans and cattle with congenital erythropoietic porphyria excrete large amounts of uroporphyrin I, and their erythrocytes have only 10 − 25% of the uroporphyrinogen III cosynthetase activity of normal erythrocytes (ROMEO and LEVIN, 1969; LEVIN, 1968b). The fox squirrel (*Sciurus niger*) normally excretes large amounts of uroporphyrin I, and the uroporphyrinogen III cosynthetase activities in its tissues are about 10% of those in the corresponding tissues of the grey squirrel, which does not excrete uroporphyrin I (LEVIN and FLYGER, 1973).

PBG deaminase activity can be measured by following the loss of PBG or the formation of uroporphyrinogen, after oxidizing it to uroporphyrin (see DAVIES and NEUBERGER, 1973). Another enzyme that metabolises PBG, PBG oxygenase, has recently been described in rat liver and brain, wheat germ and spinach chloroplasts (FRYDMAN et al., 1973a; TOMARO et al., 1973). Thus, when using crude extracts, and even partially purified enzyme (YUAN and RUSSELL, 1974) from some tissues to measure PBG deaminase, activities based solely on the loss of PBG may give falsely high values. Uroporphyrinogen III cosynthetase activity in extracts is assayed by incubating different amounts of the extracts with a partially purified preparation of PBG deaminase in the presence of PBG, and measuring the proportion of isomer I and III formed. The isomers are separated chromatographically after converting them to uroporphyrin methyl esters, coproporphyrins, or coproporphyrin methyl esters. Full details of these chromatographic methods are given by FALK (1964) and MARKS (1969).

PBG deaminase and uroporphyrinogen III cosynthetase are cytoplasmic enzymes, and they were first separated and partially purified from spinach (BOGORAD, 1958a, b) and *R. spheroides* (HOARE and HEATH, 1958). More recently, they have been purified from a number of sources including cultured soybean cells (LLAMBIAS and BATLLE, 1971a), avian erythrocytes (LLAMBIAS and BATLLE, 1971b), human erythrocytes (STEVENS et al., 1968; FRYDMAN and FEINSTEIN, 1974), bovine liver (SANCOVICH et al., 1969), and mouse spleen (LEVIN and COLEMAN, 1967; LEVIN, 1971). A PBG deaminase-uroporphyrinogen cosynthetase complex has also been extensively purified from bovine liver (SANCOVICH et al., 1969) and avian erythrocytes (LLAMBIAS and BATLLE, 1971b), suggesting that this complex exists in vivo. Additional evidence for this suggestion is the finding that the two purified enzymes from human erythrocytes readily reassociate, to form a stable complex in the absence of substrate (FRYDMAN and FEINSTEIN, 1974). Human erythrocyte PBG deaminase has a molecular weight of 25,000; the cosynthetase is considerably larger, but its exact size is not known (FRYDMAN and FEINSTEIN, 1974). The molecular weight of the avian erythrocyte PBG deaminase is about 40,000, that of the cosynthetase about 280,000, and that of the PBG deaminase-uroporphyrinogen III cosynthetase complex is about 110,000 (LLAMBIAS and BATLLE, 1971 b). These results could be accounted for if the cosynthetase forms a tetramer when separated from the deaminase.

In those mammalian tissues where PBG deaminase has been detected, the activity is generally very low, much lower than that of ALA dehydratase in the same tissue, and not very much higher than that of ALA synthetase, which is normally considered to be the rate-limiting step in heme biosynthesis. LEVIN (1968 a) could only detect activity in mouse spleen (11.2 nmol PBG used/h/mg protein); a number of other mouse tissues tested were inactive. HUTTON and GROSS (1970) found very low activity in mouse liver. They estimated it to be about $35-60$ nmol PBG used/h/g wet weight, about 10% of the activity they found in spleen. MIYAGI et al. (1971) found an activity of 22 nmol uroporphyrin formed/h/g wet weight in mouse liver, and a 10-fold lower activity in human liver. Activities in human erythrocytes of 36 nmol uroporphyrin formed/h/ml erythrocytes (SASSA et al., 1974) and 34 pmol uroporphyrin formed/h/mg protein (STRAND et al., 1972 b) have been reported. Activities in the erythrocytes (STRAND et al., 1972 b; SASSA et al., 1974) and liver (MIYAGI et al., 1971) of patients with acute intermittent porphyria are about half the normal values. It is now considered that this reduced level of the PBG deaminase is the primary genetic lesion of the heme biosynthetic pathway in this disorder. DOYLE and SCHIMKE (1969) could not detect activity in adult mouse liver, but they found high activity (2 μmol PBG used/h/g wet weight) in fetal mouse liver. The activity started to fall rapidly just before birth, reached a minimum about four days after birth, and increased again, to about 75% of the fetal value, during the first 20 days of life. These changes in activity are very similar to the ones found for ALA dehydratase (see above). Since they measured activity by following loss of PBG, it is possible that the true activity of PBG deaminase is lower than the values they give.

PBG deaminase can be visualized as catalyzing sequential reaction between the α-aminomethyl side chain of a PBG molecule with the free α-position of the next PBG molecule (head to tail condensation) to form first the dipyrrole I (Fig. 5), then a tripyrrole, and finally a linear tetrapyrrole, all of these intermediates remaining bound to the enzyme. Finally the α-aminomethyl group on the fourth PBG unit of the linear tetrapyrrole reacts with the free α-position of the first PBG unit forming a cyclic tetrapyrrole, which is released from the enzyme. Intermediates cannot normally be detected, but in the presence of high concentrations of ammonia, hydroxylamine, or methoxyamine, formation of uroporphyrinogen I by PBG deaminase is inhibited more markedly than the consumption of PBG, and intermediates accumulate (DAVIES and NEUBERGER, 1973). These intermediates appear to be linear tetrapyrroles in which the amino group of the aminomethyl side chain has been replaced by the bases added to the incubation mixture. It seems likely that they are formed by reaction between the bases and the enzyme-linear tetra-

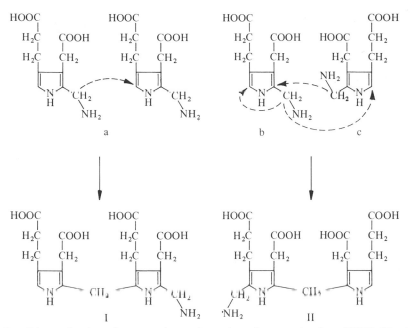

Fig. 5. Possible mechanisms for enzymic condensation of two molecules of PBG. Head-to-tail condensation (a) gives dipyrrole I. Head-to-head condensation, with either intramolecular migration (b) or intermolecular migration (c) of the aminomethyl sidechain, gives dipyrrole II

pyrrole complex, with release of the modified product into the solution. Many mechanisms have been proposed over the past 15 years to account for the inversion of one of the PBG units which occurs during formation of uroporphyrinogen III (see DAVIES et al., 1973). It has been suggested that instead of head to tail condensation, the α-aminomethyl group of one PBG molecule attacks the occupied α-position of another PBG molecule (head to head condensation), whose α-aminomethyl side chain then undergoes an intramolecular or an intermolecular migration, as shown in Figure 5 and the dipyrrole II is formed. In this dipyrrole, the two acetic acid side chains are adjacent to one another, as they are in rings A and D of uroporphyrinogen III (Fig. 3). Subsequent head to tail condensation of this dipyrrole with another two molecules of PBG followed by cyclization, would yield uroporphyrinogen III. The single head to head condensation could of course occur at the stage of formation of the di-, tri- or tetrapyrrole, or even after formation of the linear tetrapyrrole. Alternatively, three successive head to head condensations would also result in formation of a linear tetrapyrrole, which on cyclization would give uroporphyrinogen III. BATTERSBY et al. (1973) used PBG labeled with [¹³C] both in the carbon atom of the aminomethyl side chain and in the free α-carbon atom of the ring, and showed that on incorporation into uroporphyrinogen III, only one PBG unit, the one incorporated into ring D, underwent intramolecular rearrangement. Its α-aminomethyl group had migrated from its original position to the other α-carbon atom of the same pyrrole ring at some stage during the reaction (Fig. 5). That is, ring D and the γ-bridge carbon atom come from the same PBG molecule. This finding is consistent with one head to head condensation, with intramolecular rearrangement (Fig. 5), and two head-to-tail condensations before cyclization, but not with three head to head condensations.

FRYDMAN et al., (1973 b) synthesized dipyrroles I and II (Fig. 5). When incubated with PBG and PBG deaminase plus uroporphyrinogen III cosynthetase, dipyrrole I was incorporated into uroporphyrinogen I only, and dipyrrole II was incorporated into uroporphyrinogen III only. Although the incorporation of these dipyrroles into uroporphyrinogen was low, and only slightly higher in the presence of enzyme than in its absence, these results strongly suggest that the way in which the first two molecules of PBG condense on the enzyme surface determines into which isomer, I or III, they are incorporated. Additional evidence that different di- or tripyrroles are precursors of uroporphyrinogens I and III, respectively, was obtained by LLAMBIAS and BATLLE (1970, 1971 a) with the enzyme system from soybean cells. Unlike the enzyme systems from other sources, this one initially consumes PBG faster than it forms uroporphyrinogen. The intermediates have been separated from reaction mixtures. They appear to be tripyrroles. The intermediate formed in the presence of PBG deaminase is converted to uroporphyrinogen I only, when reincubated enzymically with PBG, and the intermediate formed in the presence of PBG deaminase plus uroporphyrinogen III cosynthetase is converted to uroporphyrinogen III when reincubated with enzyme and PBG.

V. Uroporphyrinogen Decarboxylase (E.C. 4.1.1.37)

Uroporphyrinogen is converted to coproporphyrinogen enzymically by decarboxylation of the four acetic acid side chains to methyl groups. Uroporphyrin is not a substrate, and the tetra- and dihydroporphyrins do not appear to be involved (MAUZERALL and GRANICK, 1958). The enzyme responsible is a cytoplasmic enzyme, and it has been demonstrated in animal, plant, and bacterial cells. It has been partially purified from a number of mammalian and avian cells, and its properties have been studied—rabbit reticulocytes (MAUZERALL and GRANICK, 1958), human erythrocytes (CORNFORD, 1964), chicken erythrocytes (BATLLE and GRINSTEIN, 1964; SAN MARTIN DE VIALE and GRINSTEIN, 1968; SAN MARTIN DE VIALE et al., 1969; TOMIO et al., 1970; GARCIA et al., 1973), and mouse spleen (ROMEO and LEVIN, 1971). The enzymes from all these sources are most active at around pH 7, have K_M values for uroporphyrinogen III of from $1-5$ µM, and there is no evidence that a cofactor, such as pyridoxal phosphate, is required, which is unusual for a decarboxylase (ROMEO and LEVIN, 1971). It seems that a single enzyme catalyzes the decarboxylation of all four acetic acid side chains. TOMIO et al. (1970) showed that the 220-fold purified enzyme from chicken erythrocytes was homogeneous on polyacrylamide gel electrophoresis, and behaved as a single protein on chromatography on Sephadex G-100. However, the reaction appears to proceed somewhat differently with enzymes from different sources. With the chicken erythrocyte enzyme (GARCIA et al., 1973) the reaction goes in two stages. The decarboxylation of the first acetic acid side chain is faster than that of the next three, and a porphyrinogen with seven carboxyl groups accumulates. With the chicken erythrocyte enzyme, the second stage of the reaction is more heat labile than the first stage, and it is also inhibited to a greater extent by Na^+ ions, a property shared by the human erythrocyte enzyme (CORNFORD, 1964). By contrast, with the spleen enzyme there is a stoichiometric conversion of uroporphyrinogen to coproporphyrinogen, and intermediates with seven, six, or five carboxyl groups do not accumulate under any of the conditions tested (ROMEO and LEVIN, 1971). The enzyme from all tissues examined decarboxylates both I and III isomers of uroporphyrinogen. With enzyme from human erythrocytes, the III isomer is decarboxylated 7.5 times faster than the I isomer (CORNFORD, 1964), with enzyme from rabbit reticulocytes (MAUZERALL and GRANICK, 1958) the III isomer is decarboxylated twice as fast as the I isomer (the II and IV isomers are also substrates), but with the mouse spleen enzyme both I and III isomers are metabolized at the same rate, and have almost identical K_M values (ROMEO and LEVIN, 1971). The reasons for these differences are not known. It seems unlikely that there is more than one active site per enzyme. More probably, the modes of binding of uroporphyrinogens I and III and their partially decarboxylated products are different in each enzyme.

Until recently, it has generally been assumed that the order of decarboxylation of the acetic acid side chains is random. STOLL et al., (1973) found that in isocoproporphyrin, a porphyrin with four carboxyl groups isolated from feces of humans with symptomatic porphyria, and of rats fed hexachlorobenzene, the propionic acid side chain on position 2 has already been decarboxylated, but the acetic acid side chain on position 5 of ring C is still intact. This finding indicates that normally this acetic acid side chain is the last one to be decarboxylated. More recently, JACKSON et al., (1975) have shown, using hemolysates of chicken erythrocytes, that decarboxylation of the acetic acid side chains of uroporphyrinogen III occurs in a sequential clockwise fashion starting with the one on ring D and ending with the one on ring C.

Uroporphyrinogen decarboxylase activity is inhibited by sulphydryl reagents such as Hg^{2+}, Cu^{2+}, iodoacetamide and p-chloromercuribenzoate, and by Mn^{2+}, and these inhibitions can be reversed by glutathione (MAUZERALL and GRANICK, 1958). Oxygen also inhibits activity probably by oxidising the substrate.

Uroporphyrinogen decarboxylase activity of mouse spleen (0.35 nmol coproporphyrin formed/h/mg protein in 25,000 g supernatant) is increased by a factor of three after treating the mice for five days with phenylhydrazine (ROMEO and LEVIN, 1971). These workers also detected activity in normal mouse liver, brain, heart, lung, testes, and kidney. In all these tissues the activity was between 0.1 and 0.3 nmol coproporphyrin formed/h/mg protein in the 25,000 g supernatant. The enzyme activity in rat liver, normally 6.5 nmol coproporphyrin/h/g wet weight, was not detectable after induction of experimental symptomatic porphyria produced by feeding the rats excess iron plus hexachlorobenzene (TALJAARD et al., 1972).

VI. Coproporphyrinogen Oxidase (E.C. 1.3.3.3)

Coproporphyrinogen oxidase catalyzes the oxidative decarboxylation of the propionate side chains on rings A and B of coproporphyrinogen III to vinyl groups (Fig. 3); the propionate groups on rings C and D are not modified. In mammalian cells, the enzyme is found only in the mitochondrion, although its exact location there is not known. The enzyme has an absolute requirement for molecular oxygen, which cannot be replaced by any of a number of other hydrogen acceptors tested (SANO and GRANICK, 1961). Highest activity is obtained in an atmosphere containing 20% (v/v) O_2 (PORRA and FALK, 1964). Because the substrate is readily oxidised by O_2, the assay is done in the presence of a reducing agent such as thioglycollate (SANO and GRANICK, 1961) or glutathione (PORRA and FALK, 1964). Both groups of researchers found that protoporphyrinogen, and not protoporphyrin, was the product of the reaction. The enzyme only acts on the III and IV isomers of coproporphyrinogen, and not on the I and II isomers (PORRA and FALK, 1964); it does not act on coproporphyrin III or on uroporphyrinogen III (SANO and GRANICK, 1961). BATLLE et al. (1965) purified the enzyme from ox liver by a factor of about 60. The enzyme had a pH optimum of 7.5 and a molecular weight of about 80,000. The K_M value for coproporphyrinogen III was 30 µM. They could find no evidence for the presence in the enzyme of an organic cofactor, and activity was not enhanced by adding known cofactors. The enzyme was inhibited reversibly by 1:10 phenanthroline and α, α'-dipyrridyl, suggesting that a tightly bound metal might be present (see also SANO and GRANICK, 1961). Pb^{2+} and Cd^{2+} inhibited activity slightly.

SANO and GRANICK (1961) assayed activity in a number of guinea pig and rabbit tissues. Highest activity was found in liver (150 nmol/h/g wet weight). Lower activities were found in bone marrow, kidney, spleen, brain, heart muscle, and pancreas. Beef thymus and chicken erythrocytes had high activity. SHANLEY et al. (1970) assayed activity in rat liver mitochondria (2.3 nmol/h/mg mitochondrial protein).

Coproporphyrinogen oxidases with pH optima, K_M values, and other properties very similar to those of the mammalian liver enzyme have been partially purified from tobacco (HSU and MILLER, 1970), Saccharomyces cerevisiae (POULSON and POLGLASE, 1974a), and R. spheroides (TAIT, 1972). S. cerevisiae (POULSON and POLGLASE, 1974a), Micrococcus denitrificans (TAIT, 1973b), and R. spheroides (TAIT, 1972) make heme when grown under anaerobic conditions. Extracts of these cells can convert coproporphyrinogen to protoporphyrinogen when incubated aerobically, or when incubated in the absence of oxygen but in the presence of S-adenosylmethionine, ATP, and $NAD(P)^+$ as hydrogen acceptor. The enzyme from S. cerevisiae has been purified (POULSON and POLGLASE, 1974a), and the same protein (molecular weight 80,000) is responsible for both aerobic and anaerobic activities. For anaerobic, but not for aerobic, activity there is an absolute requirement for a divalent metal ion such as Fe^{2+}, Co^{2+} or Mn^{2+}.

SANO and GRANICK (1961) detected a porphyrinogen with three carboxyl groups during the course of the reaction, and suggested that the propionate residues were modified one at a time. KENNEDY et al. (1970) analyzed harderoporphyrin, the three-carboxyl porphyrin found in rodent Harderian glands, and found that the single vinyl group was on ring A. This finding indicates that normally the propionate residue on ring A is modified before the one on ring B. This has been substantiated by CAVALEIRO et al. (1974) who synthesized harderoporphyrin and its isomer, which has a propionate residue on ring A and a vinyl group on ring B. The porphyrinogen of the isomer was converted to protoporphyrin by a cell-free extract of Euglena gracilis much less rapidly than was harderoporphyrinogen.

There are a number of possible mechanisms for the oxidative decarboxylation (see TAIT, 1972; DAVIES et al., 1973). GRANICK and SANO (1961) suggested that a hydride ion was removed from the β-carbon atom of the propionate side chain with simultaneous decarboxylation. Later SANO (1966), to account for the requirement for oxygen, suggested that a β-hydroxypropionate side chain was formed followed by dehydration to give an acrylate side chain, and subsequent decarboxylation to a vinyl group; alternatively the last two steps could occur by a concerted mechanism. Recent evidence rules out the formation of an acrylate side chain. ZAMAN et al. (1972) and BATTERSBY et al. (1972) showed that there is a stereospecific loss of one of the hydrogens on the β-carbon atom, but no loss of hydrogen from the α-carbon atom, of the propionate side chains. It is possible that a β-hydroxypropionate side chain is formed during the course of the oxygen-dependent reaction (SANO, 1966), but this seems less likely in the anaerobic reaction. In the anaerobic reaction, the role of S-adenosylmethionine could be to facilitate hydride ion removal from the β-carbon atom, thus initiating a concerted reaction leading directly to the vinyl group.

VII. Protoporphyrinogen Oxidase

Protoporphyrinogen is rapidly oxidized to protoporphyrin nonenzymically in the presence of oxygen, and it has generally been assumed that this is what happens in vivo. SANO and GRANICK (1961) and PORRA and FALK (1961, 1964) presented preliminary evidence that mammalian liver mitochondria contain an enzyme that oxidizes protoporphyrinogen to protoporphyrin, but no further work on this step was done until very recently. JACKSON et al. (1974) prepared coproporphyrin III labeled with tritium at the methene-bridge carbon atoms. On reduction to coproporphyrinogen III with sodium amalgam, followed by chemical reoxidation, none of the label was lost. However, after incubating the coproporphyrinogen with a chicken erythrocyte hemolysate, the protoporphyrin formed had lost half its radioactivity, showing that the oxidation of protoporphyrinogen to protoporphyrin had occurred enzymically. More recently POULSON and POLGLASE (1974b, 1975) found an oxygen-dependent protoporphyrinogen oxidase in mitochondrial extracts from Saccharomyces cerevisiae. They solubilized the enzyme and partially purified it. It has a molecular weight of 180,000, a pH optimum of 7.45, and a K_M for protoporphyrinogen IX of 4.8 µM. The enzyme is most active in the presence of GSH or dithiothreitol, and does not appear to require metal ions or other cofactors. During nonenzymic oxidation of protoporphyrinogen IX, the partially oxidized prototetrahydroporphyrin IX appears and then disappears. However, this partially oxidized intermediate cannot be detected during the enzyme reaction. The enzyme does not oxidize uroporphyrinogen I or III or coproporphyrinogen I or III. Enzyme activity is inhibited noncompetitively by heme and by hemin; 50% inhibition by 20 µM heme and by 50 µM hemin.

VIII. Heme Synthetase (E.C. 4.99.1.1)

Heme synthetase, also called ferrochelatase, catalyzes the incorporation of Fe^{2+} into protoporphyrin to form protoheme. It is located in the mitochondria of animal cells, the chloroplasts of plants, and the chromatophores of photosynthetic bacteria (cf. Lascelles, 1964; Marver and Schmid, 1972). In liver mitochondria, it is firmly attached to the inside of the inner mitochondrial membrane (Jones and Jones, 1969; McKay et al., 1969; Bugany et al., 1971), and no other cell fraction contains any activity (Jones and Jones, 1969). Protoporphyrin is formed enzymically in mitochondria (see above), and Barnes et al. (1972) have shown that Fe^{3+} is reduced to Fe^{2+} inside the inner mitochondrial membrane in proximity to the heme synthetase. Fe^{3+} is not a substrate (Porra and Jones, 1963), but Co^{2+} (Labbe and Hubbard, 1961) and Zn^{2+} are (Johnson and Jones, 1964). In addition to protoporphyrin, mesoporphyrin and deuteroporphyrin are also substrates (Johnson and Jones, 1964; Jones and Jones, 1969).

Activity can be assayed in a number of ways. The incorporation of $^{59}Fe^{2+}$ into heme, or the formation of heme, as its pyridine hemochromogen, can be measured; the disappearance of Fe^{2+} or of protoporphyrin can be measured after deproteinizing the reaction mixture; loss of porphyrin can also be followed spectrophotometrically (see Porra et al., 1967; Jones and Jones, 1969). It is difficult to obtain reproducible results using Fe^{2+} and protoporphyrin as substrates. Protoporphyrin is poorly soluble, and detergent has to be added to the assay. Fe^{2+} is readily oxidized and assays have to be done anaerobically, or in the presence of glutathione or ascorbic acid. In the presence of oxygen, these reducing agents catalyze the destruction of the protoheme formed (cf. Porra et al., 1967). For these reasons a number of authors routinely assay heme synthetase with Co^{2+} or Zn^{2+} and deuteroporphyrin or mesoporphyrin (Mazanowska et al., 1966; Jones and Jones, 1969; Barnes et al., 1971; Bugany et al., 1971; De Matteis et al., 1973). Most of the evidence is consistent with the assumption of there being a single enzyme with a broad specificity for metal ions and porphyrins (Jones and Jones, 1969; Mazanowska et al., 1966). However, Hasegawa et al. (1970) found that chelatase activities measured with Fe^{2+} and Co^{2+} in rat liver did not change in parallel after treating rats with phenobarbitone.

The enzyme has not been obtained in soluble form, and thus we know nothing about its molecular weight, and relatively little about its properties. Mazanowska et al. (1966) found that activity was markedly increased when assays with mammalian liver mitochondria were done in the presence of organic solvents. Removal of lipid from mitochondria inactivated the enzyme, and activity could be restored by adding back phospholipids. Yoshikawa and Yoneyama (1964), Sawada et al. (1969) and Takeshita et al. (1970) found that negatively charged phospholipid micelles markedly activated the avian erythrocyte enzyme. The exact role of lipid is not known. It may activate the enzyme by changing its conformation, or it may stimulate activity by solubilizing the porphyrin, or by binding with the metal ion, thus transferring it from an aqueous to a nonaqueous environment.

Formation of metalloporphyrins occurs readily under a number of conditions in the absence of cell extracts. leading some workers to doubt that there is an enzyme catalyzing this reaction (cf. Kassner and Walchak, 1973). However, conclusive evidence for an enzyme has been presented by Dailey and Lascelles (1974), who found that a mutant of *Spirillum itersonii*, which lacked membrane-bound heme synthetase activity, required heme for growth.

The heme synthetase of human bone marrow has optimum activity at pH 7.4, and the K_M values for Fe^{2+} and protoporphyrin are 17 µM and 1.8 µM respectively (BOTTOMLEY, 1968). The rat liver enzyme has optimum activity at pH 8.2, and the K_M values are similar to those for the human bone marrow enzyme (JONES and JONES, 1969; BUGANY et al., 1971). The rat liver enzyme activity is inhibited by 50% by 16 µM protoheme (JONES and JONES, 1970), and human bone marrow enzyme activity is inhibited 50% by 100 µM protoheme (BOTTOMLEY, 1968).

Heme synthetase activity, expressed as nmol cobalt deuteroporphyrin formed/min/mg mitochondrial protein, is 0.71, 0.40, 0.34, and 0.33 in rat liver, brain, kidney, and heart respectively (BARNES et al., 1971); in rat liver, the activity is about 0.4 nmol protoheme formed/min/mg mitochondrial protein (JONES and JONES, 1969). Rabbit brain, liver, and kidney have very similar activities per g of tissue, but bone marrow is less active (GIBSON and GOLDBERG, 1970). Liver mitochondria from mice are about twice as active as those from rats (DE MATTEIS et al., 1973). Heme synthetase activity has also been assayed in human liver (KAUFMAN and MARVER, 1970; NAKAO et al., 1966), and human skeletal muscle (PIMSTONE et al., 1973), where activity is the same in patients with variegate porphyria as in normal individuals, and human blood cells (LANGELAAN et al., 1970).

Heme synthetase, like ALA synthetase, ALA dehydratase, and PBG deaminase (see above), has a higher activity in fetal liver than in adult liver (FRESHNEY and PAUL, 1971). Activity increases during fetal life in the mouse, and reaches a maximum 3 days before birth. Activity falls by a factor of 2.5 during the last 3 days and reaches its lowest value at birth; the activity at birth is the same as in the adult animal.

Heme, formed by heme synthetase, moves out of mitochondria, the bulk of it probably to the microsomes (see DRUYAN and KELLY, 1972). Most of the apoproteins, including mitochondrial cytochrome c (GONZALEZ-CADAVID et al., 1971), are synthesized on cytoplasmic ribosomes, and complex with their heme groups there or in the cytoplasm. Heme appears to complex with the catalase apoprotein mainly in the peroxisomes (LAZAROW and DE DUVE, 1973 b). YODA and ISRAELS (1972) showed that export of heme from mitochondria required the presence of cell sap proteins in the surrounding medium. The heme was associated with multiple proteins, and no single carrier was identified. More recently KETTERER et al. (1974) found that ligandin, a cytoplasmic protein of liver, binds hemin with an apparent affinity constant of 10^8 M^{-1}. They suggest that this protein plays a role in removing heme from mitochondria and transporting it to the endoplasmic reticulum.

IX. Heme Oxygenase (E.C. 1.14.99.3)

Heme oxygenase is a microsomal enzyme which requires NADPH and oxygen and catalyzes the conversion of hemin and the heme of a number of hemoproteins to equimolar amounts of biliverdin IXα and carbon monoxide (TENHUNEN et al., 1968, 1969, 1970 a). Microsomal NADPH-cytochrome c reductase is also required for the reaction to occur (SCHACTER et al., 1972). The two oxygen atoms incorporated into biliverdin, and the one atom incorporated into carbon monoxide, all come from O_2 and not from water (TENHUNEN et al., 1972). The enzyme is optimally active at pH 7.4−7.5 and the K_M for hemin is 5 µM. The activities in extracts from different rat tissues, expressed as nmol of biliverdin or bilirubin formed/min/10 mg microsomal protein, are spleen 0.79, bone marrow 0.17, liver and brain 0.07, kidney 0.03, and lung 0.02 (TENHUNEN et al., 1970a). The activity in rat spleen, the major site of erythrocyte hemoglobin catabolism, is high enough to account for normal hemoglobin turnover in the whole animal (TENHUNEN et al., 1968). Heme oxygenase activity has also been assayed in chick embryo liver and heart cells (ISRAELS et al., 1974); the activity in liver is 2 − 3 times that in heart.

Protohemin IX is the best substrate, but mesohemin IX, deuterohemin IX and coprohemin I are converted to the corresponding biliverdins (TENHUNEN et al., 1969). Hemoproteins to which the heme is relatively loosely bound—methemalbumin, methemoglobin, the α- and β-chains of hemoglobin, heme-hemopexin and hemoglobin-haptoglobin complexes—are also substrates, but those hemoproteins to which the heme is firmly bound—oxyhemoglobin, carboxyhemoglobin and myoglobin—are not (TENHUNEN et al., 1969). Presumably, in the intact cell these proteins are degraded by proteolytic enzymes before their heme is released and metabolized. The biological fates of heme a, and of the covalently bound heme of cytochrome c are not known. Porphyrins and complexes of porphyrins with metals other than iron are not substrates of heme oxygenase (SCHACTER and WATERMAN, 1974).

This step appears to be the rate-limiting one in heme degradation (TENHUNEN et al., 1969), and increased activity can be induced in a number of different organs by treating rats in a variety of ways. The activity in liver increases by a factor of 2 − 3 after splenectomy, and by a factor of 2 − 7 after injecting hemoglobin or methemalbumin (TENHUNEN et al., 1970a). It is the activity in the parenchymal liver cells which increases after injecting these hemoproteins (BISSELL et al., 1971, 1972). On the other hand, infusion of heat-treated red blood cells increases enzyme activity in the sinusoidal cells of liver. Macrophages, in lung and peritoneal cavity, have high heme oxygenase activity after hemin has been injected into rats (PIMSTONE et al., 1971a), and the activity in kidney epithelial cells increases by a factor of 30 − 100 after sufficient hemoglobin has been infused intravenously to cause hemoglobinuria (PIMSTONE et al., 1971b). This increase in kidney enzyme activity is blocked by inhibitors of protein synthesis, and the enzyme appears to have a half-life of about 6 h. Increases of between 2- and 7-fold in the activity of the enzyme in liver, but not in spleen, have been observed in rats which have fasted for 72 h, after induction of hypoglycemia with insulin or mannose (these effects are reversed by glucose), and after injecting glucagon, adrenaline, or cyclic AMP (BAKKEN et al., 1972). These authors suggested that increase of heme oxygenase activity may stimulate heme turnover and hence increase bilirubin formation, which is known to occur in the whole animal after fasting and during hypoglycemia. However, another possible explanation is that hemoproteins turn over more rapidly under these conditions, and that the excess heme available for catabolism induces the increase in enzyme activity.

Involvement of cytochrome P-450 in this reaction was indicated by the marked inhibitory effect of carbon monoxide, and reversal of inhibition by light of wavelength 450 − 470 nm (TENHUNEN et al., 1972). However, the tissue distribution of heme oxygenase is different from that of the drug- and steroid-metabolizing mixed function oxidases (TENHUNEN et al., 1969). In addition, after splenectomy (TENHUNEN et al., 1970a), and after feeding $CoCl_2$ (MAINES and KAPPAS, 1974), the contents of cytochrome P-450 in rat liver do not change in parallel with the heme oxygenase activities. These findings strongly suggest that cytochrome P-450 is not involved.

YOSHIDA and KIKUCHI (1974) and YOSHIDA et al. (1974) have now solubilized and purified NADPH-cytochrome c reductase and heme oxygenase, both of which are required for heme oxygenase activity, from pig spleen, and have found that neither fraction contains significant amounts of heme. They suggest that heme binds to the apoenzyme, forming a species with the spectral properties of cytochrome P-450, and that the heme is then degraded by its own oxidative activity. A mechanism for the reaction has been proposed by YOSHIDA and KIKUCHI (1974). Hemin (Fe^{3+}) binds to heme oxygenase and is then reduced to heme (Fe^{2+}) by NADPH-cytochrome c reductase (see also TENHUNEN et al., 1972). Reaction with oxygen then forms α-hydroxyheme (α-oxyheme), and further addition of oxygen gives enzyme-biliverdin-Fe^{2+} complex and carbon monoxide. Finally, Fe^{2+} and biliverdin are released from the enzyme. KONDO et al. (1971) synthesized α-oxymesohemin and found that it was extensively converted to mesobilirubin by rats, strongly suggesting that α-oxyheme is an intermediate in the heme oxygenase reaction.

X. Biliverdin Reductase (E.C. 1.3.1.24)

LEMBERG and WYNDHAM (1936) showed that extracts of many mammalian tissues converted biliverdin to bilirubin, and that activity was stimulated by "cozymase." Liver, kidney, brain (grey matter), and spleen were the most active tissues, but muscle, heart, and lung also had some activity. SINGLETON and LASTER (1965), by following the rate of loss of biliverdin spectrophotometrically at 670 nm, found a cytoplasmic biliverdin reductase in a number of guinea pig tissues. Using biliverdin at a concentration of 60 µM, NADH was a much better cofactor than NADPH. The activity was highest in spleen and liver (approx. 1 nmol biliverdin reduced/min/mg soluble protein), and was also present in kidney, lung, brain, and intestinal mucosa. It was absent from pancreas, heart muscle, and skeletal muscle. The partially purified enzyme from liver had a pH optimum of 7.5 and K_M values of 1 µM and 240 µM for biliverdin and NADH respectively. Although the reaction did not appear to be reversible, $NADP^+$, but not NAD^+, was a strong inhibitor. By contrast, TENHUNEN et al. (1970b), using biliverdin at a concentration of 20 µM, found that biliverdin reductase activity in extracts from a number of guinea pig and rat tissues was very much higher with NADPH than with NADH. They found highest activities in rat spleen and kidney (3–4 nmol bilirubin formed/min/mg soluble protein) and slightly lower activities in liver and brain. The partially purified enzyme from rat kidney was most active at pH 7.0–7.4 and the K_M for biliverdin was 3.7 µM. Activity was markedly inhibited by Cu^{2+} and p-chloromercuribenzoate, but not by EDTA, KCN, or iodoacetate. COLLERAN and O'CARRA (1970) assayed biliverdin reductase activity in guinea pig liver extracts with NADH and NADPH, and with different concentrations of biliverdin. With biliverdin at a concentration of 25 µM, NADPH (K_M 5 µM) was more effective than NADH (K_M about 500 µM). There was competition between these cofactors, strongly suggesting that only one enzyme was present. They concluded that the apparent differences in cofactor requirement shown by the earlier workers was the result of using different concentrations of biliverdin in their assays. The K_M for biliverdin was found to be 1–2 µM in assays with NADH and 0.2 µM in assays with NADPH. Mesobiliverdin IXα and deuterobiliverdin IXα were reduced at the same rate as protobiliverdin IXα; the IXβ or IXδ isomers of protobiliverdin were reduced at less than 4% of this rate, and the IXγ isomer was inactive. O'Carra and Colleran (1971) partially purified the enzyme from guinea pig liver. The enzyme, molecular weight about 70,000, did not contain flavin, heme, or a metal, and was not inhibited by sulphydryl reagents. They showed that binding of NAD(P)H to the enzyme induced formation of a high-affinity binding site for biliverdin.

E. Conjugation of Bilirubin

Bilirubin, which is formed in most tissues, is transported bound to albumin by the serum to the liver, where one or both propionic acid side chains are esterified. The conjugated products are then excreted in the bile. Although under normal conditions the liver is responsible for conjugating all, or almost all, the bilirubin, the kidney and the digestive tract are capable of forming small amounts of conjugated bilirubin (Franco et al., 1972).

Free and conjugated bilirubins react with aryl diazonium salts (diazotised sulphanilic acid, diazotised aniline, diazotised ethyl anthranilate) to give colored products. This reaction is the one used for colorimetric determination of bilirubin in biological samples (see Lathe, 1972). These reagents react with the carbon atoms of the pyrrole rings, which are attached to the central methylene bridge carbon atom of bilirubin, forming two azodipyrrole pigments, and releasing the methylene carbon atom as formaldehyde (Hutchinson et al., 1972). When bile or serum, containing a mixture of unconjugated and mono- and di-conjugated bilirubins, reacts with one of these reagents, the resulting azodipyrroles can be separated readily by thin layer chromatography, isolated, and analyzed (see Kuenzle, 1970a, b, c; Heirwegh et al., 1970). With unconjugated bilirubin, and with bilirubin having both propionic acid side chains conjugated with the same compound, two isomeric azodipyrroles are formed; these isomers can also be separated chromatographically and analyzed (Jansen and Stoll, 1971; Compernolle et al., 1970).

It has been known for many years that bile pigment in serum can occur in at least two forms. One of these (direct reacting) reacts in the van den Bergh test (diazotized sulphanilic acid) in aqueous solution, while the other (indirect reacting) only reacts after the addition of ethanol. The chemical difference between these forms was elucidated by Lathe and his co-workers (see Billing et al., 1957; Lathe, 1972). Three bile pigments were separated from one another by reverse phase chromatography. One, which gave an indirect van den Bergh reaction, was found to be bilirubin; the other two, which were direct reacting, were found to be bilirubin β-D-monoglucuronide and bilirubin β-D-diglucuronide, with the glucuronic acid residues in ester linkage with the propionic acid side chains of bilirubin. It was thought that the compound which on analysis appeared to be bilirubin monoglucuronide might be an equimolar complex of bilirubin and its diglucuronide; however, this was disproved by Ostrow and Murphy (1970). Subsequently Jansen and Billing (1971) isolated bilirubin monoglucuronide from human and rat bile, and showed that it was present in two isomeric forms; i.e., either of the propionic acid side chains was conjugated.

Other conjugates of bilirubin have been identified in recent years, and in some species they account for a significant proportion of the conjugated bilirubin excreted in the bile. FEVERY et al. (1972a) found that in human bile 64%, and in rat bile 52%, of the bilirubin was excreted as the diglucuronide, and in man 22% and in rat 39% was excreted as the monoconjugate. In addition, small amounts of alkali-stable azodipyrroles were formed from human bile, some of which they considered might be the complex hexuronic acid conjugates isolated and identified by KUENZLE (1970a, b, c). FEVERY et al. (1972a) also found that of the total azodipyrroles formed from dog bile, 43% was the glucuronide, 30% the β-D-glucopyranoside, and 10% the β-D-xylopyranoside (see also FEVERY et al., 1971; COMPERNOLLE et al., 1971; GORDON et al., 1974). The latter two azodipyrroles were both present as mixtures of isomers. In human bile, but not in rat bile, small amounts of glucoside and xyloside were also found (FEVERY et al., 1972a). About 6% of bile pigment is present as bilirubin sulphate in man, dog, and rat (NOIR and NANET, 1974); it is not known whether it occurs as monosulphate, or disulphate, or both.

Bilirubin glucuronide is formed from bilirubin and UDPglucuronic acid, by a hepatic microsomal enzyme UDPglucuronyltransferase (UDPglucuronate glucuronyltransferase [acceptor unspecific] E.C. 2.4.1.17) (see HEIRWEGH et al., 1972; WONG, 1971a). This enzyme is firmly attached to the microsomes, and it has proved very difficult to solubilize. Hence, most of its properties have been studied with microsomes, or with preparations of them which have been treated with EDTA or a variety of detergents to increase enzyme activity (see HEIRWEGH et al., 1972; WONG, 1971a; LATHE, 1972). Liver microsomes form glucuronides of many other compounds besides bilirubin, and it is not known whether one enzyme is responsible for conjugating all the substrates, or whether there are a number of enzymes, each specific for one substrate, or for a group of related substrates.

MULDER (1972), using a preparation of rat liver microsomes activated by treatment with Triton X-100, showed that bilirubin and p-nitrophenol competitively inhibited each other's conjugation, and he concluded that both compounds were conjugated at the same active site. However, most of the evidence to date favors there being a number of different UDPglucuronyltransferases. Bilirubin-UDPglucuronyltransferase activity and transferase activity towards other substrates respond differently when isolated microsomes are treated in a number of ways (see MOWAT and ARIAS, 1970; VESSEY et al., 1973), and also when animals are treated in vivo in a number of ways (see JANSEN and HENDERSON, 1972; BOCK et al., 1973; DUVALDESTIN et al., 1975). Perhaps the most compelling evidence for there being a number of different enzymes comes from experiments with the GUNN strain of rats. These rats, and hepatic microsomal preparations from them, cannot form bilirubin glucuronides, although they can conjugate many other compounds (see MOWAT and ARIAS, 1970; JANSEN and HENDERSON, 1972). Rat liver microsomes catalyze the formation of bilirubin β-D-glucoside and bilirubin β-D-xyloside from UDPglucose and UDPxylose respectively (FEVERY et al., 1972b, c; WONG, 1971b). Interestingly, microsomal preparation from the GUNN rat cannot form either of these conjugates (FEVERY et al., 1972b), suggesting that perhaps the glucuronyl, glucosyl, and xylosyl conjugates are all formed by the same enzyme. In addition to the problem of acceptor and donor specificity of the conjugating enzyme or enzymes, there is evidence that there might be one enzyme for forming bilirubin monoglucuronide, and another enzyme for converting it to bilirubin diglucuronide (HALAC et al., 1972; JANSEN, 1974).

The first step in solving these problems has been made by GREGORY and STRICKLAND (1973) who have prepared a stable, soluble preparation of bilirubin-UDPglucuronyltransferase from rat liver microsomes. It remains to purify this preparation by the conventional techniques of protein purification, and to find out whether enzymes specific for different substrates can be separated from one another or, alternatively, whether a completely pure enzyme can be obtained which conjugates all substrates.

F. Control of Heme and Hemoprotein Biosynthesis

I. Introduction

It appears that the major factor controlling the rate of synthesis of heme in mammalian and avian cells is the rate of synthesis of ALA. The formation of ALA from succinyl CoA and glycine is the first step in the pathway leading specifically to heme, and thus it is logical that this be the rate-limiting step, and the one at which control be exerted. Evidence that it is the rate-limiting step is that only very low concentrations of ALA and other intermediates of the heme biosynthetic pathway can normally be detected in cells, that heme biosynthesis occurs more rapidly from ALA than from succinate and glycine in whole cells (DRUYAN and KELLY, 1972), and in cell-free extracts, and that ALA synthetase activity is lower than normal in cells that cannot make heme at the normal rate (cf. AOKI et al., 1974). Evidence that it is the step at which control is normally exerted is the finding that the activity, or the amount, of ALA synthetase, but not of other enzymes in the pathway, is markedly increased under conditions, such as the genetic or experimental porphyrias, where porphyrins and their precursors are synthesized at excessive rates.

Although heme is the end product of the pathway, it only plays its roles in cellular metabolism in the form of hemoproteins, and thus the synthesis of heme and the apoproteins must be coordinated, since neither accumulates in cells. The two types of cells in the body that are responsible for synthesizing the bulk of the heme are the erythropoietic cells and the liver parenchymal cells. The former account for about 80%, and the latter for about 20%, of the heme which turns over daily. However, there are major differences between these cells as regards hemoprotein synthesis and degradation. In erythropoietic cells, hemoglobin, into which most of the heme formed is incorporated, is synthesized slowly during the first 50 h out of the total 70 h taken for the proerythroblast to develop into the mature erythrocyte, i.e., while cell divisions are still occurring. After the final cell division, hemoglobin synthesis occurs rapidly, then it slows down when the cell becomes a reticulocyte, and stops when it finally matures into an erythrocyte (DENTON et al., 1975). The hemoglobin remains stable in the erythrocyte for the whole of its life, approx. 120 days in man, and the heme and globin are then broken down by the cells of the reticuloendothelial system. Thus, all that is re-

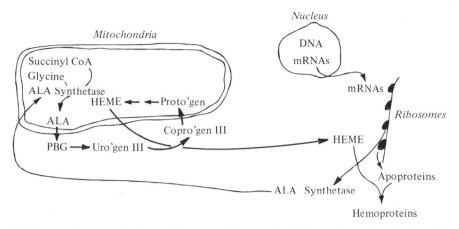

Fig. 6. Schematic representation of heme and hemoprotein biosynthesis showing how heme may regulate activity of ALA synthetase, OR, formation of ALA synthetase, and apoprotein moieties of hemoproteins

quired of any control mechanism(s) is that it be able to alter the rates of synthesis of both heme and the α- and β-globin chains in a coordinate manner at the different stages of development. By contrast, liver cells synthesize a number of hemoproteins which all have relatively short half-lives. These hemoproteins play important roles in a number of areas of intermediary metabolism, and liver cells have to be able to alter the content of one or more of these hemoproteins in response to changes in the environmental conditions, by speeding up or slowing down the rates of synthesis of both heme and the relevant apoproteins. Therefore, in liver cells, control has to be more finely poised than in erythropoietic cells. In view of the marked differences between the metabolism of hemoproteins in these two types of cells, it is possible that they may use different control mechanisms to cope with their particular requirements. Figure 6 gives an outline of some of the features which appear to be important in control.

II. Control in Erythropoietic Cells

During the early stages of development the chick embryo blastoderm contains little or no hemoglobin. However, if ALA is added, heme and hemoglobin are formed rapidly (LEVERE and GRANICK, 1965, 1967; WAINWRIGHT and WAINWRIGHT, 1966, 1967). The formation of hemoglobin, but not that of heme, was blocked by inhibitors of protein synthesis but not by inhibitors of nucleic acid synthesis, showing that the cells did not contain globin, but that they did contain messenger RNA for globin synthesis. These cells, then, have the rest of the machinery for making hemoglobin, but lack ALA synthetase. From these experiments, it was concluded that ALA synthetase is the rate-limiting step in heme biosynthesis, and that heme, acting at the ribosomal level, stimulates globin synthesis. LEVERE et al. (1967) found that a number of steroids with 5βH-configuration stimulated heme and hemoglobin synthesis in these cells, and that their action was blocked by actinomycin D, an inhibitor of RNA synthesis. These steroids had previously been found to induce the formation of ALA synthetase in chick embryo liver cells (Granick, 1966), and it was proposed that they also acted in this way in erythropoietic cells. 5βH-steroids were also shown to stimulate heme and hemoglobin synthesis in mammalian erythropoietic cells (Gorshein and Gardner, 1970; Gordon et al., 1970). Bottomley and Smithee (1969) found that erythropoietin stimulated ALA synthetase formation in rabbit bone marrow cells in vitro. Thus it would seem that steroid hormones and erythropoietin, acting independently (Gordon et al., 1970) but by a common mechanism, stimulate hemoglobin synthesis, and the development of erythropoietic cells.

Karibian and London (1965) found that addition of hemin to whole or lysed rabbit reticulocytes markedly inhibited the incorporation of glycine, but not of ALA, into heme, and also stimulated the incorporation of $[^{14}C]$-valine into newly formed hemoglobin. The incorporation of glycine into heme in rabbit reticulocytes was rapidly and markedly inhibited by inhibitors of protein synthesis (Grayzel et al., 1967). Since reticulocyte lysates can continue to make heme from glycine for several hours, even in the absence of protein synthesis, it seems that ALA synthetase does not turn over rapidly. Thus the heme that accumulates when protein synthesis is inhibited in the whole cell appears to control its own formation by inhibiting ALA synthetase activity, rather than by repressing its synthesis. These authors suggested that the rapid onset of inhibition was due to heme quickly reaching an inhibitory concentration in mitochondria, where ALA synthetase is located. Purified ALA synthetase from rabbit reticulocytes is known to be markedly inhibited by hemin (Aoki et al., 1971). An alternative role for heme has been suggested by Ponka et al. (1974) and Neuwirt et al. (1974), namely that heme regulates the transport of iron into reticulocytes. It is possible that both mechanisms operate, although which is more important is not known. At increasing concentrations of O_2 above 5% (v/v), the progressive inhibitions of heme and globin synthesis parallel one another in pigeon erythrocyte nuclei. The inhibition of globin synthesis by O_2 can be reversed by hemin, suggesting that O_2 has a primary role in controlling synthesis of heme, which in turn controls the synthesis of globin (Hammel and Bessman, 1965). A number of the enzymes of heme synthesis are known to be inhibited by O_2. All the evidence cited above is consistent with co-ordination of heme and globin synthesis being achieved by heme inhibiting its own synthesis and stimulating the synthesis of globin. Experiments with whole and lysed reticulocytes show that hemin stimulates globin formation mainly, if not solely, by preventing inhibition of initiation of its synthesis. In the absence of hemin, an inactive cytoplasmic protein is converted first to an inhibitor of peptide chain initiation, whose action is reversed by hemin, and on longer incubation to an inhibitor whose action is not reversed by hemin (cf. Gross and Rabinovitz, 1972; Balkow et al., 1973; Gross, 1974a, b). This "translational repressor" of globin synthesis has been isolated and purified from human mature erythrocytes in both hemin-reversible and hemin-irreversible forms (Freedman et al., 1974). Both forms have molecular weights of about 300,000.

Patients with iron-deficiency anaemia, or with anaemia due to lead poisoning, synthesize less α-globin than β-globin (Ben-Bassat et al., 1974; White et al., 1971; White and Harvey, 1972; White and Hoffbrand, 1974). On adding hemin to these reticulocytes, this abnormality is corrected, suggesting that hemin has a more marked stimulatory effect on initiation of the synthesis of α- than of β-globin. This conclusion is supported by the work of GIGLIONI et al. (1973) on the translation of hemoglobin mRNA from rabbit reticulocytes in Xenopus oocytes in the presence and absence of hemin.

In addition to its effects on globin synthesis, heme stimulates the formation of all other proteins formed by reticulocytes and their lysates (LODISH and DESALU, 1973; MATHEWS et al., 1973), including those programmed by added mRNA, and it also stimulates protein synthesis in nonerythroid cells (BEUZARD and LONDON, 1974). Although it is clear that the effect of hemin in controlling the rate of globin formation is of physiological importance, the significance of the stimulation of synthesis of other proteins by hemin is not yet known.

III. Control in Liver

In liver heme does not stimulate the synthesis of the protein moieties of hemoproteins. After injecting ALA or hemin into rats and mice, heme accumulates in the liver, but there is no increase in the amounts of the hemoproteins (DE MATTEIS and GIBBS, 1972; DRUYAN and KELLY, 1972). Thus, it would appear that the rates of synthesis of individual apoproteins change in response to environmental changes, and that the rate of synthesis of heme is controlled, so that sufficient is available to complex with these apoproteins (RAJAMANICKAM et al., 1975). The rate of synthesis of heme could be regulated by heme itself exercising a negative control, or by apoproteins exercising a positive control. A high concentration of heme, in excess of that bound on hemoproteins, could cause a decrease in the activity, or the amount, of the rate-limiting enzyme ALA synthetase, and a deficiency of heme, relative to the amount of apoprotein, could allow an increase. Alternatively, a high concentration of apoprotein could cause an increase in the activity, or the amount, of ALA synthetase, and absence of apoprotein could cause a decrease (cf. PADMANABAN et al., 1973).

There is much indirect evidence for the existence of regulatory heme, although it is not known where in the cell it is located, whether it occurs free in solution or bound to a protein, or whether it acts to repress formation of ALA synthetase or simply to inhibit its activity. Many of the compounds which disrupt the control of heme biosynthesis and cause a marked increase in ALA synthetase and accumulation of ALA, PBG, and porphyrins, seem to act primarily to reduce the concentration of regulatory heme in one way or another. Allylisopropylacetamide (AIA) and related compounds cause a rapid degradation of cytochrome P-450 to unknown green pigments (DE MATTEIS, 1971); phenobarbitone causes a rapid increase in formation of cytochrome P-450 (BARON and TEPHLY, 1970; RAJAMANICKAM et al., 1975); and 3,5-diethoxycarbonyl-1,4-dihydrocollidine (DDC) and griseofulvin cause a rapid fall in the activity of heme synthetase (DE MATTEIS, 1972; DE MATTEIS et al., 1973). That is, on blocking heme synthesis, or on speeding up the synthesis or breakdown of cytochrome P-450 the concentration of regulatory heme will fall rapidly, the control of ALA synthetase will be lifted, and its activity or amount will increase markedly. Additional evidence in favor of this mechanism is that when two compounds, which affect heme metabolism in different ways, are given together, the porphyrinogenic effect is much greater than when either is given alone (DE MATTEIS, 1973; DE MATTEIS and GIBBS, 1972; STEIN et al., 1970). Further support comes from the findings on acute intermittent porphyria in man (cf. MEYER and SCHMID, 1973). The primary defect in this genetic disorder is at PBG deaminase, whose activity is half the normal value. In remission, hepatic ALA synthetase is normal, but during attacks, it is markedly increased and large amounts of ALA and PBG are excreted. The simplest explanation to account for these findings is as follows. Normally, the liver can make sufficient heme for its needs even with only half the normal complement of PBG deaminase, and control is still exerted on ALA synthetase. However, when the liver has to make increased amounts of hemoproteins (probably cytochrome P-450 which has the fastest turnover, and for which much of the liver's heme is required), PBG deaminase becomes the rate-limiting step, sufficient heme cannot be made, the concentration of regulatory heme falls, and the amount, or the activity, of ALA synthetase increases. As a consequence, large amounts of ALA and PBG are made. This interpretation is supported by the finding that compounds like barbiturates, which are well known to precipitate attacks in people with acute intermittent porphyria, are porphyrinogenic in experimental animals only when heme synthesis in their liver is partially inhibited (DE MATTEIS, 1973).

It is possible that porphyrinogenic compounds can also disrupt the control of heme biosynthesis in other ways. GAJDOS and GAJDOS-TÖRÖK (1969b) found that there was a marked fall in the hepatic ATP concentration before the increase in ALA synthetase in animals given a number of different compounds. There was an inverse correlation between the ATP concentration and the amount of porphyrin produced, but no correlation between NADH concentration and porphyrin formation. That experimental porphyria might be due to a reduction in the ability of the cell to oxidise NADH was proposed by COWGER et al. (1963) (see also LABBE, 1967). More recently, BEATTIE et al. (1973) have suggested that the increase in hepatic ALA synthetase in rats caused by ethanol ingestion is due to a change in the $NADH/NAD^+$ ratio in the cell. LABBE et al. (1965) found two succinyl CoA synthetases in mouse liver, and showed that after giving animals AIA or DDC, there was a marked increase in the activity of one of them prior to an increase in ALA synthetase. They concluded that increasing the availability of succinyl CoA for ALA formation might be one of the primary effects of these compounds. PATTON and BEATTIE (1973) suggested that an increase in the ability of ALA synthetase to react with succinyl CoA, because of structural changes in the mitochondrion or conformational changes in the enzyme itself, might account for the increased activity of the enzyme in experimental porphyria.

While it seems likely that heme regulates the rate of formation of ALA, it is not known exactly how it does this. It could act at the genetic level to repress the formation of mRNA for ALA synthetase, or at the ribosomal level to inhibit the synthesis of the enzyme. Alternatively, it could act directly on the enzyme in the mitochondrion to inhibit its activity. The uncertainty arises from current inability to measure the amount of the enzyme as distinct from its activity. A change in activity, as measured in cell-free systems, could be due to a change in the number of enzyme molecules, or to a change in the activity of the enzyme molecules. Most, but by no means all, of the evidence suggests that heme regulates the rate of synthesis of the enzyme in the cell and hence its amount. This would provide a rapid means to control heme synthesis, since ALA synthetase apparently has a short half-life in liver mitochondria. Porphyrinogenic compounds, probably acting by reducing the concentration of regulatory heme, cause an increase in ALA synthetase not only in mitochondria, but also in the cytoplasm of liver cells (cf. HAYASHI et al., 1969). In chick embryo liver cells there is an increase in mitochondria only (TOMITA et al., 1974). These increases are blocked by inhibitors of RNA and protein synthesis (SASSA and GRANICK, 1970; TYRRELL and MARKS, 1972). A requirement for RNA for increase in ALA synthetase has been directly shown by HICKMAN et al. (1968) and SKEA et al. (1971); RNA isolated from the livers of porphyric animals, but not RNA from the livers of normal ones, caused an increase in ALA synthetase and in porphyrin formation when added to chick embryo liver cells. Hemin, given at the same time as porphyrinogenic compounds, stops the increase in ALA synthetase probably by acting on the ribosomes to inhibit translation of mRNA into protein (SASSA and GRANICK, 1970; TYRRELL and MARKS, 1972). If hemin is given to rats after the porphyrinogenic compound, the high activity of ALA synthetase in mitochondria falls, and the cytoplasmic activity increases (HAYASHI et al., 1972), suggesting to these authors that hemin may also block the transport of ALA synthetase to its functional site in the mitochondrion. In similar experiments with mice (GAYATHRI et al., 1973) and with chick embryo livers (TOMITA et al., 1974) hemin caused a fall in the mitochondrial ALA synthetase activity, but no rise in cytoplasmic activity.

Although regulation of the formation of ALA synthetase on the ribosomes with heme acting as an inhibitor is favored by most researchers, regulation of formation of ALA synthetase with apocytochrome P-450 acting as an inducer at the translational level has been proposed by PADMANABAN et al. (1973) to explain their own work, and that of others, on experimental porphyria in animals. To my mind, both these hypotheses are equally capable of explaining how the cell coordinates the synthesis of heme and apoproteins, and further work is required to show which is correct.

Regulation of the rate of formation of ALA synthetase on cytoplasmic ribosomes, by either of the above mechanisms, requires that enzyme molecules be constantly transported to their functional site in the mitochondrial matrix. I find it difficult to visualize how this large protein molecule can readily cross both the outer and inner mitochondrial membranes. It would be much simpler if heme were to regulate its own synthesis by inhibiting the activity of the enzyme. The activity of partially purified hepatic ALA synthetase is reversibly inhibited by low concentrations of heme, but whether inhibition occurs in the intact cell is difficult to prove. However, the subcellular organization seems to be ideal, since ALA synthetase is located in the mitochondrial matrix or even loosely bound to the inner mitochondrial membrane to which heme synthetase is also attached. If heme is made faster than it is removed, to make hemoproteins, the concentration at the site of synthesis could increase and inhibit ALA synthetase activity. Conversely, if heme is removed faster than it is synthesized the concentration at the site of synthesis would fall, the activity of ALA synthetase could increase, and hence heme could be synthesized more rapidly. The normal changes in the demand for heme might only cause relatively small changes in ALA synthetase activity. However, if the concentration of inhibitory heme were to fall markedly, either because of its rapid removal into hemoproteins or because its synthesis was blocked at some stage beyond formation of ALA, there could be a large increase in ALA synthetase activity and excessive synthesis of intermediates in the pathway. That ALA synthetase activity in mitochondria from porphyric animals is much higher than in those from normal animals, in assays with intact or only partially damaged mitochondria, could be due to their having a much lower concentration of inhibitory heme rather than a larger amount of ALA synthetase. In this respect, it is of interest that sonicated mitochondria from normal and porphyric animals both have the same high ALA synthetase activity (PATTON and BEATTIE, 1973; see also Sect. D.II). Sonication of mitochondria may remove the inhibitory heme from the vicinity of the enzyme, and allow maximum activity to be expressed, although other explanations are possible (see PATTON and BEATTIE, 1973).

While the most reasonable explanation for the effects of inhibitors of RNA and protein synthesis and of hemin in vivo is that the cell regulates the rate of synthesis of ALA synthetase, it is not impossible to explain many of these effects in terms of reversible inhibition of enzyme activity by heme. Inhibitors of protein and RNA synthesis could block the effects of porphyrinogenic compounds by inhibiting the formation of the protein moieties of hemoproteins; this could lead to accumulation of heme in mitochondria and inhibition of ALA synthetase activity. The effect of hemin in reversing the effects of porphyrinogenic compounds in vivo could be due to its being taken up rapidly by mitochondria under these conditions and inhibiting ALA synthetase activity (cf. GAYATHRI et al., 1973). The high activity of ALA synthetase in fetal liver, and the lack of effect of DDC and hemin administered in vivo (WOODS and DIXON, 1972) could be due to the fact that the partially purified fetal enzyme, unlike the adult one, is not inhibited by hemin (WOODS and MURTHY, 1975). In adult animals, whose ALA synthetase activity is inhibited by hemin, the apparent rapid turnover of the enzyme caused by inhibitors of protein synthesis could be due to inhibition of enzyme activity by heme which accumulates in mitochondria. However, the rapid turnover of the fetal enzyme (WOODS, 1974) cannot be explained in the same way since it is not inhibited by hemin.

It may be that heme regulates its own synthesis in one way only, either by inhibiting the formation of ALA synthetase, or by inhibiting the activity of the enzyme. However, it is also possible that heme functions in both these ways, and that the relative importance of each mechanism varies with the metabolic conditions in the cell.

We normally think of the biosynthetic pathway from succinyl CoA and glycine to heme as being unbranched in mammalian cells. However, both ALA and PBG can be converted enzymically to other products. If excessive amounts of ALA or PBG were converted to these products under some conditions, less of them would be available to form heme, and control of heme biosynthesis could be disrupted. ALA is transaminated (KOWALSKI et al., 1959) and oxidatively deaminated (PISANI et al., 1967) to γ, δ-dioxovaleric acid by extracts of a number of mammalian tissues. It is not known whether these enzymes metabolize a significant proportion of the ALA formed in vivo, or whether their activities change under different conditions.

Tschudy et al. (1962) found that the metabolism of ALA by alternative pathways in liver did not change in experimental porphyria. A PBG oxygenase, which converts PBG mainly to 2-hydroxy-5-oxoPBG, occurs in liver microsomes (Tomaro et al., 1973; Frydman et al., 1975). The activity of the enzyme is normally low, but on purification an inhibitor is removed, and the activity increases. In vivo the activity increases markedly after injecting small amounts of progesterone or pregnenolone into rats. Progesterone is a weak inducer of hepatic ALA synthetase in rats (Kaufman et al., 1970) and in chick embryo liver cells, but it can be metabolized to a number of 5βH steroids which are strong inducers (Granick and Sassa, 1971). There is evidence that 5βH steroids act at the nuclear level to stimulate the synthesis of mRNA, possibly that coding for ALA synthetase (Granick and Sassa, 1971; Incefy et al., 1974; Incefy and Kappas, 1974). It is also possible that progesterone, or perhaps one of its derivatives, may stimulate PBG oxygenase activity. This could cause a fall in the amount of heme synthesized, and lead to a subsequent increase in the activity or the amount of ALA synthetase. Further work is required to test the validity of this idea, but it has the merit that the primary action of 5βH steroids, like that of other porphyrinogenic compounds, would be to interfere with heme metabolism at a step beyond the control enzyme ALA synthetase.

Abbreviations

AIA	Allylisopropylacetamide
ALA	Aminolevulinic acid
ATP	Adenosine triphosphate
CoA	Coenzyme A
Cyclic AMP	Adenosine 3, 5-cyclic monophosphate
Copro'gen	Coproporphyrinogen
DDC	3,5-Diethoxycarbonyl-1,4-dihydrocollidine
DNA	Deoxyribonucleic acid
EDTA	Ethylenediaminetetraacetic acid
GSH	Glutathione (reduced)
mRNA	Messenger ribonucleic acid
NAD$^+$ (NADH)	Nicotinamide adenine dinucleotide (reduced form)
NADP$^+$ (NADPH)	Nicotinamide adenine dinucleotide phosphate (reduced form)
PBG	Porphobilinogen
UDP	Uridine diphosphate
Uro'gen	Uroporphyrinogen

References

Abboud, M.M., Jordan, P.M., Akhtar, M.: Biosynthesis of 5-aminolevulinic acid. Involvement of a retention-inversion mechanism. J. chem. Soc. chem. Commun. 643−644 (1974)

Åkeson, Å., Ehrenstein, G.v., Hevesy, G., Theorell, H.: Life span of myoglobin. Arch. Biochem. Biophys. **91**, 310−318 (1960)

Aoki, Y., Urata, G., Wada, O., Takaku, F.: Measurement of δ-aminolevulinic acid synthetase in human erythroblasts. J. clin. Invest. **53**, 1326−1334 (1974)

Aoki, Y., Wada, O., Urata, G., Takaku, F., Nakao, K.: Purification and some properties of δ-aminolevulinate (ALA) synthetase in rabbit reticulocytes. Biochem. biophys. Res. Commun. **42**, 568−575 (1971)

Aschenbrenner, V., Druyan, R., Albin, R., Rabinowitz, M.: Heme a, cytochrome c and total protein turnover in mitochondria of rat heart and liver. Biochem. J. **119**, 157 – 160 (1970)

Bakken, A.F., Thaler, M.M., Schmid, R.: Metabolic regulation of heme catabolism and bilirubin production. I. Hormonal control of hepatic heme oxygenase activity. J. clin. Invest. **51**, 530 – 536 (1972)

Balkow, K., Mizuno, S., Rabinovitz, M.: Inhibition of an initiation codon function by hemin deficiency and the hemin-controlled translational repressor in the reticulocyte cell-free system. Biochem. biophys. Res. Commun. **54**, 315 – 323 (1973)

Barnes, R., Connelly, J.L., Jones, O.T.G.: The utilization of iron and its complexes by mammalian mitochondria. Biochem. J. **128**, 1043 – 1055 (1972)

Barnes, R., Jones, M.S., Jones, O.T.G., Porra, R.J.: Ferrochelatase and δ-aminolevulinate synthetase in brain, heart, kidney, and liver of normal and porphyric rats. Biochem. J. **124**, 633 – 637 (1971)

Baron, J., Tephly, T.R.: Further studies on the relationship of the stimulatory effects of phenobarbital and 3,4-benzpyrene on hepatic heme synthesis and their effects on hepatic microsomal drug oxidations. Arch. Biochem. Biophys. **139**, 410 – 420 (1970)

Batlle, A.M. del C., Benson, A., Rimington, C.: Purification and properties of coproporphyrinogenase. Biochem. J. **97**, 731 – 740 (1965)

Batlle, A.M. del C., Ferramola, A.M., Grinstein, M.: Purification and general properties of δ-aminolevulate dehydratase of cow liver. Biochem. J. **104**, 244 – 249 (1967)

Batlle, A.M. del C., Grinstein, M.: Porphyrin biosynthesis. II. Phyriaporphyrinogen III., a normal intermediate in the biosynthesis of protoporphyrin 9. Biochim. biophys. Acta (Amst.) **82**, 13 – 20 (1964)

Battersby, A.R., Baldas, J., Collins, J., Grayson, D.H., James, K.J., McDonald, E.: Mechanism of biosynthesis of the vinyl groups of protoporphyrin IX. J. chem. Soc. chem. Commun. 1265 – 1266 (1972)

Battersby, A.R., Hunt, E., McDonald, E.: Biosynthesis of type III porphyrins: nature of the rearrangement process. J. chem. Soc. chem. Commun. 442 – 443 (1973)

Beattie, D.S., Patton, G.M., Rubin, E.: The control of δ-aminolevulinic acid synthetase in rat liver mitochondria. Effect of pyrazole on the apparent induction. Enzyme **16**, 252 – 257 (1973)

Ben-Bassat, I., Mozel, M., Ramot, B.: Globin synthesis in iron-deficiency anemia. Blood **44**, 551 – 555 (1974)

Berk, P.D., Howe, R.B., Berlin, N.I.: Disorders of bilirubin metabolism. In: Duncan's Diseases of Metabolism. Genetics and Metabolism. 7th edn. Bondy, P.K., Rosenberg, L.E. (eds.), pp. 825 – 882. Philadelphia – London – Toronto: W.B. Saunders Company 1974a

Berk, P.D., Rodkey, F.L., Blaschke, T.F., Collison, H.A., Waggoner, J.G.: Comparison of plasma bilirubin turnover and carbon monoxide production in man. J. Lab. clin. Med. **83**, 29 – 37 (1974b)

Beuzard, Y., London, I.M.: The effects of hemin and double-stranded RNA on α and β globin synthesis in reticulocytes and Krebs II ascites cell-free systems and the relationship of these effects to an initiation factor preparation Proc. nat. Acad. Sci. (Wash.) **71**, 2863 – 2866 (1974)

Billing, B.H., Cole, P.G., Lathe, G.H.: The excretion of bilirubin as a diglucuronide giving the direct van den Bergh reaction. Biochem. J. **65**, 774 – 784 (1957)

Bissell, D.M., Hammaker, L., Schmid, R.: Cellular sites of erythrocyte and hemoglobin catabolism in the liver. Blood **38**, 789 (1971)

Bissell, D.M., Hammaker, L., Schmid, R.: Hemoglobin and erythrocyte catabolism in rat liver: The separate roles of parenchymal and sinusoidal cells. Blood **40**, 812 – 822 (1972)

Bock, K.W., Fröhling, W., Remmer, H., Rexer, B.: Effects of phenobarbital and 3-methylcholanthrene on substrate specificity of rat liver microsomal UDP-glucuronyltransferase. Biochim. biophys. Acta (Amst.) **327**, 46 – 56 (1973)

Bock, K.W., Krauss, E., Fröhling, W.: Regulation of δ-aminolevulinic acid synthetase by drugs and steroids in vivo and in isolated perfused rat liver. Europ. J. Biochem. **23**, 366 – 371 (1971)

Bogorad, L.: The enzymatic synthesis of porphyrins from porphobilinogen. I. Uroporphyrin I. J. biol. Chem. **233**, 501 – 509 (1958a)

Bogorad, L.: The enzymatic synthesis of porphyrins from porphobilinogen. II. Uroporphyrin III. J. biol. Chem. **233**, 510 – 515 (1958 b)

Bottomley, S.S.: Characterization and measurement of heme synthetase in normal human bone marrow. Blood **31**, 314 – 322 (1968)

Bottomley, S.S., Smithee, G.A.: Effect of erythropoietin on bone marrow Δ-aminolevulinic acid synthetase and heme synthetase. J. Lab. clin. Med. **74**, 445 – 452 (1969)

Boveris, A., Chance, B.: The mitochondrial generation of hydrogen peroxide. General properties and effect of hyperbaric oxygen. Biochem. J. **134**, 707 – 716 (1973)

Bugany, H., Flothe, L., Weser, U.: Kinetics of metal chelatase of rat liver mitochondria. FEBS Lett. **13**, 92 – 94 (1971)

Calissano, P., Cartasegna, C., Matteini, M.: Purificazione e proprieta dell' ALA deidratasi critrocitaria umana. G. Biochim. **15**, 18 – 29 (1966)

Cavaleiro, J.A.S., Kenner, G.W., Smith, K.M.: Pyrroles and related compounds. Part XXXII. Biosynthesis of protoporphyrin IX from coproporphyrinogen III. J. chem. Soc. (Perkin I) 1188 – 1194 (1974)

Cheh, A., Neilands, J.B.: Zinc, an essential metal ion for beef liver δ-aminolevulinate dehydratase. Biochem. biophys. Res. Commun. **55**, 1060 – 1063 (1973)

Coleman, D.L.: Purification and properties of δ-aminolevulinate dehydratase from tissues of two strains of mice. J. biol. Chem. **241**, 5511 – 5517 (1966)

Colleran, E., Ó Carra, P.: Specificity of biliverdin reductase. Biochem. J. **119**, 16P – 17P (1970)

Comai, K., Gaylor, J.L.: Existence and separation of three forms of cytochrome P-450 in rat liver microsomes. J. biol. Chem. **248**, 4947 – 4955 (1973)

Compernolle, F., Jansen, F.H., Heirwegh, K.P.M.: Mass-spectrometric study of the azopigments obtained from bile pigments with diazotised ethyl anthranilate. Biochem. J. **120**, 891 – 894 (1970)

Compernolle, F., Van Hees, G.P., Fevery, F., Heirwegh, K.P.M: Mass-spectrometric structure elucidation of dog bile azopigments as the acyl glycosides of glucopyranose and xylopyranose. Biochem. J. **125**, 811 – 819 (1971)

Cooper, J.M., Thomas, P.: Cytochromes of ovary mitochondria: effect of human chorionic gonadotrophin. Biochem. J. **117**, 24P – 25P (1970)

Cornford, P.: Transformation of porphobilinogen into porphyrins by preparations from human erythrocytes. Biochem. J. **91**, 64 – 73 (1964)

Cowger, M.L., Labbe, R.F., Sewell, M.: Oxidative metabolism of tissue culture cells in the presence of porphyria inducing drugs. Arch. Biochem. Biophys. **101**, 96 – 102 (1963)

Dailey, H.A., Lascelles, J.: Ferrochelatase activity in wild type and mutant strains of *Spirillum itersonii*. Solubilization with chaotropic agents. Arch. Biochem. Biophys. **160**, 523 – 529 (1974)

Daly, J.S.F., Little, J.M., Troxler, R.F., Lester, R.: Metabolism of ^{3}H-myoglobin. Nature (Lond.) **216**, 1030 – 1031 (1967)

Davies, R.C., Gorchein, A., Neuberger, A., Sandy, J.D., Tait, G.H.: Biosynthesis of bacteriochlorophyll. Nature (Lond.) **245**, 15 – 19 (1973)

Davies, R.C., Neuberger, A.: Polypyrroles formed from porphobilinogen and amines by uroporphyrinogen synthetase of *Rhodopseudomonas spheroides*. Biochem. J. **133**, 471 – 492 (1973)

De Matteis, F.: Loss of heme in rat liver caused by the porphyrinogenic agent 2-allyl-2-isopropylacetamide. Biochem. J. **124**, 767 – 777 (1971)

De Matteis, F.: The effects of drugs on the activities of 5-aminolevulinate synthetase and other enzymes in the pathway of heme biosynthesis. Biochem. J. **130**, 52P – 53P (1972)

De Matteis, F.: Drug interactions in experimental hepatic porphyria. A model for the exacerbation by drugs of human variegate porphyria. Enzyme **16**, 266 – 275 (1973)

De Matteis, F., Abbritti, G., Gibbs, A.H.: Decreased liver activity of porphyrin-metal chelatase in hepatic porphyria caused by 3,5-diethoxycarbonyl-1,4-dihydrocollidine. Biochem. J. **134**, 717 – 727 (1973)

De Matteis, F., Gibbs, A.: Stimulation of liver 5-aminolevulinate synthetase by drugs and its relevance to drug-induced accumulation of cytochrome P-450. Studies with phenylbutazone and 3,5-diethoxycarbonyl-1,4-dihydrocollidine. Biochem. J. **126**, 1149 – 1160 (1972)

Denton, M.J., Spencer, N., Arnstein, H.R.V.: Biochemical and enzymic changes during
erythrocyte differentiation: The significance of the final cell division. Biochem. J. **146**,
205–211 (1975)

Doyle, D.: Subunit structure of δ-aminolevulinate dehydratase from mouse liver. J. biol.
Chem. **246**, 4965–4972 (1971)

Doyle, D., Schimke, R.T.: The genetic and developmental regulation of hepatic δ-aminolevulinate dehydratase in mice. J. biol. Chem. **244**, 5449–5459 (1969)

Druyan, R., De Bernard, B., Rabinowitz, M.: Turnover of cytochromes labeled with δ-aminolevulinic acid $-^3$H in rat liver. J. biol. Chem. **244**, 5874–5878 (1969)

Druyan, R., Kelly, A.: The effect of exogenous δ-aminolevulinate on rat liver heme and cytochromes. Biochem. J. **129**, 1095–1099 (1972)

Duvaldestin, P., Mahu, J.-L., Berthelot, P.: Effect of fasting on substrate specificity of rat
liver UDP-glucuronyltransferase. Biochim. biophys. Acta (Amst.) **384**, 81–86 (1975)

Ebert, P.S., Tschudy, D.P., Choudhry, J.N., Chirigos, M.A.: A simple micro method for the
direct determination of δ-amino[^{14}C]levulinic acid production in murine spleen and liver
homogenates. Biochim. biophys. Acta (Amst.) **208**, 236–250 (1970)

Falk, J.E.: Porphyrins and Metalloporphyrins. Amsterdam–London–New York: Elsevier
Publishing Co., 1964

Fanica-Gaignier, M., Clement-Metral, J.: 5-Aminolevulinic acid synthetase of *Rhodopseudomonas spheroides* Y. Purification and some properties. Europ. J. Biochem. **40**, 13–18
(1973a)

Fanica-Gaignier, M., Clement-Metral, J.: 5-Aminolevulinic acid synthetase of *Rhodopseudomonas spheroides* Y. Kinetic mechanism and inhibition by ATP. Europ. J. Biochem. **40**,
19–24 (1973b)

Feigelson, P., Dashman, T., Margolis, F.: The half-life time of induced tryptophan peroxidase
in vivo. Arch. Biochem. Biophys. **85**, 478–482 (1959)

Fevery, J., Van Damme, B., Michiels, R., De Groote, J., Heirwegh, K.P.M.: Bilirubin conjugates in bile of man and rat in the normal state and in liver disease. J. clin. Invest. **51**,
2482–2492 (1972a)

Fevery, J., Van Hees, G.P., Leroy, P., Compernolle, F., Heirwegh, K.P.M.: Excretion in dog
bile of glucose and xylose conjugates of bilirubin. Biochem. J. **125**, 803–810 (1971)

Fevery, J., Leroy, P., Heirwegh, K.P.M.: Enzymic transfer of glucose and xylose from uridine
diphosphate glucose and uridine diphosphate xylose to bilirubin by untreated and digitonin-activated preparations from rat liver. Biochem. J. **129**, 619–633 (1972b)

Fevery, J., Leroy, P., Van de Vijver, M., Heirwegh, K.P.M.: Structures of bilirubin conjugates synthesised in vitro from bilirubin and uridine diphosphate glucuronic acid, uridine
diphosphate glucose or uridine disphosphate xylose by preparations from rat liver Biochem J.
129, 635–644 (1972c)

Finelli, V.N., Murthy, L., Peirano, W.B., Petering, H.G.: δ-Aminolevulinate dehydratase, a
zinc dependent enzyme. Biochem. biophys. Res. Commun. **60**, 1418–1424 (1974)

Fleischmann, R., Mattenheimer, H., Holmes, A.W., Remmer, H.: Micromethod for the preparation of a microsomal fraction from rat and human liver by differential sedimentation.
Biochem. biophys. Res. Commun. **62**, 289–295 (1975)

Franco, D., Preaux, A.-M., Bismuth, H., Berthelot, P.: Extra hepatic formation of bilirubin
glucuronides in the rat. Biochim. biophys. Acta (Amst.) **286**, 55–61 (1972)

Freedman, M.L., Geraghty, M., Rosman, J.: Hemin control of globin synthesis. Isolation of
a hemin-reversible translational repressor from human mature erythrocytes. J. biol. Chem.
249, 7290–7294 (1974)

Freshney, R.I., Paul, J.: Measurement of aminolevulinate synthetase activity in normal mouse
liver with [2-^{14}C]-glycine. Biochim. biophys. Acta (Amst.) **220**, 594–601 (1970)

Freshney, R.I., Paul, J.: The activities of three enzymes of heme synthesis during hepatic
erythropoiesis in the mouse embryo. J. Embryol. exp. Morph. **26**, 313–322 (1971)

Frydman, R.B., Feinstein, G.: Studies on porphobilinogen deaminase and uroporphyrinogen III
cosynthetase from human erythrocytes. Biochim. biophys. Acta (Amst.) **350**, 358–373
(1974)

Frydman, R.B., Tomaro, M.L., Frydman, B., Wanschelbaum, A.: Porphobilinogen excretion
in chemical induced porphyria: Reversal by induction of porphobilinogen oxygenase.
FEBS Lett. **51**, 206–210 (1975)

Frydman, R.B., Tomaro, M.L., Wanschelbaum, A., Andersen, E.M., Awruch, J., Frydman, B.:
 Porphobilinogen oxygenase from wheat germ: Isolation, properties and products formed.
 Biochem. **12**, 5253−5262 (1973a)

Frydman, R.B., Valasinas, A., Frydman, B.: Mechanism of uroporphyrinogen biosynthesis
 from porphobilinogen. Enzyme **16**, 151−159 (1973b)

Gajdos, A., Gajdos-Török, M.: Porphyrines et Porphyries. Biochemic et clinique. Paris:
 Masson et Cie. 1969a

Gajdos, A., Gajdos-Török, M.: The quantitative regulation of the biosynthesis of porphyrins
 by intracellular ATP concentration. Biochem. Med. **2**, 372−388 (1969b)

Garcia, R.C., San Martin de Viale, L.C., Tomio, J.M., Grinstein, M.: Porphyrin biosynthesis. X. Porphyrinogen carboxylyase from avian erythrocytes. Further properties. Biochim. biophys. Acta (Amst.) **309**, 203−210 (1973)

Gayathri, A.K., Rao, M.R.S., Padmanaban, G.: Studies on the induction of δ-aminolevulinic
 acid synthetase in mouse liver. Arch. Biochem. Biophys. **155**, 299−306 (1973)

Ghazarian, J.G., Jefcoate, C.R., Knutson, J.C., Orme-Johnson, W.H., De Luca, H.F.: Mitochondrial cytochrome P-450. A component of chick kidney 25-hydroxycholecalciferol-1α-
 hydroxylase. J. biol. Chem. **249**, 3026−3033 (1974)

Gibson, K.D., Neuberger, A., Scott, J.J.: The purification and properties of δ-aminolevulic
 acid dehydrase. Biochem. J. **61**, 618−629 (1955)

Gibson, S.L.M., Goldberg, A.: Defects in heme synthesis in mammalian tissues in experimental
 lead poisoning and experimental porphyria. Clin. Sci. **38**, 63−72 (1970)

Gighoni, B., Gianni, A.M., Comi, P., Ottolenghi, S., Rungger, D.: Translational control of
 globin synthesis by hemin in Xenopus oocytes. Nature (Lond.) (New. Biol.) **246**, 99−103
 (1973)

Goldberg, A.L., Howell, E.M., Li, J.B., Martel, S.B., Prouty, W.F.: Physiological significance
 of protein degradation in animal and bacterial cells. Fed. Proc. **33**, 1112−1120 (1974)

González-Cadavid, N.F., Ortega, J.P., González, M.: The cell-free synthesis of cytochrome c
 by a microsomal fraction from rat liver. Biochem. J. **124**, 685−694 (1971)

Gordon, A.S., Zanjani, E.D., Levere, R.D., Kappas, A.: Stimulation of mammalian erythropoiesis by 5βH steroid metabolites. Proc. nat. Acad. Sci. (Wash.) **65**, 919−924 (1970)

Gordon, E.R., Dadoun, M., Goresky, C.A., Chan, T.-H., Perlin, A.S.: The isolation of an
 azobilirubin β-D-monoglucoside from dog gall-bladder bile. Biochem. J. **143**, 97−105
 (1974)

Gorshein, D., Gardner, F.H.: Erythropoietic activity of steroid metabolites in mice. Proc.
 nat. Acad. Sci. (Wash.) **65**, 564−568 (1970)

Granick, J.L., Sassa, S., Granick, S., Levere, R.D., Kappas, A.: Studies in lead poisoning.
 II. Correlations between the ratio of activated and inactivated δ-aminolevulinic acid dehydratase of whole blood and the blood lead level. Biochem. Med. **8**, 149−159 (1973)

Granick, S.: The induction in vitro of the synthesis of δ-aminolevulinic acid synthetase in
 chemical porphyria: A response to certain drugs, sex hormones and foreign chemicals.
 J. biol. Chem. **241**, 1359−1375 (1966)

Granick, S., Gilder, H.: Distribution, structure, and properties of the tetrapyrroles. Advanc.
 Enzymol. **7**, 305−368 (1947)

Granick, S., Mauzerall, D.: The metabolism of heme and chlorophyll. In: Metabolic Pathways. Greenberg, D.M. (ed.), 2nd ed., Vol. II. pp. 525−616. New York−London: Academic
 Press 1961

Granick, S., Sano, S.: Mitochondrial coproporhyrinogen oxidase and the formation of protoporphyrin. Fed. Proc. **20**, 376 (1961)

Granick, S., Sassa, S.: δ-Aminolevulinic acid synthetase and the control of heme and chlorophyll synthesis. In: Metabolic Pathways. Vogel, H.J. (ed.), 3rd ed., Vol. V, pp. 77−141.
 New York−London: Academic Press 1971

Granick, S., Urata, G.: Increase in activity of δ-aminolevulinic acid synthetase in liver mitochondria induced by feeding of 3,5-dicarbethoxy-1,4-dihydrocollidine. J. biol. Chem. **238**,
 821−827 (1963)

Grassl, M., Augsburg, G., Coy, U., Lynen, F.: Zur chemischen Konstitution des Cytohämins.
 Biochem. Z. **337**, 35−47 (1963a)

Grassl, M., Coy, U., Seyffert, R., Lynen, F.: Die chemische Konstitution des Cytohämins.
 Biochem. Z. **338**, 771−795 (1963b)

Gray, C.H., Neuberger, A., Sneath, P.H.A.: Studies in congenital porphyria. 2. Incorporation of ^{15}N in the stercobilin in the normal and in the porphyric. Biochem. J. **47**, 87–92 (1950)

Grayzel, A.I., Fuhr, J.E., London, I.M.: The effects of inhibitors of protein synthesis on the synthesis of heme in rabbit reticulocytes. Biochem. biophys. Res. Commun. **28**, 705–710 (1967)

Gregory, D.H. II, Strickland, R.D.: Solubilization and characterization of hepatic bilirubin UDP-glucuronyltransferase. Biochim. biophys. Acta (Amst.) **327**, 36–45 (1973)

Gross, M.: Control of globin synthesis by hemin. Regulation by hemin of the formation and inactivation of a translational repressor of globin synthesis in rabbit reticulocyte lysates. Biochim. biophys. Acta (Amst.) **340**, 484–497 (1974a)

Gross, M.: Control of globin synthesis by hemin. An intermediate form of the translational repressor in rabbit reticulocyte lysates. Biochim. biophys. Acta (Amst.) **366**, 319–332 (1974b)

Gross, M., Rabinovitz, M.: Control of globin synthesis in cell-free preparations of reticulocytes by formation of a translational repressor that is inactivated by hemin. Proc. nat. Acad. Sci. (Wash.) **69**, 1565–1568 (1972)

Gross, S.R., Hutton, J.J.: Induction of hepatic δ-aminolevulinic acid synthetase activity in strains of inbred mice. J. biol. Chem. **246**, 606–614 (1971)

Gurba, P.E., Sennett, R.E., Kobes, R.D.: Studies on the mechanism of action of δ-aminolevulinate dehydratase from bovine and rat liver. Arch. Biochem. Biophys. **150**, 130–136 (1972)

Halac, E., Dipiazza, M., Detwiler, P.: The formation of bilirubin mono and diglucuronide by rat liver microsomal fractions. Biochim. biophys. Acta (Amst.) **279**, 544–553 (1972)

Hammel, C.L., Bessman, S.P.: Control of hemoglobin synthesis by oxygen tension in a cell-free system. Arch. Biochem. Biophys. **110**, 622–627 (1965)

Harding, B.W., Wong, S.H., Nelson, D.H.: Carbon monoxide-combining substances in rat adrenal. Biochim. biophys. Acta (Amst.) **92**, 415–417 (1964)

Hartz, J.W., Funakoshi, S., Deutsch, H.F.: The levels of superoxide dismutase and catalase in human tissues as determined immunochemically. Clin. chim. Acta **46**, 125–132 (1973)

Hasegawa, E., Smith, C., Tephly, T.R.: Induction of hepatic mitochondrial ferrochelatase by phenobarbital. Biochem. biophys. Res. Commun. **40**, 517–523 (1970)

Hayasaka, S., Tuboi, S.: Control of δ-aminolevulinate synthetase activity in *Rhodopseudomonas spheroides*. J. Biochem. (Tokyo) **76**, 157–168 (1974)

Hayashi, N., Kurashima, Y., Kikuchi, G.: Mechanism of allylisopropylacetamide-induced increase of δ-aminolevulinate synthetase in liver mitochondria. V. Mechanism of regulation by hemin of the level of δ-aminolevulinate synthetase in rat liver mitochondria. Arch. Biochem. Biophys. **148**, 10–21 (1972)

Hayashi, N., Yoda, B., Kikuchi, G.: Mechanism of allylisopropylacetamide-induced increase of δ-aminolevulinate synthetase in liver mitochondria. IV. Accumulation of the enzyme in the soluble fraction of rat liver. Arch. Biochem. Biophys. **131**, 83–91 (1969)

Hayashi, N., Yoda, B., Kikuchi, G.: Differences in molecular sizes of δ-aminolevulinate synthetases in the soluble and mitochondrial fractions of rat liver. J. Biochem. (Tokyo) **67**, 859–861 (1970)

Heirwegh, K.P.M., Van Hees, G.P., Leroy, P., Van Roy, F.P., Jansen, F.H.: Heterogeneity of bile pigment conjugates as revealed by chromatography of their ethyl anthranilate azopigments. Biochem. J. **120**, 877–890 (1970)

Heirwegh, K.P.M., Van de Vijver, M., Fevery, J.: Assay and properties of digitonin-activated bilirubin uridine diphosphate glucuronyltransferase from rat liver. Biochem. J. **129**, 605–618 (1972)

Hickman, R., Saunders, S.J., Dowdle, E., Eales, L.: The effect of carbohydrate on δ-aminolevulinate synthetase: The role of ribonucleic acid. Biochim. biophys. Acta (Amst.) **161**, 197–204 (1968)

Hoare, D.S., Heath, H.: Intermediates in the biosynthesis of porphyrins from porphobilinogen by *Rhodopseudomonas spheroides*. Nature (Lond.) **181**, 1592–1593 (1958)

Holzer, H.: Regulation of enzymes by enzyme-catalyzed chemical modification. Advanc. Enzymol. **32**, 297–326 (1969)

Hsu, W.P., Miller, G.W.: Coproporphyrinogenase in tobacco (Nicotiana tabacum L). Biochem. J. **117,** 215 – 220 (1970)

Hutchinson, D.W., Johnson, B., Knell, A.J.: The reaction between bilirubin and aromatic diazo compounds. Biochem. J. **127,** 907 – 908 (1972)

Hutton, J.J., Gross, S.R.: Chemical induction of hepatic porphyria in inbred strains of mice. Arch. Biochem. Biophys. **141,** 284 – 292 (1970)

Incefy, G.S., Kappas, A.: Enhancement of RNA synthesis in avian liver cell cultures by a 5β-steroid metabolite during induction of δ-aminolevulinate synthase. Proc. nat. Acad. Sci. (Wash.) **71,** 2290 – 2294 (1974)

Incefy, G.S., Rifkind, A.B., Kappas, A.: Inhibition of δ-aminolevulinate synthetase induction by α-amanitin in avian liver cell cultures. Biochim. biophys. Acta (Amst.) **361.** 331 – 344 (1974)

Ip, M.M., Chee, P.Y., Swick, R.W.: Turnover of hepatic mitochondrial ornithine amino-transferase and cytochrome oxidase using [^{14}C] carbonate as tracer. Biochim. biophys. Acta (Amst.) **354,** 29 – 38 (1974)

Irving, E.A., Elliott, W.H.: A sensitive radiochemical assay method for δ-aminolevulinic acid synthetase. J. biol. Chem. **244,** 60 – 67 (1969)

Israels, L.G., Schacter, B.A., Yoda, B., Goldenberg, G.J.: δ-Aminolevulinic acid transport, porphyrin synthesis and heme catabolism in chick embryo liver and heart cells. Biochim. biophys. Acta (Amst.) **372,** 32 – 38 (1974)

Jackson, A.H., Games, D.E., Couch, P., Jackson, J.R., Belcher, R.B., Smith, S.G.: Conversion of coproporphyrinogen III to protoporphyrin IX. Enzyme **17,** 81 – 87 (1974)

Jackson, A.H., Sancovich, H.A., Ferramola, A.M., Evans, N., Games, D.E., Matlin, S.A., Elder, G.H., Smith, S.G.: Macrocyclic intermediates in the biosynthesis of porphyrins. Phil. Trans. B **273,** 119 – 134 (1975)

Jansen, F.H., Billing, B.H.: The identification of monoconjugates of bilirubin in bile as amide derivatives. Biochem. J. **125,** 917 – 919 (1971)

Jansen, F.H., Stoll, M.S.: Separation and structural analysis of vinyl- and isovinyl-azobilirubin derivatives. Biochem. J. **125,** 585 – 597 (1971)

Jansen, P.L.M.: The enzyme-catalyzed formation of bilirubin diglucuronide by a solubilized preparation from cat liver microsomes. Biochim. biophys. Acta (Amst.) **338,** 170 – 182 (1974)

Jansen, P.L.M., Henderson, P.Th.: Influence of phenobarbital treatment on p-nitrophenol and bilirubin glucuronidation in Wistar rat, Gunn rat and cat. Biochem. Pharmacol. **21,** 2457 – 2462 (1972)

Johnson, A., Jones, O.T.G.: Enzymic formation of hemes and other metalloporphyrins. Biochim. biophys. Acta (Amst.) **93,** 171 – 173 (1964)

Jones, E.A., Bloomer, J.R., Berlin, N.I.: The measurement of the synthetic rate of bilirubin from hepatic hemes in patients with acute intermittent porphyria. J. clin. Invest. **50,** 2259 – 2265 (1971)

Jones, M.S., Jones, O.T.G.: The structural organization of heme synthesis in rat liver mito-chondria. Biochem. J. **113,** 507 – 514 (1969)

Jones, M.S., Jones, O.T.G.: Permeability properties of mitochondrial membranes and the regulation of heme biosynthesis. Biochem. biophys. Res. Commun. **41,** 1072 – 1079 (1970)

Jordan, P.M., Shemin, D.: δ-Aminolevulinic acid synthetase. In: The Enzymes. Boyer, P.D. (ed.), 3rd ed., Vol. VII, pp. 339 – 356. New York – London: Academic Press 1972

Kanai, Y., Sugimura, T., Matsushima, T., Kawamura, A.: Studies on in vivo degradation of rat hepatic catalase with or without modification by 3-amino-1,2,4-triazole. J. biol. Chem. **249,** 6505 – 6511 (1974)

Kaplan, B.H.: δ-Aminolevulinic acid synthetase from the particulate fraction of liver of porphyric rats. Biochim. biophys. Acta (Amst.) **235,** 381 – 388 (1971)

Karibian, D., London, I.M.: Control of heme synthesis by feedback inhibition. Biochem. biophys. Res. Commun. **18,** 243 – 249 (1965)

Kassner, R.J., Walchak, H.: Heme formation from Fe (II) and porphyrin in the absence of ferrochelatase activity. Biochim. biophys. Acta (Amst.) **304,** 294 – 303 (1973)

Kaufman, L., Marver, H.S.: Biochemical defects in two types of human hepatic porphyria. New Engl. J. Med. **283,** 954 – 958 (1970)

Kaufman, L., Swanson, A.L., Marver, H.S.: Chemically induced porphyria: Prevention by prior treatment with phenobarbital. Science **170**, 320 – 322 (1970)

Kennedy, G.Y., Jackson, A.H., Kenner, G.W., Suckling, C.J.: Isolation, structure and synthesis of a tricarboxylic porphyrin from the Harderian glands of the rat. FEBS Lett. **6**, 9 – 12 (1970)

Ketterer, B., Tipping, E., Beale, D., Meuwissen, J., Kay, C.M.: Proteins which specifically bind carcinogens. Proceedings of XI International Cancer Congress, Florence 1974, Excerpta Medical International Congress Series No. 350, Vol. 2, pp. 25 – 29 (1975)

Kiese, M., Kurz, H., Thofern, E.: Bildung v Fermenthämin aus Protohämin durch eine hämin-bedürftige Mutante eines Mikrokokkenstammes. Biochem. Z. **330**, 541 – 544 (1958)

Kikuchi, G., Kumar, A., Talmage, P., Shemin, D.: The enzymatic synthesis of δ-amino-levulinic acid. J. biol. Chem. **233**, 1214 – 1219 (1958)

Kondo, T., Nicholson, D.C., Jackson, A.H., Kenner, G.W.: Isotopic studies of the conversion of oxophlorins and their ferrihemes into bile pigments in the rat. Biochem. J. **121**, 601 – 607 (1971)

Korinek, J., Moses, H.L.: Theophylline suppression of Δ-aminolevulinic acid synthetase induction in chick embryo and rat livers. Biochem. biophys. Res. Commun. **53**, 1246 – 1252 (1973)

Kowalski, E., Dancewicz, A.M., Szot, Z., Lipinski, B., Rosiek, O.: Studies on δ-aminolevulinic acid transamination. Acta biochim. pol. **6**, 257 – 266 (1959)

Krishnakantha, T.P., Kurup, C.K.R.: Increase in hepatic catalase and glycerol phosphate dehydrogenase activities on administration of clofibrate and clofenapate to the rat. Biochem. J. **130**, 167 – 175 (1972)

Kuenzle, C.C.: Bilirubin conjugates of human bile. Isolation of phenylazo derivatives of bile bilirubin. Biochem. J. **119**, 387 – 394 (1970a)

Kuenzle, C.C.: Bilirubin conjugates of human bile. Nuclear-magnetic resonance, infrared, and optical spectra of model compounds. Biochem. J. **119**, 395 – 409 (1970b)

Kuenzle, C.C.: Bilirubin conjugates of human bile. The excretion of bilirubin as the acyl glycosides of aldobiuronic acid, pseudoaldobiuronic acid, and hexuronosylhexuronic acid with a branched chain hexuronic acid as one of the components of the hexuronosyl-hexuronide. Biochem. J. **119**, 411 – 435 (1970c)

Labbe, R.F.: Metabolic anomalies in porphyria. The result of impaired biological oxidation? Lancet 1967 **I**, 1361 – 1364

Labbe, R.F., Hubbard, N.: Metal specificity of the iron-protoporphyrin chelating enzyme from rat liver. Biochim. biophys. Acta (Amst.) **52**, 130 – 135 (1961)

Labbe, R.F., Kurumada, T., Onisawa, J.: The role of succinyl CoA synthetase in the control of heme biosynthesis. Biochim. biophys. Acta (Amst.) **111**, 403 – 415 (1965)

Landaw, S.A., Callahan, E.W. Jr., Schmid, R.: Catabolism of heme in vivo: comparison of the simultaneous production of bilirubin and carbon monoxide. J. clin. Invest. **49**, 914 – 925 (1970)

Langelaan, D.E., Losowsky, M.S., Toothill, C.: Heme synthetase activity in human blood cells. Clin. chim. Acta **27**, 453 – 459 (1970)

Lascelles, J.: Tetrapyrrole Biosynthesis and Its Regulation. New York – Amsterdam: W.A. Benjamin, Inc. 1964

Lascelles, J., Altshuler, T.: Mutant strains of *Rhodopseudomonas spheroides* lacking δ-amino-levulinate synthase: Growth, heme and bacteriochlorophyll synthesis. J. Bact. **98**, 721 – 727 (1969)

Lathe, G.H.: The degradation of heme by mammals and its excretion as conjugated bilirubin. Essays Biochem. **8**, 107 – 148 (1972)

Lazarow, P.B., De Duve, C.: The synthesis and turnover of rat liver peroxisomes IV Biochemical pathway of catalase synthesis. J. Cell Biol. **59**, 491 – 506 (1973a)

Lazarow, P.B., De Duve, C.: The synthesis and turnover of rat liver peroxisomes. V Intracellular pathway of catalase synthesis. J. Cell Biol. **59**, 507 – 524 (1973b)

Lemberg, R., Wyndham, R.A.: Reduction of biliverdin to bilirubin in tissues. Biochem. J. **30**, 1147 – 1170 (1936)

Levere, R.D., Granick, S.: Control of hemoglobin synthesis in the cultured chick blastoderm by δ-aminolevulinic acid synthetase: Increase in the rate of hemoglobin formation with δ-aminolevulinic acid. Proc. nat. Acad. Sci. (Wash.) **54**, 134 – 137 (1965)

Levere, R.D., Granick, S.: Control of hemoglobin synthesis in the cultured chick blastoderm. J. biol. Chem. **242**, 1903 – 1911 (1967)

Levere, R.D., Kappas, A., Granick, S.: Stimulation of hemoglobin synthesis in chick blastoderms by certain 5β androstane and 5β pregnane steroids. Proc. nat. Acad. Sci. (Wash.) **58**, 985 – 990 (1967)

Levin, E.Y.: Uroporphyrinogen III cosynthetase from mouse spleen. Biochem. **7**, 3781 – 3788 (1968a)

Levin, E.Y.: Uroporphyrinogen III cosynthetase in bovine erythropoietic porphyria. Science **161**, 907 – 908 (1968b)

Levin, E.Y.: Enzymatic properties of uroporphyrinogen III cosynthetase. Biochem. **10**, 4669 – 4675 (1971)

Levin, E.Y., Coleman, D.L.: The enzymatic conversion of porphobilinogen to uroporphyrinogen catalysed by extracts of hematopoietic mouse spleen. J. biol. Chem. **242**, 4248 – 4253 (1967)

Levin, E.Y., Flyger, V.: Erythropoietic porphyria of the fox squirrel *Sciurus niger*. J. clin. Invest. **52**, 96 – 105 (1973)

Levin, W., Kuntzman, R.: Biphasic decrease of radioactive hemoprotein from liver microsomal CO-binding particles. Effect of 3-methylcholanthrene. J. biol. Chem. **244**, 3671 – 3676 (1969)

Levitt, M., Schacter, B.A., Zipursky, A., Israels, L.G.: The nonerythropoietic component of early bilirubin. J. clin. Invest. **47**, 1281 – 1294 (1968)

Lewis, M., Lee, G.R., Cartwright, G.E., Wintrobe, M.M.: Glycine decarboxylation in the porcine erythrocyte: Its relation to aminolevulinic acid synthesis. Biochim. biophys. Acta (Amst.) **141**, 296 – 309 (1967)

Llambias, E.B.C., Batlle, A.M. del C.: Uroporphyrinogen III cosynthetase. Evidence for the existence of a polypyrrolic substrate in soybean callus tissue. FEBS Lett. **6**, 285 – 288 (1970)

Llambias, E.B.C., Batlle, A.M. del C.: Studies on the porphobilinogen deaminase-uroporphyrinogen cosynthetase system of cultured soybean cells. Biochem. J. **121**, 327 – 340 (1971a)

Llambias, E.B.C., Batlle, A.M. del C.: Porphyrin Biosynthesis VIII. Avian erythrocyte porphobilinogen deaminase-uroporphyrinogen III cosynthetase, its purification, properties, and the separation of its components. Biochim. biophys. Acta (Amst.) **227**, 180 – 191 (1971b)

Lodish, H.F., Desalu, O.: Regulation of synthesis of nonglobin proteins in cell-free extracts of rabbit reticulocytes. J. biol. Chem. **248**, 3520 – 3527 (1973)

London, I.M.: The metabolism of the erythrocyte. Harvey Lect. **56**, 151 – 189 (1961)

London, I.M., West, R., Shemin, D., Rittenberg, D.: On the origin of bile pigment in normal man. J. biol. Chem. **184**, 351 – 358 (1950)

Lu, A.Y.H, West, S.B., Vore, M., Ryan, D., Levin, W.: Role of cytochrome b_5 in hydroxylation by a reconstituted cytochrome P-450 containing system. J. biol. Chem. **249**, 6701 – 6709 (1974)

Maines, M.D., Kappas, A.: Cobalt induction of hepatic heme oxygenase: with evidence that cytochrome P-450 is not essential for this enzyme activity. Proc. nat. Acad. Sci. (Wash.) **71**, 4293 – 4297 (1974)

Margolis, F.L.: Regulation of porphyrin biosynthesis in the Harderian gland of inbred mouse strains. Arch. Biochem. Biophys. **145**, 373 – 381 (1971)

Marks, G.S.: Heme and Chlorophyll. Chemical, Biochemical and Medical Aspects. London: D. Van Nostrand Company Ltd. 1969

Marver, H.S., Schmid, R.: The porphyrias. In: The Metabolic Basis of Inherited Disease. Stanbury, J.B., Wyngaarden, J.B., Fredrickson, D.S. (eds.), 3rd ed., pp. 1087 – 1140. New York: McGraw-Hill 1972

Marver, H.S., Collins, A., Tschudy, D.P., Rechcigl, M. Jr.: δ-Aminolevulinic acid synthetase II. Induction in rat liver. J. biol. Chem. **241**, 4323 – 4329 (1966a)

Marver, H.S., Tschudy, D.P., Perlroth, M.G., Collins, A.: δ-Aminolevulinic acid synthetase I. Studies in liver homogenates. J. biol. Chem. **241**, 2803 – 2809 (1966b)

Mathews, M.B., Hunt, T., Brayley, A.: Specificity of the control of protein synthesis by hemin. Nature (Lond.) (New Biol.) **243**, 230 – 233 (1973)

Mauzerall, D., Granick, S.: Porphyrin biosynthesis in erythrocytes. III. Uroporphyrinogen and its decarboxylase. J. biol. Chem. **232**, 1141 − 1162 (1958)

Mazanowska, A.M., Neuberger, A., Tait, G.H.: Effect of lipids and organic solvents on the enzymic formation of zinc protoporphyrin and heme. Biochem. J. **98**, 117 − 127 (1966)

McKay, R., Druyan, R., Getz, G.S., Rabinowitz, M.: Intramitochondrial localization of δ-aminolevulate synthetase and ferrochelatase in rat liver. Biochem. J. **114**, 455 − 461 (1969)

Meigs, R.A., Ryan, K.J.: Cytochrome P-450 and steroid biosynthesis in human placenta. Biochim. biophys. Acta (Amst.) **165**, 476 − 482 (1968)

Meyer, U.A., Marver, H.S.: Enhancement of the fractional catabolic rate of microsomal heme in chemically induced porphyria. S. Afr. J. Lab. clin. Med. **17**, 175 − 177 (1971a)

Meyer, U.A., Marver, H.S.: Chemically induced porphyria: Increased microsomal heme turnover after treatment with allylisopropylacetamide. Science **171**, 64 − 66 (1971b)

Meyer, U.A., Schmid, R.: Hereditary hepatic porphyrias. Fed. Proc. **32**, 1649 − 1655 (1973)

Miyagi, K., Cardinal, R., Bossenmaier, I., Watson, C.J.: The serum porphobilinogen, and the porphobilinogen deaminase in normal and porphyric individuals. J. Lab. clin. Med. **78**, 683 − 695 (1971)

Moore, M.R., Goldberg, A.: Normal and abnormal heme biosynthesis. In: Iron in Biochemistry and Medicine. Jacobs, A., Worwood, M. (eds.), pp. 115 − 144. London − New York: Academic Press 1974

Mowat, A.P., Arias, I.M.: Observations of the effect of diethylnitrosamine on glucuronide formation. Biochim. biophys. Acta (Amst.) **212**, 175 − 178 (1970)

Mulder, G.J.: Bilirubin and the heterogeneity of microsomal uridine diphosphate glucuronyltransferase from rat liver. Biochim. biophys. Acta (Amst.) **289**, 284 − 292 (1972)

Murthy, V.V., Woods, J.S.: Solubilization and partial purification of mitochondrial δ-aminolevulinate synthetase from fetal rat liver. Biochim. biophys. Acta (Amst.) **350**, 240 − 246 (1974)

Murty, H.S., Caasi, P.I., Brook, S.K., Nair, P.P.: Biosynthesis of heme in the vitamin E-deficient rat. J. biol. Chem. **245**, 5498 − 5504 (1970)

Muzyka, V.I.: δ-Aminolevulinic acid synthetase in grey substance of brain hemispheres (Russian). Biokhimiya **37**, 1220 − 1223 (1972) (Biochemistry—Translation by Consultants Bureau, New York, pp. 1022 − 1024)

Nakao, K., Wada, O., Kitamura, T., Vono, K., Urata, G.: Activity of aminolevulinic acid synthetase in normal and porphyric human livers. Nature (Lond.) **210**, 838 − 839 (1966)

Narisawa, K., Kikuchi, G.: Mechanism of allylisopropylacetamide-induced increase of δ-aminolevulinate synthetase in rat liver mitochondria. Biochim. biophys. Acta (Amst.) **123**, 596 − 605 (1966)

Neuberger, A.: Aspects of the metabolism of glycine and of porphyrins. Biochem. J. **78**, 1 − 10 (1961)

Neuwirt, J., Poňka, P., Borová, J.: Heme and the production of δ-aminolevulinic acid in rabbit reticulocytes. Enzyme **17**, 100 − 107 (1974)

Nicholls, P., Elliott, W.B.: The cytochromes. In: Iron in Biochemistry and Medicine. Jacobs, A., Worwood, M. (eds.), pp. 221 − 277. London − New York: Academic Press 1974

Noir, B.A., Nanet, H.: A study of the ethyl anthranilate derivatives of bilirubin sulphate. Confirmation of the existence of bilirubin sulphate conjugates in bile. Biochim. biophys. Acta (Amst.) **372**, 230 − 236 (1974)

Ó Carra, P., Colleran, E.: Properties and kinetics of biliverdin reductase. Biochem. J. **125**, 110P (1971)

Ostrow, J.D., Murphy, N.H.: Isolation and properties of conjugated bilirubin from bile. Biochem. J. **120**, 311 − 327 (1970)

Padmanaban, G., Satyanarayana Rao, M.R., Malathi, K.: A model for the regulation of δ-aminolevulinate synthetase induction in rat liver. Biochem. J. **134**, 847 − 857 (1973)

Patton, G.M., Beattie, D.S.: Studies on hepatic δ-aminolevulinic acid synthetase. J. biol. Chem. **248**, 4467 − 4474 (1973)

Pimstone, N.R., Blekkenhorst, G., Eales, L.: Enzymatic defects in hepatic porphyria. Enzyme **16**, 354 − 366 (1973)

Pimstone, N.R., Engel, P., Tenhunen, R., Seitz, P.T., Marver, H.S., Schmid, R.: Inducible heme oxygenase in the kidney: A model for the homeostatic control of hemoglobin catabolism. J. clin. Invest. **50**, 2042 − 2050 (1971 b)

Pimstone, N.R., Tenhunen, R., Seitz, P.T., Marver, H.S., Schmid, R.: The enzymic degradation of hemoglobin to bile pigments by macrophages. J. exp. Med. **133**, 1264 − 1281 (1971 a)

Pisani, W., Bonzanino, A., Coscia, G.C.: Attivitá delta-aminolevulico-ossidative degli omogenati di fegato di ratto in varie condizioni sperimentali. Boll. Soc. ital. Biol. sper. **43**, 65 − 67 (1967)

Poňka, P., Neuwirt, J., Borová, J.: The role of heme in the release of iron from transferrin in reticulocytes. Enzyme **17**, 91 − 99 (1974)

Poole, B.: The kinetics of disappearance of labeled leucine from the free leucine pool of rat liver and its effect on the apparent turnover of catalase and other hepatic proteins. J. biol. Chem. **246**, 6587 − 6591 (1971)

Porra, R.J., Falk, J.E.: Protein-bound porphyrins associated with protoporphyrin biosynthesis. Biochem. biophys. Res. Commun. **5**, 179 − 184 (1961)

Porra, R.J., Falk, J.E.: The enzymic conversion of coproporphyrinogen III into protoporphyrin IX. Biochem. J. **90**, 69 − 75 (1964)

Porra, R.J., Jones, O.T.G.: Studies on ferrochelatase. 1. Assay and properties of ferrochelatase from a pig liver mitochondrial extract. Biochem. J. **87**, 181 − 185 (1963)

Porra, R.J., Vitols, K.S., Labbe, R.F., Newton, N.A.: Studies on ferrochelatase. The effects of thiols and other factors on the determination of activity. Biochem. J. **104**, 321 − 327 (1967)

Poulson, R., Polglase, W.J.: Aerobic and anaerobic coproporphyrinogenase activities in extracts from *Saccharomyces cerevisiae*. Purification and characterization. J. biol. Chem. **249**, 6367 − 6371 (1974 a)

Poulson, R., Polglase, W.J.: Site of glucose repression of heme biosynthesis. FEBS Lett. **40**, 258 − 260 (1974 b)

Poulson, R., Polglase, W.J.: The enzymic conversion of protoporphyrinogen IX to protoporphyrin IX. Protoporphyrinogen oxidase activity in mitochondrial extracts of *Saccharomyces cerevisiae*. J. biol. Chem. **250**, 1269 − 1274 (1975)

Rajamanickam, C., Satyanarayana Rao, M.R., Padmanaban, G.: On the sequence of reactions leading to cytochrome P-450 synthesis-effect of drugs. J. biol. Chem. **250**, 2305 − 2310 (1975)

Romeo, G., Levin, E.Y.: Uroporphyrinogen III cosynthetase in human congenital erythropoietic porphyria. Proc. nat. Acad. Sci. (Wash.) **63**, 856 − 863 (1969)

Romeo, G., Levin, E.Y.: Uroporphyrinogen decarboxylase from mouse spleen. Biochim. biophys. Acta (Amst.) **230**, 330 − 341 (1971)

Sancovich, H.A., Batlle, A.M.C., Grinstein, M.: Porphyrin biosynthesis VI. Separation and purification of porphobilinogen deaminase and uroporphyrinogen isomerase from cow liver. Biochim. biophys. Acta (Amst.) **191**, 130 − 143 (1969)

San Martin de Viale, L.C., Garcia, R.C., de Pisarev, D.K., Tomio, J.M., Grinstein, M.: Studies on uroporphyrinogen decarboxylase from chicken erythrocytes. FEBS Lett. **5**, 149 − 152 (1969)

San Martin de Viale, L.C., Grinstein, M.: Porphyrin biosynthesis IV. 5- and 6-COOH porphyrinogens (Type III) as normal intermediates in heme synthesis. Biochim. biophys. Acta (Amst.) **158**, 79 − 91 (1968)

Sano, S.: 2,4-Bis(β-hydroxypropionic acid) deuteroporphyrinogen IX, a possible intermediate between coproporphyrinogen III and protoporphyrin IX. J. biol. Chem. **241**, 5276 − 5283 (1966)

Sano, S., Granick, S.: Mitochondrial coproporphyrinogen oxidase and protoporphyrin formation. J. biol. Chem. **236**, 1173 − 1180 (1961)

Sardesai, V.M., Lenaghan, R., Rosenberg, J.C.: Tissue delta-aminolevulinic acid synthetase activity in hemorrhagic shock. Biochem. Med. **6**, 366 − 371 (1972)

Sassa, S., Granick, S.: Induction of δ-aminolevulinic acid synthetase in chick embryo liver cells in culture. Proc. nat. Acad. Sci. (Wash.) **67**, 517 − 522 (1970)

Sassa, S., Granick, S., Bickers, D.R., Bradlow, H.L., Kappas, A.: A microassay for uroporphyrinogen I synthase, one of three abnormal enzyme activities in acute intermittent porphyria, and its application to the study of the genetics of this disease. Proc. nat. Acad. Sci. (Wash.) **71**, 732−736 (1974)

Satyanarayana Rao, M.R., Padmanaban, G., Muthukrishnan, S., Sarma, P.S.: Feedback inhibition of δ-aminolevulinate dehydratase by coproporphyrinogen III. Indian J. Biochem. **7**, 132−133 (1970)

Sawada, H., Takeshita, M., Sugita, Y., Yoneyama, Y.: Effect of lipid on protoheme ferrolyase. Biochim. biophys. Acta (Amst.) **178**, 145−155 (1969)

Schacter, B.A., Nelson, E.B., Marver, H.S., Masters, B.S.S.: Immunochemical evidence for an association of heme oxygenase with the microsomal electron transport system. J. biol. Chem. **247**, 3601−3607 (1972)

Schacter, B.A., Waterman, M.R.: Activity of various metalloporphyrin protein complexes with microsomal heme oxygenase. Life Sci. **14**, 47−53 (1974)

Schimke, R.T.: Control of enzyme levels in mammalian tissues. Advanc. Enzymol. **37**, 135−187 (1973)

Schimke, R.T., Doyle, D.: Control of enzyme levels in animal tissues. Ann. Rev. Biochem. **39**, 929−976 (1970)

Schmid, R.: Hyperbilirubinemia. In: The Metabolic Basis of Inherited Disease. Stanbury, J.B., Wyngaarden, J.B., Fredrickson, D.S. (eds.), 3rd ed., pp. 1141−1178. New York: McGraw-Hill 1972

Schneider, W.C.: Intracellular distribution of enzymes XIII. Enzymatic synthesis of deoxycytidine diphosphate choline and lecithin in rat liver. J. biol. Chem. **238**, 3572−3578 (1963)

Scholnick, P.L., Hammaker, L.E., Marver, H.S.: Soluble δ-aminolevulinic acid synthetase of rat liver. I . Some properties of the partially purified enzyme. J. biol. Chem. **247**, 4126−4131 (1972a)

Scholnick, P.L., Hammaker, L.E., Marver, H.S.: Soluble δ-aminolevulinic acid synthetase of rat liver. II. Studies related to the mechanism of enzyme action and hemin inhibition. J. biol. Chem. **247**, 4132−4137 (1972b)

Shanley, B.C., Zail, S.S., Joubert, S.M.: Porphyrin metabolism in experimental hepatic siderosis in the rat. Brit. J. Haemat. **18**, 79−87 (1970)

Sharma, D.C.: Aberration of porphyrin metabolism in iron-deficient anaemic rats. Biochem. J. **134**, 821−823 (1973)

Shemin, D.: Mechanism and control of pyrrole synthesis. Biochem. Soc. Symp. **28**, 75−89 (1968)

Shemin, D.: δ-Aminolevulinic acid dehydratase. In: The Enzymes. Boyer, P.D. (ed.), 3rd ed., Vol. VII, pp. 323−337. New York−London: Academic Press 1972

Singleton, J.W., Laster, L.: Biliverdin reductase in guinea pig liver. J. biol. Chem. **240**, 4780−4789 (1965)

Skea, B.R., Downie, E.D., Moore, M.R., Davidson, J.N.: Induction of δ-aminolevulate synthetase activity in cultured chick-embryo liver cells by ribonucleic acid. Biochem. J. **121**, 25P (1971)

Stein, J.A., Tschudy, D.P., Corcoran, P.L., Collins, A.: δ-Aminolevulinic acid synthetase III. Synergistic effect of chelated iron on induction. J. biol. Chem. **245**, 2213−2218 (1970)

Stevens, E., Frydman, R.B., Frydman, B.: Separation of porphobilinogen deaminase and uroporphyrinogen III cosynthetase from human erythrocytes. Biochim. biophys. Acta (Amst.) **158**, 496−498 (1968)

Stoll, M.S., Elder, G.H., Games, D.E., O'Hanlon, P., Millington, D.S., Jackson, A.H.: Isocoproporphyrin: nuclear-magnetic-resonance and mass spectral methods for the determination of porphyrin structure. Biochem. J. **131**, 429−432 (1973)

Strand, L.J., Felsher, B.F., Redeker, A.G., Marver, H.S.: Heme biosynthesis in intermittent acute porphyria: decreased hepatic conversion of porphobilinogen to porphyrins and increased delta-aminolevulinic acid synthetase activity. Proc. nat. Acad. Sci. (Wash.) **67**, 1315−1320 (1970)

Strand, L.J., Meyer, U.A., Felsher, B.F., Redeker, A.G., Marver, H.S.: Decreased red cell uroporphyrinogen I synthetase activity in intermittent acute porphyria. J. clin. Invest. **51**, 2530−2536 (1972b)

Strand, L.J., Swanson, A.L., Manning, J., Branch, S., Marver, H.S.: Radiochemical microassay for δ-aminolevulinic acid synthetase in hepatic and erythroid tissues. Analyt. Biochem. **47**, 457−470 (1972a)

Sweeney, V.P., Pathak, M.A., Asbury, A.K.: Acute intermittent porphyria. Increased ALA-synthetase activity during an acute attack. Brain **93**, 369 – 380 (1970)

Tait, G.H.: Coproporphyrinogenase activities in extracts of *Rhodopseudomonas spheroides* and *Chromatium* Strain D. Biochem. J. **128**, 1159 – 1169 (1972)

Tait, G.H.: Aminolevulinate synthetase of *Micrococcus denitrificans*. Purification and properties of the enzyme, and the effect of growth conditions on the enzyme activity in cells. Biochem. J. **131**, 389 – 403 (1973a)

Tait, G.H.: Control of aminolevulinate synthetase in *Micrococcus denitrificans*. Enzyme **16**, 21 – 27 (1973b)

Takeshita, M., Sugita, Y., Yoneyama, Y.: Relation between electrophoretic charge of phospholipids and the activating effect on protoheme ferrolyase. Biochim. biophys. Acta (Amst.) **202**, 544 – 546 (1970)

Taljaard, J.J.F., Shanley, B.C., Deppe, W.M., Joubert, S.M.: Porphyrin metabolism in experimental hepatic siderosis in the rat. III. Effect of iron overload and hexachlorobenzene on liver heme biosynthesis, Brit. J. Haemat. **23**, 587 – 593 (1972)

Tanaka, M., Bottomley, S.S.: Bone marrow Δ-aminolevulinic acid synthetase activity in experimental sideroblastic anemia. J. Lab. clin. Med. **84**, 92 – 98, (1974)

Tenhunen, R., Marver, H.S., Pimstone, N.R., Trager, W.F., Cooper, D.Y., Schmid, R.: Enzymatic degradation of heme. Oxygenative cleavage requiring cytochrome P-450. Biochem. **11**, 1716 – 1720 (1972)

Tenhunen, R., Marver, H.S., Schmid, R.: The enzymic conversion of heme to bilirubin by microsomal heme oxygenase. Proc. nat. Acad. Sci. (Wash.) **61**, 748 – 755 (1968)

Tenhunen, R., Marver, H.S., Schmid, R.: Microsomal heme oxygenase. Characterization of the enzyme. J. biol. Chem. **244**, 6388 – 6394 (1969)

Tenhunen, R., Marver, H.S., Schmid, R.: The enzymatic catabolism of hemoglobin: Stimulation of microsomal heme oxygenase by hemin. J. Lab. clin. Med. **75**, 410 – 421 (1970a)

Tenhunen, R., Ross, M.E., Marver, H.S., Schmid, R.: Reduced nicotinamide-adenine dinucleotide phosphate dependent biliverdin reductase: Partial purification and characterisation. Biochem. **9**, 298 – 303 (1970b)

Tomaro, M.L., Frydman, R.B., Frydman, B.: Porphobilinogen oxygenase from rat liver: Induction, isolation and properties. Biochem. **12**, 5263 – 5268 (1973)

Tomio, J.M., Garcia, R.C., San Martin de Viale, L.C., Grinstein, M.: Porphyrin biosynthesis. VII. Porphyrinogen carboxylase from avian erythrocytes. Purification and properties. Biochim. biophys. Acta (Amst.) **198**, 353 – 363 (1970)

Tomita, Y., Ohashi, A., Kikuchi, G.: Induction of δ-aminolevulinate synthetase in organ culture of chick embryo liver by allylisopropylacetamide and 3,5-dicarbethoxy-1,4-dihydrocollidine. J. Biochem. (Tokyo) **75**, 1007 – 1015 (1974)

Tschudy, D.P.: Porphyrin Metabolism and the porphyrias. In: Duncan's Diseases of Metabolism. Genetics and Metabolism. Bondy, P.K., Rosenberg, L.E. (eds.), 7th ed., pp. 775 – 824. Philadelphia – London – Toronto: W.B. Saunders Co. 1974

Tschudy, D.P., Marver, H.S., Collins, A.: A model for calculating messenger RNA half-life: Short-lived messenger RNA in the induction of mammalian δ-aminolevulinic acid synthetase. Biochem. biophys. Res. Commun. **21**, 480 – 487 (1965a)

Tschudy, D.P., Perlroth, M.G., Marver, H.S., Collins, A., Hunter, G.Jr., Rechcigl, M.Jr.: Acute intermittent porphyria: The first overproduction disease localized to a specific enzyme. Proc. nat. Acad. Sci. (Wash.) **53**, 841 – 847 (1965b)

Tschudy, D.P., Rose, J., Hellman, E., Collins, A., Rechcigl, M.Jr.: Biochemical studies of experimental porphyria. Metabolism **11**, 1287 – 1301 (1962)

Tyrrell, D.L.J., Marks, G.S.: Drug induced porphyrin biosynthesis V. Effect of protohemin on the transcriptional and post-transcriptional phases of δ-aminolevulinic acid synthetase induction. Biochem. Pharmacol. **21**, 2077 – 2093 (1972)

Urata, G., Granick, S.: Biosynthesis of α-aminoketones and the metabolism of aminoacetone. J. biol. Chem. **238**, 811 – 820 (1963)

Vessey, D.A., Goldenberg, J., Zakim, D.: Differentiation of homologous forms of hepatic microsomal UDP-glucuronyltransferase. II. Characterization of the bilirubin conjugating form. Biochim. biophys. Acta (Amst.) **309**, 75 – 82 (1973)

Wainwright, S.D., Wainwright, L.K.: Regulation of the initiation of hemoglobin synthesis in the blood island cells of chick embryos. I. Qualitative studies on the effects of actinomycin D and δ-aminolevulinic acid. Canad. J. Biochem. **44**, 1543 – 1560 (1966)

Wainwright, S.D., Wainwright, L.K.: Regulation of the initiation of hemoglobin synthesis in the blood island cells of chick embryos. II. Early onset and stimulation of hemoglobin formation induced by exogenous δ-aminolevulinic acid. Canad. J. Biochem. **45**, 344 – 347 (1967)

Warnick, G.R., Burnham, B.F.: Regulation of porphyrin biosynthesis. Purification and characterization of δ-aminolevulinic acid synthase. J. biol. Chem. **246**, 6880 – 6885 (1971)

Weissberg, J.B., Voytek, P.E.: Liver and red cell porphobilinogen synthase in the adult and fetal guinea pig. Biochim. biophys. Acta (Amst.) **364**, 304 – 319 (1974)

Welton, A.F., Aust, S.D.: Multiplicity of cytochrome P-450 hemoproteins in rat liver microsomes. Biochem. biophys. Res. Commun. **56**, 898 – 906 (1974)

Wetterberg, L., Marver, H.S., Swanson, A.L.: Delta-aminolevulinic acid synthetase in the Harderian gland. S. Afr. J. Lab. clin. Med. **17**, 189 – 191 (1971)

White, J.M., Brain, M.C., Ali, M.A.M.: Globin synthesis in sideroblastic anaemia. I. α and β peptide chain synthesis. Brit. J. Haemat. **20**, 263 – 275 (1971)

White, J.M., Harvey, D.R.: Defective synthesis of α and β globin chains in lead poisoning. Nature (Lond.) **236**, 71 – 73 (1972)

White, J.M., Hoffbrand, A.V.: Heme deficiency and chain synthesis. Nature (Lond.) **248**, 88 (1974)

Whiting, M.J., Elliott, W.H.: Purification and properties of solubilized mitochondrial δ-aminolevulinic acid synthetase and comparison with the cytosol enzyme. J. biol. Chem. **247**, 6818 – 6826 (1972)

Whiting, M.J., Granick, S.: Purification of δ-aminolevulinic acid synthetase (ALV-S) from chick embryo liver mitochondria. Fed. Proc. **34**, 640 (1975)

Wilson, E.L., Burger, P.E., Dowdle, E.B.: Beef-liver 5-Aminolevulinic acid dehydratase. Purification and properties. Europ. J. Biochem. **29**, 563 – 571 (1972)

Wong, K.P.: Bilirubin glucuronyltransferase. Specific activity and kinetic studies. Biochem. J. **125**, 27 – 35 (1971 a)

Wong, K.P.: Formation of bilirubin glycoside. Biochem. J. **125**, 929 – 934 (1971 b)

Woods, J.S.: Studies on the role of heme in the regulation of δ-aminolevulinic acid synthetase during fetal hepatic development. Molec. Pharmacol. **10**, 389 – 397 (1974)

Woods, J.S., Dixon, R.L.: Studies on the perinatal differences in the activity of hepatic δ-aminolevulinic acid synthetase. Biochem. Pharmacol. **21**, 1735 – 1744 (1972)

Woods, J.S., Murthy, V.V.: δ-Aminolevulinic acid synthetase from fetal rat liver: Studies on the partially purified enzyme. Molec. Pharmacol. **11**, 70 – 78 (1975)

Wu, W.H., Shemin, D., Richards, K.E., Williams, R.C.: The quaternary structure of δ-aminolevulinic acid dehydratase from bovine liver. Proc. nat. Acad. Sci. (Wash.) **71**, 1767 – 1770 (1974)

Yamamoto, T., Skanderberg, J., Zipursky, A., Israels, L.G.: The early appearing bilirubin: Evidence for two components. J. clin. Invest. **44**, 31 – 41 (1965)

Yoda, B., Israels, L.G.: Transfer of heme from mitochondria in rat liver cells. Canad. J. Biochem. **50**, 633 – 637 (1972)

Yoshida, T., Kikuchi, G.: Sequence of the reaction of heme catabolism catalyzed by the microsomal heme oxygenase system. FEBS Lett. **48**, 256 – 261 (1974)

Yoshida, T., Takahashi, S., Kikuchi, G.: Partial purification and reconstitution of the heme oxygenase system from pig spleen microsomes. J. Biochem. (Tokyo) **75**, 1187 – 1191 (1974)

Yoshikawa, H., Yoneyama, Y.: Incorporation of iron in the heme moiety of chromoproteins. In: Iron Metabolism. Gross, F. (ed.), pp. 24 – 37. Berlin – Göttingen – Heidelberg: Springer 1964

Yuan, M., Russell, C.S.: Porphobilinogen derivatives as substrates for porphobilinogenase. FEBS Lett. **46**, 34 – 38 (1974)

Zaman, Z., Abboud, M.M., Akhtar, M.: Mechanism and stereochemistry of vinyl group formation in heme biosynthesis. J. chem. Soc. chem. Commun. 1263 – 1264 (1972)

Zaman, Z., Jordan, P.M., Akhtar, M.: Mechanism and stereochemistry of the 5-aminolevulinate synthetase reaction. Biochem. J. **135**, 257 – 263 (1973)

Zuyderhoudt, F.M.J., Borst, P., Huijing, J.: Intramitochondrial localization of 5-aminolevulinate synthase induced in rat liver by allylisopropylacetamide. Biochim. biophys. Acta (Amst.) **178**, 408 – 411 (1969)

CHAPTER 2

Induction of Hepatic Hemoproteins

K.W. BOCK and H. REMMER

A. Introduction

A multitude of studies have shown that enzyme levels in animal tissues can be altered by physiological, nutritional, and hormonal manipulations, as well as by the administration of various chemicals foreign to the body. In particular, the level of a hepatic hemoprotein, microsomal cytochrome P-450, is increased by the administration of a wide variety of lipid-soluble xenobiotics (e.g., drugs, insecticides, herbicides, and carcinogenic polycyclic hydrocarbons). The induction of this cytochrome is the primary concern of this review. It is contrasted with increases in the levels of other hepatic hemoproteins, such as tryptophan pyrrolase, microsomal cytochrome b_5, mitochondrial cytochromes, and catalase.

Evidence given below indicates that the increase in the level of cytochrome P-450 is due to induction; i.e., to an increased rate of synthesis of this protein relative to its normal rate (for an operational definition of "induction" see B). Cytochrome P-450 is part of a multienzyme electron transport chain involved in the oxidation of numerous lipid-soluble drugs, as well as endogenous compounds such as cholesterol, steroid hormones, and fatty acids. Therefore, this cytochrome has attracted considerable interest. It is well known that the duration and intensity of drug action is influenced by its metabolism. Furthermore, the toxicity of many drugs can be either decreased or increased by their metabolism, e.g., ultimate carcinogens are very often produced by the cytochrome P-450 dependent oxidation reaction. A number of detailed reviews on this subject have been published recently (see references to recommended reviews).

Hemoproteins occupy key positions in the function of hepatocyte organelles. Therefore, the regulation of hemoprotein levels is often linked to the general regulation of these organelles. Table 1 lists hepatic hemoproteins, their functional location in the hepatocyte, and their biological half-lives. Hemoprotein synthesis requires coordinated heme and protein synthesis, as well as the subsequent attachment of the cofactor to the apoprotein. The final location of the hemoprotein is in most instances different from its site of synthesis. Thus, the level of liver hemoproteins may also be influenced by altering their transport from the site of synthesis, and incorporation into their functional sites within the cell. Although the role of these posttranslational events is poorly understood, it is conceivable that they may play a role in determining levels of hemoproteins in cell organelles.

The present survey is aimed at critically reviewing our still incomplete knowledge on the mechanisms regulating the levels of liver microsomal cytochrome P-450, rather than giving a complete list of chemical inducers. The complex induction phenomena which have been studied in detail with phenobarbital and 3-methyl-

Table 1. Localization and turnover of liver hemoproteins

Cell Compartment	Hemoprotein	Biological half-life	References
Cytoplasm	Tryptophan pyrrolase	2 h[a]	Schimke et al., 1965 Knox and Piras, 1967
Endoplasmic reticulum	{ Cytochrome(s) P-450	1 − 2 d[c]	Greim et al., 1970 Levin and Kuntzman, 1969
	{ Cytochrome b_5	2 d[c], 3.5 − 4 d[b]	Kuriyama et al., 1969 Greim et al., 1970 Bock and Siekevitz, 1970 Druyan et al., 1969
Peroxisomes	Catalase	2 d[b, c]	Poole et al., 1969
Mitochondria:			
Inner Membrane	Cytochrome a, a_3		
	Cytochrome b	5.5 d[c]	Druyan et al., 1969
	Cytochrome c, c_1	6.1 d[c]	Druyan et al., 1969
Outer Membrane	Cytochrome b_5	4.4 d[c]	Druyan et al., 1969

Method of study: [a] Kinetic analysis, immunochemical isolation; [b] incorporation of guanidino-^{14}C arginine; [c] ^{14}C-5-aminolevulinate incorporation.

cholanthrene as chemical inducers are contrasted with increases in the levels of other hepatic hemoproteins, especially with the increase of catalase and mitochondrial cytochromes following treatment with the hypolipidemic drug clofibrate. Changes in the levels of some of these proteins produced by nutritional and hormonal factors will also be discussed in this chapter, while the decrease in the levels of hemoproteins caused by chemical agents will be dealt with in other chapters of this volume.

B. Use of the Term Induction in Studies on Mammalian Tissues

"Induction" is commonly used in a very broad sense. Therefore, a few words on this term as it is used in the present review are necessary.

SCHOENHEIMER's concept of the "dynamic state of body constituents," developed more than 30 years ago (SCHOENHEIMER, 1942), has to be taken into consideration when induction is studied in mammalian tissues, since both the level of a protein and the time course of increase of this level will depend upon its rates of synthesis and degradation. The term induction has been defined by bacteriologists as an increase in the rate of synthesis of a specific protein, which in bacterial systems implicates the synthesis of specific mRNA (JACOB and MONOD, 1961; EPSTEIN and BECKWITH, 1968). In contrast to growing bacterial systems, where protein degradation plays a minor role in determining total enzyme levels, the levels of proteins in animal tissues in steady state are always regulated both by synthesis and degradation (SCHIMKE and DOYLE, 1970). Due to the metabolic and structural complexities of animal cells, including rapid nRNA turnover (ATTARDI et al., 1966; HARRIS, 1968) and variably stable mRNA (REVEL and HIATT, 1964; KAFATOS and REICH, 1968), a number of regulatory factors exist besides those regulating the formation of specific mRNA. Since in many instances the molecular mechanisms of the induction process are poorly understood, we use the term induction operationally according to SCHIMKE and DOYLE (SCHIMKE and DOYLE, 1970), as an increase in the ratio of the rate of protein synthesis over the rate of protein degradation. Thus, an increase in protein amount is described without mechanistic implications

Enzyme synthesis follows zero-order kinetics (PRICE et al., 1962; SCHIMKE et al., 1965). The simplest expression for the rate of protein degradation is first order, as shown by the exponential decay of in vivo labeled proteins (OMURA et al., 1967). Thus, a change in tissue content of an enzyme involving both protein synthesis and degradation can be described by:

$$dP/dt = S - kP$$

where P is the amount of a specific protein/unit weight, S the rate constant for synthesis, and k the first order rate constant of protein degradation. At any time that a steady state for the protein level exists, i.e.,

$$dP/dt = 0, \quad \text{then} \quad P = S/k$$

It is evident that P is determined by the respective values of S and k. The amount of a specific protein (P) can be increased by increasing the rate of protein synthesis or by decreasing the rate of degradation. A term often used to express the rate of degradation is the half-life ($T^1/_2$). This is defined by the following relationship:

$$T^1/_2 = \frac{\ln 2}{k}$$

where k is the rate constant of degradation.

When the level of a protein is increased by an induction process, the time taken to increase to one-half of the final steady state level is approximately equal to the half-life (BERLIN and SCHIMKE, 1965). Therefore, it is experimentally possible to estimate the half-life of a protein by following the time course of its increase to a new steady state level. The same principle is applied in pharmacokinetics, when, for example, the blood level of a drug is maintained or altered by constant intravenous infusions (GOLDSTEIN et al., 1969). Figure 1 illustrates that the time taken to reach a new steady state level of a protein depends on its rate of degradation. The enzymes listed in the figure differ greatly in their degradation rates or biological half-lives, which range from about 2 h for both tyrosine transaminase and tryptophan pyrrolase to 84 and 96 h for glutamic-alanine transaminase and arginase, respectively. Tryptophan pyrrolase and tyrosine transaminase are rapidly induced by cortisone, whereas glutamic-alanine transaminase and arginase respond more slowly. Although the time course and magnitude of induction are quite different for these enzymes, it has been calculated that the ratios of rates of synthesis under basal conditions, to rates of synthesis in cortisone-treated animals are quite similar for the various enzymes. Thus the apparent small response of an enzyme such as arginase is not a reflection of low sensitivity to the effects of cortisone but of slow turnover.

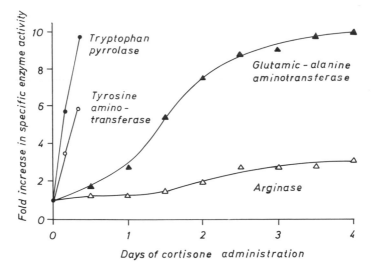

Fig. 1. Time course of increase in tryptophan pyrrolase, tyrosine aminotransferase, glutamic-alanine transaminase, and arginase with cortisone administration. Animals received 10 mg cortisone acetate every 8 h i.m. Each value is the mean of 3 animals (from BERLIN et al., 1965)

These concepts have been presented in a somewhat simplified form to facilitate an understanding of some of the processes involved in the increase of protein levels in animal tissues. Real steady state conditions do not exist in vivo. Furthermore, a number of posttranslational control factors exist which we have not considered. As has already been pointed out, hemoprotein synthesis requires coordinated heme and protein synthesis, and the attachment of the cofactor to the apoprotein, as well as the formation of the ternary complex at the functional site within the cell. (This will be discussed in more detail below.)

C. Tryptophan Pyrrolase (Dioxygenase)

Tryptophan pyrrolase, the rate-limiting enzyme in tryptophan degradation, is the first enzyme whose concentration was shown to be increased by a hormone (KNOX, 1951). It is a cytoplasmic liver hemoprotein for which two different mechanisms of induction have been clearly and conclusively characterized: (1) hormonal and (2) cofactor or substrate-type induction. This hemoprotein is present in fed rats in approximately equal proportion as holoenzyme and apoenzyme (FEIGELSON and GREENGARD, 1962; BADAWY and EVANS, 1973). Using an immunologic method, FEIGELSON and GREENGARD (1962) showed that both corticoids and tryptophan increase the concentration of tryptophan pyrrolase in rat liver. The initial effect of tryptophan was to convert inactive apoenzyme to active holoenzyme by saturation with heme. This first phase was followed by an increase in the total amount of holoenzyme. On the other hand, hydrocortisone increased both apo- and holo-enzyme. SCHIMKE et al. (1965) demonstrated that cortisone increased the rate of

synthesis of tryptophan pyrrolase without affecting its degradation, whereas tryptophan prevented almost completely the degradation of the enzyme. They proposed
that the presence of tryptophan caused the conversion of the enzyme to active
holoenzyme, which is the form resistant to degradation. Glucocorticoids cause an
hormonal type of induction, involving the synthesis of new apoenzyme, whereas
tryptophan produces a substrate or cofactor-type induction, involving a decreased
rate of degradation of preexisting apoenzyme while its normal rate of synthesis
continues.

Increased activity of tryptophan pyrrolase has also been reported after the
administration of phenobarbital, phenylbutazone (BADAWY and EVANS, 1973), and
the porphyrogen allylisopropylacetamide (MARVER et al., 1966). However it has
been shown recently that conditions leading to destruction, inhibition of synthesis,
increased utilization, and enhanced synthesis of liver heme will modify the saturation of apotryptophan pyrrolase with its heme activator. Thus, the increase in
tryptophan pyrrolase level caused by phenobarbital and phenylbutazone is not an
induction but is due to an increase in heme saturation of the enzyme (heme synthesis is increased following the administration of phenobarbital). In the case of
the porphyrogen, the increase in holo plus apotryptophan pyrrolase may be a
stress-mediated hormonal-type of induction (BADAWY and EVANS, 1973).

Interestingly, in the guinea pig, tryptophan pyrrolase is only present as the
holoenzyme and cannot be induced by corticoids. In species lacking a hormonal-
type of induction, tryptophan is more toxic (BADAWY and EVANS, 1974).

D. Cytochromes of the Endoplasmic Reticulum

I. Cytochrome(s) P-450

1. Cytochrome P-450-Dependent Monooxygenase(s)

Cytochrome P-450 is part of an electron transport chain consisting of two protein
components. Cytochrome P-450 is the terminal oxidase in this electron transport
chain, and binds lipid-soluble substrates and molecular oxygen. The second component is a NADPH-dependent flavoprotein (Fp) called cytochrome P-450 reductase, or NADPH cytochrome c reductase (cytochrome c is used as a convenient artificial electron acceptor). Several molecules of cytochrome P-450 probably form a complex with one molecule of the flavoprotein (ESTABROOK, 1971). This complex catalyzes the oxidation of a great variety of lipid-soluble chemicals of diverse structures
(aliphatic and aromatic hydrocarbons, heterocyclic compounds and their derivatives). Furthermore the oxidation of a large number of normal body constituents
such as steroid hormones, cholesterol, bile acids, fatty acids, and other lipid-soluble
endogenous compounds, is carried out by cytochrome P-450 dependent monooxygenase reactions (CONNEY and KUNTZMAN, 1971). Recent evidence suggests a
nonrigid complex between cytochromes P-450 and NADPH cytochrome P-450
reductase allowing independent lateral movement of the two proteins in the membrane. In this way one molecule of NADPH cytochrome P-450 reductase is able
to provide reducing equivalents to a number of cytochrome P-450 molecules, e.g.,

to cytochromes P-450 newly incorporated into the membrane (YANG, 1977). Random distribution and lateral diffusion has also been shown for the catalytic interaction of NADPH cytochrome b_5 reductase and cytochrome b_5 in hepatic microsomes (ROGERS and STRITTMATTER, 1974). Monooxygenase reactions have been found in most tissues of the body, but occur predominately in liver (CONNEY, 1967). As will be discussed in section 3, the substrate specificity of the microsomal monooxygenase system resides in cytochrome P-450, which consists of a family of related cytochromes with different substrate specificities. Some of these cytochrome P-450 species seem to be rather unspecific, while other probably catalyse very specific reactions such as cholesterol-7α-hydroxylation. Two specific cytochrome P-450 dependent monooxygenases are found in adrenal medulla mitochondria and catalyse cholesterol-11β-hydroxylation and cholesterol side chain cleavage (for references see CONNEY and KUNTZMAN, 1971).

For all the cytochrome P-450 dependent oxidation reactions which have been studied (including oxidation at the aromatic ring, an alkyl side chain oxidative dealkylation, N-oxidation, S-oxidation, epoxidation etc.) the following overall stoichiometry has been established:

$$XH + NADPH + H^+ + O_2 \longrightarrow XOH + NADPH^+ + H_2O \, .$$

With $^{18}O_2$ it has been demonstrated that one-half of the oxygen molecule is found in the oxidized substrate, and the rest in H_2O. Therefore the enzyme complex catalyzing this reaction has been called mixed-function oxidase (MASON et al., 1965) or monooxygenase (HAYAISHI, 1962) in contrast to dioxygenases such as tryptophan pyrrolase which incorporates both atoms of the oxygen molecule into the substrate.

The involvement of only two protein components in liver microsomal monooxygenase reactions has been recently confirmed in reconstitution experiments using purified components (VAN DER HOEVEN et al., 1974; IMAI and SATO, 1974; VAN DER HOEVEN and COON, 1974). For reconstitution of an active system a phospholipid (phosphatidylcholine) is also necessary (STROBEL et al., 1970).

Cytochrome P-450 dependent monooxygenases are of considerable pharmacological and toxicological interest for two reasons: (1) the duration and intensity of action of many drugs are largely determined by the rate at which they are metabolized in the body; (2) metabolism by the monooxygenase sometimes leads to the formation of reactive metabolites which are often carcinogens, mutagens, or responsible for other toxic side reactions of drugs (GILLETTE et al., 1974).

Most lipid-soluble compounds are bound to cytochrome P-450 leading to characteristic spectral changes (REMMER et al., 1966). Three classes of spectral changes have been observed. The type I spectral change represents the interaction of a substrate (e.g., hexobarbital, aminopyrine) with the cytochrome. Compounds such as phenacetin or n-butanol give a so-called reversed type I spectrum, which is thought to be the consequence of the displacement of an "endogenous" type I substrate from the binding site on cytochrome P-450 (SCHENKMAN et al., 1972). Alternatively, this may be a composite spectrum arising from the superimposition of substrate interactions with different species of cytochrome P-450. Type II binding spectra are thought to result from the interaction of substrates like aniline or

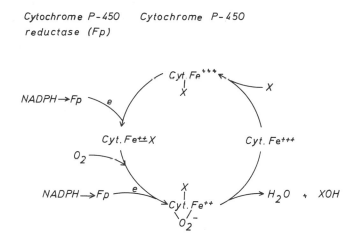

Fig. 2. Redox cycle of cytochrome P-450 during oxidation of drugs (X)

n-octylamine with the 6th coordination valency of heme iron. The bound type I substrates are subsequently oxidized in a redox cycle (Fig. 2). Two electrons are transferred stepwise to the cytochrome by the NADPH-dependent cytochrome P-450 reductase. The first electron reduces the cytochrome after a substrate is bound. The second electron activates molecular oxygen which is bound to the cytochrome after its reduction. The second electron can be provided alternatively by a NADH-dependent electron transport chain (discussed in D.II; ESTABROOK, 1971).

2. Chemical Inducers

Studies during the last two decades have firmly established that the protein components of the monooxygenase system can be induced by a great variety of chemicals. Our knowledge about this induction phenomenon stems from two lines of investigations: (1) studies on the metabolism of carcinogenic azodyes (CONNEY et al., 1956) and (2) studies on drug tolerance (REMMER, 1959). Among the first known inducers were the carcinogen 3-methylcholanthrene (CONNEY et al., 1956), and the hypnotic drug phenobarbital (REMMER, 1959). These inducing agents were later classified in distinctly different groups, as they stimulate the synthesis of two different species of cytochrome P-450, which in turn catalyze different oxidation reactions (discussed in Sect. D.I.4). Since then, an ever-growing number of compounds have been found to be potent inducing agents (Table 2). The list of compounds is not meant to be exhaustive; rather it is meant to acquaint the reader with the wide variety of compounds that have been studied.

The induced level of cytochrome P-450 is maintained as long as the inducer is present. Chronic administration of phenobarbital to rats causes the level of cytochrome P-450 to rise until a new steady state level is reached after 3 days (Fig. 3). After a single intraperitoneal injection of phenobarbital, the induced cytochrome P-450 level rapidly returns to the normal level as the inducer is eliminated from

Table 2. Compounds inducing cytochrome(s) P-450 and cytochrome P-450 dependent monooxygenase(s)

Pharmacologic action	Compound	References
Hypnotics and sedatives	Barbiturates (Phenobarbital)	Remmer, 1959
		Conney et al., 1960
	Gluthethimide	Kato and Vasanelli, 1962
		Kato et al., 1962
		Schmid et al., 1964
	Chloral hydrate	Kato and Vasanelli, 1962
		Cucinell et al., 1966
Anticonvulsants	Diphenylhydantoin	Kato and Vasanelli, 1962
		Remmer, 1962
Tranquilizer	Meprobamate	Kato et al., 1962
		Philips et al., 1962
		Douglas et al., 1963
	Chlordiazepoxide	Hoogland et al., 1966
		Kutt and McDowell, 1968
Antipsychotics	Chlorpromazine	Kato and Vasanelli, 1962
		Wattenberg and Leong, 1965
	Imipramine	Breyer, 1972
Central nervous system stimulants	Nikethamide	Brazda and Baucum, 1961
		Kato and Vasanelli, 1962
Anti-inflammatory agents	Phenylbutazone	Conney et al., 1960
		Chen et al., 1962
	Aminopyrine	Conney et al., 1960
Hypoglycemic agents	Tolbutamide	Remmer et al., 1964
	Carbutamide	Remmer et al., 1964
Antihistaminics	Orphenadrine	Conney et al., 1960
	Diphenhydramine	Kato et al., 1962
	Chlorcyclizine	Conney et al., 1961
Antibiotics	Rifampicin	Michot et al., 1970
		Remmer et al., 1973
	Griseofulvin	Wada et al., 1968
Fungicides	Clotrimazole	Tettenborn, 1970
Steroids	Spironolactone	Solymoss et al., 1969
		Stripp et al., 1970
	Pregnenolone-16-carbonitrile	Solymoss et al., 1971
Insecticides	DDT	Hart and Fouts, 1963
		Ghazal et al., 1964
	Chlordane	Hart et al., 1963
	Dieldrin	Hart et al., 1963
		Ghazal et al., 1964
	Aldrin	Hart and Fouts, 1963
	Hexachlorocyclohexane (HCH)	Hart et al., 1963
		Ghazal et al., 1964
		Koransky et al., 1964
	Hexachlorobenzene	Wada et al., 1968
		Stonard and Nenov, 1974
Carcinogenic polycyclic hydrocarbons	3-Methylcholanthrene	Conney et al., 1956
		Cramer et al., 1960
		Gelboin and Blackburn, 1964
	3,4-Benzpyrene	Conney et al., 1960
		Conney et al., 1957

Table 2 (continued)

Pharmacological action	Compound	References
Miscellaneous	TCDD	Buu-Iloi et al., 1971
		Greig and De Matteis, 1973
		Poland et al., 1974
	Polychlorinated biphenyls	Villeneuve et al., 1971
	(PCB)	Bruckner et al., 1973
	Flavones	Wattenberg et al., 1968
	Safrole	Parke et al., 1970

Abbreviations: DDT, Chlorphenothane
TCDD,2,3,7,8-tetrachlorodibenzo-p-dioxin.

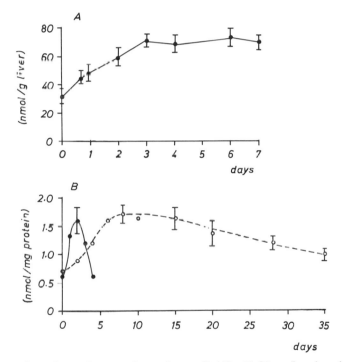

Fig. 3. Increase of rat liver microsomal cytochrome P-450. A) 80 mg/kg phenobarbital daily; determination of cytochrome P-450 in liver homogenates according to Greim, 1970. B) ●——● 80 mg/kg phenobarbital once i.p.; ○– – – –○ 200 mg/kg DDT once i.p.; determination of cytochrome P-450 in microsomes according to Omura and Sato (1964)

the body. In contrast, the insecticide DDT accumulates in body fat, and therefore inducing concentrations of DDT are maintained for a long time (Fig. 3).

Cytochrome P-450 and associated monooxygenase reactions are also induced during therapy in man (Chen et al., 1962; Cucinell et al., 1965; Kuntzman et al., 1966; MacDonald et al., 1967; Alvares et al., 1969; Ackerman and Heinrich,

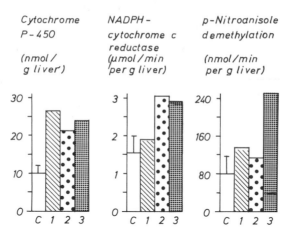

Fig. 4. Components of drug-metabolizing monooxygenase in liver biopsy specimens of patients receiving rifampicin (1,2) and diphenylhydantoin plus phenobarbital (3). C = controls ± standard deviation (n = 19); 1 = 33 y ♂, 600 mg rifampicin daily for 5 days; 2 = 30 y ♂, 600 mg rifampicin daily for 14 days; 3 = 29 y ♂, 500 mg diphenylhydantoin daily for 2 months plus 15 mg phenobarbital for 7 days before liver biopsy (from REMMER, 1973)

1970; NELSON et al., 1971; DAVIES and THORGEIRSSON, 1971; SCHOENE et al., 1972; REMMER et al., 1973; PELKONEN et al., 1974). However only after treatment with drugs which accumulate in the body can a marked increase in cytochrome P-450 be detected in liver biopsy specimens (Fig. 4).

Chemical inducers act at the cellular level, since induction of aryl hydrocarbon hydroxylase has also been demonstrated in liver cell cultures (NEBERT and GELBOIN, 1968; NEBERT and GIELEN, 1971; WHITLOCK Jr. and GELBOIN, 1974).

In order to trigger the induction process, the inducer probably has to interact with the target cell for a certain minimum time period; for example, hexobarbital does not significantly induce cytochrome P-450 in male rats; in this species, the half-life of hexobarbital in blood is only 0.5 h. However, hexobarbital does stimulate its own metabolism in dogs (T $^{1}/_{2}$ of hexobarbital = 3 h) and in man (T$^{1}/_{2}$ = 4 − 6 h) (REMMER, 1970). All the known inducers are lipid soluble compounds which interact with cytochrome P-450 to give type I spectral shifts (see Sect. D.I.1). It is therefore tempting to speculate that the inducer-binding site of the proposed receptor may have features in common with the type I binding site of cytochrome P-450. In addition to the lipid solubility of inducers, more specific structural requirements have also been described for inducing agents (POLAND and GLOVER, 1973).

3. Cytochrome P-450, One Hemoprotein or Many?

Evidences slowly accumulated that multiple forms of cytochrome P-450 exist (SLADEK and MANNERING, 1966; FROMMER et al., 1972; LU et al., 1972, 1973; NEBERT and KON, 1973). It has been recognized for quite some time that phenobarbital and 3-methylcholanthrene stimulate different oxidation reactions (CONNEY, 1967).

Phenobarbital-induced monooxygenase systems oxidize hexobarbital and amino-pyrine, whereas 3-methylcholanthrene-induced monooxygenase systems oxidize, for example, benzpyrene[1]. Treatment of rats with 3-methylcholanthrene leads to the synthesis of a form of cytochrome P-450 with altered spectral properties, which has been called cytochrome P-446 (HILDEBRANDT et al., 1968), cytochrome P-448 (ALVARES et al., 1967), or cytochrome P_1-450 (SLADEK and MANNERING, 1966). Purified cytochrome preparations from controls, and from rats treated with pheno-barbital or 3-methylcholanthrene, showed different EPR spectra (NEBERT and KON, 1973; WITMER et al., 1974), behaved differently in isoelectric focussing (CONNEY et al., 1973), and showed different molecular weights in SDS-polyacrylamide gel electrophoresis (ALVARES and SIEKEVITZ, 1973). Cytochrome P-450 fractions with different spectral properties have also been separated by diethylaminoethyl cellulose chromatography (COMAI and GAYLOR, 1973). The substrate specificity of the mono-oxygenase complex resides in the cytochrome, as demonstrated in reconstitution experiments with partially purified fractions (LU et al., 1973). The presence of multiple cytochrome P-450 species with different catalytic activities is now firmly established. Phenobarbital-inducible and β-naphthoflavone- (or 3-methylcholan-threne-) inducible forms of liver microsomal cytochromes P-450 have been separated and purified (HASHIMOTO and IMAI, 1976; HAUGEN and COON, 1976; HUANG et al., 1976; THOMAS et al., 1976; JOHNSON and MULLER-EBERHARD, 1977).

4. Studies on the Induction Mechanism of Cytochrome P-450

The induction phenomena observed in liver following treatment with pheno-barbital are complex, involving many processes besides the induction of cytochrome P-450 (see Sect. D.I.6). So far, they are by no means understood. Nevertheless a few features of the increase of cytochrome P-450 may be discussed in this section.

The induction of cytochrome P-450 and NADPH cytochrome-c reductase can be prevented by inhibition of protein synthesis at the transcriptional or transla-tional level (ERNSTER and ORRENIUS, 1965; GELBOIN, 1971; JACOB et al., 1974). Furthermore, after the administration of phenobarbital, an increased in vivo in-corporation of amino acids into cytochrome P-450 (DEHLINGER and SCHIMKE, 1972; KURIYAMA et al., 1969; ARIAS et al., 1969) and into NADPH cytochrome-c reductase has been demonstrated under conditions excluding a change in the pre-cursor pool. This was shown by determining the level of incorporation into the purified proteins. Turnover studies suggest that phenobarbital increases the level of NADPH cytochrome-c reductase, both by increasing the rate of synthesis, and decreasing the rate of degradation (JICK and SHUSTER, 1966; KURIYAMA et al., 1969). However the decrease in degradation is still debated, since phenobarbital also causes an increased reutilization of the labeled amino acids (SCHIMKE and DOYLE, 1970). An increased incorporation of heme precursors into a preparation, which contained cytochrome P-450 as the only hemoprotein, has also been shown

---

[1] The oxidation of benzpyrene—designated benzpyrene hydroxylase or aryl hydrocarbon hy-droxylase—is usually assayed fluorometrically by following the production of fluorescent phenols. However, it has been recently shown that besides a number of fluorescent phenols, various nonphenolic metabolites are formed (HOLDER et al., 1974; SELKIRK et al., 1974).

(Marver, 1969). From the relatively high amount and short biological half-life of cytochrome P-450 (Table 1), it has been estimated that most of the heme synthesized in the hepatocyte is needed for the synthesis of this cytochrome (Marver and Schmid, 1972). This may be the basis for the clinical observations that administration of inducing agents to patients with a defect in heme metabolism (e.g., acute intermittent porphyria) frequently leads to an acute porphyric attack (De Matteis and Gibbs, 1972). It has been noted that the level of the rate limiting enzyme in heme biosynthesis, δ-aminolevulinic acid synthetase, is increased after the administration of phenobarbital to fasting rats (Marver, 1969). This initial increase may not solely reflect the need for increased heme synthesis, since δ-aminolevulinic acid synthetase later decreases when cytochrome P-450 has reached the induced steady state level (Bock et al., 1971). During the induction of cytochrome P-450 by phenylbutazone, no increase of δ-aminolevulinic acid synthetase has been noticed (De Matteis and Gibbs, 1972). However, compounds known to induce drug-metabolizing enzymes in mammalian liver are very often potent inducers of δ-aminolevulinic acid synthetase in chick liver cell cultures (Granick, 1966).

A biphasic rate of loss of radioactivity has been reported in so called cytochrome P-450 particles labeled in vivo with the heme precursor δ-aminolevulinic acid (Levin and Kuntzman, 1969). Half-lives of 7 and 48 h have been determined for the two phases. However it is still debated whether the fast turnover component ($T^{1}/_{2} = 7$ h) represents a cytochrome P-450 species, or contamination by a small amount of a mobile microsomal heme pool. This heme pool is detectable after increasing heme synthesis (Druyan and Kelly, 1972). It is conceivable that the heme pool has a very high specific radioactivity shortly after pulse labeling. Therefore, it may be very difficult to distinguish between heme contamination of the cytochrome P-450 preparation, and a real incorporation of heme into the cytochrome.

Evidence for a pool of free cytochrome P-450 apoprotein has been reported. (Correia and Meyer, 1975). After phenobarbital administration, the rate of synthesis of the apoprotein is primarily increased. The apoprotein accumulates when heme synthesis is inhibited. Interestingly, it is found in "heavy" microsomes sedimenting with the mitochondrial fraction. It is known that inhibition of heme synthesis will lead to a decrease of cytochrome P-450, or prevent its induction. However, an increased rate of heme synthesis will not increase cytochrome P-450, but rather the heme pool in microsomes (Druyan and Kelly, 1972). With regard to the site of synthesis of cytochrome P-450, it has been earlier reported that after phenobarbital treatment, cytochrome P-450 and NADPH cytochrome-c reductase increase first in the rough microsomal fractions, and subsequently in smooth microsomes (Ernster and Orrenius, 1965; Dallner et al., 1966).

Detailed investigations on the induction mechanism of benzpyrene hydroxylase have been carried out in liver cell cultures (Nebert and Gielen, 1971; Whitlock Jr. and Gelboin, 1974) and in mice (Gielen et al., 1972). However, the benzpyrene hydroxylase reaction, which is induced by polycyclic hydrocarbons, is catalyzed by a form of cytochrome P-450 different from that induced by phenobarbital, as discussed in the previous section. Studies on the incorporation of ^{14}C- and ^{3}H-leucine into hepatic microsomal proteins from responsive and nonresponsive mice indicate that the enhanced formation of cytochrome P-448 and P-450 by β-naphthoflavone and phenobarbital, respectively, is primarily the result of an increased rate of de novo protein synthesis rather than a decreased degradation rate or a conversion of pre-existing polypeptides (HAUGEN et al., 1976).

In addition, mutants have been found in inbred strains of mice in which benz-pyrene hydroxylase cannot be induced by 3-methylcholanthrene (GIELEN et al., 1972; POLAND et al., 1974). These mice also lack the ability to respond to 3-methyl-cholanthrene with the formation of cytochrome P-448. However they respond normally to phenobarbital. The lack of response to 3-methylcholanthrene is not due to a mutation in the structural gene(s) necessary for benzpyrene hydroxylase synthesis, since in these strains of mice benzpyrene hydroxylase can be induced by TCDD (2,3,7,8-tetrachlorodibenzo-p-dioxin; GREIG and DE MATTEIS, 1973; POLAND et al., 1974). TCDD is a toxic contaminant formed during the commercial synthesis of the herbicide 2,4,5-trichlorophenoxyacetic acid, and is normally about 30,000 times more potent as an inducer for rat benzpyrene hydroxylase than 3-methylcholanthrene (POLAND and GLOVER, 1974). In nonresponsive mice, per-haps a mutation has occurred which results in production of an inducer-binding receptor, having a diminished affinity for aromatic hydrocarbons, but still having affinity for TCDD.

A stereospecific, high affinity binding protein for ^{3}H-TCDD (2,3,7,8-tetra-chlorodibenzo-p-dioxin) was found in hepatic cytosol of mice (POLAND et al., 1976). Low affinity specific binding was observed in nonresponsive mice. The binding affinity of 23 dibenzo-p-dioxins and dibenzofurans for this cytosol-binding species closely correlated with the potencies of these compounds as inducers of aryl hydrocarbon hydroxylase activity. The polycyclic hydrocarbons that induce hepatic hydroxylase activity competed with ^{3}H-TCDD for hepatic cytosol binding but phenobarbital, pregnenolone-16-carbonitrile, and the steroid hormones had no specific binding. These studies suggest that this binding protein may be the receptor for the induction of hepatic aryl hydrocarbon hydroxylase.

5. Factors Influencing the Induction of Cytochrome P-450

a) *Species Differences, Genetic Factors*

Inducible cytochrome P-450 dependent monooxygenases are found in most verte-brates including man (CONNEY, 1967). However, large variations in the metabolism of specific compounds and response of monooxygenase levels to inducers have been found among different species (CONNEY, 1967). This makes the extrapolation to man of data obtained in experimental animals very uncertain. Therefore great efforts are currently made to elucidate the control of cytochromes P-450 in man (GELBOIN et al., 1976; CONNEY et al., 1976).

The genetic make-up of the individuals of a population within a given species may also be important in the response to enzyme inducers. Greater than 10-fold differences in blood levels of diphenylhydantoin have been observed in epileptic patients receiving the same dose of the drug (REMMER et al., 1969). The large varia-tion in the blood level largely reflects differences in the hydroxylation rate. Similar observations have been made with nortriptyline (ALEXANDERSON et al., 1969). The individual differences in metabolism, which were obvious in fraternal twins, were not observed in identical twins, indicating the importance of genetic factors (Vessel and Page, 1968a, b; Alexanderson et al., 1969; Vessel, 1975). Since the enzyme system is not saturated under in vivo conditions, the reaction rate depends not only upon the enzyme level, but also upon substrate concentration. Hence the individual variation in drug metabolism may be caused by a number of factors, including binding proteins in the blood and tissue, as well as storage sites such as lipids. Consequently variations in rates of drug metabolism observed in man may be attributed to a multiplicity of factors. Strains of mice which do not respond to 3-methylcholanthrene have been described (Gielen et al., 1972), as discussed in section D.I.4. Recent studies with human lymphocyte cultures indicate differences in the inducibility of benzpyrene hydroxylase in man (Kellermann et al., 1973a), and these differences have been correlated with the development of lung cancer in cigarette smokers (Kellermann et al., 1973b). These studies, however, have to be confirmed. Tumorigenesis in mouse skin is probably unrelated to genetic differences in the induction of benzpyrene hydroxylase, since the constitutive level of the hydroxylase activity in the skin of these mice is thought to be sufficient to initiate chemical carcinogenesis (Nebert et al., 1972).

b) *Developmental Factors*

The level of drug metabolizing monooxygenases is low in the fetus and the newborn. It begins to increase during, or shortly after birth (Dallner et al., 1966; Conney, 1967). This may be one of the causes of the greater sensitivity of newborns to drugs. The constitutive level of benzpyrene hydroxylase, as well as its inducibility by 3-methylcholanthrene, increases after birth in mice (Gielen et al., 1972). In human fetuses, drug-metabolizing enzymes appear during the first half of pregnancy, and their activity during gestation reach about one third of those found in the adult (Gillette and Stripp, 1975).

c) *Hormonal Factors*

In contrast to most other mammalian species, including man, the level of cytochrome P-450 is sex dependent in the rat (Quinn et al., 1958; Schenkman et al., 1967). The cytochrome P-450 level is lower in female than in male rats. It can be increased in female rats by treatment with testosterone, whereas the cytochrome level in male rats is lowered after treatment with estradiol (Quinn et al., 1958). Adrenalectomy or hypophysectomy lowers, but does not abolish, the basal monooxygenase activity or its inducibility by phenobarbital (Remmer, 1972b). Treatment of male rats with thyroxine increases NADPH cytochrome-c reductase, but lowers cytochrome P-450 and hence monooxygenase (Kato and Takahashi, 1968; Mitropolous et al., 1968).

d) *Nutritional Factors*

Fasting decreases the amount of cytochrome P-450 on a whole liver weight basis (Bock et al., 1973a), and decreases the level of drug metabolizing monooxygenases (Kato and Gillette, 1965). However, when the inducer phenobarbital is present in fasting rats, cytochrome P-450 increases to higher levels than in fed rats (Greim, 1970; Bock et al., 1973). Feeding low protein diets for 2 weeks (Marshall and McLean, 1962), or fat free diets for 3 weeks (Norred and Wade, 1972), reduces drug-metabolizing monooxygenase. Furthermore, the administration of phenobarbital to rats given a low protein diet, though raising the level of cytochrome P-450, does not raise it to the value found in control rats treated with phenobarbital (MARSHALL and MCLEAN, 1962). Hence, there is a difference between the induction of cytochrome P-450 in fasting animals and in animals fed a low protein diet. Evidence was obtained that the macronutrient composition (high protein, low carbohydrate versus low protein, high carbohydrate diet) greatly influences drug oxidations in man (ALVARES et al., 1976).

6. Connection Between the Induction of Cytochrome P-450 Dependent Monooxygenase(s) and Other Effects of Inducing Agents

a) *Induction of Microsomal Enzymes and the Proliferation of Endoplasmic Reticulum Membranes*

In early studies, it was recognized that phenobarbital not only stimulates the synthesis of drug-metabolizing enzymes, but also leads to a marked proliferation of the smooth endoplasmic reticulum to which these enzymes are bound (REMMER and MERKER, 1963), and to an increase in liver mass (CONNEY et al., 1960). 3-Methylcholanthrene on the other hand, induces a smaller number of enzymes and does not lead to a significant proliferation of endoplasmic reticulum (CONNEY, 1967). Both inducing compounds stimulate not only the production of monooxygenases, but also at least two microsomal enzymes functionally linked to the monooxygenase system, UDP-glucuronyltransferase (INSCOE and AXELROD, 1960; ZEIDENBERG et al., 1967; MULDER, 1970; BOCK et al., 1973b) and epoxide hydrase (OESCH et al., 1971; OESCH, 1973). UDP-glucuronyltransferase converts a variety of lipid-soluble compounds to highly polar glucuronides, which can be actively eliminated from the cell. Very often hydroxylated products of monooxygenases are substrates of UDP-glucuronyltransferase. As with the monooxygenases, phenobarbital and 3-methylcholanthrene have selective stimulatory effects on UDP-glucuronyltransferase activities (BOCK et al., 1973b; JACOBSON et al., 1975). Epoxide hydrase converts highly reactive epoxides, formed during the oxidation of aromatic compounds, to the corresponding dihydrodiols (OESCH and DALY, 1972). The formation of a complex between epoxide hydrase and the monooxygenase system has been reported. The formation of this complex seems to be stimulated by treatment with 3-methylcholanthrene (OESCH and DALY, 1972). However, not all protein constituents of microsomal membranes are induced; e.g., glucose-6-phosphatase or nucleoside diphosphatase (REMMER and MERKER, 1963; ERNSTER and ORRENIUS, 1965) are decreased in their specific activities in microsomes after proliferation of smooth membranes. Thus, the composition of the membranes changes during proliferation. Together with the general increase in membrane proteins, both phospholipid (YOUNG et al., 1971) and cholesterol synthesis (ERIKSSON, 1973) are increased. Slight alterations in the lipid composition of the membranes have been reported (DAVISON and WILLS, 1974). Since the inducible drug-metabolizing enzymes represent a considerable proportion of the total membrane proteins of the endoplasmic reticulum, it is conceivable that the membrane proliferation might be a necessary consequence of the induction of these enzymes. A possible coupling between the induction of cytochromes P-450 and functionally coordinated proteins (such as microsomal UDP-glucuronyltransferases and epoxide hydrase, and the cytosol glutathione S-transferases) was intensely investigated because of its many toxicological implications. Similar to their differential action on cytochrome P-450, phenobarbital and 3-methylcholanthrene probably induce separate UDP-glucuronyltransferases (Bock et al., 1977). In non-responsive mice the inducibility of both aryl hydrocarbon hydroxylase and UDP-glucuronyltransferase (4-methylumbelliferone as substrate) is lost as an inherited trait. This non-responsiveness of both enzymes co-segregates in genetic crosses of responsive and non-responsive mice (Owens, 1977) suggesting a regulatory linkage between both enzymes. On the other hand, a number of examples are known in favour of an independent control of cytochromes P-450 and UDP-glucuronyltransferases (Dutton and Burchell, 1977). These conflicting observations may in part be reconciled in terms of the Britten-Davidson model as discussed by Kumaki et al., 1977. A regulatory linkage between these major phase I and II reactions may be important for the removal of toxic metabolites generated by aryl hydrocarbon hydroxylase (Nemoto and Gelboin, 1976). In contrast, the inducible epoxide hydrase does not appear to be linked with aryl hydrocarbon hydroxylase in non-responsive mice (Oesch et al., 1973).

b) *General Cell Changes Induced by Treatment with Phenobarbital*

Similar to cytochromes P-450 the organic anion binding protein, ligandin (formerly called Y-protein), is induced by both phenobarbital and 3-methylcholanthrene type chemicals. This abundant protein, constituting 5% of the soluble hepatic proteins, binds a variety of ligands noncovalently including dyes, drugs, metabolites, heme and bilirubin. Ligandin was recently identified with glutathione S-transferase B (Habig et al., 1974) and Δ^5-3-ketosteroid isomerase (Benson et al., 1977). This inducible protein with various binding and catalytic activities may have important implications in organic anion transport, drug toxicity, detoxication and carcinogenesis.

A high rate of drug-metabolism leads to marked changes in intermediary metabolism. During drug oxidation, the ratio NADPH/NAD decreases (Kunz et al., 1966b; Sies and Brauser, 1970). The need for the rapid regeneration of NADPH and UDP-glucuronic acid may be the reason for the marked stimulation of the pentose phosphate and glucuronate pathways (Kunz et al., 1966b). The general stimulation of catabolic processes is reflected by the observation that rates of gluconeogenesis from lactate (Scholz et al., 1973) and of lipogenesis from glucose are depressed during drug metabolism (Thurman and Scholz, 1973). In perfused livers of phenobarbital-treated rats, the degradation of aminopyrine consumed at a maximum 30% of the total oxygen uptake of the organ (Thurman and Scholz, 1969). Due to this large oxygen consumption by the cytochrome P-450 dependent monooxygenases, oxygen might become limiting, leading to a competition between mitochondria and microsomes for molecular oxygen. The possible interdependence between these two organelles is further suggested by the observation that, during active drug metabolism, mitochondria are often surrounded by endoplasmic reticulum membranes (Moldeus et al., 1973).

It has been shown that the number of mitochondria and peroxisomes is increased in liver after treatment with phenobarbital (STRÄUBLI et al., 1969). In addition the amounts of mitochondrial and peroxisomal enzymes increase approximately corresponding to the increase in liver weight (KUNZ et al., 1966b). This may be connected with the large oxygen consumption by the induced cytochrome P-450 systems. In addition, an enlargement of lysosomes as well as an increase in the level of lysosomal proteases has also been reported (HORNEF, 1970).

The rate of synthesis of albumin, the major secretory protein of the liver, does not seem to be increased after phenobarbital (MATERN et al., 1972). Thus, phenobarbital does not increase the synthesis of all proteins in the hepatocyte.

c) *Liver Growth*

Liver growth can be the result of an increase in the size (hypertrophy) or number (hyperplasia) of cellular elements. In the liver, many different stimuli are known to increase the rate of DNA synthesis without subsequent cell division, leading to an increased proportion of polyploid nuclei. These polyploid nuclei, however, are always euploid unless the cell has undergone malignant transformation. Some authors have classified the increase in the proportion of polyploid nuclei in the liver as hyperplasia (BARKA and POPPER, 1967).

A number of compounds which stimulate drug metabolism (e.g., phenobarbital and hexachlorocyclohexanes) lead to liver growth. In addition to the induction of drug-metabolizing enzymes and proliferation of smooth endoplasmic reticulum, a marked increase in DNA synthesis, in mitotic index and in the formation of polyploid nuclei, has been noticed after treatment with various stereoisomers of hexachlorocyclohexane (KORANSKY et al., 1966; SCHULTE-HERMANN et al., 1968; SCHULTE-HERMANN, 1974). Thus liver growth is due to hypertrophy as well as hyperplasia. Increase in DNA synthesis and mitotic index, leading to an increase in ploidy pattern, is less marked after treatment with phenobarbital. Thus liver growth after phenobarbital is mainly due to the hypertrophy resulting from the factors described under a and b. There are a number of compounds which stimulate liver growth without markedly inducing the levels of drug-metabolizing enzymes, e.g., the hypolipidemic drug nafenopin, (BECKETT et al., 1972; REDDY et al., 1973), and the anesthetic halothane (KUNZ et al., 1966a, b; PLATT and COCKRILL, 1969). Hence, there is certainly no strict correlation between an increase in the levels of drug-metabolizing enzymes and liver growth.

7. Reversibility of Induction Phenomena

The increased liver weight returns to normal when the administration of the inducer ceases. This observation has been made with barbiturates (KUNZ et al., 1966a; SCHLICHT et al., 1968; ARGYRIS and MAGNUS, 1968; OWEN et al., 1971; BOLENDER and WEIBEL, 1973), DDT (FITZHUGH and NELSON, 1947) and 3-methylcholanthrene (ARGYRIS and LAYMAN, 1969). The rate at which liver enlargement recedes seems to be closely related to the rate of elimination of the inducer. Liver weights in rats and mice return to normal levels within a few days when inducers with relatively short biological half-lives, such as phenobarbital, are used (KUNZ et al., 1966a;

SCHLICHT et al., 1968; ARGYRIS and MAGNUS, 1968). The return to the normal state takes weeks when compounds with a longer biological half-life, such as DDT (FITZHUGH and NELSON, 1947), 3-methylcholanthrene, or TCDD (POLAND and GLOVER, 1973) are used. After termination of treatment with DDT (1000 ppm in the diet), the increase in liver mass and cell enlargement were still clearly seen at 2 weeks; they were less distinct at $4-6$ weeks, and after $8-10$ weeks had completely disappeared (FITZHUGH and NELSON, 1947). No gross alterations of cellular constituents have been noticed in the regression phase (SCHLICHT et al., 1968). The increased amount of endoplasmic reticulum membranes returns to normal after cessation of phenobarbital treatment, the excess membranes being removed within 5 days, as shown by quantitative electron microscopy (BOLENDER and WEIBEL, 1973). During the regression phase, an increase in volume (800%) and number (96%) of autophagic vacuoles occurred. Similarly, the increase in ploidy pattern after phenobarbital treatment is fully reversible (SCHAUDE, 1972).

II. Cytochrome b_5

Cytochrome b_5 is a constituent of endoplasmic reticulum membranes, as well as outer mitochondrial membranes (SOTTOCASA et al., 1967) and membranes of the Golgi complex of hepatocytes (FLEISCHER et al., 1971; FARQUHAR et al., 1974). Only the role of microsomal (i.e., endoplasmic reticulum) cytochrome b_5 will be discussed.

Microsomal cytochrome b_5 is one of the best characterized microsomal proteins with respect to its protein structure and its attachment to the membrane (SPATZ and STRITTMATTER, 1971; SATO et al., 1969). However, its function is still debated. Cytochrome b_5 is part of an NADH-dependent electron transport chain which provides electrons both for a steroyl-CoA desaturase system (HOLLOWAY et al., 1963; GELLHORN and BENJAMIN, 1964; OSHINO et al., 1966), and for cytochrome P-450-dependent monooxygenase reactions (Fig. 5). The involvement of

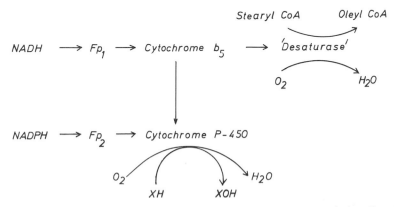

Fig. 5. Role of cytochrome b_5 in liver microsomal electron transport chains. Fp_1: Cytochrome b_5 reductase or NADH cytochrome-c reductase. Fp_2: Cytochrome P-450 reductase or NADPH cytochrome c-reductase. XH: lipophilic chemical. The terminal oxidase in the desaturase system (*"Desaturase"*), which has been called "cyanide sensitive factor" (OSHINO et al., 1966), has recently been characterized as a nonheme iron protein (STRITTMATTER et al., 1974)

cytochrome b_5 in drug metabolism has been demonstrated by several lines of evidence: NADH acts synergistically in drug metabolism, and during drug oxidation the steady state of reduction of cytochrome b_5 is lowered (HILDEBRANDT and ESTABROOK, 1971; CORREIA and MANNERING, 1973a, b). Furthermore, addition of antibodies to cytochrome b_5 blocks the flow of electrons to cytochrome P-450 (MANNERING et al., 1974). From these studies it has been concluded that the second electron required in the monooxygenase reaction (Figs. 2, 5) can be donated by NADH by cytochrome b_5. Another role of the NADH-dependent electron transport chain in drug metabolism has been postulated: certain compounds (e.g., perfluoro-n-hexane) will bind to cytochrome P-450 (and stimulate oxygen uptake) without the incorporation of the active oxygen into the xenobiotic. This phenomenon has been called "uncoupling" (WHITE-STEVENS and KAMIN, 1970; ULLRICH and DIEL, 1971; NARASIMHULU, 1971). The active oxygen may be reduced to water by the NADH cytochrome b_5 system instead of being liberated as hydrogen peroxide (STAUDT et al., 1974).

Evidence for differential turnovers of the heme and protein moieties of cytochrome b_5 has been obtained (Table 1) by simultaneous in vivo labeling of the heme moiety with ^{3}H-5-aminolevulinate and the protein moiety with guanidino-^{14}C-arginine (BOCK and SIEKEVITZ, 1970). This finding confirms earlier studies in which the heme and protein moiety had been separately labeled (KURIYAMA et al., 1969; GREIM et al., 1970). Hence, at least for this cytochrome, an exchange of the heme moiety in vivo is suggested. This notion has been confirmed in other studies (DRUYAN et al., 1973). There is also evidence for a cytochrome b_5 apoprotein pool in microsomes, equivalent to about 5% of the cytochrome present in the membrane (NEGISHI and OMURA, 1970; HARA and MINIKAMI, 1970). The amount of cytochrome b_5 increases after treatment with phenobarbital. This increase is slight in the rat, but marked in the rabbit (REMMER and MERKER, 1963). It has been demonstrated that in the rat the increase of cytochrome b_5 is due to decreased degradation (KURIYAMA et al., 1969).

E. Catalase

Catalase represents about 11 – 16% of total peroxisomal protein (LEIGHTON et al., 1969). Its biological half-life has been estimated to be about 2 days (POOLE et al., 1969). A detailed study of its synthesis has been reported by LAZAROW and DE DUVE (1973a, b). Their conclusions are schematically shown in Figure 6 in order to demonstrate how complicated the posttranslational pathway of hemoprotein synthesis can be. The apoprotein of catalase is synthesized by cytoplasmic polysomes and subsequently appears in the peroxisome, where heme is attached, probably to a monomeric intermediate, which then aggregates to form the active catalase. The biological half-lives of the apomonomer, monomer, and tetramer have been determined to be 49 min, 17 min, and 3100 min respectively. The apomonomer and monomer have been estimated to represent 1.6% and 0.5% of total catalase.

Electron microscopic studies revealed a marked proliferation of hepatic peroxisomes after treatment with the hypolipidemic drugs clofibrate (BEST and DUNCAN, 1964; AZARNOFF et al., 1965; HESS et al., 1965; PLATT and THORP, 1966; SALVADOR

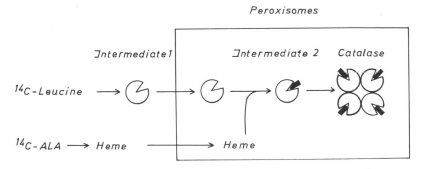

Fig. 6. Topology of catalase biosynthesis. ^{14}C-leucine and ^{14}C-5-aminolevulinic acid (ALA) have been used to label intermediates. Representation of intermediate 2 as a subunit is hypothetical (from LAZAROW and DE DUVE, 1973b)

et al., 1970; REDDY et al., 1970, 1973; BECKETT et al., 1973) and nafenopin (BECKETT et al., 1972; REDDY et al., 1973). This proliferation was associated with a 27% increase in catalase and a 58% decrease in peroxisomal urate oxidase (GEAR et al., 1974). However, the proliferation of peroxisomes cannot yet be linked to the hypocholesterolemic action of these drugs (HAVEL and KANE, 1973). There is an even more pronounced increase in mitochondrial constituents, as discussed in the following section. Recently a fatty acyl-CoA oxidizing system was described in rat liver peroxisomes which is enhanced by clofibrate (LAZAROW and DE DUVE, 1976). The existence of this system may provide a plausible explanation of the action of clofibrate on peroxisomes and on lipid metabolism. Furthermore, unlike phenobarbital which induces ligandin in liver cytosol, the hypolipidemic drugs clofibrate and nafenopin increase the Z-protein in liver cytosol which binds fatty acids and may play a role in their esterification and/or intracellular translocation (FLEISCHNER et al., 1975). The binding of hypolipidemic drugs to Z may interfere with these processes and thereby reduce plasma triglyceride concentrations.

F. Mitochondrial Cytochromes

The respiratory chain in inner mitochondrial membranes contains cytochromes b, cc_1, and as the terminal oxidase, cytochrome aa_3. Studies with yeasts have demonstrated that the complicated pathways of synthesis of these cytochromes involve both nuclear and mitochondrial gene products (SCHATZ and MASON, 1974). Cytochrome-c is unique in that the heme moiety is covalently attached to the apoprotein (FALK, 1964). The biological half-lives of these cytochromes are longer than those of the other hepatic hemoproteins (Fig. 1). Studies on the mode of action of the hypolipidemic drugs clofibrate and nafenopin revealed marked increases in number of mitochondria (and hence in the total amounts of mitochondrial cytochromes), together with increases of the levels of other mitochondrial enzymes such as glycerolphosphate dehydrogenase which is increased 6-fold (WESTERFELD et al., 1968; HESS et al., 1965; GEAR et al., 1974). The content of cytochromes aa_3, b, c_1, and c in mitochondria does not significantly change during the doubling of total mitochondria which occurs within 10—20 days of treatment of rats with clofibrate (GEAR et al., 1974). The above mitochondrial changes resemble those observed after thyroxine treatment (WESTERFELD et al., 1968; REITH et al., 1973; HAVEL and KANE, 1973), and part of the effects of clofibrate and nafenopin have been ascribed to an increase of free thyroxine, which is released by these hypolipidemic drugs from the plasma proteins (HAVEL and KANE, 1973). However, the concomitant proliferation of peroxisomes, seen after treatment with the hypolipidemic drugs, cannot be related to the action of thyroxine. The increase of mitochondrial cytochromes by hypolipidemic drugs, which accompanies the increase in total mitochondria, is probably not a primary reaction to these drugs, but more likely a consequence of secondary adaptations.

G. Summary of Conclusions

Liver hemoproteins function at key positions in many organelles of the hepatocyte. Only a few facets of their complicated biosynthetic pathways have been elucidated. Their induction in response to a variety of chemicals has been described.

The induction of tryptophan pyrrolase is discussed as an example of both hormonal and substrate or cofactor type induction. The marked induction of cytochrome(s) P-450 by a great variety of lipid-soluble chemicals is of considerable pharmacological interest because drug metabolism may decrease or increase both drug toxicity and activity. Phenobarbital and 3-methylcholanthrene, the first compounds which were shown to cause an induction of drug-metabolizing enzymes, have been classified as different types of inducing agents. They differentially stimulate the synthesis of various forms of cytochrome P-450. The induction of cytochrome(s) P-450 by inducing agents probably represents one of the key processes in a complex chain of adaptive events which finally lead to the proliferation of endoplasmic reticulum membranes and to liver growth. These complex processes are reversible.

In contrast to the induction of cytochrome(s) P-450, the induction of microsomal cytochrome b_5 by phenobarbital, and the increases of peroxisomal catalase and of mitochondrial cytochromes by the hypolipidemic drug clofibrate are not primary events, but are probably "secondary adaptations."

The induction of cytochrome(s) P-450, the primary concern of this review, still leaves us with more questions than answers. Cell culture systems and genetically nonresponsive mice may help to elucidate the interaction of a wide variety of chemicals with a hypothetical receptor which initiates the cascade of events leading to induction of drug-metabolizing enzymes, proliferation of membranes, and liver growth. Recent progress in the purification of cytochrome P-450 (purification being very often the rate limiting step in our knowledge of protein function) will help to resolve the problems of multiplicity and unspecificity of drug metabolizing enzymes. Comparative studies on the regulation of these enzyme systems in liver and extrahepatic tissues will clarify the role of these enzymes in pharmacokinetics and drug toxicity.

Recommended Reviews

Brodie, B.B., Gillette, J.R. (eds.): Concepts in Biochemical Pharmacology, Handbook of
  Experimental Pharmacology, Vol. 28, Part 2. Berlin – Heidelberg – New York: Springer
  1971
Conney, A.H.: Pharmacological implications of microsomal enzyme induction. Pharmacol.
  Rev. **19**, 317 – 366 (1967)
Conney, A.H., Burns, J.J.: Metabolic interactions among environmental chemicals and drugs.
  Science **178**, 576 – 586 (1972)
Gillette, J.R.: Biochemistry of drug oxydation and reduction by enzymes in hepatic endo-
  plasmic reticulum. Advanc. Pharmacol. **4**, 219 – 261 (1966)
Havel, R.J., Kane, J.P.: Drugs and lipid metabolism. Ann. Rev. Pharmacol. **13**, 287 – 308
  (1973)
Kuntzman, R.: Drug and enzyme induction. Ann. Rev. Pharmacol. **9**, 21 – 36 (1969)
Remmer, H.: Induction of drug metabolizing enzyme system in the liver. Europ. J. clin.
  Pharmacol. **5**, 116 – 136 (1972)
Schimke, R.T., Doyle, D.: Control of enzyme levels in animal tissues. Ann. Rev. Biochem.
  39, 929 – 976 (1970)
Schulte-Hermann, R.: Induction of liver growth by xenobiotic compounds and other stimuli.
  Critical Reviews in Toxicology **3**, 97 – 158 (1974)

References

Ackermann, E., Heinrich, I.: Die Aktivität der N- und O-Demethylase in der Leber des Menschen. Biochem. Pharmacol. **19**, 327 – 342 (1970)
Alexanderson, E., Price Evans, D.A., Sjöqvist, F.: Steady-state plasma levels of nortriptyline
  in twins: Influence of genetic factors and drug therapy. Brit. med. J. **1969 IV**, 764 – 768
Alvares, A.P., Anderson, K.E., Conney, A.H., Kappas, A.: Interactions between nutritional
  factors and drug biotransformations in man. Proc. nat. Acad. Sci. (Wash.) **73**, 2501 – 2504
  (1976)
Alvares, A.P., Schilling, G., Levin, W., Kuntzman, R.: Studies on the induction of CO-binding pigments in liver microsomes by phenobarbital and 3-methylcholanthrene. Biochem.
  biophys. Res. Commun. **29**, 521 – 526 (1967)
Alvares, A.P., Schilling, G., Levin, W., Kuntzman, R., Brand, L., Mark, L.C.: Cytochromes
  P-450 and b5 in human liver microsomes. Clin. Pharmacol. Ther. **10**, 655 – 659 (1969)
Alvares, A.P., Siekevitz, P.: Gel electrophoresis of partially purified cytochromes P-450 from
  liver microsomes of variously treated rats. Biochem. biophys. Res. Commun. **54**, 923 – 929
  (1973)
Argyris, T.S., Layman, D.L.: Liver growth associated with the induction of demethylase
  activity after injection of 3-methylcholanthrene in immature rats. Cancer Res. **29**, 549 – 553
  (1969)
Argyris, T.S., Magnus, D.: The stimulation of liver growth and demethylase activity following
  phenobarbital treatment. Develop. Biol. **17**, 187 – 201 (1968)
Arias, I.M., Doyle, D., Schimke, R.T.: Studies on the synthesis and degradation of proteins
  of the endoplasmic reticulum of rat liver. J. biol. Chem. **244**, 3303 – 3315 (1969)
Attardi, C., Parnas, H., Hwang, M.I.H., Attardi, B.: Giant-size rapidly labeled nuclear ribo-
  nucleic acid and cytoplasmic messenger ribonucleic acid in immature duck erythrocytes.
  J. molec. Biol. **20**, 145 – 182 (1966)
Azarnoff, D.L., Tucker, D.R., Barr, G.A.: Studies with ethylchlorophenoxyisobutyrate (clo-
  fibrate). Metabolism **14**, 959 – 965 (1965)
Badawy, A.A.B., Evans, M.: The effects of chemical porphyrogens and drugs on the activity
  of rat liver tryptophan pyrrolase. Biochem. J. **136**, 885 – 892 (1973)
Badawy, A.A.B., Evans, M.: Guinea pig liver tryptophan pyrrolase. Biochem. J. **138**, 445 – 451
  (1974)

Barka, T., Popper, H.: Liver enlargement and drug toxicity. Medicine (Baltimore) **46**, 103 – 108 (1967)

Beckett, R.B., Weiss, R., Stitzel, R.E., Cenedella, R.J.: Studies on the hepatomegaly caused by the hypolipidemic drugs nafenopin and clofibrate. Toxicol. appl. Pharmacol., **23**, 42 – 53 (1972)

Benson, A.M., Talalay, P., Keen, J.H., Jakoby, W.B.: Relationship between the soluble glutathione-dependent Δ^5-3-ketosteroid isomerase and the glutathione S-transferases of the liver. Proc. nat. Acad. Sci. (Wash.) **74**, 158 – 162 (1977)

Berlin, C.M., Schimke, R.T.: Influence of turnover rates on the responses of enzymes to cortisone. Molec. Pharmacol. **1**, 149 – 156 (1965)

Best, M.M., Duncan, C.H.: Hypolipemia and hepatomegaly from ethylchlorophenoxyiso-butyrate (CPIP) in the rat. J. Lab. clin. Med. **64**, 634 – 642 (1964)

Bock, K.W., Clausbruch, U.C.v., Josting, D., Ottenwälder, H.: Separation and partial purification of two differentially inducible UDP-glucuronyltransferases from rat liver. Biochem. Pharmacol. **26**, 1097 – 1100 (1977)

Bock, K.W., Fröhling, W., Remmer, H.: Influence of fasting and hemin on microsomal cytochromes and enzymes. Biochem. Pharmacol. **22**, 1557 – 1564 (1973a)

Bock, K.W., Fröhling, W., Remmer, H., Rexer, B.: Effects of phenobarbital and 3-methylcholanthrene on substrate specificity of rat liver microsomal UDP-glucuronyltransferase. Biochim. biophys. Acta (Amst.) **327**, 45 – 56 (1973b)

Bock, K.W., Krauss, E., Fröhling, W.: Regulation of δ-aminolevulinic acid synthetase by drugs and steroids in vivo and in isolated perfused rat liver. Europ. J. Biochem. **23**, 366 – 371 (1971)

Bock, K.W., Siekevitz, P.: Turnover of heme and protein moieties of rat liver microsomal cytochrome b_5. Biochem. biophys. Res. Commun. **41**, 374 – 380 (1970)

Bolender, R.P., Weibel, E.R.: A morphometric study of the removal of phenobarbital induced membranes from hepatocytes after cessation of treatment. J. Cell Biol. **56**, 746 – 761 (1973)

Boyd, G., Grimwade, A., Lawson, M.: Studies on rat liver microsomal 7α hydroxylase. Europ. J. Biochem. **37**, 334 – 340 (1973)

Brazda, F.G., Baucum, R.: The effect of nikethamide on the metabolism of pentobarbital by liver microsomes of the rat. J. Pharmacol. exp. Ther. **132**, 225 – 298 (1961)

Breyer, U.: Perazine, chlorpromazine, and imipramine as inducers of microsomal drug metabolism Naunyn-Schmiedeberg's Arch. Pharmacol. **272**, 277 – 288 (1972)

Bruckner, J.V., Khanna, K.L., Cornish, H.H.: Biological responses of the rat to polychlorinated biphenyls. Toxicol. appl. Pharmacol. **24**, 434 – 448 (1973)

Buu-Hoï, N.P., Hien, D., Saint-Ruf, G., Servoin-Sidoine, J.: Propriétés cancéromimétiques de la tétrachloro-2,3,7,8-dibenzo-p-dioxine. C. R. Acad. Sci. (Paris), Ser. D **272**, 1447 – 1450 (1971)

Chen, W., Vrindten, P.A., Dayton, P.G., Burns, J.J.: Accelerated aminopyrine metabolism in human subjects pretreated with phenylbutazone. Life Sci. **1**, 35 – 39 (1962)

Comai, J., Gaylor, J.L.: Existence and separation of three forms of cytochrome P-450 from rat liver microsomes. J. biol. Chem. **248**, 4947 – 4955 (1973)

Conney, A.H.: Pharmacological implications of microsomal enzyme induction. Pharmac. Rev. **19**, 317 – 366 (1967)

Conney, A.H., Davison, C., Gastel, R., Burns J.J.: Adaptive increases in drug metabolizing enzymes induced by phenobarbital and other drugs. J. Pharmacol. exp. Ther. **130**, 1 – 8 (1960)

Conney, A.H., Kapitulnik, J., Levin, W., Dansette, P., Jerina, D.: Use of drugs in the evaluation of carcinogen metabolism in man. In: Screening Tests in Chemical Carcinogenesis. Montesano, R., Bartsch, H., Tomatis, L. (eds.). International Agency for Research on Cancer (IARC), Scientific Publications No. 12, pp. 319 – 336 (1976)

Conney, A.H., Kuntzman, R.: Metabolism of normal body constituents by drug-metabolizing enzymes in liver microsomes. In: Handbook of Experimental Pharmacology. Brodie, B.B., Gillette, J.R. (eds.). Vol. 28, Part 2, pp. 401 – 421. Berlin – Heidelberg – New York: Springer 1971

Conney, A.H., Lu, A.Y.H., Levin, W., Smogys, A., West, S., Jacobson, M., Ryan, D., Kuntzman, R.: Effect of enzyme inducers on substrate specificity of the cytochrome P-450's. Drug Metab. Dispos. **1**, 199 – 209 (1973)

Conney, A.H., Michaelson, I.A., Burns, J.J.: Stimulatory effect of chlorcyclizine on barbiturate metabolism. J. Pharmacol. exp. Ther. **132,** 202–206 (1961)

Conney, A.H., Miller, E.C., Miller, J.A.: The metabolism of methylated aminoazo dyes. V. Evidence for induction of enzyme synthesis in the rat by 3-methylcholanthrene. Cancer Res. **16,** 450–456 (1956)

Conney, A.H., Miller, E.C., Miller, J.A.: Substrate-induced synthesis and other properties of benzpyrene hydroxylase in rat liver. J. biol. Chem. **228,** 753–766 (1957)

Correia, M.A., Mannering, G.J.: Reduced diphosphopyridine nucleotide synergism of the reduced triphosphopyridine nucleotide-dependent mixed-function oxidase system of hepatic microsomes. Effects of activation and inhibition of the fatty acyl coenzyme A desaturation system. Molec. Pharmacol. **9,** 455–469 (1973a)

Correia, M.A., Mannering, G.J.: Reduced diphosphopyridine nucleotide synergism of the reduced triphosphopyridine nucleotide-dependent mixed-function oxidase system of hepatic microsomes. Role of the type I drug-binding site of cytochrome P-450. Molec. Pharmacol. **9,** 470–485 (1973b)

Correia, M.A., Meyer, U.A.: Apocytochrome P-450: Reconstitution of functional cytochrome with hemin in vitro. Proc. nat. Acad. Sci. (Wash.) **72,** 400–404 (1975)

Cramer, J.W., Miller, J.A., Miller, E.C.: The hydroxylation of the carcinogen 2-acetylamino-fluorene by rat liver: Stimulation by pretreatment in vivo with 3-methylcholanthrene. J. biol. Chem. **235,** 250–256 (1960)

Cucinell, S.A., Conney, A.H., Sansur, M., Burns, J.J.: Drug interactions in man. Lowering effect of phenobarbital on plasma levels of bishydroxycoumarin (dicumarol) and diphenyl-hydantoin (dilantin). Clin. Pharmacol. Ther. **6,** 420–424 (1965)

Cucinell, S.A., Odessky, L., Weiss, M., Dayton, P.G.: The effect of chloralhydrate on bis-hydroxycoumarin metabolism. J. Amer. med. Ass. **197,** 366–368 (1966)

Dallner, G., Siekevitz, P., Palade, G.E.: Biogenesis of endoplasmic reticulum membranes. Synthesis of constitutive microsomal enzymes in developing rat hepatocytes. J. Cell Biol. **30,** 97–117 (1966)

Davies, D.S., Thorgeirsson, S.S.: Mechanism of hepatic drug oxidation and its relationship to individual differences in rates of oxidation in man. Ann. N.Y. Acad. Sci. **179,** 411–420 (1971)

Davison, S.C., Wills, E.D.: Studies on the lipid composition of the rat liver endoplasmic reti-culum after induction with phenobarbitone and 20-methylcholanthrene. Biochem. J. **140,** 461–468 (1974)

Dehlinger, P.J., Schimke, R.T.: Effects of phenobarbital, 3-methylcholanthrene and hematin on the synthesis of protein components of rat liver microsomal membranes. J. biol. Chem. **247,** 1257–1264 (1972)

De Matteis, F., Gibbs, A.: Stimulation of liver 5-aminolevulinate synthetase by drugs and its relevance to drug-induced accumulation of cytochrome P-450. Biochem. J. **126,** 1149–1160 (1972)

Douglas, J.F., Ludwig, B.J., Smith, N.: Studies on the metabolism of meprobamate. Proc. Soc. exp. Biol. (N.Y.) **112,** 436–439 (1963)

Druyan, B., De Bernard, B., Rabinowitz, M.: Turnover of cytochromes labeled with δ-amino-levulinic acid-^{3}H in rat liver. J. biol. Chem. **244,** 5874 (1969)

Druyan, R., Jakovcic, S., Rabinowitz, M.: Studies of cytochrome synthesis in rat liver. Bio-chem. J. **134,** 377–385 (1973)

Druyan, R., Kelly, A.: The effect of exogenous δ-aminolevulinate on rat liver heme and cyto-chromes. Biochem. J. **129,** 1095–1099 (1972)

Dutton, G.J., Burchell, B.: Newer aspects of glucuronidation. In: Progress in Drug Metabolism Bridges, J.W., Chasseaud, L.F. (eds.), Vol. 2, pp. 1–70. London: Wiley 1977

Epstein, W., Beckwith, J.R.: Regulation of gene expression. Ann. Rev. Biochem. **37,** 411–436 (1968)

Eriksson, L.C.: Studies on the biogenesis of endoplasmic reticulum in the liver cell. Acta path. microbiol. scand., Sect. B, Suppl. 239 (1973)

Ernster, L., Orrenius, S.: Substrate-induced synthesis of the hydroxylating enzyme system of liver microsomes. Fed. Proc. **24,** 1190–1199 (1965)

Estabrook, R.W.: Cytochrome P-450—Its function in the oxidative metabolism of drugs.

In: Handbook of Experimental Pharmacology. Brodie, B.B., Gillette, J.R. (eds.). Vol. 28, Part 2, pp. 264–284. Berlin–Heidelberg–New York: Springer 1971

Falk, J.E.: Porphyrins and Metalloporphyrins. Amsterdam–London–New York: Elsevier Publ. Comp. 1964

Farquhar, M.G., Bergeron, J.J.M., Palade, G.E.: Cytochemistry of Golgi fractions prepared from rat liver. J. Cell Biol. **60**, 8–25 (1974)

Feigelson, P., Greengard, O.: Immunochemical evidence for increased titers of liver tryptophan pyrrolase during substrate and hormonal enzyme induction. J. biol. Chem. **237**, 3714–3717 (1962)

Fitzhugh, O.G., Nelson, A.A.: The chronic oral toxicity of DDT. J. Pharmacol. exp. Ther. **89**, 18–30 (1947)

Fleischer, S., Fleischer, B., Azzi, A., Chance, B.: Cytochrome b₅ and P 450 in liver cell fractions. Biochim. biophys. Acta (Amst.) **225**, 194–200 (1971)

Fleischner, G., Meijer, D.K.F., Levine, W.G., Gatmaitan, Z., Gluck, R., Arias, I.M.: Effect of hypolipidemic drugs, nafenopin and clofibrate, on the concentration of ligandin and Z protein in rat liver. Biochem. biophys. Res. Commun. **67**, 1401–1407 (1975)

Frommer, U., Ullrich, V., Staudinger, H., Orrenius, S.: The monooxygenation of n-heptane by rat liver microsomes. Biochim. biophys. Acta (Amst.) **280**, 487–494 (1972)

Gear, A.R.L., Albert, A.D., Bednarek, J.M.: The effect of the hypocholesterolemic drug clofibrate on liver mitochondrial biogenesis. J. biol. Chem. **249**, 6495–6504 (1974)

Gelboin, H.V.: Mechanisms of induction of drug metabolism enzymes. In: Handbook of Experimental Pharmacology. Brodie, B.B., Gillette, J.R. (eds.). Vol. 28, Part 2, pp. 431–451. Berlin–Heidelberg–New York: Springer 1971

Gelboin, H.V., Blackburn, N.R.: The stimulatory effect of 3-methylcholanthrene on benzpyrene hydroxylase activity in several rat tissues. Inhibition by actinomycin D and puromycin. Cancer Res. **24**, 356–360 (1964)

Gelboin, H.V., Okuda, T., Selkirk, J., Nemoto, N., Yang, S.K., Wiebel, F.J., Whitlock, Jr., J.P., Rapp, H.J., Bast, Jr., R.C.: Benzo(a)-pyrene metabolism; Enzymatic and liquid chromatographic analysis and application to human liver, lymphocytes and monocytes. In: Screening Tests in Chemical Carcinogenesis. Montesano, R., Bartsch, H., Tomatis, L. (eds.). International Agency for Research on Cancer (IARC), Scientific Publications No. 12, pp. 225–247 (1976)

Gellhorn, A., Benjamin, W.: The intracellular localization of an enzymatic defect of lipid metabolism in diabetic rats. Biochim. biophys. Acta (Amst.) **84**, 167–175 (1964)

Ghazal, A., Koransky, W., Portig, J., Vohland, H.W., Klempau, I.: Beschleunigung von Entgiftungsreaktionen durch verschiedene Insektizide. Naunyn-Schmiedebergs Arch. exp. Path. Pharmak. **249**, 1–10 (1964)

Gielen, J.E., Goujon, F.M., Nebert, D.W.: Genetic regulation of aryl hydrocarbon hydroxylase induction. II. Simple mendelian expression in mouse tissues in vivo. J. biol. Chem. **247**, 1125–1137 (1972)

Gillette, J.R., Mitchell, J.R., Brodie, B.B.: Biochemical mechanisms of drug toxicity. Ann. Rev. Pharmacol. **14**, 271–288 (1974)

Gillette, J.R., Stripp, B.: Pre-and postnatal enzyme capacity for drug metabolite production. Fed. Proc. **34**, 172–178 (1975)

Goldstein, A., Aronow, L., Kalman, S.M.: Zero order absorption, first order elimination: The plateau principle. In: Principles of Drug Action, pp. 292–317. New York: Harper and Row 1969

Granick, S.: The induction in vitro of the synthesis of δ-aminolevulinic acid synthetase in chemical porphyria: A response to certain drugs, sex hormones, and foreign chemicals. J. biol. Chem. **241**, 1359–1375 (1966)

Greig, J.B., De Matteis, F.: Effects of 2,3,7,8-tetrachloro-dibenzo-p-dioxin on drug metabolism and hepatic microsomes of rats and mice. Environ. Health Perspec., Exp. Issue **5**, 211–219 (1973)

Greim, H.: Synthesesteigerung und Abbauhemmung bei der Vermehrung mikrosomaler Cytochrome P-450 und b-5 durch Phenobarbital. Naunyn-Schmiedeberg's Arch. Pharmakol. **266**, 261–275 (1970)

Greim, H., Schenkman, J.B., Klotzbücher, M., Remmer, H.: The influence of phenobarbital on the turnover of hepatic microsomal cytochrome b-5 and cytochrome P-450 hemes in the rat. Biochim. biophys. Acta (Amst.) **201**, 20−25 (1970)

Habig, W.H., Papst, M.J., Fleischner, G., Gatmaitan, Z., Arias, I.M., Jacoby, W.B.: The identity of glutathione S-transferase B with ligandin, a major binding protein of liver. Proc. Nat. Acad. Sci. (Wash.) **71**, 3879−3882 (1974)

Hara, T., Minakami, S.: Presence of apo-cytochrome b_5 in microsomes. Incorporation of radioactive heme to the cytochrome in vitro. J. Biochem. (Tokyo) **67**, 741−743 (1970)

Harris, H.: Nucleus and Cytoplasm. London: Oxford Univ. Press 1968

Hart, L.G., Fouts, J.R.: Effects of acute and chronic DDT administration on hepatic microsomal drug metabolism in the rat. Proc. Soc. exp. Biol. (N.Y.) **114**, 388−396 (1963)

Hart, L.G., Shultice, R.W., Fouts, J.R.: Stimulatory effects of chlordane on hepatic microsomal drug metabolism in the rat. Toxicol. appl. Pharmacol. **5**, 371−386 (1963)

Hashimoto, C., Imai, Y.: Purification of a substrate complex of cytochrome P-450 from liver microsomes of 3-methylcholanthrene-treated rabbits. Biochem. biophys. Res. Commun. **68**, 821−827 (1976)

Haugen, D.A., Coon, M.J.: Properties of electrophoretically homogeneous phenobarbital-inducible and β-naphthoflavone-inducible forms of liver microsomal cytochrome P-450. J. biol. Chem. **251**, 7929−7939 (1976)

Haugen, D.A., Coon, M.J., Nebert, D.W.: Induction of multiple forms of mouse liver cytochrome P-450. J. biol. Chem. **251**, 1817−1827 (1976)

Havel, R.J., Kane, J.P.: Drugs and lipid metabolism. Ann. Rev. Pharmacol. **13**, 287−308 (1973)

Hayaishi, O.: Oxygenases. New York: Academic Press 1962

Hess, R., Stäubli, W., Riess, W.: Nature of the hepatomegalic effect produced by ethylchlorophenoxyisobutyrate in the rat. Nature (Lond.) **208**, 856−858 (1965)

Hildebrandt, A., Estabrook, R.W.: Evidence for the participation of cytochrome b_5 in hepatic microsomal mixed-function oxidation reactions. Arch. Biochem. biophys. **143**, 66−79 (1971)

Hildebrandt, A., Remmer, H., Estabrook, R.W.: Cytochrome P-450 of liver microsomes, one pigment or many. Biochem. biophys. Res. Commun. **30**, 607−612 (1968)

Holder, G., Yagi, H., Dansette, P., Jerina, D.M., Levin, W., Lu, A.Y.H., Conney, A.H.: Effects of inducers and epoxide hydrase on the metabolism of benzo(a) pyrene by liver microsomes and a reconstituted system: Analysis by high pressure liquid chromatography. Proc. nat. Acad. Sci. (Wash.) **71**, 4356−4360 (1974)

Holloway, P.W., Peluffo, P., Wakil, S.J.: On the biosynthesis of dienoic fatty acid by animal tissues. Biochem. biophys. Res. Commun. **12**, 300−304 (1963)

Hoogland, D.R., Miya, T.S., Bousquer, W.F.: Metabolism and tolerance studies with chlordiazepoxide-2-^{14}C in the rat. Toxicol. appl. Pharmacol. **9**, 116−123 (1966)

Hornef, W.: Quantitative changes of the activity of lysosomal enzymes in the induced rat liver. Naunyn-Schmiedeberg's Arch. Pharmak. **266**, 361−362 (1970)

Huang, M.-T., West, S.B., Lu, A.Y.H.: Separation, purification and properties of multiple forms of cytochrome P-450 from the liver microsomes of phenobarbital-treated mice. J. biol. Chem. **251**, 4659−4665 (1976)

Imai, J., Sato, R.: A gel-electrophoretically homogeneous preparation of cytochrome P-450 from liver microsomes of phenobarbital-pretreated rabbits. Biochem. biophys. Res. Commun. **60**, 8−14 (1974)

Inscoe, J.K., Axelrod, J.: Some factors affecting glucuronide formation in vitro: J. Pharm. exp. Ther. **129**, 128−131 (1960)

Jacob, F., Monod, J.: Genetic regulatory mechanisms in the synthesis of proteins. J. molec. Biol. **3**, 318−356 (1961)

Jacob, S.T., Scharf, M.B., Vessel, E.S.: Role of RNA in induction of hepatic microsomal mixed function oxidases. Proc. nat. Acad. Sci. (Wash.) **71**, 704−707 (1974)

Jacobson, M.M., Levin, W., Conney, A.H.: Studies on bilirubin and steroid glucuronidation by rat liver microsomes. Biochem. Pharmacol. **24**, 655−662 (1975)

Jick, H., Shuster, L.: The turnover of microsomal reduced nicotinamide adenine nucleotide phosphate-cytochrome c reductase in the livers of mice treated with phenobarbital. J. biol. Chem. **241**, 5366−5369 (1966)

Johnson, E.F., Muller-Eberhard, U.: Resolution of two forms of cytochrome P-450 from liver microsomes of rabbits treated with 2,3,7,8-tetrachlorodibenzo-p-dioxin. J. biol. Chem. **252,** 2839 – 2845 (1977)

Kafatos, F.C., Reich, J.: Stability of differentiation—specific and nonspecific messenger RNA in insect cells. Proc. nat. Acad Sci. (Wash.) **60,** 1458 – 1465 (1968)

Kato, R., Chiesara, E., Vasanelli, P.. Increased activity of microsomal strychnine metabolizing enzyme induced by phenobarbital and other drugs. Biochem. Pharmacol. **11,** 913 – 922 (1962)

Kato, R., Gillette, J.R.: Effect of starvation on NADPH-dependent enzymes in liver microsomes of male und female rats. J. Pharmacol. exp. Ther. **150,** 279 – 284 (1965)

Kato, R., Takahashi, A.: Thyroid hormone and activities of drug-metabolizing enzymes and electron transport systems of rat liver microsomes. Molec. Pharmacol. **4,** 109 – 120 (1968)

Kato, R., Vasanelli, P.: Induction of increased meprobamate metabolism in rats pretreated with some neurotropic drugs. Biochem. Pharmacol. **11,** 779 – 794 (1962)

Kellermann, G., Cantrell, E., Shaw, C.R.: Variations in extent of aryl hydrocarbon hydroxylase induction in cultured human lymphocytes. Cancer Res. **33,** 1654 – 1656 (1973 a)

Kellermann, G., Shaw, C.R., Luyten-Kellermann, M.: Aryl hydrocarbon hydroxylase inducibility and bronchogenic carcinoma. New Engl. J. Med. 934 – 937 (1973 b)

Knox, W.E.: Two mechanisms which increase in vivo the liver tryptophan peroxidase activity: Specific enzyme adaptation and stimulation of the pituitary-adrenal system. Brit. J. exp. Path. **32,** 462 – 469 (1951)

Knox, W.E., Piras, M.M.: Tryptophan pyrrolase of liver. Conjugation in vivo during cofactor induction by tryptophan analogues. J. biol. Chem. **242,** 2959 – 2965 (1967)

Koransky, W., Magour, S., Merker, H.J., Schlicht, I., Schulte-Hermann, R.: Influence of inducing substances on growth of liver and microsomal electron transport systems. Proceedings Third International Pharmacological Meeting, Vol. 4, p. 55. New York: Pergamon Press 1966

Koransky, W., Portig, J., Vohland, H.W., Klempau, I.: Aktivierung von Mikrosomenenzymen durch Hexachlorcyclohexan-Isomere. Naunyn-Schmiedebergs Arch. exp. Path. Pharmakol. **247,** 61 – 67 (1964)

Kumaki, K., Jensen, N.M., Shire, J.G.M., Nebert, D.W.: Genetic difference in induction of cytosol reduced-NAD(P): menadione oxidoreductase and microsomal aryl hydrocarbon hydroxylase in the mouse. J. biol. Chem. **252,** 157 – 165 (1977)

Kuntzman, R., Mark, L.C., Brand, L., Jacobson, M., Levin, W., Conney, A.H.: Metabolism of drugs and carcinogens by human liver enzymes. J. Pharmacol. exp. Ther. **152,** 151 – 156 (1966)

Kunz, W., Schaude, G., Schimasseck, H., Schmid, W., Siess, M.: Stimulation of liver growth by drugs, II. Biochemical analysis. Proceedings European Society for the Study of Drug Toxicity, Excerpta Medica Foundation, Amsterdam., 7, 138 – 153 (1966 a)

Kunz, W., Schaude, G., Schmid, W., Siess, M.: Stimulation of liver growth by drugs, I. Morphological analysis. Proceedings European Society for the Study of Drug Toxicity, Excerpta Medica Foundation, Amsterdam, **7,** 113 – 137 (1966 b)

Kuriyama, Y., Omura, T., Siekevitz, P., Palade, G.E.: Effects of phenobarbital on the synthesis and degradation of the protein components of rat liver microsomal membranes. J. biol. Chem. **244,** 2017 – 2026 (1969)

Kutt, H.W., McDowell, F.: Management of epilepsy with diphenylhydantoin sodium. J. Amer. med. Ass. **203,** 969 – 974 (1968)

Lazarow, P.B., De Duve, C.: The synthesis and turnover of rat liver peroxisomes. Biochemical pathway of catalase synthesis. J. Cell Biol. **59,** 491 – 506 (1973 a)

Lazarow, P.B., De Duve, C.: The synthesis and turnover of rat liver peroxisomes. Intracellular pathway of catalase synthesis. J. Cell Biol. **59,** 507 – 524 (1973 b)

Lazarow, P.B., De Duve, C.: A fatty aryl-CoA oxidizing system in rat liver peroxisomes; enhancement by clofibrate, a hypolipidemic drug. Proc. nat. Acad. Sci. (Wash.) **73,** 2043 – 2046 (1976)

Leighton, F., Poole, B., Lazarow, P.B., De Duve, C.: The synthesis and turnover of rat liver peroxisomes. Fractionation of peroxisome proteins. J. Cell Biol. **41,** 521 – 535 (1969)

Levin, W., Kuntzman, R.: Biphasic decrease of radioactive hemoprotein from liver microsomal carbon monoxide-binding particles. Effect of phenobarbital and chlordane. Molec. Pharmacol. **5,** 499 – 506 (1969)

Lu, A.Y.H., Kuntzman, R., West, S., Jacobson, M., Conney, A.H.: Reconstituted liver micro-somal enzyme system that hydroxylates drugs, other foreign compounds, and endogenous substrates. Role of the cytochrome P-450 and P-448 fractions in drug and steroid hydroxy-lations. J. biol. Chem. **247**, 1727–1734 (1972)

Lu, A.Y.H., Levin, W., West, S.B., Jacobson, M., Ryan, D., Kuntzman, R., Conney, A.H.: Reconstituted liver microsomal enzyme system that hydroxylates drugs, other foreign compounds, and endogenous substrates. Different substrate specificities of the cytochrome P-450 fractions from control and phenobarbital-treated rats. J. biol. Chem. **248**, 456–460 (1973)

MacDonald, M.G., Robinson, D.S., Jaffe, J.S., Sylvester, D.: The effects of phenobarbital, glutethimide, and chloral betaine on plasma half-life and anticoagulant action of warfarin in man. Pharmacologist **9**, 191–196 (1967)

Mannering, G.J., Kuwahara, S., Omura, T.: Immunochemical evidence for the participation of cytochrome b_5 in the NADH synergism of the NADPH-dependent mono-oxidase system of hepatic microsomes. Biochem. biophys. Res. Commun. **57**, 476–481 (1974)

Marshall, J.W., McLean, A.E.M.: The effect of oral phenobarbitone on hepatic microsomal cytochrome P-450 and demethylation activity in rats fed normal and low protein diets. Biochem. Pharmacol. **18**, 153–157 (1962)

Marver, H.S.: The role of heme in the synthesis and repression of microsomal protein. In: Microsomes and Drug Oxidations. Gillette, J.R., Conney, A.H., Cosmides, C.J., Estabrook, R.W., Fouts, J.R., Mannering, G.J. (eds.), pp. 495–511. New York: Academic Press 1969

Marver, H.S., Schmid, R.: The prophyrias. In: Metabolic Basis of Inherited Desease. Stanbury, J.B., Wyngaarden, J.B., Fredrickson, D.S. (eds.), pp. 1087–1140. New York: McGraw-Hill Book Co. 1972

Marver, H.S., Tschudy, D.P., Perlroth, M.G.: Coordinate synthesis of heme and apoenzyme in the formation of tryptophan pyrrolase. Science **154**, 501–502 (1966)

Mason, H.S., North, J.C., Vanneste, M.: Microsomal mixed function oxidations. The meta-bolism of xenobiotics. Symposium of electron transport systems in microsomes. Fed. Proc. **24**, 1172–1180 (1965)

Matern, S., Fröhling, W., Bock, K.W.: Albumin synthesis in isolated perfused livers from phenobarbital pretreated rats. Naunyn-Schmiedeberg's Arch. Pharmacol. **273**, 242–247 (1972)

Michot, F., Bürgi, M., Büttner, J.: Rimactan (Rifampicin) und Anticoagulantientherapie. Schweiz. med. Wschr. **100**, 583–584 (1970)

Mitropoulos, K.A., Suzuki, M., Myant, N.B., Danielsson, H.: Effects of thyroidectomy and thyroxine treatment on the activity of 12α-hydroxylase and of some components of micro-somal electron transfer chains in rat liver. FEBS Ltrs. **1**, 13–15 (1968)

Moldeus, P.W., Young-Nam, C., Cinti, D.L., Schenkman, J.B.: Hepatic organelle interaction. Mitochondrial modification of microsomal drug metabolism. J. biol. Chem. **248**, 8574–8584 (1973)

Mulder, G.J.: The effect of phenobarbital on the submicrosomal distribution of uridine diphosphate glucuronyltransferase from rat liver. Biochem. J. **117**, 319–324 (1970)

Narasimhulu, S.: Uncoupling of oxygen activation from hydroxylation in the steroid C-21 hydroxylase of bovine adrenocortical microsomes. Arch. Biochem. Biophys. **147**, 384–390 (1971)

Nebert, D.W., Benedict, W.F., Gielen, J.E., Oesch, F., Daly, J.W.: Aryl hydrocarbon hydroxy-lase, epoxide hydrase, and 7,12-dimethylbenz(a)anthracene-produced skin tumorigenesis in the mouse. Molec. Pharmacol. **8**, 374–379 (1972)

Nebert, D.W., Gelboin, H.V.: Substrate-inducible microsomal aryl hydroxylase in mammalian cell culture. Assay and properties of induced enzyme. J. biol. Chem. **243**, 6242–6249 (1968)

Nebert, D.W., Gielen, J.E.: Aryl hydrocarbon hydroxylase induction in mammalian liver cell culture. J. biol. Chem. **246**, 5199–5206 (1971)

Nebert, D.W., Kon, H.: Genetic regulation of aryl hydrocarbon hydroxylase induction. Specific changes in spin state of cytochrome P-450 from genetically responsive animals. J. biol. Chem. **248**, 169–178 (1973)

Negishi, M., Omura, T.: Presence of apo-cytochrome b_5 in microsomes from rat liver. J. Biochem. **67**, 745 – 747 (1970)

Nelson, E.B., Raj, P.P., Belfi, K.J., Masters, B.S.S.: Oxidative drug metabolism in human liver microsomes. J. Pharmacol. exp. Ther. **178**, 580 – 588 (1971)

Nemoto, N., Gelboin, H.V.: Enzymatic conjugation of benzo(a)pyrene oxides, phenols and dihydrodiols with UDP-glucuronic acid. Biochem. Pharmacol. **25**, 1221 – 1226 (1976)

Norred, W.P., Wade, A.E.: Dietary fatty acid-induced alterations of hepatic microsomal drug-metabolizing enzymes. Biochem. Pharmacol. **21**, 2887 – 2897 (1972)

Oesch, F.: Mammalian epoxide hydrases: Inducible enzymes catalysing the inactivation of carcinogenic and cytotoxic metabolites derived from aromatic and olefinic compounds. Xenobiotica **3**, 305 – 340 (1973)

Oesch, F., Daly, J.: Conversion of naphthaline to trans naphthaline dihydrodiol: Evidence for the presence of a coupled aryl monooxygenase-epoxide hydrase system in hepatic microsomes. Biochem. biophys. Res. Commun. **46**, 1713 – 1720 (1972)

Oesch, F., Jerina, D.M., Daly, J.: A radiometric assay for hepatic epoxide hydrase activity with (7-^{3}H) styrene oxide. Biochim. biophys. Acta (Amst.) **227**, 685 – 697 (1971)

Oesch, F., Morris, N., Daly, J.W., Gielen, J.E., Nebert, D.W.: Genetic expression of the induction of epoxide hydrase and aryl hydrocarbon hydroxylase activities in the mouse by phenobarbital or 3-methylcholanthrene. Molec. Pharmacol. **9**, 692 – 696 (1973)

Omura, T., Sato, R.: The carbon monoxide-binding pigment of liver microsomes. J. biol. Chem. **239**, 2370 – 2385 (1964)

Omura, T., Sato, R., Cooper, D.Y., Rosenthal, O., Estabrook, R.W.: Function of cytochrome P-450 in microsomes. Fed. Proc. **24**, 1181 – 1189 (1965)

Omura, T., Siekevitz, P., Palade, G.E.: Turnover of constituents of the endoplasmic reticulum membranes of rat hepatocytes. J. biol. Chem. **242**, 2389 – 2396 (1967)

Oshino, N., Imai, Y., Sato, R.: Electron-transfer mechanism associated with fatty acid desaturation catalyzed by liver microsomes. Biochim. biophys. Acta (Amst.) **128**, 13 – 28 (1966)

Owen, N.V., Griffing, W.J., Hoffman, D.G., Gibson, W.R., Anderson, R.C.: Effects of dietary administration of 5-(3,4-dichlorophenyl)-5-ethylbarbituric acid (dichlorophenobarbital) to rats. Emphasis on hepatic drug-metabolizing enzymes and morphology. Toxicol. appl. Pharmacol. **18**, 720 – 733 (1971)

Owens, I.S.: Genetic regulation of UDP-glucuronyltransferase. Induction by polycyclic aromatic compounds in mice. J. biol. Chem. **252**, 2827 – 2833 (1977)

Parke, D.V., Rahman, H.: The induction of hepatic microsomal enzymes by safrole. Biochem. J. **119**, 53P – 54P (1970)

Pelkonen, O., Kaltiala, E.H., Larmi, T.K.I., Kärki, N.T.: Cytochrome P-450-linked monooxygenase system and drug-induced spectral interactions in human liver microsomes. Chem. biol. Interact. **9**, 205 – 216 (1974)

Phillips, B.M., Miya, T.A., Yim, G.K.W.: Studies on the mechanism of meprobamate tolerance in the rat. J. Pharmacol. exp. Ther. **135**, 223 – 229 (1962)

Platt, D.S., Cockrill, B.L.: Biochemical changes in rat liver in response to treatment with drugs and other agents. II. Effects of halothane, DDT, and other chlorinated hydrocarbons, thioacetamide, dimethylnitrosamine and ethionine. Biochem. Pharmacol. **18**, 445 – 457 (1969)

Platt, D.S., Thorp, J.M.: Changes in the weight and composition of the liver in the rat, dog, and monkey, treated with ethylchlorophenoxyisobutyrate. Biochem. Pharmacol. **15**, 915 – 925 (1966)

Poland, A., Glover, E.: Chlorinated dibenzo-p-dioxins: Potent inducers of δ-aminolevulinic acid synthetase and aryl hydrocarbon hydroxylase. A study of the structure-activity relationship. Molec. Pharmacol. **9**, 736 – 747 (1973)

Poland, A.P., Glover, E.: Comparison of 2,3,7,8-tetrachlorodibenzo-p-dioxin, a potent inducer of aryl hydrocarbon hydroxylase, with 3-methylcholanthrene. Molec. Pharmacol. **10**, 349 – 359 (1974)

Poland, A., Glover, E., Kende, A.S.: Stereospecific, high affinity binding of 2,3,7,8-tetrachlorodibenzo-p-dioxin by hepatic cytosol. J. biol. Chem. **251**, 4936 – 4946 (1976)

Poland, A.P., Glover, E., Robinson, J.R., Nebert, D.E.: Genetic expression of aryl hydro-carbon hydroxylase activity. Induction of monooxygenase activities and cytochrome P_1-450 formation by 2,3,7,8-tetrachlorodibenzo-p-dioxin in mice genetically "nonresponsive" to other aromatic hydrocarbons. J. biol. Chem. **249**, 5599 — 5606 (1974)

Poole, B., Leighton, F., De Duve, C.: The synthesis and turnover of rat liver peroxisomes. Turnover of peroxisome proteins. J. Cell Biol. **41**, 536 — 546 (1969)

Price, V.E., Sterlin, W.R., Tarantola, V.A., Hartley, R.W., Jr., Rechcigl, M., Jr.: The kinetics of catalase synthesis and destruction in vivo. J. biol. Chem. **237**, 3468 — 3475 (1962)

Quinn, G.P., Axelrod, J., Brodie, B.B.: Species, strain, and sex differences in metabolism of hexobarbitone, amidopyrine, antipyrine and aniline. Biochem. Pharmacol. **1**, 152 — 159 (1958)

Reddy, J., Chiga, M., Bunyaratvej, S., Svoboda, D.: Microbodies in experimentally altered cells. VII. CPJB-induced hepatic microbody proliferation in the absence of significant catalase synthesis. J. Cell Biol. **44**, 226 — 234 (1970)

Reddy, J., Svoboda, D., Azarnoff, D.: Microbody proliferation in liver induced by nafenopin, a new hypolipidemic drug: Comparison with CPIB. Biochem. biophys. Res. Commun. **52**, 537 — 543 (1973)

Reith, A., Brdiczka, D., Nolte, J., Staudte, H.W.: The inner membrane of mitochondria under influence of triiodothyronine and riboflavin deficiency in rat heart muscle and liver. Exp. Cell Res. **77**, 1 — 14 (1973)

Remmer, H.: Der beschleunigte Abbau von Pharmaka in den Lebermikrosomen unter dem Einfluß von Luminal. Naunyn-Schmiedeberg's Arch. exp. Path. Pharmakol. **235**, 279 — 290 (1959)

Remmer, H.: Drug Tolerance. CIBA Foundation Symp. on Enzymes and Drug Action, p. 276. London: 1962

Remmer, H.: The role of the liver in drug metabolism. Amer. J. Med. **49**, 617 — 629 (1970)

Remmer, H.: Induction of drug metabolizing enzyme system in the liver. Europ. J. clin. Pharmacol. **5**, 116 — 136 (1972a)

Remmer, H.: The induction of the enzymic "detoxication" system in liver cells. Rev. Canad. Biol. **31**, 193 — 222 (1972b)

Remmer, H., Hirschmann, J., Greiner, I.: Die Bedeutung von Kumulation und Elimination für die Dosierung von Phenytoin (Diphenylhydantoin) Dtsch. med. Wschr. **94**, 1265 — 1272 (1969)

Remmer, H., Merker, H.-J.: Drug-induced changes in the liver endoplasmic reticulum: Associa-tion with drug-metabolizing enzymes. Science **142**, 1657 — 1658 (1963)

Remmer, H., Schenkman, J., Estabrook, R.W., Sasame, H., Gillette, J., Narasimhulu, S., Cooper, D.Y., Rosenthal, O.: Drug interactions with hepatic microsomal cytochrome. Molec. Pharmacol. **2**, 187 — 190 (1966)

Remmer, H., Schoene, B., Fleischmann, R.A.: Induction of the unspecific microsomal hydroxy-lase in the human liver. Drug Metabolism and Disposition **1**, 224 — 230 (1973)

Remmer, H., Siegert, M., Merker, H.-J.: Vermehrung arzneimittelabbauender Enzyme durch Tolbutamid. Naunyn-Schmiedeberg's Arch. exp. Path. Pharmakol. **249**, 71 — 84 (1964)

Revel, M., Hiatt, H.H.: The stability of liver messenger RNA. Proc. nat. Acad. Sci. (Wash.) **51**, 810 — 818 (1964)

Rogers, M.J., Strittmatter, P.: The binding of reduced nicotinamide adenine dinucleotide-cytochrome b_5 reductase to hepatic microsomes. J. biol. Chem. **249**, 5565 — 5569 (1974)

Salvador, R.A., Haber, S., Atkins, C., Gommi, B.W., Welch, R.M.: Effect of clofibrate and 1-methyl-1-piperidyl-bis-(p-chlorophenoxy) acetate (Sandoz 42-343) on steroid and drug metabolism by rat liver microsomes. Life Sci. **9**, 397 — 400 (1970)

Sato, R., Nishibayashi, H., Ito, A.: Characterization of two hemoproteins of liver microsomes. In: Microsomes and Drug Oxidations. Gillette, J.R., Conney, A.H., Cosmides, C.J., Estabrook, R.W., Fouts, J.R., Mannering, G.J. (eds.), pp. 111 — 128. New York: Academic Press 1969

Schatz, G., Mason, T.L.: The biosynthesis of mitochondrial proteins. Ann. Rev. Biochem. **43**, 51 — 87 (1974)

Schaude, G.: Cytologische Differenzierung des normalen und des fremdstoffinduzierten Leber-wachstums bei der weißen Maus. Habilitationsschrift, Marburg, 1972

Schenkman, J.B., Cinti, D.L., Orrenius, S., Moldeus, P., Kraschnitz, R.: The nature of the reversed type I (modified type II) spectral change in liver microsomes. Biochemistry 11, 4243−4251 (1972)

Schenkman, J.B., Frey, I., Remmer, H., Estabrook, R.W.: Sex differences in drug metabolism by rat liver microsomes. Molec. Pharmacol. 3, 516−525 (1967)

Schimke, R.T., Doyle, D.: Control of enzyme levels in animal tissues. Ann. Rev. Biochem. 39, 929−976 (1970)

Schimke, R.T., Sweeney, F.W., Berlin, C.M.: The roles of synthesis and degradation in the control of rat liver tryptophan pyrrolase. J. biol. Chem. 240, 322−331 (1965)

Schlicht, I., Koransky, W., Magour, S., Schulte-Hermann, R.: Größe und DNS-Synthese der Leber unter dem Einfluß körperfremder Stoffe. Naunyn-Schmiedeberg's Arch. exp. Path. Pharmakol. 261, 26−41 (1968)

Schmid, K., Cornu, F., Imhof, P., Keberle, H.: Die biochemische Deutung der Gewöhnung an Schlafmittel. Schweiz. med. Wschr. 94, 235−240 (1964)

Schoene, B., Fleischmann, R.A., Remmer, H., v. Oldershausen, H.F.: Determination of drug metabolizing enzymes in needle biopsies of human liver. Europ. J. clin. Pharmacol. 4, 65−73 (1972)

Schoenheimer, R.: Dynamic State of Body Constituents. Cambridge: Harvard Univ. Press 1942

Scholz, R., Hansen, W., Thurman, R.G.: Interaction of mixed-function oxidation with biosynthetic processes. Inhibition of gluconeogenesis by aminopyrine in perfused rat liver. Europ. J. Biochem. 38, 64−72 (1973)

Schulte-Hermann, R.: Induction of liver growth by xenobiotic compounds and other stimuli. Critical Reviews in Toxicology 3, 97−158 (1974)

Schulte-Hermann, R., Thom, R., Schlicht, I., Koransky, W.: Zahl und Ploidiegrad der Zellkerne der Leber unter dem Einfluß körperfremder Stoffe. Naunyn-Schmiedebergs Arch. exp. Path. Pharmakol. 261, 42−58 (1968)

Selkirk, J.K., Croy, R.G., Roller, P.P., Gelboin, H.V.: High-pressure liquid chromatographic analysis of benzo(a)pyrene metabolism and covalent binding and the mechanism of action of 7,8-benzoflavone and 1,2-epoxy-3,3,3-trichloropropane. Cancer Res. 34, 3474−3480 (1974)

Sies, H., Brauser, B.: Interaction of mixed function oxidase with its substrates and associated redox transitions of cytochrome P-450 and pyridine nucleotides in perfused rat liver. Europ. J. Biochem. 15, 531−540 (1970)

Sladek, N.E., Mannering, G.J.: Evidence for a new P-450 hemoprotein in hepatic microsomes from methylcholanthrene treated rats. Biochem. biophys. Res. Commun. 24, 668−674 (1966)

Solymoss, B., Classen, H.G., Varga, S.: Increased hepatic microsomal activity induced by spironolactone and other steroids. Proc. Soc. exp. Biol. (N.Y.) 132, 940−942 (1969)

Solymoss, B., Werringloer, J., Toth, S.: The influence of pregnenolone-16α-carbonitrile on hepatic mixed-function oxygenases. Steroids 17, 427−433 (1971)

Sottocasa, L., Kuylenstierna, B., Ernster, L., Bergstrand, A.: An electron-transport system associated with the outer membrane of liver mitochondria. J. Cell Biol. 32, 415−438 (1967)

Spatz, L., Strittmatter, P.: A form of cytochrome b_5 that contains an additional hydrophobic sequence of 40 amino acid residues. Proc. nat. Acad. Sci. (Wash.) 68, 1042−1046 (1971)

Stäubli, W., Hess, R., Weibel, E.R.: Correlated morphometric and biochemical studies on the liver cell. Effects of phenobarbital on rat hepatocytes. J. Cell Biol. 42, 92−112 (1969)

Staudt, H., Lichtenberger, F., Ullrich, V.: The role of NADH in uncoupled microsomal monooxygenations. Europ. J. Biochem. 46, 99−106 (1974)

Stonard, M.D., Nenov, P.Z.: Effect of hexachlorobenzene on hepatic microsomal enzymes in the rat. Biochem. Pharmacol. 23, 2175−2183 (1974)

Stripp, B., Hamrick, M., Zampaglione, N.: Effect of spironolactone treatment of rats on the oxidation of drugs by liver microsomes. Fed. Proc. 29, 346, 571 (1970)

Strittmatter, P., Spatz, L., Corcoran, D., Rogers, M.J., Setlow, B., Redline, R.: Purification and properties of rat liver microsomal stearyl coenzyme A desaturase. Proc. nat. Acad. Sci. (Wash.) 71, 4565−4569 (1974)

Strobel, H.W., Lu, A.Y.H., Heidema, J., Coon, M.J.: Phosphatidylcholine requirement in the enzymatic reduction of hemoprotein P-450 and in fatty acid, hydrocarbon, and drug hydroxylation. J. biol. Chem. **245,** 4851 – 4854 (1970)

Tettenborn, D.: Toxicität und enzyminduzierende Aktivität von Clotrimazol. Naunyn-Schmiedeberg's Arch. Pharmakol. **266,** 468 (1970)

Thomas, P.E., Lu, A.Y.H., Ryan, D., West, S.B., Kawalek, J., Lewin, W.: Multiple forms of rat liver cytochrome P-450. J. biol. Chem. **251,** 1385 – 1391 (1976)

Thurman, R.G., Scholz, R.: Mixed function oxidation in perfused rat liver. The effect of aminopyrine on oxygen uptake. Europ. J. Biochem. **10,** 459 – 467 (1969)

Thurman, R.G., Scholz, R.: Interaction of mixed-function oxidation with biosynthetic processes. Inhibition of lipogenesis by aminopyrine in perfused rat liver. Europ. J. Biochem. **38,** 73 – 78 (1973)

Ullrich, V., Diehl, H.: Uncoupling of monooxygenation and electron transport by fluorocarbons in liver microsomes. Europ. J. Biochem. **30,** 509 – 512 (1971)

Van der Hoeven, T.A., Coon, M.J.: Preparation and properties of partially purified cytochrome P-450 and reduced nicotinamide adenine dinucleotide phosphate-cytochrome P-450 reductase from rabbit liver microsomes. J. biol. Chem. **249,** 6302 – 6310 (1974)

Van der Hoeven, T.A., Haugen, D.A., Coon, M.J.: Cytochrome P-450 purified to apparent homogeneity from phenobarbital-induced rabbit liver microsomes: catalytic activity and other properties. Biochem. biophys. Res. Commun. **60,** 569 – 575 (1974)

Vesell, E.S.: Pharmacogenetics. Biochem. Pharmacol. **24,** 445 – 450 (1975)

Vesell, E.S., Page, J.G.: Genetic control of drug levels in man: phenylbutazone. Science **159,** 1479 – 1480 (1968 a)

Vesell, E.S., Page, J.G.: Genetic control of drug levels in man: antipyrine. Science **161,** 72 – 73 (1968 b)

Villeneuve, D.C., Grant, D.L., Phillips, W.E.J., Clark, M.L., Clegg, D.J.: Effects of PCB administration on microsomal enzyme activity in pregnant rabbits, Bull. environ. Contam. Toxicol. **6,** 120 (1971)

Wada, O., Yano, Y., Urata, G., Nakao, K.: Behavior of hepatic microsomal cytochromes after treatment of mice with drugs known to disturb porphyrin metabolism in liver. Biochem. Pharmacol. **17,** 595 – 603 (1968)

Wattenberg, L.W., Leong, J.L.: Effects of phenothiazines on protective systems against polycyclic hydrocarbons. Cancer Res. **25,** 365 – 370 (1965)

Wattenberg, L.W., Page, M.A., Leong, J.L.: Induction of increased benzpyrene hydroxylase activity by flavones and related compounds. Cancer Res. **28,** 934 – 937 (1968)

Westerfeld, W.R., Richert, D.A., Ruegamer, W.R.: The role of the thyroid hormone in the effect of p-chlorophenoxyisobutyrate in rats. Biochem. Pharmacol. **17,** 1003 – 1016 (1968)

White-Stevens, R.H., Kamin, H.: Uncoupling of oxygen activation from hydroxylation in a bacterial salicylate hydroxylase. Biochem. biophys. Res. Commun. **38,** 882 – 889 (1970)

Whitlock, J.P., Jr., Gelboin, H.V.: Aryl hydrocarbon (benzo(a)pyrene) hydroxylase induction in rat liver cells in culture. J. biol. Chem. **249,** 2616 – 2623 (1974)

Witmer, C., Remmer, H., Nehls, R., Krauss, P., Snyder, R.: Optical and EPR spectra of microsomal hemoproteins. Fed. Proc. **33,** 587 (1974)

Yang, C.S.: Interactions between solubilized cytochrome P-450 and hepatic microsomes. J. biol. Chem. **252,** 293 – 298 (1977)

Young, D.L., Powell, C., McMillan, W.O.: Phenobarbital-induced alterations in phosphatidylcholine and triglyceride synthesis in hepatic endoplasmic reticulum. J. Lipid Res. **12,** 1 – 8 (1971)

Zeidenberg, P., Orrenius, S., Ernster, L.: Increase in levels of glucuronylating enzymes and associated rise in activities of mitochondrial oxidative enzymes upon phenobarbital administration in the rat. J. Cell Biol. **32,** 528 – 531 (1967)

CHAPTER 3

Inhibition of Liver Hemoprotein Synthesis*

Thomas R. Tephly

A. Introduction

The synthesis of heme is an important process for the mammalian organism since heme serves as a prosthetic group for a critically important class of proteins, the hemoproteins. These are involved in several metabolic processes with some of them capable of adaptation to the changes in the environment. Whereas most prosthetic groups of proteins are preformed and derived from dietary sources, the heme moiety is synthesized entirely in the animal organism through a complex metabolic pathway which is subjected to efficient control. When heme is ultimately formed in the mitochondrion there is a requirement for its transport to the sites of protein synthesis and then for transport of hemoproteins from assembly sites to their functional sites. These latter processes are still largely unknown. Because of the multifarious nature of the heme biosynthetic pathway and of its interrelation with other metabolic systems, the synthesis of hemoproteins is sensitive to inhibition at numerous attack sites. The purpose of this chapter is to summarize the effects of certain substances which inhibit both the heme biosynthetic process in vivo and the synthesis of certain hepatic hemoproteins after treatment of animals in vivo. Since the effect of chemicals on heme biosynthesis and breakdown is a dominant theme which runs through each chapter of this book, attention will be given only to those aspects which do not form the theme of other chapters. Certain speculations are offered concerning mechanisms of inhibiton which may have more general relevance to other potential inhibitors. No attempt is made to discuss the effect of inhibitors of protein synthesis and the mechanism by which this class of agents affects heme biosynthesis.

A growing number of scientists are becoming aware of the importance of the mechanism of toxicity of agents which act by affecting heme metabolism. It is hoped that through an understanding of the mechanism of action of these agents more rational treatment of chemical toxicity can occur. That an insight into the basic physiology and potential disease processes should also result is implicit.

* Supported in part by USPHS Grant GM 12675.

This work was conducted at: The Department of Pharmacology, The University of Michigan, Ann Arbor, Michigan, and The Toxicology Center, Department of Pharmacology, The University of Iowa, Iowa City, Iowa 52242 U.S.A.

B. Agents Inhibiting Heme Biosynthesis and Hepatic Hemoprotein Synthesis

I. 3-Amino-1,2,4-triazole

The herbicide, 3-amino-1,2,4-triazole (aminotriazole) is a potent inhibitor of catalase activity in vivo (HEIM et al., 1956; MARGOLIASH and NOVOGRODSKY, 1958; and TEPHLY et al., 1961) and has a pronounced and rather selective inhibitory effect on catalase activity in vitro. Very few other enzymes have been shown to be affected either in vitro or in vivo. TSCHUDY and COLLINS (1957) showed that aminotriazole inhibits hepatic δ-aminolevulinic acid (ALA) dehydratase (E.C. 4.2.1.24), the enzyme catalyzing the second step of heme biosynthesis. Large doses were required for inhibition of the enzyme but aminotriazole is relatively non-toxic and could therefore be given in high doses. Even though the enzyme inhibited is supposed not to be rate-limiting, its inhibition might conceivably lead to a decrease in the rate of heme and hemoprotein synthesis. This is not unlike the situation where lead accumulation leads to accumulation of ALA due to the inhibition of ALA dehydratase. The consequences of that inhibition are well recognized (ALVARES et al., 1975; GOLDBERG, 1972; and MEYER and MAXWELL, 1976).

KATO (1967) reported that the administration of aminotriazole to rats markedly decreased the activities of certain drug metabolizing enzymes and the content of cytochrome P-450 in hepatic microsomes but had no effect on the content of cytochrome b_5. Aminotriazole also inhibited the induction by phenobarbital of cytochrome P-450 and certain drug metabolizing enzymes. He concluded that these effects were due to inhibition of the biosynthesis of cytochrome P-450. However, there was no direct evidence of the effects of aminotriazole on heme biosynthesis and the doses which were employed in that study were extremely high and could have conceivably produced certain nonspecific effects, such as general inhibition of protein synthesis. BARON and TEPHLY (1969a) studied the effect of aminotriazole on the rate of incorporation of both ^{14}C-ALA and ^{59}Fe into microsomal heme. They showed that aminotriazole decreased the incorporation of both heme precursors into microsomal heme and inhibited the stimulation of ^{59}Fe incorporation into microsomal heme produced by phenobarbital administration. The induction of rat hepatic microsomal cytochrome P-450 and of microsomal N-demethylation of ethylmorphine, norcodeine and 3-methyl-4-monomethylaminoazobenzene produced by phenobarbital was also inhibited by aminotriazole. Aminotriazole had no effect on the induction of the hepatic microsomal flavoprotein, NADPH-cytochrome c redutase by phenobarbital and neither did aminotriazole have any effect on the rate of incorporation of amino acids into microsomal protein.

Similar results have been obtained (BARON and TEPHLY, 1969b) when benzpyrene was used as an inducing agent. The rate of [2-^{14}C]glycine incorporation into hepatic microsomal heme was stimulated by benzpyrene and this enhancement was prevented by the administration of aminotriazole. The increase in ALA synthetase (BARON and TEPHLY, 1969b) was not prevented by aminotriazole treatment. These authors concluded that the effects of aminotriazole in preventing the induction of hepatic microsomal cytochrome P-450 was due to an inhibition of heme biosynthesis at the level of ALA dehydratase and not to inhibition of protein biosynthesis. This pattern of effects has been used as a model to test other compounds which may exert effects on heme biosynthesis without affecting protein synthesis.

WOODS (1974) has recently investigated the effect of aminotriazole on ALA synthetase activity in rat liver. He found that in the adult rat ALA synthetase doubled in the mitochondria within 3 h of treatment with aminotriazole. Since the stimulation of ALA synthetase is thought to represent an increased synthesis of the enzyme protein, Woods concluded that aminotriazole does not inhibit liver protein synthesis and that it stimulates the formation of ALA synthetase by decreasing the formation of the ultimate product, heme. WOODS (1974) also showed a significant decrease in fetal mitochondrial ALA synthetase activity following aminotriazole treatment. A reversal of the aminotriazole-induced decrease in mitochondrial ALA synthetase activity in fetal liver was produced by the administration of hemin when it was administered one hour after aminotriazole injection. It is conceivable, therefore, that aminotriazole inhibits protein synthesis in fetal liver.

Another possibility for the action of aminotriazole is through its wellknown goitrogenic effect (STRUM and KARNOVSKY, 1971). The indirect effect of aminotriazole through an action of the thyroid gland is unlikely, however, since amino triazole loses its ability to inhibit heme biosynthesis within $2-3$ days of administration (BARON and TEPHLY, 1969a), and the effect of aminotriazole on the thyroid gland persists through this period of time (STRUM and KARNOVSKY, 1971).

RAISFELD et al. (1970) showed that although increases in cytochrome P-450 and drug hydroxylase activity produced by phenobarbital alone were prevented by administration of aminotriazole together with phenobarbital, the increases in membranes of endoplasmic reticulum, observed by electron microscopy and measured by microsomal phospholipid, were comparable in animals receiving phenobarbital alone or in combination with aminotriazole. Aminotriazole did not, by itself, produce proliferation of endoplasmic reticulum membranes. Therefore, in the presence of an inducer such as phenobarbital, interference with cytochrome P-450 biosynthesis by aminotriazole does not affect induction of the formation of membranes of the hepatic endoplasmic reticulum. These results suggest that induced increases of cytochrome P-450 and of the membranes of endoplasmic reticulum are controlled by separate mechanisms.

Although aminotriazole has been widely used as an inhibitor of heme biosynthesis and as a method of decreasing microsomal cytochrome P-450, its action is limited to only about $24-48$ h after injection of single high doses in rats (3 g/kg) (BARON and TEPHLY, 1969a). This loss of effectiveness may be partly explained by its mechanism of inhibition of ALA dehydratase. We have observed that the inhibition of ALA dehydratase is partially competitive and its inhibitor constant is very high (about 80 mM). However, radioisotopic measurements after ^{14}C-aminotriazole administration (3 g/kg) showed liver concentrations of aminotriazole (and/or its metabolites) of about 5 mmol/kg of liver. If the inhibition of ALA dehydratase accounts for the effect of aminotriazole on heme biosynthesis, then this effect would be expected to last only until the steady state concentration of ALA becomes sufficient to overcome the aminotriazole effect. When phenobarbital is injected simultaneously with aminotriazole, there is a marked induction of ALA synthetase, an event which would tend to increase the steady state level of ALA and, in time, overcome the inhibition of ALA dehydratase. In the control animal an induction of ALA synthetase may also occur following the inhibition of heme synthesis through a reduction of the feedback control of heme on ALA synthetase. While aminotriazole has been useful in the past in inhibiting hemoprotein synthesis, more effective agents are now available and should be used instead.

II. The Effect of Metals on Heme Biosynthesis

Lead is known to exert a profound effect on heme biosynthesis (Goldberg, 1972 and Meyer and Maxwell, 1976). Its effects on the terminal step in heme biosynthesis, that catalyzed by protoheme ferrolyase (EC 4.99.1.1, ferrochelatase) have been described (Labbe and Hubbard, 1961, and Tephly et al., 1971). The details and mechanisms of lead inhibition of heme biosynthesis will be covered elsewhere in this book. Labbe and Hubbard (1961) showed the inhibition of this enzyme by a number of metals and the inhibitory effect of 3,5-diethoxycarbonyl-1,4-dihydrocollidine (DDC) has been studied by Onisawa and Labbe (1963), Tephly et al. (1971) and De Matteis et al. (1973). The properties and characteristics of ferrochelatase have been extensively examined by Nishida and Labbe (1959), Labbe and Hubbard (1959, 1961). Porra and Jones (1963a, 1963b), Porra et al. (1967) and Jones and Jones (1968, 1969). Recently, Wagner and Tephly (1975) have studied the inhibition of ferrochelatase by certain metals in vitro and have shown the capacity of several metals to lower certain hemoprotein levels after administration of these metals in vivo (Wagner et al., 1976). Labbe and Hubbard (1961) and Jones and Jones (1968) have suggested that ferrochelatase activity and cobalt cheletase activity reflect the activity of a common enzyme. On the other hand, Tephly et al. (1971) have shown that it is possible to alter the activity of one without changing the activity of the other. For example, they showed a differential metal inhibition on the two chelatase activities in certain rat organs and also an induction of ferrochelatase activity by phenobarbital without an effect on cobalt chelatase activity in rat liver. In addition, these workers were unable to show an effect of DDC on cobalt chelatase activity while they showed an effect of DDC on ferrochelatase activity. These results conflict with results obtained by De Matteis et al. (1973) who observed an inhibition of cobalt chelatase activity by DDC. The latter workers used a spectrophotometric method which was developed by Jones and Jones (1969) and which employs mesoporphyrin and Co^{++} as substrates and it is possible, therefore, that these differences in results may reflect differences in assay conditions. More work is required to establish with certainty whether cobalt chelatase and ferrochelatase reflect one or several enzyme activities.

1. The Inhibition of Liver Heme Synthesis by Cobalt

Cobaltous chloride administration in vivo produces a marked decrease in hepatic microsomal heme concentration and, as was seen previously with aminotriazole, cobaltous chloride prevents increases in heme content of hepatic microsomes brought on by administration of phenobarbital (Tephly et al., 1973). Through the appropriate use of cobaltous chloride and phenobarbital in vivo it has been possible to adjust the hepatic microsomal content of heme and cytochrome P-450 to

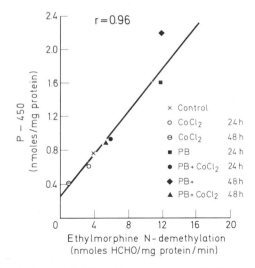

Fig. 1. The relation of cytochrome P 450 to the metabolism of ethylmorphine. (By permission of the authors and publishers, Academic Press. Reprinted from TEPHLY and HIBBELN, 1971)

almost any desired level. When this is done and when a representative drug metabolic reaction is studied, a linear relationship between cytochrome P-450 concentration and ethylmorphine N-demethylation is observed (Fig. 1). That the intercept
does not go through the origin is interpreted to mean that there is a certain pool
of cytochrome P-450, measurable but incapable of participating in the catalysis of
ethylmorphine N-demethylation. Although further studies will be needed to determine this with certainty, recent observations in several laboratories (COMAI and
GAYLOR, 1973; GLAUMANN, 1970; and KAWALEK and LU, 1975) show that several
forms of cytochrome P-450 exist in hepatic microsomes. TEPHLY and HIBBELN (1971)
have shown the effect of cobaltous chloride pretreatment on hexobarbital metabolism in perfused rat liver and others have used cobalt treatment to show the role
of cytochrome P-450 in participation of the conversion of certain drugs to toxic
metabolites (MITCHELL et al., 1973a; POTTER et al., 1973).

    That cobaltous chloride is acting on the biosynthesis of heme rather than on
the protein biosynthetic process is suggested by numerous results. Cobaltous
chloride administration leads to slight increases in NADPH-cytochrome c reductase
activity of hepatic microsomes (TEPHLY et al., 1973); ^{14}C-leucine incorporation
into hepatic microsomes is increased after cobaltous chloride administration; livers
of rats treated with cobaltous chloride contain more microsomal protein per gram
of liver than control animals (TEPHLY et al., 1973); and cobaltous chloride treatment leads to increases in heme oxygenase activity (MAINES and KAPPAS, 1974)
and ALA synthetase activity (MEYER and MAXWELL, 1976), two effects which
are thought to require de novo protein synthesis. That heme oxygenase is increased
by cobalt treatment (MAINES and KAPPAS, 1974) suggests that cobalt may also act
through an increased heme breakdown in vivo. Figure 2 shows the effect of cobalt
treatment on the rate of incorporation and subsequent loss of ^{14}C-ALA in hepatic
microsomal heme. While a dramatic effect on incorporation is seen, effects of cobalt

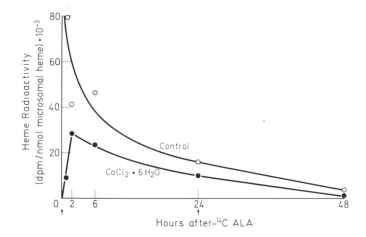

Fig. 2. The effect of cobaltous chloride administration on the incorporation of ^{14}C-amino-levulinic acid (ALA) into and subsequent loss from microsomal heme. ^{14}C-ALA, 10 µCi, was injected into Sprague-Dawley rats at zero time and cobaltous chloride, 60 mg/kg, was injected s.c. at the arrows as described by Tephly et al. (1973). Microsomal heme was extracted as described by Baron and Tephly (1969a)

on breakdown are not evident. Similar results were reported by Nakamura et al. (1975). However, De Matteis and Gibbs (1975) report an effect of cobalt on hepatic heme breakdown.

Although cobaltous chloride could be acting at numerous steps in the heme biosynthetic pathway, one hypothesis concerning its inhibition is that it effects the last step in heme biosynthesis, that catalyzed by ferrochelatase activity. Cobaltous chloride may be acting as an alternate substrate for ferrochelatase, but it has not been possible thus far to isolate from the urine, blood, or various organs of the rat a complex of cobalt and protoporphyrin IX. Therefore, it would appear that cobalt does not easily form a chelate with protoporphyrin IX in vivo in the rat, although it does so in vitro.

Recent studies have been performed which deal with possible mechanisms of inhibition of ferrochelatase by cobaltous chloride. We have shown that cobalt does not compete with iron for ferrochelatase. In the presence of either ascorbic acid or reduced glutathione (GSH) cobalt is an effective inhibitor of ferrochelatase activity, but, if cupric ion is added to an anaerobic system containing GSH and a solubilized preparation of ferrochelatase, there is a reversal of cobalt inhibition of ferrochelatase (Wagner and Tephly, 1975). Since copper can regulate the Michaelis constant of iron with ferrochelatase in the presence of GSH (Wagner et al., 1976) we interpret the copper effect as an allosteric regulatory effect on the enzyme. Cobalt thus appears to attack at the allosteric site of copper-GSH regulation site on the enzyme, and, thereby, facilitates the iron interaction with ferrochelatase. The inhibition of ferrochelatase by lead is also reversed by added Cu^{++} in the presence of GSH in vitro (Wagner and Tephly, 1975). These findings suggest a possible role of copper in heme biosynthesis in vivo. It is well known that copper deficiency can alter normal erythropoiesis (Lee et al., 1968; Vilter et al., 1974).

In studies where ferrochelatase has been measured in copper deficiency states and found to be normal, the ferrochelatase assays employed have been performed in the presence of rather high iron concentrations (VILTER et al., 1974). No effect of copper on ferrochelatase is seen at high iron concentrations because copper decreases the K_m for iron and has no effect on the V_{max} (WAGNER et al., 1976). Ascorbic acid is also able to regulate iron utilization by ferrochelatase as shown by GOLDBERG and his colleagues (GOLDBERG, 1959; LOCHHEAD and GOLDBERG, 1959, 1961) who suggested a possible role of ascorbic acid and sulfhydryl compounds in the physiologic regulation of heme biosynthesis.

It is also possible that cobalt or lead inhibit ferrochelatase by a nonspecific effect at sulfhydryl moieties or by reacting specifically with GSH. However, this explanation is less than satisfactory because Hg^{++} is not a very potent inhibitor of ferrochelatase in spite of its reactivity with sulfhydryl groups. Also, cobalt is a more potent inhibitor of ferrochelatase when ascorbic acid is used as a reducing agent than when GSH is used.

It might be tempting to speculate that cobalt inhibits respiration of tissue and that this mechanism accounts for the inhibition of heme biosynthesis. Indeed, several enzymes are inhibited at concentrations of 10^{-3} M (LAFORET und THOMAS, 1955). However, even at this very high concentration certain sulfhydryl-dependent and sulfhydryl-independent enzymes are not inhibited (LAFORET and THOMAS, 1955). LAFORET and THOMAS (1955) have shown that heme biosynthesis in erythroid cells is inhibited at concentrations that have no effect on oxygen consumption. LEVY et al. (1950) tested a number of enzymes in homogenates of rat liver and kidney for sensitivity to cobalt. Both oxidative and non-oxidative as well as sulfhydryl-dependent and sulfhydryl-independent enzymes were included in their study. Aerobic and anaerobic conditions were employed and high concentrations of cobaltous ions were used (10^{-3} M). They found that only two out of four sulfhydryl-dependent enzymes and only two out of five sulfhydryl-independent enzymes were markedly inhibited. Other have shown that cobalt treatment in vivo (1.25 mg/rat) causes a depression in respiration of the liver (DINGLE et al., 1962) 21 h after injection. These authors attribute this effect to accumulation of cobalt in mitochondria. However, cobalt exerts an effect on ALA incorporation into hepatic microsomal heme (Fig. 2) at a time when there should be a minimal effect on respiration.

Since cobalt is taken up in mitochondria (DINGLE et al., 1962) one might question whether its effects could be due to an interference with the uptake of iron or other key substrates by mitochondria. However, at least as far as ferrochelatase is concerned, inhibition occurs equally well with solubilized enzyme as with mitochondrial preparations (WAGNER et al., 1976).

Recent studies have shown that the effects of cobalt are not limited to cytochrome P-450, but extend to other liver hemoproteins, and that here again inhibition of heme synthesis is involved. YASUKOCHI et al. (1974) have found that the administration of cobaltous chloride to rats causes a decrease in hepatic catalase activity. They observed that the incorporation of ^{14}C-glycine into catalase heme was decreased by cobaltous chloride injections, but that incorporated into catalase protein remained unchanged. Furthermore, they found an inhibition of the rate of incorporation of ^{14}C-ALA into catalase heme with no effect on the rate of incorporation of ^{3}H-leucine in catalase protein. The initial rate of leucine incorporation into mitochondrial and cytosol catalase was markedly decreased. The degradation rate of catalase protein was not altered by treatment with cobalt. Recently, our laboratory has also shown that cobaltous chloride administration leads to marked decreases in hepatic catalase activity and SWEENEY (1976) has reported decreases in hepatic catalase activity following cobaltous chloride administration. Other studies show that although cobaltous chloride administration leads to marked effects on microsomal heme content, there was only a slight effect on the level of mitochondrial heme (WAGNER and TEPHLY, 1973). These observations may reflect the rate of turnover of certain hemoproteins; that is, cobaltous chloride affects those hemoproteins whose turnover is most rapid and fails to alter significantly those hemoproteins with longer half-lives.

It has recently been reported by NAKAMURA et al. (1975) and DE MATTEIS and GIBBS (1975) that cobalt treatment leads to marked and rapid decreases in ALA synthetase activity. These results have been confirmed in our laboratory. Thus, not only is there a potential block at ferrochelatase, but there is a potential block at ALA synthetase which would lead to decreased flux of substrates to ferrochelatase.

2. Effect of Manganese and Cadmium

LABBE and HUBBARD (1961) have shown that manganese is a potent inhibitor of ferrochelatase activity. They suggest that Mn^{++} does not react with the sulfhydryl portion of the ferrochelatase and that Mn^{++} inhibited non-competitively with respect to Fe^{++}. Recent studies by WAGNER et al. (1976) showed that manganese was a potent inhibitor of ferrochelatase activity and when administered to rats in vivo produced a marked decrease in the concentration of hepatic microsomal cytochrome P-450 and also reduced the activity of hepatic catalase. The ratio of potency of cobalt to manganese with respect to the inhibition of ferrochelatase resembles the ratio of potency of the two metals, cobalt and manganese, in their ability to decrease hepatic microsomal cytochrome P-450 levels. On the basis of these studies WAGNER et al. (1976) have suggested that these two metals exert their effects on heme biosynthesis and hepatic microsomal cytochrome P-450 through their actions at ferrochelatase.

It has been shown by COTZIAS and his co-workers (BERTINCHAMPS et al., 1966; MAYNARD and COTZIAS, 1955; and PAPAVASILIOU et al., 1966) that manganese is taken up by liver, accumulated in mitochondria and excreted in the bile and feces. Since ferrochelatase is located in mitochondria the effects of manganese on hepatic ferrochelatase activity may be insured by its uptake into mitochondria. One might also predict that the extent and duration of action of manganese may be longer than that of cobalt since the extent of manganese uptake is greater than that of cobalt (GREENBERG et al., 1943).

Because of the effect of metals, such as lead, cobalt, and manganese, on ferrochelatase activity, heme biosynthesis and hepatic microsomal cytochrome P-450 synthesis, one can predict that other metals or agents which affect ferrochelatase activity should inhibit heme biosynthesis and hepatic hemoprotein synthesis. For example, it has recently been reported that cadmium administration to rats leads to prolonged effects of drugs which are metabolized by hepatic microsomal mixed function oxidases (JOHNSTON et al., 1975). This is probably due to an effect of cadmium on hepatic microsomal cytochrome P-450 since cadmium treatment does produce a decrease in hepatic microsomal cytochrome P-450 (HADLEY et al., 1974). The effect of cadmium on ferrochelatase has not been investigated.

III. Role of Agents Which Affect the Availability of Glycine

The first step in the synthesis of heme, the condensation of succinyl-CoA with glycine to form δ-aminolevulinic acid (ALA) is catalyzed by mitochondrial ALA synthetase (EC 2.3.1.37). This enzyme is generally considered to be the rate-limiting enzyme of heme biosynthesis and its induction by drugs such as phenobarbital (BARON and TEPHLY, 1970) and polycyclic hydrocarbons (BARON and TEPHLY, 1969 b; BARON and TEPHLY, 1970) and by porphyrinogenic agents such as DDC or AIA is well known. PIPER et al. (1973) have examined the possibility of regulating the available hepatic concentrations of glycine and thereby affecting the overall rate of synthesis of hepatic heme. Three observations encouraged these attempts: (1) SCHOLNICK et al. (1972) showed that the Michaelis constant (K_m) of glycine for hepatic ALAs was high (10 mM); (2) BRAY et al. (1955) showed that hippurate synthesis may be regulated by the availability of glycine in vivo, and finally, (3) liver was known to contain high activity of glycine acyltransferase in mitochondria (KIELLEY and SCHNEIDER, 1950; SCHACHTER and TAGGART, 1954).

TEPHLY et al. (1973) studied the effect of p-aminobenzoic acid (PABA) on hepatic microsomal cytochrome P-450 concentrations and on the metabolism of ethylmorphine. PABA treatment of rats significantly lowered cytochrome P 450 levels and ethylmorphine N-demethylation in hepatic microsomes without affecting hepatic microsomal NADPH-cytochrome c reductase activity. Furthermore, PABA injected at a dose of 1 g/kg at 12-h intervals reversed the induction of hepatic microsomal cytochrome P-450 brought about by phenobarbital treatment (40 mg/kg, daily). The induction of NADPH-cytochrome c reductase activity by phenobarbital was not reversed by the treatment with PABA. Hence, these results resemble those obtained with aminotriazole and cobaltous chloride in that it was possible to regulate heme biosynthesis and hepatic microsomal cytochrome P-450 levels with agents that can alter heme biosynthesis and at the same time not alter the effects on other hepatic microsomal components of electron transport such as NADPH-cytochrome c reductase.

PIPER et al. (1973) have also reported that the experimental porphyria induced in the rat by the porphyrogenic agent, DDC, can be reversed by sodium benzoate or PABA treatment. DDC, through its inhibition of ferrochelatase activity and induction of ALA synthetase activity, produced a marked experimental porphyria characterized by elevated urinary excretion of heme precursors, ALA, porphobilinogen (PBG) and porphyrins as well as by elevated levels of tissue and blood porphyrins. The administration of benzoate or PABA markedly decreased the urinary excretion of heme precursors and lowered the level of tissue and blood porphyrins. To show that the action of these agents was dependent on glycine, exogenous glycine was injected. The administration of glycine prevented the reversal of the porphyrias affected by benzoate or PABA. It should be recalled that the metabolic product resulting from glycine conjugation with a benzoic acid derivative yields hippuric acid derivatives, compounds that are known to be rapidly excreted by the kidney. The metabolites have no effect on heme biosynthesis (Piper et al., 1973). Therefore, benzoate or PABA, both excellent substrates of glycine acyltransferase, promote the diversion of glycine from the heme biosynthetic pathway in the liver to hippurates, products which are rapidly excreted in the urine.

These results also suggest a possible treatment for acute hepatic porphyrias in man. The use of PABA in diseases such as scleroderma has been reported where doses of up to 12 g of PABA administered daily apparently yield no adverse effects (Zarafonetis, 1962). This type of treatment would probably be only useful for hepatic porphyrias since the liver contains high levels of glycine acyltransferase whereas other organs apparently contain much less activity.

IV. Effect of Acetate on Heme Biosynthesis

As indicated above, glycine administration reversed the effects of benzoate on heme biosynthesis. Piper et al. (1973) noted that although glycine reversed the prevention of experimental porphyria produced by benzoate it was less effective in counteracting the effect of PABA on the experimental porphyria. One possible explanation for this observation was that PABA was, to a certain extent, acylated and that the acylation process itself could regulate, to some degree, the synthesis of heme precursors possibly through an effect on the available hepatic concentrations of coenzyme A. These authors therefore studied the effect of acetate, an agent known to react with coenzyme A, on porphyria produced by DDC, on hepatic microsomal cytochrome P-450 levels, on microsomal ethylmorphine N-demethylation and NADPH-cytochrome c reductase activities. They found that acetate treatment could reverse the experimental porphyria (Piper and Tephly, 1974). However, unlike the other agents considered previously (aminotriazole, cobaltous chloride and benzoate) acetate was not only capable of reversing the inductive effect of phenobarbital on cytochrome P-450 and ethylmorphine N-demethylation, but also had a significant effect on the stimulation by phenobarbital of NADPH-cytochrome c reductase activity (Piper and Tephly, 1974). Acetate treatment decreased ALA synthetase activity in vivo in DDC-induced, porphyric rats and acetate would also decrease ALA synthetase activity in vitro when added to hepatic homogenates (Piper and Tephly, 1974). The effect of acetate on ALA synthetase activity in vitro could be partially reversed by the addition of succinate (Piper and Tephly, 1974). Glycine had no effect on the inhibition of ALA synthetase produced by acetate. The authors speculated that agents which may increase the utilization of CoA in vivo may have an effect on heme biosynthesis, possibly by decreasing the availability of CoA and, subsequently, of succinyl-CoA. Sulfanilamide is known to react with acetyl-CoA through its conversion to acetylsulfanilamide. This agent was also shown to be effective in decreasing the urinary excretion of porphyrins in DDC-treated rats. The finding that the inhibition of ALA synthetase activity caused in vitro by the addition of acetate could be reversed by succinate, is also compatible with their suggestion. However, the finding that acetate treatment also affected the stimulation of NADPH-cytochrome c reductase caused by phenobarbital cannot be readily explained with a depletion of CoA.

The effect of glucose administration on the synthesis of ALA synthetase is well known. Bonkowsky et al. (1973) have recently studied the effects of numerous substances known to be intermediary metabolites of glucose on ALA synthetase activity. They showed that glycerol and fructose were as effective as glucose in inhibiting the synthesis of ALA synthetase. However, they did not report on the effects of acetate. It is possible that acetate, also a key metabolic intermediate of glucose metabolism, may be responsible for the "glucose effect." It may also be possible that the "glucose effect" is due, at least in part, to a regulation of the steady state level of succinyl-CoA. Thus, several agents which might be expected to increase the utilization of CoA may indirectly be altering the level of succinyl-CoA available for the heme biosynthetic process and ultimately control the rate of heme biosynthesis. Because succinyl-CoA is a metabolite central to both Krebs cycle and heme biosynthesis, the regulation of heme biosynthesis by intermediary metabolism of glucose can be expected. Because numerous drugs are acetylated, certain drugs may play an important role through their metabolic demand. This demand may have adverse effects in the individual with hepatic porphyria since a tendency to reduce the rate of heme synthesis leads to marked increases in hepatic ALA synthetase. Once the drug level is reduced, a marked overstimulation of heme biosynthesis could occur and, in a porphyric patient, this would have disastrous results.

C. Conclusions

The heme biosynthetic system is effectively regulated and may be perturbed by exogenous factors like chemicals. Marked effects are seen, usually under extraordinary circumstances, such as in genetic diseases or under exposure or treatment conditions with certain drugs and chemicals. This chapter dealt with some substances such as herbicides, metals, and drugs that disturb the equilibrium of heme biosynthesis and produce changes in hemoproteins, primarily those of the hepatic endoplasmic reticulum. Certain speculations were made concerning the mechanisms by which these agents alter heme biosynthesis in the liver with the view that, although the exact mechanisms may not be known at this time, by studying them we may ultimately arrive at a better understanding of chemical toxicities, of regulation of the substrate flux to heme, and possibly also of the therapeutic measures for toxic states or diseases.

Abbreviations

ALA	δ-Aminolevulinic acid
NADPH	Reduced nicotinamide adenine dinucleotide phosphate
GSH	Reduced glutathione
K_m	Michaelis constant
V_{max}	Maximal velocity
AIA	Allylisopropylacetamide
DDC	3,5-Diethoxycarbonyl-1,4-dihydrocollidine
PABA	p-Aminobenzoic acid
CoA	Coenzyme A

References

Alvares, A.P., Kapelner, S., Sassa, S., Kappas, A.: Drug metabolism in normal children, lead-poisoned children, and normal adults. Clin. Pharm. Ther. **17**, 179 – 183 (1975)

Baron, J., Tephly, T.R.: Effect of 3-amino-1,2,4-triazole on the induction of rat hepatic microsomal oxidases, cytochrome P-450 and NADPH-cytochrome c reductase by phenobarbital. Molec. Pharmacol. **5**, 10 – 20 (1969 a)

Baron, J., Tephly, T.R.: The role of heme synthesis during the induction of hepatic microsomal cytochrome P-450 and drug metabolism produced by benzpyrene. Biochem. biophys. Res. Commun. **36**, 526 – 532 (1969 b)

Baron, J., Tephly, T.R.: Further studies on the relationship of the stimulatory effects of phenobarbital and 3,4-benzpyrene on hepatic heme synthesis to their effects in hepatic microsomal drug oxidations. Arch. Biochem. Biophys. **139**, 410 – 420 (1970)

Bertinchamps, A.J., Miller, S.T., Cotzias, G.C.: Interdependence of routes excreting manganese. Amer. J. Physiol. **211**, 217 – 224 (1966)

Bonkowsky, H.L., Collins, A., Doherty, J.M., Tschudy, D.P.: The glucose effect in rat liver: studies of δ-aminolevulinate synthetase and tyrosine aminotransferase. Biochim. biophys. Acta (Amst.) **320**, 561 – 576 (1973)

Bray, H.G., Humphris, B.G., Thorpe, W.V., White, K., Wood, P.B.: Kinetic studies on the metabolism of foreign organic compounds. 6. Reactions of some nuclear substituted benzoic acids, benzamides and toluenes in the rabbit. Biochem. J. **59**, 162 – 167 (1955)

Comai, K., Gaylor, J.L.: Existence and separation of three forms of cytochrome P-450 from rat liver microsomes. J. biol. Chem. **248**, 4947 – 4955 (1973)

Dingle, J.T., Heath, J.C., Webb, M., Daniel, M.: The biological action of cobalt and other metals II. The mechanism of the respiratory inhibition produced by cobalt in mammalian tissues. Biochim. biophys. Acta (Amst.) **65**, 34 – 46 (1962)

De Matteis, F., Abbritti, G., Gibbs, A.: Decreased liver activity of porphyrin-metal chelatase in hepatic porphyria caused by 3,5-diethyoxycarbonyl-1,4-dihydrocollidine. Studies in rats and mice. Biochem. J. **134**, 717 – 727 (1973)

De Matteis, F., Gibbs, A.H.: Proceedings of the International Porphyrin Meeting, Sannas, Finland 1975

Glaumann, H.: Chemical and enzymatic composition of microsomal subfractions from rat liver after treatment with phenobarbital and 3-methylcholanthrene. Chem.-Biol. Interactions **2**, 369 – 380 (1970)

Goldberg, A.: The enzymic formation of heme by the incorporation of iron into protoporphyrin; importance of ascorbic acid, ergothioneine and glutathione. Brit. J. Haemat. **5**, 150 – 157 (1959)

Goldberg, A.: Lead poisoning and heme biosynthesis. Brit. J. Haemat. **23**, 521 – 524 (1972)

Greenberg, D.M., Copp, D.H., Cuthbertson, E.M.: Studies in mineral metabolism with the aid of artificial radioactive isotopes. VII. The distribution and excretion, particularly by way of the bile, of iron, cobalt, and manganese. J. biol. Chem. **147**, 749 – 756 (1943)

Hadley, W.M., Miya, T.S., Bousquet, W.F.: Cadmium inhibition of hepatic drug metabolism in the rat. Toxicol. appl. Pharmacol. **28**, 384 – 391 (1974)

Heim, W.G., Applemen, D., Pyfrom, H.T.: Effects of 3-amino-1,2,4-triazole (AT) on catalase and other compounds. Amer. J. Physiol. **186**, 19 – 23 (1956)

Johnston, R.E., Miya, T.S., Schnell, R.C.: Cadmium potentiation of drug response-role of the liver. Biochem. Pharm. **24**, 877 – 881 (1975)

Jones, M.S., Jones, O.T.G.: Evidence for the location of ferrochelatase on the inner membrane of rat liver mitochondria. Biochem. biophys. Res. Commun. **31**, 977 – 982 (1968)

Jones, M.S., Jones, O.T.G.: The structural organization of heme synthesis in rat liver mitochondria. Biochem. J. **113**, 507 – 514 (1969)

Kato, R.: Effect of administration of 3-aminotriazole on the activity of microsomal drug-metabolizing enzyme systems of rat liver. Jap. J. Pharmacol. **17**, 56 – 64 (1967)

Kawalek, J.C., Lu, A.Y.H.: Reconstituted liver microsomal enzyme system that hydroxylates drugs, other foreign compounds, and endogenous substances VIII. Different catalytic activities of rabbit and rat cytochromes P-448. Molec. Pharmacol. **11**, 201 – 210 (1975)

Kielley, R.K., Schneider, W.C.: Synthesis of p-aminohippuric acid by mitochondria of mouse liver homogenates. J. biol. Chem. **187**, 869 – 880 (1950)

Labbe, R.F.: An enzyme which catalyzes the insertion of iron into protoporphyrin. Biochim. biophys. Acta (Amst.) **31**, 589 – 590 (1959)

Labbe, R.F., Hubbard, N.: Metal specificity of the iron-protoporphyrin chelating enzyme from rat liver. Biochim. biophys. Acta (Amst.) **52**, 130 – 135 (1961)

Laforet, M.T., Thomas E.D.: The effect of cobalt on heme synthesis by bone marrow in vitro. J. biol. Chem. **218**, 595 – 598 (1955)

Lee, G.R., Cartwright, G.E., Wintrobe, M.M.: Heme biosynthesis in copper deficient swine. Proc. Soc. exp. Biol. (N.Y.) **127**, 977 – 981 (1968)

Levy, H., Levison, F., Schade, A.L.: The effect of cobalt on the activity of certain enzymes in homogenates of rat tissue. Arch. Biochem. Biophys. **27**, 34 – 40 (1950)

Lochhead, A.C., Goldberg, A.: Transfer of iron to protoporphyrin for heme biosynthesis, role of ascorbic acid and glutathione. Lancet **1959 II**, 271 – 272

Lochhead, A.C., Goldberg, A.: The enzymic formation of heme by human and rat tissues. Biochem. J. **78**, 146 – 150 (1961)

Maines, M.D., Kappas, A.: Cobalt induction of hepatic heme oxygenase; with evidence that cytochrome P-450 is not essential for this enzyme activity. Proc. nat. Acad. Sci. (Wash.) **71**, 4293 – 4297 (1974)

Margoliash, E., Novogrodsky, A.: A study of the inhibition of catalase by 3-amino-1,2,4-triazole. Biochem. J. **68**, 468 – 475 (1958)

Maynard, L.S., Cotzias, G.C.: The partition of manganese among organs and intracellular organelles of the rat. J. biol. Chem. **214**, 489 – 495 (1955)

Meyer, U.A., Maxwell, J.D.. Mechanism of drug sensitivity in hepatic porphyria. In: Porphyrins in Human Diseases. Doss (ed.). Basel, Switzerland: Karger 1976

Mitchell, J.R., Jollow, D.J., Gillette, J.R., Brodie, B.B.: Drug metabolism as a cause of drug toxicity. Drug Metab. Dispos. **1**, 418 – 423 (1973b)

Mitchell, J.R., Jollow, D.J., Potter, W.Z., Davis, D.C., Gillette, J.R., Brodie, B.B.: Acetaminophen-induced hepatic necrosis. I. Role of drug metabolism. J. Pharmacol exp. Ther. **187**, 185 194 (1973a)

Nakamura, M., Yasukochi, Y., Minakami, S.: Effect of cobalt on heme biosynthesis in rat liver and spleen. J. Biochem. **78**, 373 – 380 (1975)

Nishida, G., Labbe, R.F.: Heme biosynthesis. On the incorporation of iron into protoporphyrin. Biochim. biophys. Acta (Amst.) **31**, 519 – 524 (1959)

Onisawa, J., Labbe, R.F.: Effects of diethyl-1,4-dihydro-1,4,6-trimethylpyridine-3,5-dicarboxylate on the metabolism of porphyrins and iron. J. biol. Chem. **238**, 724 – 727 (1963)

Papavasiliou, P.S., Miller, S.T., Cotzias, G.C.: Role of liver in regulating distribution and excretion of manganese. Amer. J. Physiol. **211**, 211 216 (1966)

Piper, W.N., Condie, L.W., Tephly, T.R.: The role of substrates for glycine acyltransferase in the reversal of chemically induced porphyria in the rat. Arch. Biochem. Biophys. **159**, 671 – 677 (1973)

Piper, W.N., Tephly, T.R.: The reversal of experimental porphyria and the prevention of induction of hepatic mixed-function oxidase by acetate. Arch. Biochem. Biophys. **164**, 351 – 356 (1974)

Porra, R.J., Jones, O.T.G.: Studies on ferrochelatase. I. Assay and properties of ferrochelatase from a pig-liver mitochondrial extract. Biochem. J. **87**, 181 – 185 (1963a)

Porra, R.J., Jones, O.T.G.: Studies on ferrochelatase. II. An investigation of the role of ferrochelatase in the biosynthesis of various heme prosthetic groups. Biochem. J. **87**, 186 – 191 (1963b)

Porra, R.J., Vitols, K.S., Labbe, R.F., Newton, N.A.: Studies on ferrochelatase. The effects of thiols and other factors on the determination of activity. Biochem. J. **104**, 321 – 327 (1967)

Potter, W.Z., Davis, D.C., Mitchell, J.R., Jollow, D.J., Gillette, J.R., Brodie, B.B.: Acetaminophen-induced hepatic necrosis. III. Cytochrome P-450-mediated covalent binding in vitro. J. Pharmacol. exp. Ther. **187**, 203 – 210 (1973)

Raisfeld, I., Bacchin, P., Hutterer, F., Schaffner, F.: The effect of 3-amino-1,2,4-triazole on the phenobarbital-induced formation of hepatic microsomal membranes. Molec. Pharmacol. **6**, 231 – 239 (1970)

Schachter, D., Taggart, J.V.: Glycine N-acylase: purification and properties. J. biol. Chem. **208**, 263 – 275 (1954)

Scholnick, P.L., Hammaker, L.E., Marver, H.S.: Soluble δ-aminolevulinic acid synthetase of rat liver. J. biol. Chem. **247,** 4132–4137 (1972)

Strum, J.M., Karnovsky, M.J.: Aminotriazole goiter. Fine structure and localization of thyroid peroxidase activity. Lab. Invest. **24,** 1–12 (1971)

Sweeney, G.D.: Hepatic catalase activity during states of altered heme synthesis. In: Porphyrins in Human Diseases. Doss (ed.). Basel, Switzerland: Karger 1976

Tephly, T.R., Hasegawa, E., Baron, J.: Effect of drugs on heme synthesis in the liver. Metabolism **20,** 200–214 (1971)

Tephly, T.R., Hibbeln, P.: The effect of cobalt chloride administration on the synthesis of hepatic microsomal cytochrome P-450. Biochem. biophys. Res. Commun. **42,** 589–595 (1971)

Tephly, T.R., Mannering, G.J., Parks, R.E. Jr.: Studies on the mechanism of inhibition of liver and erythrocytic catalase activity by 3-amino-1,2,4-triazole (AT). J. Pharmacol. exp. Ther. **134,** 147–151 (1961)

Tephly, T.R., Webb, D., Trussler, P., Kniffen, F., Hasegawa, E., Piper, W.: The regulation of heme synthesis related to drug metabolism. Drug Metab. Dispos. **1,** 259–266 (1973)

Tschudy, D.P., Collins, A.: Effect of 3-amino-1,2,4-triazole on δ-aminolevulinic acid dehydrase activity. Science **126,** 168 (1957)

Vilter, R.W., Bozian, R.C., Hess, E.V., Zellner, D.C., Petering, H.G.: Manifestations of copper deficiency in a patient with systemic sclerosis on intravenous hyperalimentation. New Engl. J. Med. **291,** 188–191 (1974)

Wagner, G.S., Dinamarca, M.L., Tephly, T.R.: Studies on ferrochelatase activity: role in regulation of hepatic heme biosynthesis. In: Porphyrins in Human Diseases. Doss (ed.). pp. 111–122. Basel, Switzerland: Karger, 1976

Wagner, G.S., Tephly, T.R.: The role of ferrochelatase in the regulation of heme synthesis by drugs and metals. Pharmacologist **15,** 170 (1973)

Wagner, G.S., Tephly, T.R.: A possible role of copper in the regulation of heme biosynthesis through ferrochelatase. Cytochromes P-450 and b_5. Cooper, Rosenthal, Snyder, Witmer (eds.), pp. 343–354. New York: Plenum Pub. Corp. 1975

Woods, J.S.: Studies on the role of heme in the regulation of δ-aminolevulinic acid synthetase during fetal hepatic development. Molec. Pharmacol **10,** 389–397 (1974)

Yasukochi, Y., Nakamura, M., Minakami, S.: Effect of cobalt on the synthesis and degradation of hepatic catalase in vivo. Biochem. J. **144,** 455–464 (1974)

Zarafonetis, C.J.D.: Treatment of localized forms of scleroderma. Amer. J. med. Sci. **243,** 147–158 (1962)

Loss of Liver Cytochrome P-450 Caused by Chemicals

Damage to the Apoprotein and Degradation of the Heme Moiety

F. De Matteis

A. Introduction

The most common response of the liver to the administration of foreign chemicals is an increase in the concentration of its hemoproteins (especially that of cytochrome P-450); this is one aspect of the more general adaptive response, usually referred to as induction of the drug-metabolizing system, which has been dealt with by Bock and Remmer in Chapter 2. There are cases, however, in which a chemical causes a decrease rather than an increase in the concentration of the hemoproteins of the liver, and this may result from an inhibition of their formation, from an increase in the rate of their degradation, or, finally, from a combination of these two mechanisms. Compounds which are thought to act by inhibiting heme synthesis have been discussed by Tephly in Chapter 3. The purpose of this paper is to consider in detail the effects of those chemicals that increase the rate of degradation of heme and hemoproteins in the liver. In the discussion of these effects, one particular hemoprotein—cytochrome P-450—will figure prominently. This is partly because this hemoprotein has attracted a great deal of interest in the last few years, and it is also easy to measure, so it has been extensively studied in several laboratories; also, cytochrome P-450 is particularly liable to toxic damage by a number of chemicals, apparently much more liable than the other hemoproteins of the liver, including the other cytochrome of the endoplasmic reticulum, cytochrome b_5. This is due to the properties peculiar to cytochrome P-450 of interaction with several classes of potentially toxic chemicals. These properties, listed in Table 1, are briefly considered below.

Firstly, cytochrome P-450 plays a central role in drug oxidation. This hemoprotein is the terminal oxidase and possibly also the binding site for several chemicals which are oxidized in the liver to reactive derivatives. These reactive metabolites will be produced at the P-450 site or very near it, so it is not surprising that the hemoprotein may be an early target of their toxic action.

Secondly, the unusual structural properties of cytochrome P-450, in which one of the co-ordination valencies of the iron of the heme moiety is saturated by a thiol ligand from the apoprotein (see for example Stern and Peisach, 1974; Yu and Gunsalus, 1974), must be considered. This sulphur ligand is responsible not only for the spectral characteristics of the hemoprotein (unusual for a cytochrome of the b type), but also, apparently, for its stability and function, since oxidation of this thiol group or its blockade by sulphydryl reagents converts P-450 to the so-called P-420, an unstable derivative deprived of functional activity. This thiol group may then provide a site for the toxic effect of heavy metals and other sulphydryl reagents on P-450, although their interaction with other SH groups in the

Table 1. Several properties of cytochrome P-450 which make it a preferential target for the toxic action of several chemicals

Property of cytochrome P-450	Type of lesion	Example of chemicals involved
Terminal oxidase and binding site for the activation of foreign chemicals	Damage to either heme or apoprotein moieties by reactive metabolites	AIA CS$_2$
Organisation of hemoprotein within the hydrophobic environment of the membrane of endoplasmic reticulum	Conversion of P-450 to P-420 and destruction of the heme moiety during lipid peroxidation	CCl$_4$? Fe ? Pb
Presence of a SH ligand from the apoprotein to the Fe of heme. Other SH groupings in the apoprotein and in the membrane	Blockage of SH groupings; conversion of P-450 to P-420, followed by loss of heme	Heavy metals and other SH reagents
Heme moiety may serve as a substrate for heme oxygenase	Increased breakdown of heme moiety	Co, ? Heme ? Fe, ? Pb and other metals

apoprotein or in the membrane may also be expected to result in loss of stability and enzymatic activity.

Thirdly, consider the organization of the hemoprotein within the hydrophobic environment of the membrane of the endoplasmic reticulum. The structural integrity of the membrane is apparently necessary for the normal structure and function of cytochrome P-450, since detergents, lipolytic enzymes, etc., convert P-450 to P-420. In addition, the close proximity of the hemoprotein to the phospholipids and the several components of the electron transport chain of the endoplasmic reticulum provides an explanation for the preferential destruction of the heme of this hemoprotein, which is observed in the course of lipid peroxidation of the membranes.

Finally, consider the ability of the heme moiety of the cytochrome to serve as a substrate for heme oxygenase, presumably after dissociation from the apoprotein. This may result in an increased turnover of the heme of cytochrome P-450 and contribute to the loss of hemoprotein seen under conditions where the activity of heme oxygenase is markedly stimulated, for example, after cobalt treatment.

More than one of these mechanisms may be involved in the action of a single chemical, and in some cases the relative contribution of the various mechanisms to the overall effect on the hemoprotein is not clear. Nevertheless, for reasons of convenience, the action of many chemicals will be discussed below under a single mechanism on the somewhat arbitrary assumption that one mechanism plays a predominant role.

B. Loss of Liver Cytochrome P-450 Caused by Chemicals Which Require Metabolic Conversion to Reactive Derivatives

Three main classes of chemicals can be distinguished: 1) allyl-containing compounds, such as 2-allyl-2-isopropylacetamide (AIA); 2) certain sulphur-containing chemicals, such as carbon disulphide (CS_2), and 3) carbon tetrachloride (CCl_4). Even though activation through metabolism appears to be essential for the effect of the these chemicals on cytochrome P-450, there are important differences between the three classes in the nature of the primary target, in the extent of the liver lesion which accompanies the effect on P-450 and also, most likely, in the underlying mechanism of their toxicity. AIA appears to affect primarily the heme moiety of the cytochrome, CS_2 its protein moiety, whereas with CCl_4 the lesion is more widespread and extends to other constituents of the membranes and of the cell leading to liver cell necrosis.

I. 2-Allyl-2-isopropylacetamide and Related Drugs

Allyl-containing acetamides and barbiturates have long been known to cause increased formation of porphyrins in the liver of experimental animals (see the following chapter on the experimental porphyrias). Their ability to promote rapid loss of liver cytochrome P-450 has been recognized more recently. Although most of the work on the destruction of cytochrome P-450 has been carried out with AIA, several other allyl-containing barbiturates and acetamides are similarly active (see Sect. I.3).

1. Loss of Pre-existing Cytochrome P-450

WADA et al. (1968) and WATERFIELD et al. (1969) first described a decline in cytochrome P-450 concentration following administration of AIA to mice and rabbits, respectively. No attempt was made by these authors to establish whether the decrease was due to inhibition of cytochrome synthesis, to loss of existing pigment, or to interference by the drug with the development of the characteristic spectrum with carbon monoxide. In order to distinguish between these possibilities, the decrease in the cytochrome P-450 concentration after a single dose of AIA was studied in rats that, at the time of administration of the drug, had a greatly increased concentration of cytochrome P-450 in their liver microsomes, because they had been pretreated with phenobarbitone (DE MATTEIS, 1970; 1971a). The rate of the decrease caused by AIA in these animals was found to be much more rapid than that obtained after nearly complete inhibition of liver protein synthesis by cycloheximide, suggesting that inhibition of cytochrome synthesis alone could not explain the fast rate of loss seen after AIA. The loss of cytochrome P-450 caused by AIA was accompanied by a loss of microsomal heme, demonstrating conclusively that there was a loss of the existing cytochrome (DE MATTEIS, 1970).

In contrast with the marked loss of microsomal cytochrome P-450 and heme observed after administration of AIA to phenobarbitone-treated rats, the cytochrome b_5 and protein content of the microsomal fraction and glucose-6-phosphatase activity of the liver did not change. This indicated that the decrease of cytochrome P-450 was not produced through a general effect on the endoplasmic reticulum leading to a loss of all components of the microsomal fraction but was more likely to result from a specific effect on cytochrome P-450. The data discussed below, in fact, suggest that AIA may preferentially affect the heme moiety of the cytochrome.

2. Conversion of Heme into Unidentified "Green Pigments"

The decline in cytochrome P-450 concentration caused by AIA in vivo was found to be affected by treatments known to alter the activity of microsomal drug-metabolizing enzymes (see Sect. I.3). Using these different pretreatment conditions, the amount of cytochrome P-450 lost was closely related to a loss of microsomal heme, determined as the pyridine hemochrome. In addition, when the liver hemes were prelabelled with either $[^3H]$- or $[^{14}C]$-5-aminolevulinate or with $[^{59}Fe]$-ferrous ascorbate before administration of the drug, on treatment with AIA there was not only a loss of cytochrome P-450 and of chemically determinable heme from the liver microsomes but also a corresponding loss of radioactivity from the hemin isolated in a crystalline form from the liver homogenate. The loss of radioactivity was most pronounced in the hemin isolated from the liver microsomes and preferentially concerned heme of rapid turnover rate (DE MATTEIS, 1971; 1973).

In similar experiments, an increased destruction of microsomal heme has been reported after administration of AIA by MEYER and MARVER (1971) and by LEVIN et al. (1972a), who described a loss of heme radioactivity from a microsomal fraction treated so that cytochrome P-450 was the only hemoprotein.

The fall in cytochrome P-450 and in heme concentration caused by AIA in the liver microsomes was also accompanied by a characteristic brown-green discolouration of the whole liver, which was particularly intense in the microsomal fraction (DE MATTEIS, 1971). In 1955, SCHWARTZ and IKEDA described a discolouration of the liver of rats and rabbits given either AIA or the related drug allyl-isopropyl-acetylurea (Sedormid), and they extracted and partially characterized certain "green pigments" responsible for this abnormal colour. The significance of these pigments remained obscure, although SCHWARTZ and IKEDA suggested that they might be porphyrin-like intermediates on the pathway to heme. Our results suggested, on the other hand, that the abnormal pigments might arise from some chemical change in existing heme. There are now several lines of evidence which support the latter interpretation, and they can be summarized as follows.

Firstly, a clear correlation exists between loss of cytochrome P-450 heme and degree of brown-green discolouration of the microsomes, when comparing the effect of AIA in rats pretreated in different ways. Thus, pretreatment of the animals with agents, such as phenobarbitone and DDT, which stimulate the activity of the liver drug-metabolizing system, will increase both the loss of heme and the degree of discolouration of the microsomes produced by a single dose of AIA; whereas, pretreatment with SKF 525-A (an inhibitor of the drug-metabolizing system) will reduce the intensity of both these effects (DE MATTEIS, 1971).

Secondly, production of "green pigments" can be demonstrated in vitro as a result of the action of AIA on either the post-mitochondrial supernatant of the liver homogenate or the isolated microsomal fraction. Under these conditions there is a corresponding destruction of P-450 heme, but no significant de novo synthesis of porphyrins takes place (DE MATTEIS, 1971; UNSELD and DE MATTEIS, 1975).

Finally, the most conclusive evidence that the "green pigments" originate from pre-existing heme (rather than from free porphyrins or their precursors) is afforded by isotopic experiments carried out both in vivo and in vitro. In the first experiment

(DE MATTEIS, 1971), the liver hemes of phenobarbitone-induced rats were pre-lebelled with radioactive 5-aminolaevulinate given before administration of the drug, and the distribution of the label was studied between heme and the fraction known from the work of SCHWARTZ to contain the "green pigments". The heme pools were labelled by giving 5-amino[4-^{14}C]laevulinate 26 h and [G-^{3}H]5-amino-laevulinate 2 h before the drug. Animals killed 1 h after the administration of AIA showed a considerable loss of the radioactivity of both isotopes in the heme isolated from the liver homogenates, and a corresponding increase in the radio-activity of both isotopes was recovered in the "green pigment" fraction. The loss of ^{3}H radioactivity from heme was greater than that of ^{14}C, suggesting that rapidly turning-over heme might be preferentially destroyed by AIA. In agreement with this interpretation, when the order of administration of the two labelled 5-amino-laevulinates was inverted, a greater loss of ^{14}C (as compared with that of ^{3}H) was found (DE MATTEIS, 1973).

In contrast to the results obtained by prelabelling heme with [^{3}H]- and [^{14}C]-5-aminolaevulinate, when the liver hemes were prelabelled with ^{59}Fe, no increase was noted in the radioactivity of the "green pigments" fraction after administra-tion of AIA, suggesting that these derivatives of heme (or at least that fraction recovered after SCHWARTZ's isolation procedure involving extraction into strong acid) have lost most of their iron.

In more recent work (UNSELD and DE MATTEIS, 1975), two additional ap-proaches have been followed in order to isolate the "green pigments", one of them involving a milder extraction procedure. The pigments have then been partially characterized by fluorescence and absorption spectroscopy and their relationship to preformed heme again investigated by isotopic studies. The first technique in-volved extraction of the liver microsomes with 10% acetic acid in acetone followed by column chromatography of the extract on dibutylaminohydroxypropyl Sephadex LH-20 in the acetate form, a gel with anion-exchange properties (ALME and NYSTROM, 1971), which is capable of separating unesterified porphyrins according to their number of carboxyl groups (Fig. 1). The microsomal extracts after incuba-tion with AIA in vitro (or after treatment of rats with AIA in vivo) showed, in addition to the normal brown band of heme, a more rapidly eluted green band. Both bands exhibited a strong absorption around 400 nm, but neither of them fluoresced when excited at around 400 nm. In experiments in which the liver heme had been prelabelled with 5-amino[4-^{14}C]laevulinate, [^{14}C]-labelling was seen in both bands; treatment with AIA caused a loss of radioactivity and also of absorb-ance at 400 nm from the heme band and a corresponding gain in both absorbance and radioactivity in the "green pigment" fraction (Fig. 2).

The "green pigments" could also be separated from heme by thin-layer chromato-graphy of a chloroform extract after methylation of the whole liver. In this system, AIA-treatment resulted in the appearance of several green bands, all of which showed red fluorescence under u.v. light. The most intense of these, when extracted into chloroform, exhibited a visible spectrum of the aetio-type and when excited at 416 nm fluoresced with a maximum of 654 nm. The absorbance maxima of this pigment showed a shift towards the red when compared with those of protopor-phyrin (Table 2), similar to what has been reported for porphyrins bearing elec-tronwithdrawing substituents in their 2 and 4 positions. In experiments involving

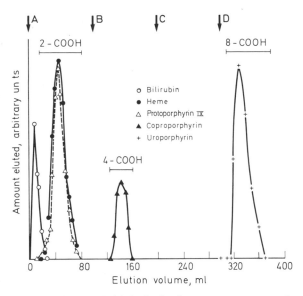

Fig. 1. Differential elution of several biologically important tetrapyrroles from a column (10 cm long, 1 cm internal diameter) of dibutylaminohy roxypropyl-Sephadex LH 20 in the acetate form. The various compounds were applied dissolved in 0.5 ml of 10% glacial acetic acid in acetone. Elution was with 10% acetic acid in acetone (↑A), followed by 20% acetic acid in acetone (↑B), 20% acetic acid in methanol (↑C), and 40% acetic acid in methanol (↑D) (Poole, T.W. and De Matteis, F., unpublished)

prelabelling of liver heme with 5-amino[4-^{14}C]laevulinate, [^{14}C]radioactivity was found to be associated with both heme and green-pigment bands on thin-layer chromatography. However, whereas on the control plate more than 90% of the total radioactivity was present in heme, this was less than 40% after AIA treatment, when a further 48% of radioactivity was present in the green-pigment bands.

Therefore, the isotopic studies showed a close correlation between the loss of label from pre-existing heme and the gain of radioactivity in "green pigment" fractions when they were separated by either 1) the technique of Schwartz and Ikeda (1955), or the more recently employed techniques of 2) thinlayer chromatography and 3) column chromatography. However, red fluorescence and an aetio-type spectrum, compatible with free porphyrins (rather than metallo-porphyrins), were only observed when the "green pigments" were obtained by techniques 1) and 2) above, which involve treatment with strong acid[1]; they were not seen when they were isolated by technique 3) involving the relatively mild procedure of colum chromatography, unless they were subsequently subjected to treatment with strong acid (Unseld and De Matteis, 1975). It seems likely, therefore, that the column pigment(s) are an intermediary between heme and the porphyrin-like struc-

---

[1] Fluorescence and absorption data compatible with free porphyrins have also been reported by Schwartz and Ikeda (1955) and by McDonagh et al. (1976) for "green pigments" isolated by extraction with 7.5 N HCl. In fact, the absorption spectrum reported by the latter authors for two of their pigments appears identical to the aetio-type spectrum exhibited by our major band on thin-layer chromatography.

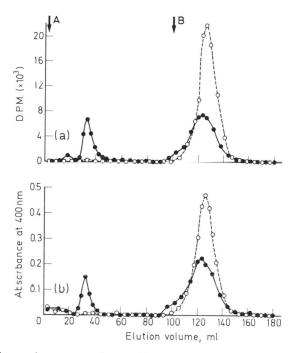

Fig. 2a and b. Column chromatography on dibutylaminohydroxypropyl-Sephadex LH 20 of extracts of microsomal pellet after incubation with NADPH and AIA (●) or with NADPH alone (○). Elution was with 5% acetic acid in acetone (↑A), followed by 10% acetic acid in acetone (↑B). Fractions were examined for (a) disintegrations per minute after prelabelling with 5-amino[4-¹⁴C]laevulinate and (b) absorption at 400 nm (from UNSELD and DE MATTEIS 1975 reproduced by permission of S. Karger AG, Basel)

Table 2. Absorption maxima of main green pigment obtained by thin-layer chromatography of a CHCl₃ extract after methylation of livers from AIA-treated rats. Comparison with the methyl esters of two authentic porphyrins

Pigment	Type of spectrum	Absorbance maxima (nm) in CHCl₃	References
Protoporphyrin	Aetio	407, 505, 541, 575, 630	FALK, 1964
Main Green Pigment	Aetio	416, 512, 546, 592, 650	UNSELD and DE MATTEIS, 1975
2:4-Diformyldeutero-porphyrin	Aetio	? , 525, 562, 595, 651	LEMBERG and FALK, 1951

tures which are produced by more vigorous chemical treatment. The former may still contain iron in a loosely bound form; the iron may then be lost upon treatment with strong acid (see also DE MATTEIS, 1971a), and this would result in the appearance of fluorescence and of an aetio-type spectrum. These concepts are summarized in Fig. 3, where the relationship of the two main types of green pigments to each other and to preformed heme are schematically represented. More

$$\text{Heme} \xrightarrow[\text{acetamide}]{\text{2-allyl-2-isopropyl-}} \begin{array}{c}\text{modified heme} \\ \text{(column pigment)}\end{array} \xrightarrow[\text{acids}]{\text{strong}} \begin{array}{c}\text{modified} \\ \text{porphyrins}\end{array} + \text{Fe}$$

(t.l.c. pigments)

Fig. 3. Hypothetic relationship of the two main types of green pigments to each other and to preformed heme (after De Matteis and Unseld, 1976)

support for this concept has recently been obtained (Unseld and De Matteis, unpublished) by prelabelling the liver heme with ^{59}Fe; on treatment with AIA, there was a loss of label from heme and a gain of radioactivity in association with the green band isolated by the mild procedure of column chromatography, but the [^{59}Fe] radioactivity was largely lost from the "green pigments" on treatment with strong acid encountered in the process of methylation.

In experiments involving prelabelling of liver heme with 5-amino[4-^{14}C]laevulinate, at least 60% of the total nonheme radioactivity of the liver from treated rats could be recovered in pigments with a porphyrin-like spectrum after thin-layer chromatography (De Matteis and Unseld, 1976). It can therefore be concluded that the bulk of the derivatives of heme produced by the action of AIA still retain the closed tetrapyrrolic structure. On the other hand, Landaw et al. (1970) reported that AIA-treated rats given [2-^{14}C]glycine exhaled strongly labelled CO, which might be expected to be produced from the cleavage of any of the four methine bridges of heme. This may indicate that a small proportion of the heme that is attacked by AIA may in the process undergo cleavage or, alternatively, that opening of the ring does not take place during conversion of heme into green pigments but at a later stage during their further metabolism.

3. Importance of the Allyl Group and Role of the Drug-Metabolizing Activity of the Liver

Results obtained with several acetamides and barbiturates chemically related to AIA indicate the importance of the allyl group in the molecule of these drugs for both destruction of cytochrome P-450 and conversion of heme to "green pigments" (Abbritti and De Matteis, 1971). The way in which the allyl group is implicated is not yet known. However, evidence has been obtained both in vivo and in vitro (De Matteis, 1971 a; Abbritti and De Matteis, 1971) which suggests (even though it does not conclusively prove) that the allyl group may require conversion by way of drug metabolism into an active agent which is, in turn, responsible for heme destruction. The first line of evidence is represented by the finding that the effect of AIA on cytochrome P-450 is influenced by treatments known to alter the activity of the microsomal drug-metabolizing system. Pretreatment of rats with either phenobarbitone or DDT, which stimulate drug metabolism in the liver microsomal fraction, greatly increased the loss of cytochrome P-450 caused by AIA, whereas compound SKF-525 A, an inhibitor of drug-metabolizing enzymes, decreased the loss. The second line of evidence is given by results obtained in vitro. When rat-liver microsomes were incubated with either AIA or an allyl-containing analogue of AIA, a loss of cytochrome P-450 and a brown-green discolouration of the micro-

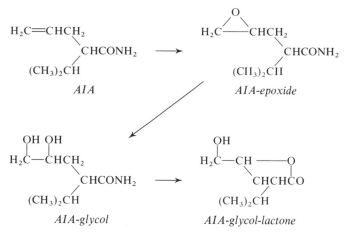

Fig. 4. Metabolism of AIA in the rat (after DOEDENS, 1971)

somal pellet were observed only when NADPH, the co-factor essential for metabolism of drugs by the microsomes, was also present. These results have been confirmed and extended by LEVIN et al. (1972b and 1973a), who have also found that the allyl group is essential for the destruction of cytochrome P-450 heme by several barbiturates. They also suggested that the allyl group may require metabolism to some reactive derivative in order to cause destruction of heme, and, in support of this, have reported the following additional evidence: In a purified reconstituted microsomal system secobarbital, an allyl-containing barbiturate was found to cause destruction of P-450 in the presence of NADPH only when cytochrome P-450 reductase and a purified lipid fraction were also present. All these constituents must be present simultaneously for a drug to be metabolized.

If metabolism of the allyl group is in fact involved, what is then the reactive metabolite? An epoxide would be an attractive candidate (DE MATTEIS, 1973; LEVIN et al., 1973a), since it is known that olefins can be oxidized to epoxides (DALY, 1971), and that certain epoxides are alkylating agents under physiological conditions. DOEDENS (1971) has studied the metabolism of AIA by the rat and has obtained strong evidence that AIA is metabolized to an epoxide (Fig. 4). Similarly, secobarbital and other allyl-containing barbiturates (FOREMAN and MAYNERT, 1970; HARVEY et al., 1972) have been reported to be metabolized to epoxides. It is possible, then, that epoxides are involved in the destruction of cytochrome P-450 heme by these allyl-containing drugs. However, no direct evidence for this role of epoxides has yet been obtained.

Recent findings (IVANETICH et al., 1975) indicate that Fluroxene (2,2,2-trifluoroethyl vinyl ether), an anaesthetic containing the unsaturated vinyl grouping, can also cause destruction of cytochrome P-450 both in vivo and in vitro. As previously shown for the AIA group of drugs, the unsaturated grouping is specifically required for this effect, the destruction of P-450 is stimulated by pretreatment with phenobarbitone, and the effect in vitro requires the presence of NADPH. IVANETICH et al. (1975) also suggest the possible activation of the unsaturated grouping to a reactive epoxide.

4. Possible Mechanisms Underlying the Loss of Heme

The exact mechanism by which destruction of heme and conversion of heme to green pigments are brought about by AIA is not known. Several possibilities were considered (De Matteis, 1971), and it is now useful to re-examine these in the light of the more recent evidence (Unseld and De Matteis, 1975; De Matteis and Unseld, 1976; McDonagh et al., 1976) on the nature of the "green pigments". First, the drug or a derivative therefrom (by becoming bound to components of the membrane and altering it) might expose the cytochrome P-450 heme to coupled oxidation by endogenously occurring reductants, such as ascorbate or NADPH. This mechanism would be expected to result, however, in cleavage of the tetra-pyrrolic ring at one of the methine bridges, which would then result in the evolution of carbon monoxide, as has been reported in the coupled oxidation of heme or hemoproteins (Schmid and McDonagh, 1975); in contrast, the recent isotopic and spectral data on the "green pigments" suggest that most of these derivatives of heme retain the closed tetrapyrrolic structure.

A second possibility is that the structure of heme might be altered by peroxides (derived from either the drug itself or components of the membranes, such as lipids), if these were produced as a result of the metabolism of AIA. Levin et al. (1973b) have obtained evidence which suggests that lipid peroxidation is not involved in the degradation of heme caused by secobarbital, and Schacter et al. (1973) have concluded that the degradation of heme which takes place during lipid peroxidation is accompanied by cleavage of one methene bridge of heme to generate carbon monoxide, a mechanism of degradation which would not be compatible with the type of pigments obtained by the action of AIA. However, there is no conclusive evidence that the carbon monoxide produced during lipid peroxidation does in fact originate from heme, and Levin's data do not exclude the possibility that AIA might produce a selective attack on the structure of heme through reactive species like peroxides or free radicals.

Another possibility is that a reactive derivative of AIA might itself become attached to heme and change its structure. This would explain the spectral changes observed in the green pigments which exhibited a shift towards longer wavelengths (as compared with protoporphyrin) and possibly also the reduced affinity for iron of the modified heme. If most of the molecule of the drug becomes attached to the porphyrin of heme, this would change its solubility characteristics and might account for the very high HCl number which has been reported for the "green pigments" (Schwartz and Ikeda, 1955). On this basis, it would be more difficult to explain the presence of several bands of "green pigments" on thin-layer chromatography, unless the binding of AIA on to heme would take place at different sites, or, once the binding had occurred, subsequent modifications of the chemical structure might take place. This possibility can be tested by finding out whether radioactivity from labelled AIA can be recovered in the purified "green pigments".

II. Carbon Disulphide and Other Sulphur-Containing Chemicals

When carbon disulphide (CS_2) was administered to starved male rats, there was a rapid loss of cytochrome P-450 from the liver microsomes and reduction in the activity of the drug-metabolizing enzymes of the liver (BOND and DE MATTEIS, 1969; FREUNDT and DREHER, 1969). These changes were observed in the absence of any histological lesion. However, when the rats were pretreated with pheno-barbitone in order to stimulate the activity of the liver drug-metabolizing enzymes, administration of CS_2 caused not only a greater loss of cytochrome P-450 (as observed with AIA) but also accumulation of water in the liver a few hours later (BOND and DE MATTEIS, 1969) and, histologically, marked hydropic degenerative changes in the centrilobular zones of the liver (BOND et al., 1969; MAGOS and BUTLER, 1972).

The potentiation of the liver toxicity of CS_2 by pretreatment with pheno-barbitone has been interpreted to indicate that a metabolite of CS_2, rather than CS_2 itself, may be the real toxic agent responsible for the loss of cytochrome P-450 and for the other liver changes considered above (BOND and DE MATTEIS, 1969); a concept in favour of which a number of experimental findings have been obtained in the last three years. In addition, several other sulphur-containing chemicals have recently been found to cause loss of liver cytochrome P-450 and, under appropriate conditions, changes in liver histology. These chemicals share some characteristic features of oxidative metabolism with CS_2 and may be acting by a similar mechanism.

1. Oxidative Desulphuration of CS_2

When a single dose of $[^{14}C]$-labelled CS_2 was administered to intact rats, it was found (DE MATTEIS and SEAWRIGHT, 1973) that CS_2 was partially metabolized to CO_2, and that the extent of conversion to CO_2 was directly related, under a number of experimental conditions, to the amount of cytochrome P-450 present in the liver at the time of CS_2 administration. A correlation was found between the extent of conversion of CS_2 to CO_2 and the degree of toxic liver changes caused by CS_2 (loss of cytochrome P-450 at 2 h and increase in liver water with histologically demonstrable hydropic degeneration at 24 h); phenobarbitone pretreatment, de-signed to enhance the severite of the liver injury, also significantly increased the oxidation of CS_2 to CO_2; both toxicity and oxidative metabolism were decreased by pretreatment with a small "ineffective" dose of CS_2, and both of them were greater in male than in female rats. In addition, CS_2 was also found to cause loss of cytochrome P-450 in vitro when microsomes were incubated aerobically in its presence, but it could only do this markedly when NADPH (the cofactor essential for metabolising chemicals by the mixed-function oxidase system) was also present. All these findings (DE MATTEIS and SEAWRIGHT, 1973) were compatible with the hypothesis of a toxic metabolite of CS_2, even though they do not conclusively prove it. More direct evidence for a toxic derivative is discussed below.

The conversion of CS_2 to CO_2 can be considered as a two-stage desulphura-tion reaction (Fig. 5) analogous to other oxidative desulphurations involving con-version of either P=S to P=O or of C=S to C=O (O'BRIEN, 1961). A typical example is the conversion of parathion to paraoxon which takes place mostly in the liver, is also stimulated by previous treatment with phenobarbitone (POORE and NEAL, 1972), and is catalysed by the microsomal mixed function oxidase system (DAVISON, 1955; O'BRIEN, 1959; NEAL, 1967). PTASHNE et al. (1971) have recently

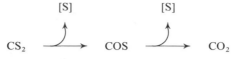

Fig. 5. Proposed pathway of CS_2 oxidative desulphuration (after De Matteis and Seawright 1973). Both sulphur atoms released during the oxidative process are shown in brackets to indicate that they are highly reactive species

suggested a mechanism for the oxidative metabolism of parathion involving the production of free reactive sulphur in the atomic state. By analogy, it has been suggested that CS_2 could give rise to elemental sulphur in two stages through the mono-oxygenated intermediate COS (Fig. 5), and that reactive sulphur liberated at the two stages of the oxidative desulphuration may become bound to cellular components and initiate toxic changes in the liver (De Matteis and Seawright, 1973).

Recent findings provide support for this hypothesis, concerning both the pathway of CS_2 oxidation and also the possible involvement of reactive sulphur in its liver toxicity. When liver microsomes were incubated with either [14]C- or ^{35}S-labelled CS_2 in the presence of NADPH (under conditions, that is, where loss of cytochrome P-450 was observed), labelled sulphur became covalently bound to the microsomes (De Matteis, 1974; Dalvi et al., 1974). Although some increase of ^{14}C binding (over the values obtained on incubation without NADPH) was also observed, the binding of ^{35}S was greatly in excess of that of ^{14}C, indicating that sulphur itself became bound. An even greater excess of ^{35}S over ^{14}C radioactivity was found in the trichloroacetic acid washings from microsomes incubated with NADPH, and some excess of ^{35}S radioactivity was also seen in the organic solvent washings (De Matteis, 1974). In contrast, when fraction V from bovine plasma was substituted for the microsomes, no ^{35}S radioactivity in excess of ^{14}C radioactivity could be demonstrated in either the precipitate or the washings thereof. These observations clearly indicate that on incubation with liver microsomes and NADPH, CS_2 was actively desulphurated, and that a portion of the sulphur liberated became covalently bound to the microsomes or converted to a compound which could then react with the microsomes so as to leave sulphur attached to them. Since ^{35}S radioactivity was found in excess of ^{14}C radioactivity in all fractions, it can also be concluded that most of the corresponding carbon must have been lost from the incubation mixture, probably as the volatile oxidation products COS and CO_2 (see below). Also, since less than 20% of the total recovered "free" sulphur was found bound to the microsomal precipitate, it is clear that, at least under the conditions of our experiments, covalent binding of sulphur to the microsomal precipitate cannot be taken as a quantitative measure of the total desulphuration of CS_2.

The nature of the "free" sulphur in the trichloroacetic acid washings (whether covalently bound to acid-soluble organic molecules or present in an inorganic form) remains to be elucidated. Some information has recently been obtained by Catignani and Neal (1975) on the form in which some of the sulphur is covalently bound to the macromolecules of the microsomes. This will be discussed later, in Section II. 3. Also in favour of the hypothesis outlined in Fig. 5 is the finding that when microsomes were incubated with CS_2 in the presence of NADPH, the production of

COS—the postulated mono-oxygenated intermediate in CS_2 oxidation—could be demonstrated (DALVI et al., 1974).

Finally, COS itself could cause loss of cytochrome P-450 when incubated with liver microsomes in the presence of NADPH. Under these conditions, some of its sulphur became covalently bound to the microsomes (DALVI et al., 1975), while—presumably—the corresponding carbon was fully oxidized to CO_2. These observations are compatible with the two-stage desulphuration of CS_2 outlined in Fig. 5 and demonstrate that both atoms of sulphur present in CS_2 can be liberated in a reactive (and potentially toxic) form.

2. Loss of Cytochrome P-450 During Oxidative Desulphuration of Parathion and of Other Sulphur-Containing Chemicals. Liver Toxicity of Phosphorothionates

In previous works (NAKATSUGAWA and DAHM, 1967; NAKATSUGAWA et al., 1968; POORE and NEAL, 1972), it has been reported that during the oxidative desulphuration of parathion, sulphur became covalently bound to the microsomes. The possible toxicologic significance of this finding had not been suspected. WILLIAMS (1959) had already suggested, however, that oxidative desulphuration might be implicated in the toxic effects of phenylthiourea in the rabbit, and preliminary findings (DE MATTEIS and SEAWRIGHT, 1973) indicated that, like CS_2, phosphorothionates could also cause loss of cytochrome P-450 and hydropic degeneration in rat liver.

These effects have now been found to be shared by several chemicals, which are oxidatively desulphurated by the liver microsomes. In one study (DE MATTEIS, 1974), three pairs of drugs were examined in vitro, each pair consisting of a compound containing sulphur (as either P=S or C=S) and the corresponding oxygen analogue. All three sulphur-containing drugs (parathion, phenylthiourea, and 1-naphthylisothiocyanate) caused loss of cytochrome P-450 in the presence of NADPH, whereas the oxygen-containing analogues (paraoxon, phenylurea and 1-naphthylisocyanate) were all inactive. In addition, the loss of cytochrome P-450 caused by parathion could be inhibited by piperonyl butoxide and by replacing air with N_2, and stimulated by either NADH or, to a larger extent, by NADPH (DE MATTEIS, 1974). These same factors have been reported to inhibit and stimulate, respectively, the oxidative desulphuration of parathion to paraoxon in vitro and the covalent binding of sulphur to microsomes which accompanies it (NAKATSUGAWA and DAHM, 1967; NAKATSUGAWA et al., 1968).

The liver effects of an analogue of parathion, such as O,O-diethyl, O-phenyl phosphoro-thionate (SV_1), which possesses a low general toxicity and can therefore be administered to rats in large doses, have also been studied in vivo (SEAWRIGHT et al., 1976). When SV_1 is administered to rats that have previously been dosed with phenobarbitone, it causes—like CS_2—loss of cytochrome P-450 and centrilobular changes in the liver. Phenobarbitone pretreatment is essential for the liver histological lesion to appear, and the lesion is characterized by marked hydropic changes; necrotic cells are uncommon, and fat infiltration is only modest. In all these respects, the SV_1-induced liver lesion is similar to that caused by CS_2 and different from that produced by CCl_4. Loss of cytochrome P-450 has also been reported on incubation of liver microsomes with several other sulphur-containing chemicals in vitro or after their administration to rats in vivo; several of these chemicals were also found to cause histologically demonstrable liver lesions (Hunter and Neal, 1974).

It can therefore be concluded that a similar lesion, characterized by loss of cytochrome P-450 and centrilobular degenerative changes, is produced in rat liver by several compounds containing sulphur as either C=S (like CS_2) or as P=S (like phosphorothionates). Reactive sulphur liberated during the oxidative desulphuration of CS_2 and of a phosphorothionate may become bound to cellular components in vivo and initiate in this way toxic changes in the liver.

3. Possible Mechanisms Underlying the Loss of Cytochrome P-450 Caused by Sulphur-Containing Chemicals. Nature of the Primary Target Within the Hemoprotein

The effect of CS_2 on cytochrome P-450 was found to be specific, or at least preferential, for this cytochrome; there was no or only a slight loss of cytochrome b_5, of total microsomal protein, or of glucose-6-phosphatase activity. In addition, the loss of cytochrome P-450 was very rapid, indicating that it was more likely to result from some change caused by CS_2 in the pre-existing cytochrome rather than from inhibition of cytochrome synthesis (Bond and De Matteis, 1969). In both these respects, the effect of CS_2 is quite similar to that of AIA.

An important difference between these two chemicals is provided, however, by the behaviour of the total heme content of the microsomes. After administration of AIA, the loss of cytochrome P-450 was accompanied by a corresponding loss of microsomal heme as measured by the pyridine hemochrome (see Sect. I. 2); in clear contrast, there was a marked loss of cytochrome P-450 in the first few hours after CS_2 administration, but the loss of heme was relatively small, and the microsomal pellet did not acquire the brown-green discolouration which accompanies the increased degradation of heme under the influence of AIA (Bond and De Matteis, 1969; De Matteis, 1973). These observations suggest that CS_2 does not like AIA, act, by promoting a primary loss of the heme moiety of the cytochrome.

A significant increase in the 420 nm absorption was noted when microsomes from CS_2-treated rats were reduced with dithionite and treated with carbon monoxide. Therefore, as a consequence of CS_2 treatment, there may have been a small increase in cytochrome P-420 (at least relative to the concentration of cytochrome P-450). In no case, however, was the P-420 peak high enough to account for the lost P-450. Therefore, most of the heme of the cytochrome P-450 which had been lost was still present in the microsomal membranes but was apparently unable to develop a characteristic spectrum on reduction and treatment with carbon monoxide. This could either be because the heme cannot bind carbon monoxide (if for example CS_2 or a metabolite were to become bound instead) or because CS_2 has caused some alteration in the protein moiety of the cytochrome leading, to a reduction of its 450 nm absorption, even though the heme moiety can still react with carbon monoxide (Bond and De Matteis, 1969). A third possibility in which both mechanisms above may be simultaneously at play has been considered by Dalvi et al. (1975), who suggest that alterations in the structure of the apoprotein (due to covalent binding of reactive sulphur) may affect the reduction of heme or its availability to the carbon monoxide ligand indirectly, perhaps by a steric mechanism. More work is required to determine which of these possible mechanisms is in fact involved in the loss of cytochrome P-450 caused by CS_2, but the original suggestion (BOND and DE MATTEIS, 1969) that the apoprotein is the primary target of the action of this chemical on cytochrome P-450 is compatible with the following recent finding.

Nearly half of the total sulphur bound to the microsomes can be released as thiocyanate on incubation with cyanide (CATIGNANI and NEAL, 1975). This has been interpreted to indicate that a portion of the sulphur released during the metabolism of CS_2 reacts with the sulphydryl groups of cysteine residues in the microsomal protein to form a hydrodisulphide.

III. Loss of Cytochrome P-450 Heme Caused by Carbon Tetrachloride in Rat Liver

Since the detailed report that carbon tetrachloride (CCl_4) given to rats will cause a centrilobular liver necrosis (CAMERON and KARUNARATNE, 1936), very many investigations have appeared on chemical and morphologic changes caused in the liver by this chemical. Most of these are beyond the scope of this paper, where only the changes in microsomal heme components (caused by CCl_4) have been considered.

SMUCKLER et al. (1967) first reported that after CCl_4 administration there was a rapid loss of cytochrome P-450, and that this was paralleled by a decreased activity of the microsomal oxidative demethylation, although there was no early change in cytochrome b_5. These findings have been confirmed by several authors. In addition, GREENE et al. (1969) and LEVIN et al. (1972a) showed that the loss of cytochrome P-450 was accompanied by a corresponding loss of microsomal heme (measured by the pyridine hemochrome or by the radioactivity recovered as purified microsomal heme, respectively). LEVIN et al. (1972a) also found that, as with AIA, the degradation products of heme were still largely present in the washed microsomes isolated after CCl_4 treatment. The labelled breakdown products were not characterized, but they did not appear to impart the same green colour to the microsomes as did AIA treatment. This may indicate that even though AIA and CCl_4 both induce a rapid loss of heme of cytochrome P-450, they may do so by a different mechanism. The extent of the microsomal damage appears to be greater with CCl_4 where, in contrast with what is found after administering AIA, a rapid loss of microsomal protein (LEVIN et al., 1972a) and of glucose-6-phosphatase activity (RECKNAGEL and LOMBARDI, 1961) is also observed. The possible significance of microsomal lipid peroxidation in causing the loss of heme (see also Sect. C) and the extensive membrane damage seen after CCl_4 is briefly considered below.

There is evidence that, as discussed for AIA and CS_2, the activity of the drug-metabolizing system is important also for the destruction of cytochrome P-450 caused by CCl_4. Thus, prior stimulation of the drug-metabolizing system with phenobarbitone (SASAME et al., 1968) increased the loss of cytochrome P-450 caused by CCl_4, whereas pretreatment with aminotriazole, which reduces the activity of the system (BARON and TEPHLY, 1969) afforded protection (DE TORANZO et al.,

1975). These findings suggested that activation of CCl_4 through metabolism was involved in the destruction of cytochrome P-450, a concept already put forward by Butler (1961) for liver toxicity of CCl_4 in general and supported by the findings of McLean and McLean (1966). Seawright and McLean (1967), Garner and McLean (1969), and others. The most favoured view is that the first step in the metabolic activation is a cleavage of the chlorine-carbon bond generating a reactive species, probably a trichloromethyl radical (Butler, 1961; Fowler, 1969). This can then either react with a hydrogen donor to form $CHCl_3$ (Uehleke et al., 1973) or become covalently bound to components of the microsomes, such as proteins and lipids (reviewed by Shah and Carlson, 1975) and initiate a chain reaction of peroxidation of the membrane polyunsaturated fatty acids; this lipid peroxidation may overcome the antioxidant defences of the liver and therefore diffuse in an autocatalytic fashion, producing extensive membrane damage and cell death (Recknagel, 1967; Slater, 1972). One point of disagreement among different authors is whether activation of CCl_4 to the trichloromethyl radical takes place at the cytochrome P-450 locus (McLean, 1967; Reiner and Uehleke, 1971) or at the site of the flavoprotein NADPH-cytochrome c reductase (Slater and Sawyer, 1971; Shah and Carlson, 1975).

Another point of dispute is whether covalent binding of reactive metabolites of CCl_4 to the microsomes is sufficient to cause the loss of cytochrome P-450 and the other disruptive changes in the membranes (De Toranzo et al., 1975), or whether lipid peroxidation is an obligatory prerequisite for these effects. The latter possibility appears more likely in view of the finding that under conditions where lipid peroxidation is prevented, for instance in presence of EDTA (Uehleke et al., 1973) or of anaerobiosis (Recknagel et al., 1975), CCl_4 is metabolized by liver microsomes, and covalent binding of its metabolite(s) is observed without any loss of cytochrome P-450 or of glucose-6-phosphatase activity. Also in favour of the importance of lipid peroxidation are the findings—to be discussed in Section C—that a loss of cytochrome P-450 heme and of glucose-6-phosphatase is also observed in the absence of CCl_4, when lipid peroxidation is allowed to take place either in isolated microsomes or in intact liver cells incubated in vitro. Therefore, it appears probable that the role of metabolism of CCl_4 is to produce a free radical initiator of lipid peroxidation, while the ensuing peroxidation of the lipids is responsible for the loss of heme and of the other membrane constituents. The mechanism by which lipid peroxides cause loss of heme will also be discussed in Section C.

C. Increased Breakdown of the Heme of Liver Cytochrome P-450 Associated with Lipid Peroxidation

I. Lipid Peroxidation in vitro

In the course of a study on the effect of 2-allyl-2-isopropylacetamide on cytochrome P-450, it was found that when either microsomes or post-mitochondrial supernatants of liver were incubated aerobically in the presence of NADPH, there was a loss of cytochrome P-450 (De Matteis, 1970 and 1971a). It was subsequently

found (DE MATTEIS, 1972) that the rate of loss of cytochrome P-450, observed
in vitro under these conditions, varied according to the species and to the nutritional state of the animal and correlated with the formation of lipid peroxide;
both lipid peroxidation and loss of cytochrome were greater with either mouse or
rat microsomes than with rabbit microsomes (see also LEVIN et al., 1973b), and
both were stimulated by a 24 h starvation. In addition, both required NADPH,
could be stimulated by the addition of $FeSO_4$ or NADH (the latter only in the
presence of NADPH), and completely prevented by two iron chelators, EDTA and
desferrioxamine (DE MATTEIS and SPARKS, 1973).

Loss of cytochrome P-450 during lipid peroxidation was also observed by
SCHACTER et al. (1972, 1973) and by LEVIN et al. (1973b), who reported a corresponding loss of microsomal heme as determined either by the pyridine hemochrome reaction or by a loss of radioactivity from microsomal heme prelabelled
with ^{3}H-5-aminolaevulinate given in vivo. SCHACTER et al. (1973) also found that
the evolution of CO, already reported by NISHIBAYASHI et al. (1968) during microsomal lipid peroxidation, takes place in an amount very nearly equimolar to the
heme lost; they concluded that there was degradation of the heme molecule by
cleavage of the tetrapyrrole ring at only one of the methene bridges. No further
characterization of the breakdown products was attempted.

REINER et al. (1972) also reported that the loss of microsomal cytochrome
P-450 could be initiated by the action of lipoxygenase from soybean on linoleic
acid when both were added to the microsomes in the incubation mixture, while
FONG et al. (1973) showed that, when lysosomes were incubated together with
microsomes, free radical-like species produced during the oxidation of NADPH
by the microsomes could be responsible for peroxidative changes in the membrane
of the lysosomes, leading to their lysis. These observations seem to me of great
interest, as they suggest that the peroxidative chain reaction can spread from the
microsomal membranes to lipid components present on their outside and, vice
versa, from the outside to components of the membranes, a phenomenon of possible great significance in the diffusion of the peroxidative damage in the cell
in vivo.

II. Lipid Peroxidation in vivo

There is evidence that starvation and iron are capable of increasing the degradation of liver heme not only in vitro but also in vivo. Animals subjected to a short-
term starvation showed a significant loss of liver cytochrome P-450 but no change
in either glucose-6-phosphatase or NAD glycohydrolase when these components
were all compared on a whole-liver basis (BOCK et al., 1973). Administration of a
single large dose of iron (as iron-dextran) to rats which were subsequently starved
for 24 h led to a further loss of cytochrome P-450 over that caused by starvation
alone (DE MATTEIS and SPARKS, 1973). In addition, both starvation and iron treatment stimulated the activity of the rate-limiting enzyme of heme biosynthesis,
5-aminolaevulinate synthetase, without any significant increase in liver porphyrin
concentration, a finding which was compatible with an increased rate of liver heme
turnover in both these conditions (DE MATTEIS and SPARKS, 1973). Direct evidence
for this was sought by prelabelling the liver hemes with radioactive 5-aminolaevuli-

nate and by studying the loss of radioactivity caused by starvation or iron overload in the following 24 h (De Matteis, 1975); iron treatment clearly enhanced the degradation of liver heme in vivo; starvation may have also increased the rate of liver heme turnover in vivo, but the effect was small and the results not conclusive. The possibility was considered that both starvation and iron might increase the peroxidation of lipids of microsomal membranes in vivo, as they do in vitro, and that this might then result in an increased rate of liver heme breakdown.

There is no conclusive evidence that under these conditions the peroxidation of lipids is increased in the liver of the intact animal in vivo. This is suggested, however, by several lines of indirect evidence. After starvation the amount of thiobarbituric acid-positive material (a commonly used index of lipid peroxidation) was increased in the liver homogenate (Chvapil et al., 1973). Wills (1972) has reported that after administration of a large dose of iron to mice in vivo, there was a small but significant reduction of oxidative demethylation activity and, when the microsomes obtained from the liver of these animals were incubated in vitro, an increased rate of lipid peroxidation. The difficulty there was to be sure that these changes in lipid peroxidation and microsomal drug metabolism were also present in vivo and were not merely artefacts produced during the preparation of the tissue or during the incubation. After administration of CCl_4, however, when similar changes in lipid peroxide content and drug-metabolizing activity have been found in liver microsomes isolated from poisoned animals, more direct evidence for in vivo lipid peroxidation has recently been provided by the finding that ethane, a degradation product of certain fatty acid peroxides, was exhaled by the intact animal in vivo (Riely et al., 1974). The exhalation of ethane could be markedly reduced by administering vitamin E to CCl_4-poisoned animals (Hafeman and Hoekstra, 1975), an agent which can prevent lipid peroxidation in vitro (Tappel, 1972; McCay et al., 1972).

In isolated surviving hepatocytes incubated in vitro, iron markedly stimulated lipid peroxide accumulation when the cell glutathione content was depleted, for example, by treatment with diethylmaleate (Högberg et al., 1975). This is of interest since during starvation, when the rate of lipid peroxidation may increase in the liver, the liver glutathione content is decreased (Jaeger et al., 1973; Tateishi et al., 1974). Högberg (1975) has also reported the presence of small amounts of malondialdchyde (a degradation product of lipid peroxide) in surviving hepatocytes, even when no exogenous iron was added. This also suggests that a limited amount of lipid peroxidation may be of normal occurrence in vivo, especially when the cellular levels of antioxidants, like reduced glutathione (GSH), are decreased.

III. Mechanisms Underlying the Production and Decomposition of Lipid Peroxides and the Associated Destruction of Heme

The enzymic initiation of lipid peroxidation and its relationship to the mechanism of drug metabolism are being actively investigated by several groups of workers, and the picture to date is far from clear. In this discussion, the emphasis will be placed on those points which appear to have been more clearly established and, particularly, on the possible mechanism by which lipid peroxidation may lead to increased heme breakdown.

The relationship of lipid peroxidation to drug metabolism will be considered first. There are a number of similarities between the two processes. Both of them can be carried out in vitro by isolated liver microsomes in the presence of O_2 and NADPH; components of the electron transport system of the microsomes, such as the flavoprotein NADPH-cytochrome-c reductase, are required in both cases, and an activated form of oxygen (see below) may be involved in both reactions. In addition, under certain conditions, reducing equivalents from NADH can apparently be utilized for both processes. The main difference—apart from the ultimate fate of oxygen which is oxidation of polyunsaturated fatty acids in one case and oxidation of lipid-soluble drugs in the other—is that lipid peroxidation requires a loosely bound pool of microsomal iron, whereas drug-metabolism apparently does not. When this pool of iron is chelated, for example by EDTA, lipid peroxidation is completely prevented (WILLS, 1969a), but microsomal oxidation of drugs is not inhibited (KAMATAKI and KITAGAWA, 1973). Since lipid peroxidation can be very effectively stimulated by ferrous iron in the absence of NADPH (BELOFF-CHAIN et al., 1965), it is likely that the function of the flavoprotein (PEDERSON et al., 1973), is to provide the reducing equivalents from NADPH to the ferric iron, reducing it to the ferrous state; Fe^{2+} would then initiate the peroxidation of lipids, possibly through the formation (during the reoxidation of Fe^{2+} by oxygen) of a reactive intermediate, such as the perferryl ion, FeO_2^{2+} (PEDERSON and AUST, 1975).

Under conditions where lipid peroxidation and drug-metabolism can both take place, for example, when microsomes are incubated aerobically in the presence of NADPH but without an excess of iron chelators, the intensity of one process is inversely related to that of the other. An increased rate of lipid peroxidation will cause a decrease in drug-metabolizing activity (WILLS, 1969b; KAMATAKI and KITAGAWA, 1973) and, conversely, when drug-metabolism is stimulated, for example, by adding to the system a drug which can be readily metabolized, the extent of lipid peroxidation will be reduced (ORRENIUS et al., 1964). The first effect results largely from the progressive inactivation of cytochrome P-450 and of other components of the drug-metabolizing system during the peroxidative damage of the membranes (LEVIN et al., 1973b; HÖGBERG et al., 1973). The second may reflect in part the fact that both processes draw reducing equivalents from the same electron transport system and may therefore compete (ORRENIUS et al., 1964); another possible explanation is the production during the metabolism of drugs of metabolites with antioxidant properties, which will inhibit lipid peroxidation (PEDERSON and AUST, 1974).

The relationship of lipid peroxidation to heme and hemoproteins is a complex one. There is evidence from studies conducted with simplified systems, where both the heme and the lipid components are in a soluble form, that heme can catalyse formation of lipid peroxides as well as their decomposition, and that in the process, part of the heme becomes degraded (TAPPEL, 1955; KOKATNUR et al., 1966; HAUROWITZ et al., 1973). How relevant are these observations to the situation in the microsomes, where both lipids and hemoproteins are membrane bound? There is no evidence that the heme of the microsomes is required for the initiation of lipid peroxidation (NILSSON et al., 1964; PEDERSON et al., 1973), but recent findings suggest that cytochrome P-450 may be involved both in the decomposition of lipid peroxides (HRYCAY and O'BRIEN, 1971) and also in the generation of lipid per-

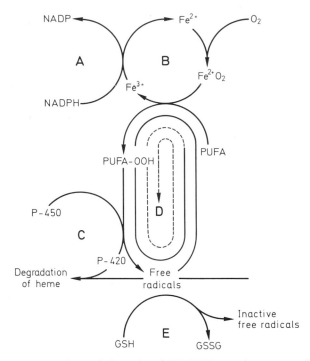

Fig. 6. Schematic representation of the role of NADPH-cytochrome *c* reductase (A), non-heme iron (B), cytochrome P-450 (C), and GSH peroxidase (E) in the generation and inactivation of lipid peroxides. The chain reaction of lipid peroxide propagation is also illustrated (D). In the process, poly-unsaturated fatty acids (PUFA) are converted to hydroperoxides (PUFA-OOH), and these and the heme of cytochrome P-450 are then degraded (see text)

oxides from organic peroxides (RADTKE and COON, 1974). Both these reactions are of a peroxidative type and are accompanied by a substantial destruction of heme. HRYCAY and O'BRIEN (1971) have proposed a mechanism for the peroxidative breakdown of lipid peroxides in which the first step is the oxidation by the lipid peroxide of the thiol ligand of the heme of cytochrome P-450 to produce the high-spin form of P-420, a very powerful peroxidase. The latter can then decompose the lipid peroxide, producing free radical intermediates which are then responsible for destruction of heme (Fig. 6). HRYCAY and O'BRIEN (1971) have also shown that various hydrogen donors, such as N,N,N',N'-tetramethyl-*p*-phenylenediamine (TMPD), or GSH can protect the hemoprotein from destruction, presumably by inactivating the oxidizing species involved in the breakdown of heme.

In summary (Fig. 6), nonheme iron appears to be the main site of initiation of lipid peroxidation, whereas cytochrome P-450 may be involved (after conversion to P-420) in the breakdown of both lipid peroxides and heme and also possibly in the diffusion of the peroxidative damage through the generation of new lipid peroxides. Protective agents like GSH may act by preventing conversion of P-450 to P-420 and also by inactivating and destroying peroxides and free radical species involved in the oxidative damage to components of the membrane, the latter effect occurring mostly in conjunction with the selenium containing enzyme, glutathione peroxidase (ROTRUCK et al., 1973; LITTLE and O'BRIEN, 1968).

A limited and controlled amount of lipid peroxidation may have a physiological role to play in the liver cell in vivo. Recent studies (KADLUBAR et al., 1973; RAHIMTULA and O'BRIEN, 1975; HRYCAY et al., 1975; ELLIN and ORRENIUS, 1975) have shown that cytochrome P-450 can utilize certain organic hydroperoxides for the hydroxylation of several drugs, steroids, and fatty acids, all of which are normally metabolized by the microsomal mixed-function oxidase system. Whether lipid peroxides can also be utilized in this and similar reactions is not known. It is possible that lipid peroxidation may have a role in the normal turnover of the membranes of the endoplasmic reticulum, and HRYCAY and O'BRIEN (1971) have suggested that degradation of cytochrome P-450 during lipid peroxidation may account for the high rate of turnover of this hemoprotein one observes in the liver under normal conditions (LEVIN and KUNTZMAN, 1969).

Tissue damage of different degrees may be expected to occur whenever the peroxidative process exceeds the antioxidant defences of the body. This may result either from an excess of a prooxidant (like exogenous iron or CCl_4), or from a deficiency of a body constituent with antioxidant properties: vitamin E in vitamin E deficiency (TAPPEL, 1972; HAFEMAN and HOEKSTRA, 1975) and shortage of GSH or inosine (JOSE et al., 1973) in starvation; and decreased activity of glutathione peroxidase in selenium deficiency (ROTRUCK et al., 1973; SCOTT et al., 1974). Administration of certain metals may also be expected to result in decreased content of GSH and may be responsible for loss of cytochrome P-450, partly through increased lipid peroxidation. This will be discussed in the following section.

D. Loss of Liver Cytochrome P-450 Caused by the Administration of Various Metals

I. Increased Rate of Liver Heme Turnover and Stimulation of Heme Oxygenase

Iron is not the only metal capable of causing loss of liver cytochrome P-450 when administered to the whole animal in vivo. A similar effect has been reported after adminstering cobaltous chloride (TEPHLY and HIBBELN, 1971), lead nitrate (SCOPPA et al., 1973), and also salts of the following metals: manganese, nickel, copper, zinc, mercury (MAINES and KAPPAS, 1975a), and cadmium (HADLEY et al., 1974). A decreased concentration of liver cytochrome P-450 has also been described after administration of methylmercury (LUCIER et al., 1973). There is evidence that several of these metals inhibit the synthesis of heme in the liver; lead, for example, is an inhibitor of 5-aminolaevulinate dehydratase (SCOPPA et al., 1973) and possibly also of the chelatase, whereas cobalt inhibits both the formation of 5-aminolaevulinate (NAKAMURA et al., 1975; DE MATTEIS and GIBBS, 1976) and also the incorporation of 5-aminolaevulinate into heme (TEPHLY et al., 1973), the latter effect probably by competing with iron for protoporphyrin (DE MATTEIS and GIBBS, 1976). So it is likely that, as discussed by TEPHLY and by SASSA in Chapters 3 and 11, respectively, the decrease in cytochrome P-450 concentration caused by these two metals may result in part from an inhibition of the synthesis of the heme moiety of the hemoprotein.

There is also evidence, however, that cobalt and lead, as well as methylmercury, stimulate the turnover of liver heme in vivo, and this effect probably contributes significantly to the loss of hemoprotein reported after the administration of these agents. Thus, rats given a single dose of cobaltous chloride showed a few hours later a stimulation of the activity of heme oxygenase (the rate-limiting enzyme of heme degradation) when this enzyme was assayed with liver preparations in vitro (MAINES and KAPPAS, 1975b). The following findings (DE MATTEIS and GIBBS, 1976) demonstrated that under these conditions the rate of liver heme breakdown was also increased in vivo: 1) in rats given cobalt the biliary excretion of bilirubin was nearly doubled, as compared with control values; 2) after cobalt treatment more radioactivity from 5-amino[4-^{14}C]-laevulinate appeared in the bile as bilirubin and less remained in the liver; 3) the time course of the uptake and loss of radioactivity in the liver heme of intact rats given labelled 5-aminolaevulinate also indicated accelerated heme turnover after cobalt treatment; 4) finally, cobalt was found to cause loss of radioactivity from prelabelled liver hemoproteins, suggesting that the heme of cytochrome P-450 itself may become degraded at a faster rate after administration of this metal. This latter finding is similar to what has been reported after administration of iron-dextran, which also stimulated markedly the activity of liver heme oxygenase (DE MATTEIS, 1975).

Similar findings of a stimulation of liver heme oxygenase and of increased rate of heme turnover in vivo have been reported after administration of several other metals which are known to decrease the concentration of cytochrome P-450 in the liver. When rats were poisoned with methylmercury (LUCIER et al., 1973) or with lead nitrate (PENNING and SCOPPA, 1975), and the rate of decline of heme radioactivity was studied in a microsomal fraction containing cytochrome P-450 as the only hemoprotein, this was found to be considerably greater than in control animals, suggesting that the rate of turnover of cytochrome P-450 was accelerated under these conditions. PENNING and SCOPPA (1975) also found that microsomes isolated from the liver of lead-poisoned animals, when incubated in the presence of NADPH, could form malondialdehyde and degrade cytochrome P-450 in vitro at rates significantly greater than those seen with control microsomes. In addition, a single dose of alpha-tocopherol given to lead-poisoned rats markedly decreased the loss of cytochrome P-450 due to lead treatment. These observations suggested the possible involvement of lipid peroxidation in the degradation of cytochrome P-450 caused by lead in vivo.

Recent findings have indicated that like cobalt and iron, mercury, lead, manganese, nickel, copper, zinc, and cadmium will also stimulate the activity of liver heme oxygenase (MAINES and KAPPAS, 1975a; 1976). Therefore, all these metals have two properties in common: they stimulate the rate of heme degradation in the liver, and they cause loss of cytochrome P-450. Before discussing the possible ways in which these two effects may be related, it is necessary to consider some additional experimental conditions where low levels of liver cytochrome P-450 have been described in association with a stimulation of heme oxygenase in the liver.

II. Other Experimental Conditions Where Stimulation of Heme Oxygenase is Seen in Association with Decreased Levels of Cytochrome P-450

One of these conditions is starvation, where, as discussed in Sections C I and C II, the rate of degradation of the heme moiety of cytochrome P-450 increases in vitro and possibly also in vivo, and the total amount of cytochrome decreases in the liver. BAKKEN et al. (1972) have reported a two- to three-fold stimulation of heme oxygenase after starvation and have obtained evidence that starvation may act by an hormonal mechanism involving glucagon and/or epinephrine through the mediation of cyclic AMP. Cyclic AMP itself was found to be effective in stimulating heme oxygenase when given to rats in vivo. It may be relevant to point out in this connection that cyclic AMP given intraperitoneally to rats has been reported in another study (WEINER et al., 1972) to cause a rapid inhibition of the liver metabolism of hexobarbitone both in the intact animal and in the isolated perfused liver, and that in further work (ROSS et al., 1973) carried out however with larger doses of cyclic AMP given over a longer experimental period, the nucleotide was also found to cause a depression of cytochrome P-450.

Loss of cytochrome P-450 is accompanied by stimulation of heme oxygenase in the experiments of BISSELL et al. (1974) on primary cultures of rat hepatocytes and also in intact rats. In the culture system, the heme oxygenase activity rose four to six fold during the first 24 h of incubation, and the increase in enzyme activity was preceded by a fall of cytochrome P-450 to about 15% of the initial level. In the animal experiments, the heme of liver cytochrome P-450 was pre-labelled with 5-amino-[5-^{14}C]-laevulinate, and 18 h later a stimulator of liver heme oxygenase (either heme, hemoglobin or endotoxin) was given; this resulted in an increased degradation of cytochrome P-450 heme (measured either by the exhalation of ^{14}CO or directly by a loss of radioactivity from the heme isolated from liver cytochrome P-450) before a stimulation of heme oxygenase activity could be demonstrated. It is important to stress that in these studies degradation of P-450 heme preceeded the stimulation of heme oxygenase, a point of some significance to which I will come back later.

III. Possible Mechanisms by Which Loss of Cytochrome P-450 and Stimulation of Heme Oxygenase may be Related

Before discussing the mechanisms involved in the stimulation of heme oxygenase, there are two main areas of uncertainty which need to be considered. Firstly, heme oxygenase is apparently a constituent of both the parenchymal and reticuloendothelial types of liver cells (BISSELL et al., 1972; HUPKA and KARLER, 1973), and it is not known for certain whether the stimulation of heme oxygenase, which one finds in liver homogenates under the various experimental conditions considered in Sections D I and D II, reflects an increased activity of the enzyme in the RE cells, in the parenchymal cells, or in both. The second point, which is not entirely clear, is whether heme is necessarily involved as the ultimate effective stimulus in the induction of heme oxygenase (also after administration of nonheme inducers, like cobalt and endotoxin) or whether the enzyme can also be stimulated by some other mechanism in which heme is not involved. In the discussion which follows, the assumptions will be made that 1) the stimulation of heme oxygenase is mediated either by heme itself or by an inducer closely related to heme, and 2) that the stimulation takes place (like the loss of cytochrome P-450) mostly in the parenchymal cells of the liver. At the present state of knowledge both these assumptions seem to me quite justified.[2]

The correlation which has been reported under a number of experimental conditions between loss of cytochrome P-450 and stimulation of heme oxygenase, suggests strongly that these two effects may be causally related (see BISSELL et al., 1974). If they are in fact related, this may be in one of two different ways. An increased degradation of cytochrome P-450 may somehow lead to an increased activity of heme oxygenase, possibly by making more heme available for the induction of the enzyme, or, conversely, the increased heme oxygenase activity may lead to increased degradation of the heme of cytochrome P-450 and therefore to loss of the hemoprotein. In these two mechanisms, the heme of cytochrome P-450 can therefore be visualized mainly as an inducer or as a substrate for heme oxygenase.

1. The Heme of Cytochrome P-450 as an Inducer for Heme Oxygenase

In the experiments by BISSELL et al. (1974), evidence was obtained that the loss of cytochrome P-450 (in the tissue culture studies) or the increased turnover of its heme moiety (in the whole animal experiments) both preceeded the stimulation of heme oxygenase. SCHMID and MCDONAGH (1975) have recently commented on these findings and have proposed as an explanation that the apoprotein of cytochrome P-450 may be the site of heme degradation (i.e., heme oxygenase) in the microsomes, a concept originally proposed by O'CARRA and COLLERAN (1969). According to this concept, cytochrome P-450 (the complete hemoprotein containing its full heme complement) is not directly involved in the catabolism of heme to bile pigments (see YOSHIDA et al., 1974; MAINES and KAPPAS, 1974), but when the hemoprotein is stripped of its heme moiety, then the free apoprotein may serve as a catalytic centre for heme breakdown by a coupled oxidation mechanism. It is not clear, however, in what way the apoprotein must differ so that it can either accept heme and retain it to form the complete hemoprotein or act on it as a substrate and degrade it to a bile pigment. Also, as previously pointed out (DE MATTEIS, 1971b), the finding that the stimulation of heme oxygenase by heme requires protein synthesis (PIMSTONE et al., 1971) is more easily compatible with a de novo synthesis of new enzyme protein than with O'CARRA and COLLERAN's concept of a pre-existing site made available for heme cleavage. Finally, the recent finding by YOSHIDA et al. (1974) that heme oxygenase can be almost completely separated by column chromatography from the CO-binding hemoprotein may indicate that the enzyme is a microsomal component unrelated to the cytochrome.

---

[2] Compatible with the assumption that the stimulation takes place in the parenchymal liver cells are the observations that starvation (BAKKEN et al., 1972) and cobalt (MAINES and KAPPAS, 1974) do not stimulate the heme oxygenase in the spleen (which is very rich in RE cells), and also the finding that a stimulation of the enzyme follows a decline in P-450 levels in cultures of hepatocytes (BISSELL et al., 1974) where contamination by reticuloendothelial cells should be minimal.

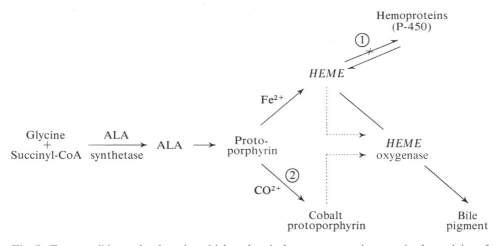

Fig. 7. Two possible mechanisms by which a chemical may cause an increase in the activity of heme oxygenase. (*1*) A primary lesion of the microsomes may divert endogenous heme towards breakdown to bile pigments and substrate mediated induction of heme oxygenase (at the expense of heme being incorporated or retained in a hemoprotein structure). (*2*) A metal, for example cobalt, may become incorporated into protoporphyrin instead of iron, giving rise to a heme-like compound. If this were not readily broken down to bilirubin, it could provide an effective and sustained stimulus for the induction of heme oxygenase. Broken arrows indicate stimulation of enzyme activity. ALA : 5-aminolaevulinate

The following explanation can be proposed to account for the decrease in cytochrome P-450 leading to the stimulation of heme oxygenase, on the basis of a specific microsomal induceable enzyme distinct from the apoprotein of cytochrome P-450 (DE MATTEIS, 1975). The early loss of cytochrome P-450 may involve either a loss of apoprotein binding sites or a reduction in their affinity for heme. This will entail two main consequences: 1) some of the heme of the pre-existing cytochrome P-450 will itself be released (see also BISSELL and HAMMAKER, 1976), and 2) probably more important, a smaller proportion of the heme which is newly made in the liver cell will be accepted and stabilized in a hemoprotein structure. As a result, the amount of heme available for degradation and for induction of heme oxygenase will increase [Fig. 7, (*1*)]. There is evidence, some of which has been discussed already, that under in vitro conditions starvation and iron can increase the peroxidative damage of the microsomal membranes, and that sulphydryl reagents, such as heavy metals, can convert P-450 to P-420 (MURAKAMI and MASON, 1967), an unstable derivative with less affinity for heme (MAINES et al., 1974). If these agents produced similar effects in vivo, and if they did so at an early stage, before the stimulation of heme oxygenase, then this would be compatible with the hypothetical mechanism outlined above. Endotoxin, a stimulator of heme oxygenase, has been reported to cause a number of early microsomal changes when administered to rats (VAINIO, 1973). Compatible with the mechanism discussed above is also the finding that agents like 3,5-diethoxycarbonyl-1,4-dihydrocollidine, and aminotriazole do not stimulate heme oxygenase (ROTHWELL et al., 1973; MAINES and KAPPAS, 1975b) (even though they cause a decrease in cytochrome P-450), since they would not be expected to provide more heme for a substrate-mediated induction of the enzyme, as both of them inhibit heme synthesis. Also compatible with the model illustrated in Fig. 7 (*1*) is the finding that AIA causes a decrease in the activity of heme oxygenase (Rothwell et al., 1973; Maines and Kappas, 1975b). This compound stimulates heme degradation by an alternative pathway which may divert heme from the physiologic breakdown to bile pigments and from its control of heme oxygenase activity.

The experimental findings obtained by Bissell et al. (1974) when hemin or hemoglobin were used to induce heme oxygenase require further comment. With these two inducers, the exogenous heme itself would be expected to provide a sufficient stimulus for heme oxygenase induction. The loss of radioactivity observed from prelabelled microsomal heme prior to the stimulation of heme oxygenase need not indicate that microsomal heme had to be released and broken down in order for the induction of the enzyme to take place. Another explanation is that microsomal heme can exchange with the "free" heme pool, and that under conditions (as after administration of large amounts of exogenous heme) where the latter pool enlarges or turns over rapidly, more radioactivity will be "washed out" of the microsomes down the degradation pathway. The findings by Abbritti and De Matteis (1973) of an apparent migration of heme radioactivity from the microsomes to the cell sap when rats with prelabelled liver heme were given large doses of unlabelled 5-aminolaevulinate, provides evidence for such an exchange in vivo.

An exception to the mechanism of induction of heme oxygenase considered above is provided by the liver effects of cobaltous chloride. With this agent, a loss of radioactivity from prelabelled liver heme was also seen but only after (and not before) the induction of heme oxygenase (De Matteis and Unseld, 1976). Therefore, increased heme turnover may be a consequence of the induction of heme oxygenase by cobalt (see below), but is unlikely to be responsible for it. An early change caused by cobalt treatment (before the stimulation of heme oxygenase) was, however, the accumulation in the liver of a relatively stable compound which could be labelled with radioactive 5-aminolaevulinate and had solubility properties similar to those of authentic cobalt-protoporphyrin; the possibility has therefore been considered that cobalt may be incorporated into protoporphyrin in preference to the normal metal substrate, iron, and may thereby give rise to cobalt-protoporphyrin in the liver in vivo (De Matteis and Gibbs, 1976). There is chemical and biochemical evidence (Jackson and Jackson, 1974; Schacter and Waterman, 1974) that cobalt-protoporphyrin is not readily broken down to bile pigments, and it is therefore possible (De Matteis and Gibbs, 1976) that the accumulation of this heme-like compound in the liver cell may provide an effective and sustained stimulus for the induction of heme oxygenase [Fig. 7 (*2*)]. Compatible with this interpretation is the finding that exogenous cobalt-protoporphyrin, when given to the intact rat in vivo, could induce liver heme oxygenase. Even though this effect has been interpreted to result from the action of cobalt liberated in an inorganic form from the cobalt-protoporphyrin (Maines and Kappas, 1975b), the possibility still exists that it is cobalt-protoporphyrin itself which is active.

In the above discussion, the assumption has been made that heme itself, or a heme-like compound, acts as the inducer of heme oxygenase. It must be stressed however that the involvement in the stimulation of heme oxygenase by cobalt and other agents of a mechanism unrelated to heme cannot be discounted altogether.

2. The Heme of Cytochrome P-450 as a Substrate for Heme Oxygenase

Isotopic studies indicate that the turnover of heme is increased in the liver of animals given either cobalt or one of several other metals (iron, lead, or methylmercury) at a time when the activity of liver heme oxygenase is stimulated. Under these conditions, there is evidence that the turnover of the heme of cytochrome P-450 itself may be increased. These observations, which have been considered in Section D I, raise two interesting questions.

First, in what way can the heme of cytochrome P-450 serve as a substrate for heme oxygenase? This is probably best explained by assuming that the heme of cytochrome P-450 can exchange with another heme pool (possibly a "free" heme pool) which can itself be accepted as a substrate for heme oxygenase. Under conditions where either the size of this latter pool is increased or its rate of turnover accelerated, more radioactivity might be expected to be lost from cytochrome P-450 and converted to bile pigments. In the case of agents which cause an instability of cytochrome P-450 (for example, by converting it to P-420 or by promoting a damage of its hydrophobic environment through lipid peroxidation), this may be an additional factor in facilitating the release of heme from the hemoprotein into a pool which can be readily degraded by heme oxygenase.

The second question is whether an increased activity of heme oxygenase can by itself cause—through increased degradation of heme—a loss of liver cytochrome P-450. This is possible, but no conclusive evidence can be offered about this point, as the various agents which stimulate heme oxygenase may also effect the level of cytochrome P-450 in some other way, for example, by inhibiting heme synthesis or by damaging the apoprotein or its environment in the membranes.

Abbreviations

AIA	2-Allyl-2-isopropylacetamide
DDT	1,1,1-Trichloro-2,2-bis-(p-chlorophenyl)-ethane
GSH	Reduced glutathione
SKF 525-A	2-Diethylaminoethyl 3,3-diphenyl-propylacetate
SV_1	O,O-diethyl, O-phenyl phosphorothionate
NADH	Reduced nicotinamide adenine dinucleotide
NADPH	Reduced nicotinamide adenine dinucleotide phosphate

References

Abbritti, G., De Matteis, F.: Decreased levels of cytochrome P-450 and catalase in hepatic porphyria caused by substituted acetamides and barbiturates. Importance of the allyl group in the molecule of the active drugs. Chem. biol. Interact. **4**, 281 – 286 (1971)

Abbritti, G., De Matteis, F.: Effect of 3,5-diethoxycarbonyl-1,4-dihydrocollidine on degradation of liver haem. Enzyme **16**, 196 – 202 (1973)

Alme, B., Nystrom, E.: Preparation of lipophilic anion exchangers from chlorohydroxypropylated sephadex and cellulose. J. Chromat. **59**, 45 – 52 (1971)

Bakken, A.F., Thaler, M.M., Schmid, R.: Metabolic regulation of heme catabolism and bilirubin production I. Hormonal control of hepatic heme oxygenase activity. J. clin Invest. **51**, 530 – 536 (1972)

Baron, J., Tephly, T.R.: The role of heme synthesis during the induction of hepatic microsomal cytochrome P-450 and drug metabolism produced by benzpyrene. Biochem. biophys. Res. Commun. **36**, 526 – 532 (1969)

Beloff-Chain, A., Serlupi-Crescenzi, G., Catanzaro, R., Venettacci, D., Balliano, M.: Influence of iron on oxidation of reduced nicotinamide-adenine-dinucleotide phosphate in rat-liver microsomes. Biochim. biophys. Acta (Amst.) **97**, 416 – 421 (1965)

Bissell, D.M., Guzelian, P.S., Hammaker, L.E., Schmid, R.: Stimulation of hepatic heme oxygenase and turnover of cytochrome P-450 may be related. Fed. Proc. **33**, 1246 (1974)

Bissell, D.M., Hammaker, L.E.: Cytochrome P-450 heme and the regulation of hepatic heme oxygenase activity. Arch. Biochem. Biophys. **176**, 91 – 102 (1976)

Bissell, D.M., Hammaker, L., Schmid, R.: Hemoglobin and erythrocyte catabolism in rat liver: The separate role of parenchymal and sinusoidal cells. Blood **40**, 812 – 822 (1972)

Bock, K.W., Frohling, W., Remmer, H.: Influence of fasting and hemin on microsomal cytochromes and enzymes. Biochem. Pharmacol. **22**, 1557 – 1564 (1973)

Bond, E.J., Butler, W.H., De Matteis, F., Barnes, J.M.: Effects of carbon disulphide on the liver of rats. Brit. J. industr. Med. **26**, 335 – 337 (1969)

Bond, E.J., De Matteis, F.: Biochemical changes in rat liver after administration of carbon disulphide, with particular reference to microsomal changes. Biochem. Pharmacol. **18**, 2531 – 2549 (1969)

Butler, T.C.: Reduction of carbon tetrachloride in vivo and reduction of carbon tetrachloride and chloroform in vitro by tissues and tissue constituents. J. Pharmac. exp. Ther. **134**, 311 – 319 (1961)

Cameron, G.R., Karunaratne, W.E.: Carbon tetrachloride in relation to liver regeneration. J. Path. Bact. **42**, 1 – 21 (1936)

Catignani, G.L., Neal, R.A.: Evidence for the formation of a protein bound hydrodisulfide resulting from the microsomal mixed function oxidase catalyzed desulfuration of carbon disulfide. Biochem. biophys. Res. Commun. **65**, 629 – 636 (1975)

Chvapil, M., Ryan, J.N., Elias, S.L., Peng, Y.M.: Protective effect of zinc on carbon tetra-chloride-induced liver injury in rats. Exp. molec. Path. **19**, 186 – 196 (1973)

Dalvi, R.R., Hunter, A.L., Neal, R.A.: Toxicological implications of the mixed-function oxidase catalysed metabolism of carbon disulphide. Chem. biol. Interact. **10**, 347 – 361 (1975)

Dalvi, R.R., Poore, R.E., Neal, R.A.: Studies of the metabolism of carbon disulfide by rat-liver microsomes. Life Sci. **14**, 1785 – 1796 (1974)

Daly, J.: Enzymatic oxidation of carbon. In: Concepts in Biochemical Pharmacology, Part 2, Handbook of Experimental Pharmacology, Vol. 28. Brodie, B.B. and Gillette, J.R. (eds.). Berlin – Heidelberg – New York: Springer 1971

Davison, A.N.: The conversion of sehradan (OMPA) and parathion into inhibitors of cholinesterase by mammalian liver. Biochem. J. **61**, 203 – 209 (1955)

De Matteis, F.: Rapid loss of cytochrome P-450 and heme caused in the liver microsomes by the porphyrogenic agent 2-allyl-2-isopropylacetamide. Febs Lett. **6**, 343 – 345 (1970)

De Matteis, F.: Loss of heme in rat liver caused by the porphyrogenic agent 2-allyl-2-iso-propylacetamide. Biochem. J. **124** 767 – 777 (1971 a)

De Matteis, F.: Contribution to the discussion of the paper by Pimstone, N.R. et al. S. Afr. J. Lab. clin. Med. **17**, 173 (1971 b)

De Matteis, F.: Mechanisms of induction of hepatic porphyria by drugs. In: Proc. 5th Int. Congr. Pharmacology, San Francisco, **2**, 89 – 99 (1972)

De Matteis, F.: Drug-induced destruction of cytochrome P-450. Drug Metab. Dispos. **1**, 267 – 272 (1973)

De Matteis, F.: Covalent binding of sulfur to microsomes and loss of cytochrome P-450 during the oxidative desulfuration of several chemicals. Molec. Pharmacol. **10**, 849 – 854 (1974)

De Matteis, F.: Iron-dependent degradation of liver heme in vivo. In: Proceedings of the International Porphyrin Meeting, Freiburg, May 1 – 4, 1975. Basel: S. Karger 1976

De Matteis, F., Gibbs, A.H.: The effect of cobaltous chloride on liver heme metabolism in the rat. Evidence for inhibition of heme synthesis and for increased heme degradation. Ann. clin. Res. **8**, Suppl. 17, 193 – 197 (1976)

De Matteis, F., Seawright, A.A.S.: Oxidative metabolism of carbon disulphide by the rat. Effect of treatments which modify the liver toxicity of carbon disulphide. Chem. biol. Interact. **7**, 375 – 388 (1973)

De Matteis, F., Sparks, R.G.: Iron-dependent loss of liver cytochrome P-450 heme in vivo and in vitro. Febs Lett. **29**, 141 – 144 (1973)

De Matteis, F., Unseld, A.: Increased liver heme degradation caused by foreign chemicals. A comparison of the effects of 2-allyl-2-isopropylacetamide and cobaltous chloride. Biochem. Soc. Trans. **4**, 205–209 (1976)

De Toranzo, E.G.D., Diaz Gomez, M.I., Castro, J.A.: Mechanism of in vivo carbon tetrachloride-induced liver microsomal cytochrome P-450 destruction. Biochem. biophys. Res. Commun. **64**, 823–828 (1975)

Doedens, D.J.: Metabolic fate of the porphyrogenic drug allylisopropylacetamide. Diss. Abstr. Part B Sci. Eng. **32**, 2901 (1971)

Ellin, A., Orrenius, S.: Hydroperoxide-supported cytochrome P-450-linked fatty acid hydroxylation in liver microsomes. Febs Lett. **50**, 378–381 (1975)

Falk, J.E.: Porphyrins and metalloporphyrins. BBA Libr. Vol. 2, p. 232. Amsterdam: Elsevier 1964

Fong, K., McKay, P.B., Poyer, J.L., Keele, B.B., Misra, H.: Evidence that peroxidation of lysosomal membranes is initiated by hydroxyl free radicals produced during flavin enzyme activity. J. biol. Chem. **248**, 7792–7797 (1973)

Foreman, R.L., Maynert, E.W.: A tetrahydrofuropyrimidine as a metabolite of secobarbital. Pharmacologist **12**, 255 (1970)

Fowler, J.S.L.: Carbon tetrachloride metabolism in the rabbit. Brit. J. Pharmacol. **37**, 733–737 (1969)

Freundt, K.J., Dreher, W.: Inhibition of drug metabolism by small concentrations of carbon disulphide. Naunym-Schmiedebergs Arch. Pharmakol. exp. Path. **263**, 208–209 (1969)

Garner, R.C., McLean, A.E.M.: Increased susceptibility to carbon tetrachloride poisoning in the rat after pretreatment with oral phenobarbitone. Biochem. Pharmacol. **18**, 645–650 (1969)

Greene, F.E., Stripp, B., Gillette, J.R.: The effect of carbon tetrachloride on heme components and ethylmorphine metabolism in rat liver microsomes. Biochem. Pharmacol. **18**, 1531–1533 (1969)

Hadley, W.M., Miya, R.S., Bousquet, W.F.: Cadmium inhibition of hepatic drug metabolism in the rat. Toxicol. appl. Pharmacol. **28**, 284–291 (1974)

Hafeman, D.F., Hoekstra, W.F.: Protection by vitamin E and selenium against lipid peroxidation in vivo as measured by ethane evolution. Fed. Prod. **34**, 939 (1975)

Harvey, D.J., Glazener, L., Stratton, C., Johnson, D.B., Mill, R.M., Horning, E.C., Horning, M.G.: Detection of epoxides of allyl-substituted barbiturates in rat urine. Res. Commun. chem. Path. Pharmacol. **4**, 247–260 (1972)

Haurowitz, F., Groh, M., Gansinger, G.: Mechanism and kinetics of the hemin-catalyzed oxidation of linoleate in the oil-water interface. J. biol. Chem. **248**, 3810–3818 (1973)

Högberg, J.: Iron induced lipid peroxidation in rat liver. A study on mechanisms and consequences. Dissertation, Karolinska Institutet, Stockholm 1975

Högberg, J., Bergstrand, A., Jakobsson, S.V.: Lipid peroxidation of rat-liver microsomes. Its effect on the microsomal membrane and some membrane-bound microsomal enzymes. Europ. J. Biochem. **37**, 51–59 (1973)

Högberg, J., Orrenius, S., Larson, R.E.: Lipid peroxidation in isolated hepatocytes. Europ. J. Biochem. **50**, 595–602 (1975)

Hrycay, E.G., Gustafsson, J., Ingelman-Sundberg, M., Ernster, L.: Sodium periodate, sodium chlorite, and organic hydroperoxides as hydroxylating agents in hepatic microsomal steroid hydroxylation reactions catalyzed by cytochrome P-450. Febs Lett. **56**, 161–165 (1975)

Hrycay, E.G., O'Brien, P.J.: Cytochrome P-450 as a microsomal peroxide utilizing a lipid peroxide substrate. Arch. Biochem. Biophys. **147**, 14–27 (1971)

Hunter, A., Neal, R.A.: Response of the hepatic mixed function oxidase system to thionosulfur-containing compounds. Pharmacologist **16**, 239 (1974)

Hupka, A.L., Karler, R.: Biotransformation of ethylmorphine and heme by isolated parenchymal and reticuloendothelial cells of rat liver. J. reticuloendoth. Soc. **14**, 225–241 (1973)

Ivanetich, K.M., Marsh, J.A., Bradshaw, J.J., Kaminsky, L.S.: Fluroxene (2,2,2-trifluoroethyl vinyl ether) mediated destruction of cytochrome P-450 in vitro. Biochem. Pharmacol. **24**, 1933–1936 (1975)

Jackson, A.H., Jackson, J.R.: Unpublished work quoted by Jackson, A.H. Heme catabolism. In: Iron in Biochemistry and Medicine. Jacobs, A., Worwood, M. (eds.), pp. 145–182. London–New York: Academic Press 1974

Jaeger, R.J., Conolly, R.B., Murphy, S.D.: Diurnal variations of hepatic glutathione concentration and its correlation with 1,1-dichloroethylene inhalation toxicity in rats. Res. Commun. chem. Path. Pharmacol. **6**, 465 – 471 (1973)

Jose, P.J., Slater, T.F., Sawyer, B.C.: The effects of starvation on rat liver microsomal inosine concentrations, reduced nicotinamide-adenine dinucleotide-linked lipid-peroxidation system and other microsomal enzymes. Biochem. Soc. Trans. **1**, 939 – 941 (1973)

Kadlubar, F.F., Morton, K.C., Ziegler, D.M.: Microsomal-catalyzed hydroperoxide-dependent C-oxidation of amines. Biochem. biophys. Res. Commun. **54**, 1255 – 1261 (1973)

Kamataki, T., Kitagawa, H.: Effects of lipid peroxidation on activities of drug-metabolizing enzymes in liver microsomes of rats. Biochem. Pharmacol. **22**, 3199 – 3207 (1973)

Kokatnur, M.G., Bergan, J.G., Draper, H.H.: Observations on the decomposition of hemin by fatty acid hydroperoxides. Proc. Soc. exp. Biol. (N.Y.) **123**, 314 – 317 (1966)

Landaw, S.A., Callahan, E.W. Jr., Schmid, R.: Catabolism of heme in vivo: comparison of the simultaneous production of bilirubin and carbon monoxide. J. clin. Invest. **49**, 914 – 925 (1970)

Lemberg, R., Falk, J.E.: Comparison of heme *a*, the dichroic heme of heart muscle, and of porphyrin *a* with compounds of known structure. Biochem. J. **49**, 674 – 683 (1951)

Levin, W., Jacobson, M., Kuntzman, R.: Incorporation of radioactive δ-aminolevulinic acid into microsomal cytochrome P-450. Selective breakdown of the hemoprotein by allylisopropylacetamide and carbon tetrachloride. Arch. Biochem. Biophys. **148**, 262 – 269 (1972a)

Levin, W., Jacobson, M., Sernatinger, E., Kuntzman, R.: Breakdown of cytochrome P-450 heme by secobarbital and other allyl-containing barbiturates. Drug. Metab. Dispos. **1**, 275 – 284 (1973a)

Levin, W., Kuntzman, R.: Biphasic decrease of radioactive hemoprotein from liver microsomal CO-binding particles. Effect of 3-methylcholanthrene. J. biol. Chem. **244**, 3671 – 3676 (1969)

Levin, W., Lu, A.Y.H., Jacobson, M., Kuntzman, R., Poyer, J.L., McCay, P.B.: Lipid peroxidation and the degradation of cytochrome P-450 heme. Arch. Biochem. Biophys. **158**, 842 – 852 (1973b)

Levin, W., Sernatinger, E., Jacobson, M., Kuntzman, R.: Destruction of cytochrome P-450 by secobarbital and other barbiturates containing allyl groups. Science **176**, 1341 – 1343 (1972b)

Little, C., O'Brien, P.J.: An intracellular GSH-peroxidase with a lipid peroxide substrate. Biochem. biophys. Res. Commun. **31**, 145 – 150 (1968)

Lucier, G.W., Matthews, H.B., Brubaker, P.E., Klein, R., McDaniel, O.S.: Effects of methylmercury in microsomal mixed-function oxidase components of rodents. Molec. Pharmacol. **9**, 237 – 246 (1973)

Magos, L., Butler, W.H.: Effect of phenobarbitone and starvation on hepatotoxicity in rats exposed to carbon disulphide vapour. Brit. J. industr. Med. **29**, 95 – 98 (1972)

Maines, M.D., Anders, M.W., Muller-Eberhard, U.: Studies on heme transfer from microsomal hemoproteins to heme-binding plasma proteins. Molec. Pharmacol. **10**, 204 – 213 (1974)

Maines, M.D., Kappas, A.: Cobalt induction of hepatic heme oxygenase; with evidence that cytochrome P-450 is not essential for this enzyme activity. Proc. nat. Acad. Sci. (Wash.) **71**, 4293 – 4297 (1974)

Maines, M.D., Kappas, A.: Regulation of hepatic heme metabolism by metals. International Porphyrin Meeting, Freiburg, May 1 – 4 1975. Abstracts page 9 (1975a)

Maines, M.D., Kappas, A.: Cobalt stimulation of heme degradation in the liver. Dissociation of microsomal oxidation of heme from cytochrome P-450. J. biol. Chem. **250**, 4171 – 4177 (1975b)

Maines, M.D., Kappas, A.: Studies on the mechanism of induction of heme oxygenase by cobalt and other metal ions. Biochem. J. **154**, 125 – 131 (1976)

McCay, P.B., Pfeifer, P.M., Stipe, W.H.: Vitamin E protection of membrane lipids during electron transport functions. Ann. N.Y. Acad. Sci. **203**, 62 – 73 (1972)

McDonagh, A.F., Pospisil, R., Meyer, U.A.: Degradation of hepatic heme to porphyrins and oxophlorins in rats treated with 2-allyl-2-isopropylacetamide. Biochem. Soc. Trans. **4**, 297 – 298 (1976)

McLean, A.E.M.: Effect of hexane and carbon tetrachloride on microsomal cytochrome (P-450). Biochem. Pharmacol. **16**, 2030 – 2033 (1967)

McLean, A.E.M., McLean, E.K.: The effect of diet and 1,1,1-trichloro-2,2-bis-(p-chlorophenyl)-ethane (DDT) on microsomal hydroxylating enzymes and on sensitivity of rats to carbon tetrachloride poisoning. Biochem. J. **100**, 564 – 571 (1966)

Meyer, U.A., Marver, H.S.: Chemically induced porphyria. Increased microsomal heme turn-over after treatment with allylisopropylacetamide. Science **171**, 64 – 66 (1971)

Murakami, K., Mason, H.S.: An electron spin resonance study of microsomal Fe$_x$. J. biol. Chem. **2421**, 1102 – 1110 (1967)

Nakamura, M., Yasukochi, Y., Minakami, S.: Effect of cobalt on heme biosynthesis in rat liver and spleen. J. Biochem. (Tokyo) **78**, 373 – 380 (1975)

Nakatsugawa, T., Dahm, P.A.: Microsomal metabolism of parathion. Biochem. Pharmacol. **16**, 25 – 38 (1967)

Nakatsugawa, T., Tolman, N.M., Dahm, P.A.: Degradation and activation of parathion analogues by microsomal enzymes. Biochem. Pharmacol. **17**, 1517 – 1528 (1968).

Neal, R.A.: Studies on the metabolism of diethyl-4-nitrophenylphosphorothionate (parathion) in vitro. Biochem. J. **103**, 183 – 191 (1967)

Nilsson, R., Orrenius, S., Ernster, L.: The TPNH-dependent oxidation of luminol catalyzed by rat liver microsomes. Biochem. biophys. Res. Commun. **17**, 303 – 309 (1964)

Nishibayashi, H., Omura, T., Sato, R., Estabrook, R.W.: Comments on the absorption spectra of hemoprotein P-450. In: Structure and Function of Cytochromes. Okunuki, K., Kamon, M.D., Sekuzu, I. (eds.), pp. 658 – 665. Baltimore – Manchester: University Park Press 1968

O'Brien, R.D.: Activation of thionophosphates by liver microsomes. Nature (Lond.) **183**, 121 – 122 (1959)

O'Brien, R.D.: Desulfuration. In: Proc. 1st Intern. Pharmacol. Meeting, Stockholm, **6**, 111 – 119 (1961)

O'Carra, P., Colleran, E.: Heme catabolism and coupled oxidation of hemoproteins. Febs Lett. **5**, 295 – 298 (1969)

Orrenius, S., Dallner, G., Ernster, L.: Inhibition of the TPNH-linked lipid peroxidation of liver microsomes by drugs undergoing oxidative demethylation. Biochem. biophys. Res. Commun. **14**, 329 – 334 (1964)

Pederson, T.C., Aust, S.D.: Relationship between reduced nicotinamide adenine dinucleotide phosphate-dependent lipid peroxidation and drug hydroxylation in rat liver microsomes. Biochem. Pharmacol. **23**, 2467 – 2469 (1974)

Pederson, T.C., Aust, S.D.: The mechanism of liver microsomal lipid peroxidation. Biochim. biophys. Acta (Amst.) **385**, 232 – 241 (1975)

Pederson, T.C., Buege, J.A., Aust, S.D.: Microsomal electron transport. The role of reduced nicotinamide adenine dinucleotide phosphate-cytochrome c reductase in liver microsomal lipid peroxidation. J. biol. Chem. **248**, 7134 – 7141 (1973)

Penning, W., Scoppa, P.: Breakdown of cytochrome P-450 in acute lead poisoning. IUPHAR Satellite Symposium on Active Intermediates: Formation, Toxicity and Inactivation, Turku, Finland, July 26 – 27, 1975, Abstracts p. 41

Pimstone, N.R., Engel, P., Tenhunen, R., Seitz, P.T., Marver, H.S., Schmid, R.: Further studies of microsomal heme oxygenase: mechanism for stimulation of enzyme activity and cellular localization. S. Afr. J. Lab. clin. Med. **17**, 169 – 173 (1971)

Poore, R.E., Neal, R.A.: Evidence for extrahepatic metabolism of parathion. Toxicol. appl. Pharmacol. **23**, 759 – 768 (1972)

Ptashne, K.A., Wolcott, R.M., Neal, R.A.: Oxygen-18 studies on the chemical mechanisms of the mixed function oxidase catalysed desulfuration and dearylation reactions of parathion. J. Pharmacol. exp. Ther. **179**, 380 – 385 (1971)

Radtke, H.E., Coon, M.J.: Role of cytochrome P-450 in lipid peroxidation and peroxide-dependent drug hydroxylation. Fed. Proc. **33**, 588 (1974)

Rahimtula, A.D., O'Brien, P.J.: Hydroperoxide dependent O-dealkylation reactions catalyzed by liver microsomal cytochrome P-450. Biochem. biophys. Res. Commun. **62**, 268 – 275 (1975)

Recknagel, R.O.: Carbon tetrachloride hepatotoxicity. Pharmacol. Rev. **19**, 145 – 208 (1967)

Recknagel, R.O., Glende, E.A. Jr., Hruszkewycz, A.M.: New data supporting an obligatory role for lipid peroxidation in carbon tetrachloride induced loss of aminopyrine demethylase, cytochrome P-450 and glucose-6-phosphatase. IUPHAR Satellite Symposium on Active Intermediates: Formation, Toxicity and Inactivation, Turku, Finland, July 26 – 27, 1975, Abstracts, P. 26

Recknagel, R.O., Lombardi, B.: Studies of biochemical changes in subcellular particles of rat liver and their relationship to a new hypothesis regarding the pathogenesis of carbon tetrachloride fat accumulation. J. biol. Chem. **236**, 564 – 569 (1961)

Reiner, O., Athanassopoulos, S., Hellmer, K.H., Murray, R.E., Uehleke, H.: Bidlung von Chloroform aus Tetrachlorkohlenstoff in Lebermikrosomen, Lipidperoxidation und Zerstörung von Cytochrom P-450. Arch. Toxikol. **29**, 219 – 233 (1972)

Reiner, O., Uehleke, H.: Bindung von Tetrachlorkohlenstoff an reduziertes mikrosomales Cytochrom P-450 und an Häm. Hoppe-Seylers Z. physiol. Chem. **352**, 1048 – 1052 (1971)

Riely, C.A., Cohen, G., Lieberman, M.: Ethane evolution: A new index of lipid peroxidation. Science **183**, 208 – 210 (1974)

Ross, W.E., Simrell, C., Oppelt, W.W.: Sex-dependent effects of cyclic AMP on the hepatic mixed function oxidase system. Res. Commun. chem. Path. Pharmacol. **5**, 319 – 332 (1973)

Rothwell, J.D., Lacroix, S., Sweeney, G.D.: Evidence against a regulatory role for heme oxygenase in hepatic synthesis. Biochim. biophys. Acta (Amst.) **304**, 871 – 874 (1973)

Rotruck, J.T., Pope, A.L., Ganther, H.E., Swanson, A.B., Hafeman, D.G., Hoekstra, W.G.: Selenium biochemical role as a component of glutathione peroxidase. Science **179**, 588 – 590 (1973)

Sasame, H.A., Castro, J.A., Gillette, J.R.: Studies on the destruction of liver microsomal cytochrome P-450 by carbon tetrachloride administration. Biochem. Pharmacol. **17**, 1759 – 1768 (1968)

Schacter, B.A., Marver, H.S., Meyer, U.A.: Hemoprotein catabolism during stimulation of microsomal lipid peroxidation. Biochim. biophys, Acta (Amst.) **279**, 221 – 227 (1972)

Schacter, B.A., Marver, H.S., Meyer, U.A.: Heme and hemoprotein catabolism during stimulation of microsomal lipid peroxidation. Drug Metab. Dispos. **1**, 286 – 290 (1973)

Schacter, B.A., Waterman, M.R.: Activity of various metalloporphyrin protein complexes with microsomal heme oxygenase. Life Sci. **14**, 47 – 53 (1974)

Schmid, R., McDonagh, A.F.: The enzymatic formation of bilirubin. Ann. N.Y. Acad. Sci. **244**, 533 – 552 (1975)

Schwartz, S., Ikeda, K.: Studies of porphyrin synthesis and interconversion, with special reference to certain green porphyrins in animals with experimental hepatic porphyria. In: Ciba Found, Symp.: Porphyrin Biosynthesis and Metabolism. Wolstenholme, G.E.W. (ed.), pp. 209 – 226. London: J. and A. Churchill Ltd. 1955

Scoppa, P., Roumengous, M., Penning, W.: Hepatic drug-metabolizing activity in lead-poisoned rats. Experientia (Basel) **29**, 970 – 972 (1973)

Scott, M.L., Noguchi, T., Combs, G.F. Jr.: New Evidence concerning mechanisms of action of vitamin E and selenium. Vitam. Horm. **32**, 429 – 444 (1974)

Seawright, A.A., Hrdlicka, J., De Matteis, F.: The hepatotoxicity of O,O-diethyl, O-phenyl phosphorothionate (SV$_1$) for the rat. Brit. J. exp. Path. **57**, 16 – 22 (1976)

Seawright, A.A., McLean, A.E.M.: The effect of diet on carbon tetrachloride metabolism. Biochem. J. **105**, 1055 – 1060 (1967)

Shah, H.C., Carlson, G.P.: Alteration by phenobarbital and 3-methylcholanthrene of functional and structural changes in rat liver due to carbon tetrachloride inhalation. J. Pharmacol. exp. Ther. **193**, 281 – 292 (1975)

Slater, T.F.: Free Radical Mechanisms in Tissue Injury. London: Pion Ltd. 1972

Slater, T.F., Sawyer, B.C.: The stimulatory effects of carbon tetrachloride on peroxidative reactions in rat liver fractions in vitro. Interaction sites in the endoplasmic reticulum. Biochem. J. **123**, 815 – 821 (1971)

Smuckler, E.A., Arrenius, E., Hultin, T.: Alterations in microsomal electron transport, oxidative N-demethylation and azo-dye cleavage in carbon tetrachloride and dimethylnitrosamine-induced liver injury. Biochem. J. **103**, 55 – 64 (1967)

Stern, J.O., Peisach, J.: A model compound study of the CO-adduct of cytochrome P-450. J. biol. Chem. **249**, 7495−7498 (1974)

Tappel, A.L.: Unsaturated lipid oxidation catalyzed by hematin compounds. J. biol. Chem. **217**, 721−733 (1955)

Tappel, A.L.: Vitamin E and free radical peroxidation of lipids. Ann. N.Y. Acad. Sci. **203**, 12−28 (1972)

Tateishi, N., Higashi, T., Shinya, S., Naruse, A., Sakamoto, Y.: Studies on the regulation of glutathione level in rat liver. J. Biochem. **75**, 93−103 (1974)

Tephly, T.R., Hibbeln, P.: The effect of cobalt chloride administration on the synthesis of hepatic microsomal cytochrome P-450. Biochem. biophys. Res. Commun. **42**, 589−595 (1971)

Tephly, T.R., Webb, C., Trussler, P., Knitten, F., Hasegawa, E., Piper, W.: The regulation of heme synthesis related to drug metabolism. Drug Metab. Dispos. **1**, 259−265 (1973)

Uehleke, H., Hellmer, K.H., Tabarelli, S.: Binding of ^{14}C-carbon tetrachloride to microsomal proteins in vitro and formation of $CHCl_3$ by reduced liver microsomes. Xenobiotica **3**, 1−11 (1973)

Unseld, A., De Matteis, F.: Isolation and partial characterisation of green pigments produced in rat liver by 2-allyl-2-isopropylacetamide. In: Proceedings of the International Porphyrin Meeting, Freiburg, May 1−4, 1975. Basel: S. Karger 1976

Vainio, H.: Defective drug metabolism in rat liver in endotoxin shock. Ann. Med. exp. Biol. Finn. **51**, 63−68 (1973)

Wada, O., Yano, Y., Urata, G., Nakao, K.: Behaviour of hepatic microsomal cytochromes after treatment of mice with drugs known to disturb porphyrin metabolism in liver. Biochem. Pharmacol. **17**, 595−603 (1968).

Waterfield, M.D., Del Favero, A., Gray, C.H.: Effect of 1,4-dihydro-3,5-dicarbethoxycollidine on hepatic microsomal heme, cytochrome b_5 and cytochrome P-450 in rabbits and mice. Biochim, biophys. Acta (Amst.) **184**, 470−473 (1969)

Weiner, M., Buterbaugh, G.G., Blake, D.A.: Inhibition of hepatic drug metabolism by cyclic 3′,5′-adenosine monophosphate. Res. Commun. chem. Path. Pharmacol. **3**, 249−263 (1972)

Williams, R.T.: Detoxication Mechanisms, 2nd, ed., p. 181. London: Chapman and Hall Limited 1959

Wills, E.D.: Lipid peroxide formation in microsomes. The role of non-heme iron. Biochem. J. **113**, 325−332 (1969a)

Wills, E.D.: Lipid peroxide formation in microsomes. Relationship of hydroxylation to lipid peroxide formation. Biochem. J. **113**, 333−341 (1969b)

Wills, E.D.: Effects of iron overload on lipid peroxide formation and oxidative demethylation by the liver endoplasmic reticulum. Biochem. Pharmacol. **21**, 239−247 (1972)

Yoshida, T., Takahashi, S., Kikuchi, G.: Partial purification and reconstitution of the heme oxygenase system from pig spleen microsomes. J. Biochem. **75**, 1187−1191 (1974)

Yu, C. A., Gunsalus, I.C.: Cytochrome P-450 cam. II. Interconversion with P-420. J. biol. Chem. **249**, 102−106 (1974)

Hepatic Porphyrias

Caused by
2-Allyl-2-isopropylacetamide, 3,5-Diethoxycarbonyl-1,4-dihydrocollidine, Griseofulvin and Related Compounds

F. De Matteis

A. Introduction

I. The Concept of Porphyria

The liver is an important site of synthesis of heme, which is then utilized as the prosthetic groups for the various hepatic cytochromes and hemoproteins (see chapter by TAIT for a detailed coverage of these aspects). Under normal conditions the intermediates of the pathway (the porphyrins and their precursors 5-amino-levulinate and porphobilinogen) accumulate or are excreted only in very small amounts. This indicates clearly that the biosynthetic pathway is very efficiently regulated to provide the amount of heme required for the turnover of the various hemoproteins of the liver cell with little waste of the intermediates. There are con-ditions, however, in which the control mechanism breaks down and far more por-phyrin and earlier precursors are synthesized than are turned into heme, so that they accumulate and are excreted in excess. These conditions are known as por-phyrias. The hepatic porphyrias, where the liver is the site of the metabolic ab-normality, should therefore be regarded as disorders of the regulation of liver heme biosynthesis.

II. Drugs and Liver Porphyrin Metabolism: Two Types of Interaction

It has been known for some time that drugs could be implicated in deranging the metabolism of porphyrins in the liver of both humans and experimental animals. In fact, much of what is known of the regulation of the pathway and some of what is known about the biosynthetic pathway itself has been obtained through the study of the effect of drugs in the hepatic porphyria of man and experimental animals.

Drugs can stimulate the activity of the pathway in the liver in one of two basically different ways. They can either cause a condition of porphyria in the liver of the *normal* individual or the *normal* experimental animal, in the absence of a genetic disposition to this metabolic disorder (effect 1, Table 1); or they can merely exacerbate a condition of porphyria in an individual carrier of the genetic defect of acute porphyria in a latent state (effect 2, Table 1). A very clear distinc-tion must be made between these two types of undesirable response to drugs. Only a few drugs can stimulate the formation of porphyrins in the normal liver and all

Table 1. Drugs and liver porphyrin metabolism: two types of interaction

Effect	Effective drugs	Property required for effect	
		Lipid solubility	Special chemical grouping
1. Induction of porphyria in the *normal* liver of man and experimental rodent	Few (allyl-containing compounds, DDC, griseofulvin)	Yes	Yes
2. Exacerbation of human *genetic* acute porphyria	Many (phenylbutazone, barbiturates, other sedatives, etc.)	Yes	No

of these have some degree of chemical specificity, as shown by the presence of certain chemical groupings which are associated with the activity. In contrast, drugs which can exacerbate the condition of acute porphyria in genetically disposed individuals are very many (Wetterberg, 1976) and do not possess any specific chemical constitution: the only property that they appear to share is a high degree of lipid solubility. A possible explanation for this difference will be provided later in this article and also, in more detail, in the article by Maxwell and Meyer.

The main purpose of this chapter is to discuss the mechanisms involved in the production of porphyria in the normal liver of man and experimental animals. Only those drugs will be considered which can lead to a marked stimulation of the pathway with accumulation of the early intermediates. The emphasis will be placed on experimental studies conducted in vivo in the whole animal, especially in rodents, the liver of which appears to resemble that of normal humans in its response to porphyria-inducing drugs. An attempt will be made to summarize the present position rather than provide a comprehensive coverage of the literature, for which the reader is referred to several recent reviews (Tschudy and Bonkowsky, 1972; Granick and Sassa, 1971; Meyer and Schmid, 1977). This is a complicated field of study, where in spite of recent advances from several laboratories there are still many points which require elucidation. The mechanisms involved will therefore be considered in terms of simplified models as these, in the author's opinion, provide a satisfactory background for the discussion of the available data and also a suitable starting point for future experimental work.

III. The Induction of Porphyria by Drugs in the Normal Liver

Drugs which induce porphyria in the liver of the normal experimental animal belong to four main groups (Fig. 1). They are either derivatives of a branched aliphatic acetamide or barbiturate, containing at least one unsaturated side chain, or they are compounds chemically related to either collidine or griseofulvin. When one of these chemicals is administered to a suitable experimental animal, there is within a few minutes or a few hours a marked increase in the excretion of porphyrins and their precursors, which can also be demonstrated in excess in the liver. The distribution of the intermediate of the pathway within the body as well as meta-

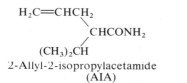

2-Allyl-2-isopropylacetamide
(AIA)

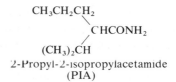

2-Propyl-2-isopropylacetamide
(PIA)

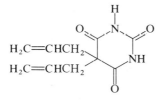

5,5-Diallylbarbituric acid

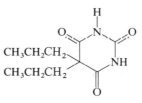

5,5-Dipropylbarbituric acid

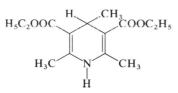

3,5-Diethoxycarbonyl-1,4-dihydrocollidine
(DDC)

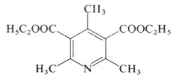

3,5-Diethoxycarbonylcollidine
(DC)

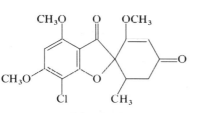

Griseofulvin

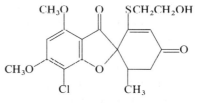
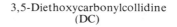

HET-griseofulvin

Fig. 1. Four classes of compounds which induce hepatic porphyria in rodents. For each porphyrogenic compound, the structure of a closely related analog which does not cause porphyria is also shown

bolic studies which will be referred to in some detail later, indicate that the liver is the main—if not the only—site of production of these pigments. Quantitative considerations show quite clearly that the increased excretion of porphyrins and their precursors cannot be due merely to a block in their further utilization along the pathway, but must represent a marked increase in their rate of formation by the liver. The same general picture of hepatic overproduction of the intermediates of the pathway is seen with all active drugs with the important difference that the main intermediate which accumulates and is excreted varies according to the drugs.

Thus protoporphyrin is the main product with both DDC and griseofulvin; while with AIA and allyl-containing barbiturates and related drugs, a mixture of different porphyrins accumulate. Therefore any attempt at discussing the mechanism by which these drugs induce porphyria must take into account two basic facts: 1) that the drugs stimulate the formation of intermediates of the pathway in the liver, and 2) that the biochemical picture can show differences according to the drug.

B. The Mechanism of Induction of Porphyria by Drugs

I. Stimulation of 5-Aminolevulinate Synthetase (ALA-S)

An important step forward in our understanding of the mechanism of action of these drugs has been the appreciation of the importance of the first enzyme of the pathway (ALA-S) in the regulation of porphyrin and heme synthesis. There are two main reasons why this enzyme plays a key role in the regulation of heme synthesis. The first is that under normal conditions its activity appears to be rate-limiting in the overall pathway. This is best illustrated by the observation that an increased supply of ALA will increase both in vivo and in vitro the liver synthesis of porphyrins and heme (Scott, 1955; Granick, 1966; Doss, 1969; De Matteis and Gibbs, 1972; Druyan and Kelly, 1972), while an increased supply of the precursors of ALA will not. A comparison of the activities of the various enzymes of the pathway (as measured with liver preparations, in vitro) is also compatible with ALA-S being normally the rate-limiting step (De Matteis, 1975).

The second reason why ALA-S is considered important in the regulation of the pathway is that this enzyme is the site where heme—the end product—exercises a negative feedback control on its own synthesis (Fig. 2). It is not yet clear whether the feedback control exercised by heme on ALA-S involves changes in the amount of enzyme formed by the protein-synthesizing apparatus (end-product repression; Granick, 1966), changes in the activity of the enzyme (end-product inhibition; Burnham and Lascelles, 1963) or both. These possibilities will be discussed in some detail later (Section B. 1.3).

In agreement with the concept that in porphyria there is an increased production of intermediates in the liver, Granick and Urata (1963) first showed that the activity of the rate-limiting enzyme of the pathway, ALA-S, is markedly increased in the liver of animals treated with DDC; a finding later extended to hepatic porphyria caused by AIA (Marver et al., 1966), allyl-containing barbiturates (Abbritti and De Matteis, 1971), and griseofulvin (Nakao et al., 1967), Granick (1966) suggested that these drugs increase the activity (and amount) of ALA-S by interacting with the portion of a specific aporepressor protein which normally binds heme and by competing with heme for this site (mechanism number 2, in Fig. 2). Heme would then be prevented from combining with the aporepressor and the operator gene for ALA-S would be kept open for a continous synthesis of the respective messenger-RNA and of the enzyme protein. This would ultimately result in an increased formation of ALA and of porphyrins which would tend to accumulate in the liver giving rise to the chemical picture of porphyria. An interference by the drugs with the formation of the "repressor heme" would not account,

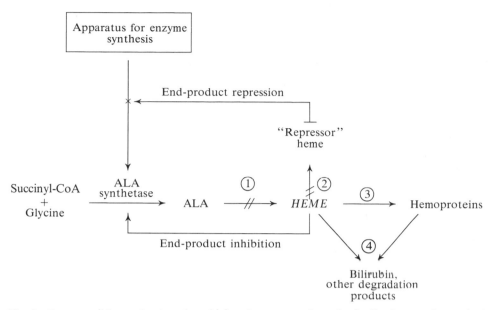

Fig. 2. Four possible mechanisms by which a drug may reduce the feedback control exercised by heme at the level of ALA-S: *1*) inhibition of heme synthesis; *2*) inhibition of the formation of "repressor" heme (GRANICK, 1966); *3*) increased rate of heme utilization; *4*) increased rate of heme degradation. Only mechanisms 1 and 4 will lead to a loss of liver heme and, of these, mechanism No. 1 may be expected to be associated with a greater accumulation of the intermediates of the pathway

however, for the difference in biochemical picture which are seen in rodents after administration of different drugs, neither would it provide a satisfactory explanation for the loss of liver heme which is seen in association with the increased ALA-S activity (see below). In addition, even though heme can counteract the stimulatory effect of drugs on ALA-S (GRANICK, 1966; MARVER, 1969), dose-response experiments in tissue culture provide no evidence that drugs and heme compete for the same site (CREIGHTON et al., 1971).

1. Interference by Drugs with the Regulation of the Pathway Through Loss of Liver Heme. The "Specific" Effect

An alternative mechanism by which griseofulvin, DDC, AIA, and allyl-containing barbiturates might interfere with the feedback control of heme and stimulate markedly the activity of ALA-S is provided by the recent findings from several laboratories that these drugs all cause a loss of heme from the liver. For example after a single dose of AIA to the rat, there is a rapid loss of a microsomal hemoprotein, cytochrome P-450 and a corresponding decrease in the total heme content of the liver at the time when the activity of the ALA-S is rising. Liver heme content, as measured by the levels of its major hemoprotein, cytochrome P-450, and activity of ALA-S behave in time in a reciprocal fashion (Fig. 3), as might be expected if loss of liver heme was causally related to the stimulation of the enzyme

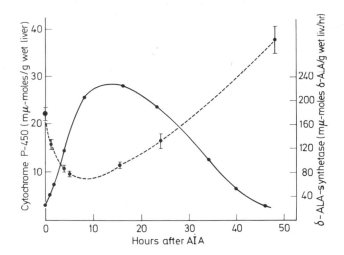

Fig. 3. The effect of a single dose of 2-allyl-2-isopropylacetamide on microsomal cytochrome P-450 levels and ALA-S activity of the liver homogenates. P-450 levels (●---●) are given as averages (± S.E.M.) of the values observed in four animals. The data on ALA-S activity (●——●) are from Marver et al. (1966). (Reproduced from De Matteis (1970), with permission) mission)

(De Matteis, 1970). A loss of cytochrome P-450 has also been reported in rats, rabbits and mice after administration of the other porphyrogenic compounds DDC, griseofulvin and allyl-containing barbiturates (Wada et al., 1968; Waterfield et al., 1969; Sweeney et al., 1971; Abbritti and De Matteis, 1971). In clear contrast, after administration to rodents of one of several drugs which do not cause hepatic porphyria, such as phenylbutazone, phenobarbitone and the nonporphyrogenic analogues of AIA, DDC and griseofulvin (see Section B.I.1.a), no loss of liver cytochrome P-450 heme is observed (this is, on the contrary, usually increased) and the ALA-S activity is stimulated only marginally. All these findings strongly suggest the importance of the loss of liver heme for the marked stimulation of ALA-S seen in porphyria.

There are two main mechanisms by which a drug might decrease the concentration of liver heme: by promoting destruction of heme, or by inhibiting its synthesis (mechanisms Nos. 4 and 1, respectively, in Fig. 2).

a) *Increased Destruction of Liver Heme Caused by Allyl-Containing Acetamides and Barbiturates*

In the case of AIA, allyl-barbiturates and other allyl-containing drugs the loss of liver heme is due to increased destruction and conversion into certain unidentified green pigments, an effect already described in detail in Chapter 4. The microsomal fraction is by far the most important site of heme destruction, probably because allyl-containing compounds have to be converted by the microsomal drug-metabolizing system to reactive derivatives in order to cause heme degradation (De Matteis, 1971a; Levin et al., 1973). Within the microsomes the effect of AIA appears to be confined to the heme of cytochrome P-450: not only are the total

protein content, glucose-6-phosphatase activity and cytochrome b_5 concentration
of the microsomes unaffected by AIA treatment (DE MATTEIS, 1971a), but the
apoprotein of cytochrome P-450 itself [rendered free from its heme complement
by the migration of the green pigments into the cell sap (DE MATTEIS, 1973a)]
remains largely unchanged. This is suggested by the finding that it can accept
exogenous heme in vitro to "reconstitute" the full, heme-containing cytochrome
(SARDANA et al., 1976). If a similar process of reconstitution takes place in vivo,
this may have important implication for the overall effect of AIA on the regulation
of liver heme biosynthesis. The apoprotein of cytochrome P-450 may then be
visualized as a catalytic center for AIA-dependent degradation of heme, not only
of the heme already present on the apoprotein at the time of drug administration,
but also of newly synthesized heme which would be subsequently accepted by the
free apoprotein and converted to green pigments.[1] Newly formed heme would then
be diverted into the degradation pathway, away from its regulatory function on
ALA-S (and on heme oxygenase) and also from its utilization for synthesis of
other hemoproteins, such as a catalase and tryptophan pyrrolase (see later). This
may account for the observation that a loss of rapidly labeled heme is also seen
from the cytosol and from the crude mitochondrial fraction of treated animals
(DE MATTEIS, 1973a) and also for the finding that exogenous heme given to perfused
livers treated with AIA is degraded to abnormal products (LANDAW et al., 1970;
LIEM and MULLER-EBERHARD, 1976). This mechanism would also account for the
marked increase in ALA-S activity, a response necessary to sustain the accelerated
heme turnover (see also LABBE, HANAWA and LOTTSFELDT, 1961), with the intermediates of the pathway accumulating since they are produced in amounts exceed-
ing the capacity of the respective enzymes.

b) *Inhibition of Liver Heme Synthesis Caused by DDC and Griseofulvin*

In the case of DDC there is also some degree of liver heme destruction (ABBRITTI
and DE MATTEIS, 1973), but inhibition of liver heme synthesis may be more important in causing the loss of liver heme and the stimulation of ALA-S activity.
A rapid loss in activity of porphyrin-metal chelatase (the enzyme which converts
protoporphyrin into heme) is caused by this drug in liver mitochondria, before
any increase in either the activity of ALA-S or in liver porphyrin concentration
(Fig. 4): an increase in liver porphyrin concentration and in ALA-S activity is
first seen when the activity of the chelatase, measured spectrophotometrically with
Co^{2+} and mesoporphyrin as substrates or isotopically with Fe^{59} and protoporphyrin, is decreased by about 70%. Also in agreement with the concept that the
inhibition of the chelatase is specifically involved in the stimulation of ALA-S
by this drug is the finding (Fig. 5) that mice, which are more sensitive than rats to
the effect of DDC on the activity of ALA-S and liver porphyrin content, are also
more sensitive with respect to the decrease in chelatase activity. In both species
an approximately 70% decrease in chelatase activity is accompanied by an increase
in liver porphyrin content and this is achieved by 5 mg DDC/kg body wt. in mice
and by 25 mg/kg in rats.

---

[1] Recent studies (REIN et al., 1976) suggest that the heme of cytochrome P-450 is not deeply
embedded in the apoprotein in a heme pocket as for other hemoproteins, but is exposed to
the outside environment. This may facilitate access of free heme to the apoprotein heme site.

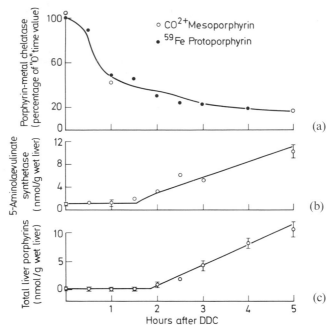

Fig. 4a–c. Effect of a single dose of 3,5-diethoxycarbonyl-1,4-dihydrocollidine on (a) the porphyrin-metal chelatase, (b) the ALA-S activity and (c) the total porphyrin concentration of rat liver. Rats were starved for 24 h, then given an IP dose of drug (100 mg/kg) and their starvation continued. The chelatase activity is expressed as a percentage of the zero-time values of either the Co^{2+} mesoporphyrin chelatase of isolated mitochondria ($\circ$; each point is the mean of four observations) or of the incorporation of ^{59}Fe into protoporphyrin by liver homogenates ($\bullet$; each point is the mean of two observations). Reproduced from De Matteis et al. (1973), with permission of the *Biochemical Journal*

There are two findings, however, that suggest that some other mechanism apart from the decrease in chelatase activity may be involved in the stimulation of ALA-S by DDC. The first is that, in the rat experiment of Fig. 4, both the activity of ALA-S and the concentration of porphyrins show a gradual decrease after 5 h, even though the chelatase activity remains very low. The second is the observation (Fig. 5) that in both rats and mice the administration of DDC in doses larger than the minimum porphyrogenic doses mentioned above is followed by a gradual increase in ALA-S activity and in porphyrin concentration without a further decrease in chelatase activity. Therefore DDC may have two actions (De Matteis et al., 1973; De Matteis and Gibbs, 1975): a specific one related to the effect on the chelatase and an additional "potentiation" action. The latter may be the "non-specific" effect (see later) common to several lipid-soluble drugs.

Inhibition of liver heme synthesis may also be important in the stimulation of ALA-S and in the production of porphyria by griseofulvin. When fed in the diet to mice, this drug also caused a rapid loss of activity of the chelatase. Furthermore, griseofulvin inhibited the chelatase much more effectively in the mouse where it caused a marked stimulation of the synthetase, than in the rat where it caused only a slight increase in ALA-S activity (Table 2). Since the rat showed signifi-

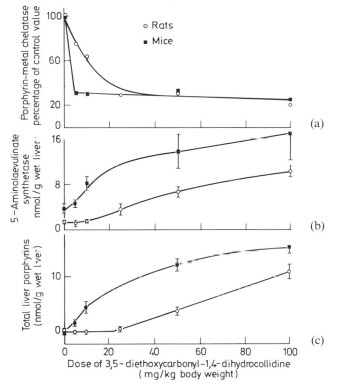

Fig. 5a—c. Effect of treating rats or mice with 3,5-diethoxycarbonyl-1,4-dihydrocollidine on (a) the porphyrin-metal chelatase activity, (b) the ALA-S activity and (c) the total porphyrin concentration of the liver. Rats (O) and mice (■) were starved for 24 h, then given 3,5-di-ethoxycarbonyl-1,4 dihydrocollidine IP and killed 5 h later. Reproduced from DE MATTEIS et al. (1973), with permission of the *Biochemical Journal*

cantly higher blood concentration of griseofulvin (Table 2), its lack of response cannot be due to impaired absorption of the drug or to rapid metabolic disposal, but must represent a diminished sensitivity of this species to the specific effect of the drug on the chelatase. This is also suggested by the observation that with a different porphyrogenic drug, AIA, the rat—not the mouse—is the more sensitive species (DE MATTEIS et al., 1973).

As originally suggested by ONISAWA and LABBE (1963) and by LOCKHEAD et al. (1967), a block in heme synthesis at the level of the chelatase explains the accumulation of large amounts of protoporphyrin which are seen in DDC and griseofulvin porphyria. Inhibition of heme synthesis at one of several steps in the biosynthetic chain has also been reported in three varieties of human porphyria and in hexachlorobenzene experimental porphyria (see chapters by MAXWELL and MEYER and by ELDER) and also in porphyrin-accumulating mutants of *Escherichia coli* (POWELL et al., 1973). In all these cases, the major intermediate which accumulates is (as in DDC and griseofulvin porphyria) that immediately before the enzyme which is deficient and in most cases an increased activity of ALA-S has also been found. Therefore inhibition of heme synthesis provides a satisfactory explanation

Table 2. Species differences in the liver response to the porphyrogenic activity of griseofulvin. Male rats and mice were given powdered diet containing, where appropriate, griseofulvin at a concentration of 1%. Results given are means ± S.E.M. of at least four observations. (Data from De Matteis and Gibbs, 1975)

Species	Treatment (and duration)	Liver ALA-S (nmol/min/g)	Total liver porphyrins (nmol/g)	Liver por- phyrin-metal chelatase (nmol/min/ mg mitoch. prot.)	Blood griseo- fulvin levels (µg/ml)
Mouse	None (control)	1.33 ± 0.16	<0.06	1.90 ± 0.05	—
	Griseofulvin (3 days)	8.87 ± 0.38^a	70.1 ± 8.8	0.45 ± 0.05^a	3.5 ± 0.24
Rat	None (control)	0.77 ± 0.22	<0.06	0.89 ± 0.05	—
	Griseofulvin (3 days)	—	0.59 ± 0.06	—	$7.8 \pm 1.18^*$
	Griseofulvin (10 days)	1.82 ± 0.18^a	0.16 ± 0.01	0.60 ± 0.03^a	—

[a] $P<0.01$, when compared with corresponding control values.
[*] $P<0.02$, when compared with corresponding values in mice.

not only for the stimulation of ALA-S (through failure of the heme feedback mechanism), but also for the differences in biochemical picture between the various types of porphyrias.

c) *Requirement for Specific Chemical Structures*

Previous work has established the existence of a structural requirement for the induction of porphyria by all four classes of compounds considered here. Thus the presence of at least one allyl substituent was found to be essential for the induction of porphyria by AIA, allyl-containing barbiturates and related drugs (Goldberg and Rimington, 1955; Stich and Decker, 1955). DDC, but not its oxidized derivative (DC), was found to be porphyrogenic (Marks et al., 1965). Finally, in the griseofulvin group of drugs, isogriseofulvin was found to be much more active than griseofulvin, but its 2'-β-hydroxyethyl thioether analog of griseofulvin (HET-griseofulvin) completely inactive (De Matteis, 1966).

It has been found more recently (Abbritti and De Matteis, 1971; De Matteis, 1975; De Matteis and Gibbs, 1975) that these differences in porphyrogenic activity can be correlated with corresponding differences in ability to stimulate markedly ALA-S activity and to cause depletion of liver heme (by one of the two specific effects considered above, namely increased heme destruction or inhibition of heme synthesis). When comparing AIA and diallyl-barbiturate with their saturated analogs, PIA and dipropyl-barbiturate, only the allyl-containing drugs caused marked stimulation of ALA-S and loss of cytochrome P-450 heme with the appearance of green pigments, the products of the abnormal degradation of heme (Table 3). Similarly, in the DDC and griseofulvin classes of drugs, the same structural requirements for the induction of ALA-S also applied to the loss of chelatase activity: compare in Table 4 the effects of DDC, griseofulvin, and isogriseofulvin with those of the corresponding analogs DC and HET-griseofulvin.

It is unlikely that the lack of porphyrogenic activity of the inactive analogs is due to their rapid metabolic disposal, as PIA and DC were still inactive when

Table 3. Importance of the allyl group in the molecule of substituted acetamides and barbiturates for the stimulation of liver ALA-S and for the degradation of the heme of liver cytochrome P-450 to green pigments. Starved female rats were given a single dose of substituted acetamides orally or of barbiturates intraperitoneally and killed 15 h later. Results given (mean ± S.E.M. of at least four observations) are from ABBRITTI and DE MATTEIS (1971)

Treatment and dose (ml/kg or mmol/kg)	Liver ALA-S (nmol/min/g)	Liver cytochrome P-450 (nmol/g)	Intensity of brown-green color of microsomal pellet
Control (oil, 10 ml)	3.06 ± 0.33	22.4 ± 0.8	—
AIA (2.1 mmol)	7.9 ± 0.7^a	15.8 ± 0.8^a	+ +
PIA (2.1 mmol)	3.37 ± 0.37	30.3 ± 2.0^a	—
Control (saline, 10 ml)	2.0 ± 0.16	23.9 ± 0.4	—
Diallylbarbituric acid (0.4 mmol)	6.37 ± 1.0^a	19.2 ± 0.7^a	+
Dipropylbarbituric acid (0.4 mmol)	2.8 ± 0.5	25.8 ± 1.8	—

[a] $P < 0.01$, when compared with corresponding control values.

Table 4. Loss of liver porphyrin-metal chelatase activity and induction of hepatic porphyria caused by drugs of the DDC and Griseofulvin groups. Requirements of special chemical structures for both effects. Starved male rats were given a single oral dose of either DDC or DC and killed between 4 and 5 h later. Male mice were given access to diets containing, where appropriate, one of the drugs at a concentration of 1%. Results are expressed as means ± S.E.M. of at least three observations or as the values obtained in individual observations. (Data from DE MATTEIS, 1975 and DE MATTEIS and GIBBS, 1975)

Species	Treatment and dose (or duration)	Liver ALA-S activity (nmol/min/g)	Liver porphyrins (nmol/g)	Mitochondrial porphyrin-metal chelatase (nmol/min/mg protein)
Rat	Oil, 10 ml/kg	1.44 ± 0.08	$0.13 + 0.02$	$0.90; 0.78$
	DDC, 100 mg/kg	10.68 ± 1.30^c	10.68 ± 1.30^c	0.26 ± 0.01^c
	DC, 100 mg/kg	—	<0.06	$1.00; 1.00$
	DC, 250 mg/kg	$2.3; 3.1$	$0.18; 0.38$	$0.77; 0.78$
Mouse	None	1.33 ± 0.16	<0.06	1.90 ± 0.05
	Griseofulvin (0.7 days)	2.20 ± 0.18^b	0.12 ± 0.04	1.64 ± 0.10^a
	Griseofulvin (3 days)	8.87 ± 0.38^c	70.1 ± 8.8	0.45 ± 0.05^c
	Isogriseofulvin (0.7 days)	2.83 ± 0.33^b	3.11 ± 1.3	0.96 ± 0.01^c
	HET-griseofulvin (3 days)	$2.86 \pm 0.27^{b*}$	<0.06	$2.17 \pm 0.09^*$

[a] $P < 0.05$, [b] $P < 0.01$, [c] $P < 0.001$, when compared with corresponding control values.
* $P < 0.001$, when compared with corresponding values obtained in mice given griseofulvin for 3 days.

given in doses sufficiently high to cause prolonged hypnosis. In addition their lack of activity cannot be due to their failure to reach the liver in sufficiently high concentrations for the following reasons: 1) they caused a slight stimulation of ALA-S and this effect could not be increased significantly by giving them in very large amounts; 2) they affected the concentration of cytochrome P-450 in the liver, but they increased it—rather than decreasing it; 3) when given together with a small dose of DDC they all potentiated the stimulation of ALA-S and the induction of porphyria caused by the former drug (see later).

It can therefore be concluded that a marked stimulation of ALA-S activity and the accumulation of the intermediates of the pathway are only seen with a few drugs which are lipid soluble and *also* possess certain *specific* chemical structures responsible for the loss of liver heme (either by inhibiting heme synthesis or by increasing its degradation). Many other lipid-soluble drugs, including the nonporphyrogenic analogs considered above, cannot cause accumulation of the intermediates of the pathway when given on their own. However they can all potentiate the porphyria caused by DDC or AIA by a *nonspecific* potentiation effect related to their property of lipid solubility. This second effect will be considered in detail in Section B.I.2.

d) *Heme Pools Depleted in Porphyria. Importance of Heme with Rapid Turnover*

In addition to regulating its own synthesis at the level of ALA-S, heme can also control its own degradation by regulating the activity of heme oxygenase, for which it can act as an inducer (SCHMID and MCDONAGH, 1975). So heme appears to be involved in two separate feedback mechanisms which operate in opposite directions: a negative feedback at the level of the rate-limiting enzyme of heme synthesis and a positive feedback on the rate-limiting enzyme of heme degradation. Accordingly, under conditions where the concentration of liver (free) heme increases, the activity of ALA-S will tend to be diminished, whereas heme oxygenase will be stimulated and the opposite effect will be expected for both enzymes when the concentration of (free) heme decreases. In either case the changes of both enzymes are those expected to bring the concentration of liver (free) heme back to normal.

On account of the uncertainties which still exist on the detailed mechanism of these feedback controls, it is not yet possible to define the identity and intracellular localization of the pool(s) of heme which are responsible for the regulation of the two enzymes. On purely theoretic grounds, the "regulatory" heme can be visualized as a relatively small heme pool with a rapid turnover rate, into which newly synthesized heme is fed and out of which heme is drawn for combination with the apoproteins of the various hemoproteins or for degradation. It could be free heme or one or more pools in rapid equilibrium with free heme (DE MATTEIS, 1975; GRANICK et al., 1975). According to this model schematically represented in Figure 6, the apoproteins of the hemoproteins, the regulatory systems for ALA-S and heme oxygenase, and the pathways of heme degradation (to either bile pigments or to the abnormal green pigments) may all compete with each other for the same pool of regulatory heme with rapid turnover.

Evidence that porphyrogenic drugs deplete the regulatory heme is provided by the findings that they markedly stimulate ALA-S and that this effect can be prevented or reversed by the administration of exogenous heme (BISSELL and HAMMAKER, 1976), which presumably gets access to (and therefore replenishes) the depleted pool. Administration of exogenous heme is also followed by stimulation of liver heme oxygenase (BISSELL and HAMMAKER, 1976) and by increased liver production of bile pigments (SNYDER and SCHMID, 1965; LANDAW et al., 1970; LIEM

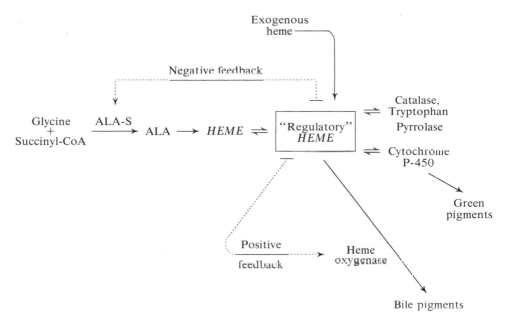

Fig. 6. A model of regulation of liver heme metabolism centered on the "regulatory" heme

and MULLER-EBERHARD, 1976) and this too is compatible with the model described in Figure 6. In addition, if the regulatory pool is depleted in porphyria, one would expect the following: 1) drugs like AIA might preferentially destroy heme with rapid turnover. 2) They might decrease the conversion of liver heme to bile pigments and cause an inhibition of heme oxygenase, as the heme which is rapidly degraded to green pigments would be lost to the normal pathway of degradation to bile pigments and also to the positive feedback control on heme oxygenase. 3) A depletion of hemoproteins other than cytochrome P-450 might also follow their administration, since (according to the model) their heme is also derived from the intermediary regulatory pool. There is some evidence for each of these and they will be discussed now, in turn.

1. In order to ascertain the approximate rate of turnover of the heme which is destroyed by AIA, the liver heme pools were dually labeled by giving to the same rat both [^{14}C]- and [^{3}H]-labeled ALA (DE MATTEIS, 1973a). The times of administration of the two labels (2 h and 26 h) were chosen so that, when AIA was administered, [^{3}H] and [^{14}C] would be expected to be present in different proportions in heme pools of appreciably different rates of turnover. The loss of radioactivity caused by AIA from heme was greater for the isotope given 2 h before the drug than for that given 26 h before, and this was observed both in the microsomes and in the cell sap, irrespective of the order in which the two isotopes were given. It was concluded that in both fractions heme with rapid turnover was preferentially affected.

2. The conversion of exogenous administered heme to bilirubin was decreased by AIA administration (LANDAW et al., 1970; LIEM and MULLER-EBERHARD, 1976)

as was that of liver heme labeled in vivo by [2-^{14}C]-glycine (Landaw et al., 1970). In addition, in three different studies administration of AIA to rats 12 − 24 h before killing caused a 50% decrease in liver heme oxygenase activity (Rotwell et al., 1973; Maines and Kappas, 1975; Maines et al., 1976). This suggests that the endogenous inducer of heme oxygenase, or regulatory heme may have been depleted by AIA.

3. A loss of catalase activity has been reported following administration of all the porphyrogenic compounds considered here, AIA and the closely related drug Sedormid (Schmid et al., 1955; Price et al., 1962), DDC (Ginsburg and Dowdle, 1963; Haeger-Aronsen, 1962), griseofulvin (De Matteis and Rimington, 1963) and allyl-containing barbiturates (Abbritti and De Matteis, 1971). In contrast, the nonporphyrogenic PIA and dipropyl barbiturate did not cause this effect.

The heme saturation of tryptophan pyrrolase was also significantly reduced by all the porphyrogenic compounds (Badawy and Evans, 1973a), whereas phenobarbitone increased the saturation of the enzyme by heme (Badawy and Evans, 1973b). Since tryptophan pyrrolase has a rapid rate of turnover (Schimke et al., 1965; Badawy and Evans, 1975) these findings are also compatible with the concept that in porphyria there is a depletion of a rapid-turnover pool of heme out of which heme can be utilized for the saturation of apotryptophan pyrrolase.

The effects of AIA and of the related drug Sedormid on liver catalase require further comment. The kinetics of decline of either the enzyme activity or of the immunochemically determined enzyme protein following treatment with these drugs strongly suggest that they inhibit the synthesis of the hemoprotein (Price et al., 1962; Kawamata et al., 1975a). Therefore it is not likely that the heme of catalase is directly destroyed by AIA as is that of cytochrome P-450. It is more likely that heme, as an essential constituent of catalase, is required for the formation of the hemoprotein and that under conditions in which there is a depletion of the precursor heme pool, heme supply may become rate limiting. Compatible with this view are the following findings: in vivo the incorporation of precursors of proteins into purified catalase was not significantly inhibited by Sedormid, whereas that of precursors of heme was markedly depressed (Schmid et al., 1955; Kawamata et al., 1975b); after either AIA or Sedormid, purified catalase contained excess protein when compared with the enzymatic activity (Kawamata et al., 1975a; Baird et al., 1976) suggesting that the enzyme was present to a larger extent than normally (Lazarow and De Duve, 1973) in an inactive, heme-free form. These findings have been interpreted as reflecting an interference by the drugs with the association of heme to the protein moiety or a drug-induced alteration of enzyme structure leading to loss of activity. They are in my view compatible with the model outlined in Figure 6, as they can be more easily explained by a rapid destruction of the precursor pool of heme (and conversion to green pigments), so that the supply of heme to catalase may become limiting. It is possible that the apoprotein of catalase which accumulates in excess in a heme-free form may slow down further synthesis of the enzyme protein or itself undergo rapid degradation. Either of these two mechanisms could explain why the protein of catalase (as determined by precipitation with antibodies, Kawamata et al., 1975a) also declines following treatment with these drugs.

2. The Action Related to the Property of Lipid Solubility of Drugs.
The Nonspecific Effect in the Stimulation of ALA-S

The first hint that the property of lipid solubility of inducing drugs was important in the stimulation of ALA-S was obtained in studies carried out in the cell-culture system devised by GRANICK (1966). Chicken embryo liver cells cultured in vitro can be made porphyric by a large number of drugs (see chapter by MARKS). In this system there is no requirement for the specific chemical groupings associated with production of porphyria in the liver of rodents, such as the allyl group in the AIA and barbiturates series of compounds (RACZ and MARKS, 1969; DE MATTEIS, 1971 b): the only property that the inducing drugs appear to share is a high degree of lipid solubility (DE MATTEIS, 1968) and this property can be correlated with the porphyrogenic activity (DE MATTEIS, 1971 b; MURPHY et al., 1975). In these respects the culture system resembles more closely the liver of patients with genetic porphyria (Table 1) than that of normal humans and experimental rodents (DE MATTEIS, 1971 b).

In order to explain these differences in sensitivity to drugs it was suggested (DE MATTEIS, 1971 b) that in both the porphyric patient and the cultured chicken liver, the hepatocyte may already intrinsically possess a lability in the regulation of the heme biosynthetic pathway that makes its ALA-S very sensitive to stimulation by a large variety of lipid soluble drugs. In the livers of normal humans and experimental rodents this lability must first be produced (either by increasing the rate of heme turnover or by causing a partial block in heme biosynthesis) for them to become sensitive to the stimulation of the pathway by a lipid-soluble compound. Support for this concept is provided by the results of studies on drug interaction in the experimental porphyria of the rodents.

a) Drug Interactions in Experimental Porphyria

In rodents, drugs like phenylbutazone and phenobarbitone stimulate ALA-S only slightly without causing accumulation of the intermediates of the pathway. However either of them, when given together with a relatively small dose of DDC, becomes very effective in stimulating ALA-S and causes an even greater porphyria (DE MATTEIS and GIBBS, 1972; DE MATTEIS, 1973 b; BOCK et al., 1973). Under these conditions the liver production of ALA is so large that the two subsequent enzymes of the pathway, ALA dehydratase and uroporphyrinogen synthetase, become rate limiting, and both ALA and PBG accumulate in excess in the liver (Table 5). This property of stimulating the porphyria caused by DDC is shared by a large number of lipid-soluble compounds, including the nonporphyrogenic analogs of either AIA, DDC, or griseofulvin (DE MATTEIS, 1973 b; DE MATTEIS and GIBBS, 1975), all of which are relatively ineffective when given on their own. As discussed before (Section B.I.1.b) this property may also be shown by DDC itself (and AIA) by virtue of their own lipid solubility, particularly when they are given at relatively high doses.

It will be noticed from Table 5 that the effect of giving phenylbutazone together with DDC (on either the activity of ALA-S or on the accumulation of the intermediates of the pathway) is far greater than the sum of the effects observed when

Table 5. Potentiation by either phenylbutazone or phenobarbitone of porphyria caused by DDC. Male rats were fasted for 24 h then given DDC intraperitoneally and at the same time either phenylbutazone or phenobarbitone orally and killed 15−16 h later. Results given are the averages of two observations or the means ± S.E.M. of at least four observations. (Data are from De Matteis, 1973b)

Given		Liver ALA-S activity (nmol/min/ g)	Liver content (nmol/g)		
Intraperitoneally (ml/kg or mg/kg)	Orally (ml/kg or mg/kg)		ALA	PBG	Total porphyrins
Oil, 10 ml	Oil, 10 ml	2.12 ± 0.33	<50	<6	0.09 ± 0.02
DDC, 100 mg	Oil, 10 ml	4.51 ± 0.49	<50	<6	2.8 ± 0.52
Oil, 10 ml	Phenylbutazone, 150 mg	5.85 ± 1.03	<50	<6	0.2 ± 0.05
DDC, 100 mg	Phenylbutazone, 150 mg	17.50 ± 0.9	131.6 ± 13	129.0 ± 8.7	8.6 ± 1.3
Oil, 10 ml	Phenobarbitone, 50 mg	3.2	<50	<6	0.15
DDC, 100 mg	Phenobarbitone, 50 mg	16.7	159	90	9.70

the two drugs were given individually. In dose-response experiments (De Matteis, 1973b) it was found that doses of DDC at least five times greater were required in the absence of phenylbutazone to obtain the same stimulation of ALA-S observed when the two drugs were given together. These results indicate some kind of synergism between the two drugs or potentiation effect and suggest that DDC and phenylbutazone (or another lipid-soluble drug) may lead to a stimulation of ALA-S through two different mechanisms.

As discussed in Section B.I.1, DDC interferes with the regulation of the pathway by lowering the concentration of heme available for control of ALA-S (the "specific" effect). It has been suggested (De Matteis, 1971b; De Matteis and Gibbs, 1972) that this specific action of drugs like DDC and AIA is also responsible for increasing the sensitivity of the liver ALA-S to a number of lipid-soluble compounds. The following findings are compatible with this interpretation: 1) AIA, which, like DDC, possesses the specific property of lowering the concentration of liver heme, also makes ALA-S very sensitive to the stimulatory effect of phenobarbitone (De Matteis, 1973b; Padmanabam et al., 1973). 2) Lower doses of DDC are required in mice than in rats to produce maximal inhibition of the chelatase (see Section B.I.1.b); correspondingly lower doses of DDC are also required in mice to increase the sensitivity of ALA-S to phenylbutazone (De Matteis, 1973b). 3) Other agents that produce inhibition of heme synthesis in either chicken embryo liver cells or in the liver of the intact rodent will also increase synergistically the response of ALA-S to lipid-soluble drugs (Strand et al., 1972; Sinclair and Granick, 1975; Maxwell and Meyer, 1976a; Sinclair in preparation). 4) Finally, in patients with genetic porphyria a partial block in liver heme biosynthesis is present already, intrinsically, as a result of the genetic defect (see chapter by Maxwell and Meyer). This may explain why in these patients the liver ALA-S is unusually sensitive to stimulation by a number of lipid-soluble drugs (De Matteis, 1973b; Maxwell and Meyer, 1976a, b).

It can therefore be concluded that the specific effect of certain drugs in interfering with the regulation of the pathway renders the liver ALA-S very sensitive to a second drug action, the nonspecific effect. The first effect is characteristic only of the porphyrogenic drugs, those capable of increasing the rate of liver heme degradation or of inhibiting its synthesis; the second is a feature of many compounds—porphyrogenic and nonporphyrogenic alike—which have in common the property of lipid solubility.

b) *Possible Mechanisms Underlying the Nonspecific Effect*

More difficult to define is the mechanism underlying the nonspecific effect, that associated with the property of lipid solubility. Two possibilities have been considered (DE MATTEIS, 1971 b).

1. The effect may be related to the property that many lipid-soluble drugs possess of stimulating the formation of the apoprotein of cytochrome P-450 (DE MATTEIS and GIBBS, 1972; PADMANABAN et al., 1973), for which some direct evidence has recently been obtained (CORREIA and MEYER, 1975; RAJAMANICKAM et al., 1975). This would then result in an increased utilization of heme for the formation of the cytochrome (mechanism No. 3 in Fig. 2) out of the intermediary pool of "regulatory" heme (Fig. 6). Under normal conditions, when there is no excessive degradation of heme and the synthesis of heme is unimpaired, a considerable accumulation of cytochrome P-450 is observed after phenylbutazone or phenobarbitone, with either small or no changes in the activity of ALA-S. This suggests that the amount of ALA and heme which is normally made by the liver is sufficient to meet the increased demand for enhanced P-450 formation (without big changes in the level of regulatory heme) or that, if any increased quantity of ALA must be made, it need only be a small amount. When, however, the regulatory heme is already partially depleted by a drug like AIA or DDC (through increased heme destruction or inhibited heme synthesis) the same stimulus to increased heme utilization may lead to a further marked depletion of the regulatory pool and therefore ultimately to a marked stimulation of ALA-S.

2. Alternatively, the nonspecific effect associated with lipid solubility may be in some way related to the property that many lipid-soluble drugs possess of stimulating the synthesis of several liver proteins and of increasing the size of the liver. Perhaps lipid-soluble drugs activate by some unknown basic mechanism the synthesis of the messenger-RNAs for several enzyme proteins, including that for ALA-S. Direct and indirect evidence for increased liver synthesis of messenger-type RNA has been obtained after administering several lipid-soluble drugs, including phenobarbitone, DDC and AIA (GELBOIN et al., 1967; PIPER and BOUSQUET, 1968; NAWATA and KATO, 1973; DEL FAVERO et al., 1975; SARDANA et al., 1975; MOSES et al., 1976). SINCLAIR (in preparation) has recently suggested that the effect on ALA-S of lipid-soluble drugs may be mediated through induced synthesis of the messenger-RNA for this enzyme, a suggestion in keeping with the experimental findings of SASSA and GRANICK (1970), TYRRELL and MARKS (1972), and TOMITA et al. (1974).

Both possible mechanisms considered above for the nonspecific effect of lipid-soluble drugs (increased synthesis of apocytochrome P-450 leading to increased ALA-S activity and direct effect of the drugs on the synthesis of ALA-S itself) require protein synthesis (see later). The main difference between the two is that the first also involves depletion of regulatory heme, whereas the second does not. Direct measurements of the concentration of liver free heme are not yet possible, but some information about this concentration can be gained indirectly from the activity of heme-dependent enzymes, such as catalase and tryptophan pyrrolase, since, according to the model described in Figure 6, the heme necessary for their synthesis would be expected to be drawn from the intermediary regulatory pool. Sweeney (1976) has recently studied the effect of DDC given either on its own or in combination with phenobarbitone on the activity of liver catalase and found that when the two drugs were given together (under conditions, that is, where the induction of ALA-S was markedly potentiated) the catalase activity was also considerably decreased. This finding suggested that a further depletion of the precursor regulatory pool may have taken place as a result of phenobarbitone administration and is therefore more readily compatible with the first mechanism considered above, that involving accumulation of cytochrome P-450. This conclusion is based, however, on the assumptions that the decreased catalase activity observed under these conditions reflects only decreased rate of catalase synthesis and that the decreased rate of synthesis is entirely due to limited supply of heme, two points for which as yet there is no direct experimental evidence.

3. Possible Role of Drug Metabolism and of Protein Synthesis in the Stimulation of ALA-S Caused by Drugs

The way in which the two main effects of drugs which have been considered above (the specific and nonspecific effects) interact with each other to produce the stimulation of ALA-S is far from clear. In Figure 7 certain possibilities are illustrated in a scheme which may facilitate an understanding of the results discussed below.

The stimulation of ALA-S caused by DDC could be prevented by prior administration to the rat of either an inhibitor of drug-metabolizing enzymes (SKF 525-A) or of an inhibitor of protein synthesis (cycloheximide). An important difference was that SKF 525-A also prevented the inhibition of the chelatase, whereas cycloheximide did not (De Matteis et al., 1973). Similar results have been obtained with AIA: here again either inhibitor could prevent the stimulation of ALA-S, but only SKF 525-A could also prevent the destruction of liver heme (De Matteis, 1971a; Satyanarayana Rao et al., 1972).

These results suggest that the effect of DDC and AIA on liver heme synthesis and degradation (the specific effect) is not the only factor involved in the stimulation of ALA-S: there is also a requirement for an additional factor or effect which can be prevented by cycloheximide. An attempt is made below to explain the results obtained with the two inhibitors in terms of the model described in Fig. 7 and also to discuss in the light of the model the role of drug metabolism and of protein synthesis for the stimulation of ALA-S caused by drugs.

The effect of SKF 525-A could be explained by an interference with the uptake of the porphyria-inducing drugs either by the liver itself or, within the liver, by the relevant site of action. However Satyanarayana Rao et al. (1972) have shown that the uptake of AIA by the liver and by the liver microsomal fraction was not inhibited by SKF 525-A. Alternatively, the effect of this inhibitor may indicate that both AIA and DDC need to be converted by way of drug-metabolism to some active derivative in order to cause destruction of liver heme or inhibition of the

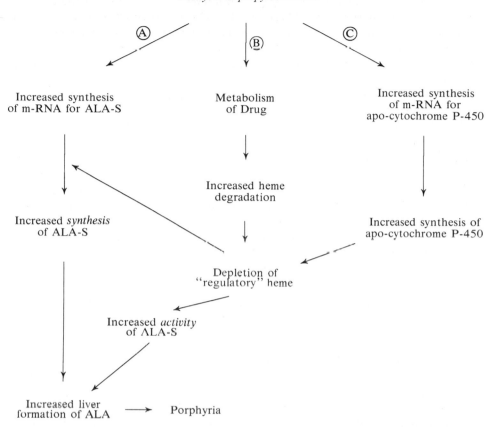

Fig. 7. Possible ways in which the specific and nonspecific effect of drugs interact with each other to produce the stimulation of ALA-S. The specific effect (pathway B) is produced only by the porphyrogenic drugs (like AIA, illustrated here), may require metabolism of the drug to an active derivative, and is inhibited by SKF 525-A. The nonspecific effect (involving pathways A and/or C) is produced by many lipid-soluble drugs (porphyrogenic and nonporphyrogenic alike), requires protein synthesis, and is inhibited by cycloheximide

chelatase, respectively (pathway B in Fig. 7). The following evidence is compatible with this latter possibility. First, results obtained in vitro suggest that metabolism of the allyl group may be required for the destruction of liver heme by either AIA (DE MATTEIS, 1971a), or allyl-containing barbiturates (LEVIN et al., 1973). Second, in newborn rats, which have a low activity of liver drug-metabolizing enzymes (KATO et al., 1964), DDC and AIA did not increase ALA-S (see also WOODS and DIXON, 1972) and only caused a slight inhibition of the chelatase (DE MATTEIS, 1975) and no change in heme degradation (PADMANABAN et al., 1973). In addition, if metabolism of AIA, allyl-barbiturates, DDC and griseofulvin to some active derivative was important for the destruction of heme and for the inhibition of the chelatase, then this might provide an explanation for the structural requirements for activity, which have been described in all four classes of compounds (see

Section B.I.1.c); and also for the species differences in response to these drugs, which can be very marked (De Matteis et al., 1973; De Matteis and Gibbs, 1975). All these lines of evidence are indirect, however, and until the postulated metabolites are actually isolated and tested for their activity, the problem of the metabolic activation of drugs for the production of the specific effect must be considered unresolved.

The role of drug-metabolism in porphyria is further complicated by the existence of data in the literature which suggest an opposite effect. Thus Marks and coworkers have reported that in the chick embryo an increased rate of metabolism of AIA, DDC, or other drugs can be correlated with a decreased porphyrogenic activity (Racz and Marks, 1972; Marks et al., 1973; Murphy et al., 1975). Similarly, Kaufman et al. (1970) have found in rats that pretreatment with phenobarbitone increased the rate of metabolism of AIA but diminished its property of stimulating ALA-S. Can these two opposite effects of drug-metabolism be reconciled? A possible explanation is provided by the involvement of two basically different mechanisms in the stimulation of ALA-S by drugs. Although metabolism of the porphyrogenic drugs may be necessary to produce the specific effect of destroying heme or inhibiting the chelatase (pathway B in Fig. 7), it will also divert the drugs away from their nonspecific effect (pathways A and C in Fig. 7), for which lipid solubility is required and where the parent compounds—rather than their metabolites—are probably involved. In the chick embryo cell cultures, where AIA and other drugs work entirely (or almost entirely) through the nonspecific effect related to their lipid solubility (De Matteis, 1971b; Murphy et al., 1975), increased metabolism will of course result in decreased porphyrogenic activity. In the liver of the intact rodents, where AIA stimulates ALA-S by producing both the specific and the nonspecific effect, it is possible that when the rate of metabolism of the drug is large enough to interfere markedly with the nonspecific effect, then the stimulation of ALA-S may also be diminished, even though destruction of heme is still taking place (see also Maxwell and Meyer, 1976b).

Let us now turn to consider the effect of cycloheximide and the role of protein synthesis. The ability of cycloheximide and of other inhibitors of protein synthesis to prevent the induction of ALA-S has been known for some time and the simplest explanation for this effect (Granick, 1966) is that the changes in ALA-S activity reflect changes in the amount of the enzyme protein which is synthesized de novo under the influence of the porphyrogenic drugs. Whiting and Granick (1976) have recently determined immunochemically the amount of enzyme protein present in chick embryo liver mitochondria during both induction of ALA-S by porphyrogenic drugs and the inhibition of this effect caused by hemin. They concluded that changes in enzyme activity observed under both conditions are entirely due to corresponding changes in amount of enzyme protein and that these are achieved primarily through stimulation or inhibition of the rate of synthesis of the enzyme; protein degradation plays no significant role in the process. If the same applies to the liver of the intact rodent, can both the specific and the nonspecific effect of drugs be brought together at the level of an increased synthesis of ALA-S? Perhaps—as discussed before—the lipid-soluble effect of drugs results primarily in increased synthesis of the messenger-RNA for several liver enzyme proteins, including that for ALA-S (pathway A in Fig. 7); whereas heme depletion may lead more specifically to an increased translation of the messenger-RNA for ALA-S. There is some evidence that in the chick embryo system the effect of heme is at the level of translation (SASSA and GRANICK, 1970; STRAND et al., 1972; TYRRELL and MARKS, 1972) and PADAMANABAN et al. (1973) have similarly suggested that in rat liver the concentration of heme may control the rate of synthesis of ALA-S by regulating the translation of its messenger-RNA. This scheme would explain why the specific and nonspecific effects discussed above interact with each other in a synergistic fashion to produce the stimulation of ALA-S. Both pathways A and B (Fig. 7) would be leading to increased synthesis of ALA S, but through two different actions, one at the transcriptional, the other at the translational stage of protein synthesis.

It cannot be excluded, however, that protein synthesis may be related to the activity of ALA-S in some other, less direct way. For example, if in the liver of rodents the activity of ALA-S was subjected to direct inhibition by a free heme pool in vivo, lipid-soluble drugs by increasing heme utilization may cause a depletion of the regulatory pool and indirectly lead to a stimulation of the activity of ALA S. This might result from an increased synthesis of the messenger-RNA for cytochrome P-450 (JACOB et al., 1974) and from an accumulation of the apocytochrome P-450 (pathway C in Fig. 7). This second scheme will also provide a possible explanation for the effect of cycloheximide: by inhibiting the synthesis of the apoprotein of cytochromes, the inhibitor might conceivably increase the concentration of free heme and lead to an inhibition of the enzyme (DE MATTEIS, 1975).[2] It could also explain the synergistic interaction between the specific and nonspecific effects of drugs in the stimulation of ALA-S, as both pathways B and C (Fig. 7) lead to a depletion of regulatory heme, but through different mechanisms.

Therefore, the results obtained with cycloheximide do not necessarily exclude the possibility that, in rodents, porphyrogenic drugs may increase the activity of ALA-S. Although most authors favor the hypothesis of an increased amount of enzyme, the possibility of changes in its activity should also be considered, for the following reasons:

1. A direct inhibition of rat liver ALA-S by heme has been documented with partially purified preparations of the enzyme (KAPLAN, 1971; SCHOLNICK et al., 1972; WHITING and ELLIOTT, 1972).

2. The heme-forming enzyme (chelatase) is in close association with the ALA-S at or n ar the mitochondrial inner membrane (MCKAY et al., 1969; ZUYDERHOUDT et al., 1969; JONES and JONES, 1969), an arrangement ideally suited to a direct control of the activity of the synthetase by the concentration of heme at the very site of heme synthesis.

3. Liver mitochondria obtained from normal rodents and—to a lesser extent— mitochondria obtained after treatment with porphyrogenic drugs showed an apparent increase in ALA-S activity in vitro when they were subjected to ultrasounds or to repeated freezing and thawing, or when their extracts were further diluted (GAYATHRI et al., 1973; PATTON and BEATTIE, 1973), suggesting that these treatments may have altered the distribution or concentration of an endogenous inhibi-

---

[2] Recent results (ABOUL-EL-MAKAREM and BOCK, 1976) suggest that cycloheximide, by inhibiting utilization of heme for the synthesis of hemoproteins, may cause accumulation of heme in a free, rapidly degradable, form.

tor. Furthermore, in mixing experiments, control mitochondria were found to inhibit the ALA-S activity of "porphyric" mitochondria, a property associated with the insoluble fraction of the mitochondrial homogenate and not affected by heating at 100°C for 5 min (Irving and Elliott, 1969). These results suggest a heat-stable inhibitor of ALA-S: the inhibitor might be present in relatively large amounts in the control mitochondria where the ALA-S activity is very low.

4. When rats were treated with cobaltous chloride (De Matteis and Gibbs, 1977) there was a marked loss of hepatic ALA-S activity, an effect probably mediated through inhibition of the activity of the enzyme rather than interference with its rate of synthesis. Cobalt treatment also caused formation in the liver of a stable compound with solubility properties similar to those of cobalt-protoporphyrin. It is possible therefore that this hemelike compound may be responsible for diminishing ALA-S activity by a mechanism similar to that involved in the feedback inhibition of the enzyme by heme.

In conclusion, the nonspecific effect involved in the stimulation of ALA-S by drugs may be mediated either by an increased synthesis of ALA-S itself or by increased formation of the apoprotein of cytochrome P-450. Either mechanism would require protein synthesis and therefore provides an explanation for the ability of cycloheximide to inhibit the induction of ALA-S and porphyria. The specific effect, on the other hand, may require metabolic activation of the drugs to a derivative responsible for destruction of heme or inhibition of the chelatase. It is uncertain at present whether depletion of heme affects ALA-S by increasing the synthesis of the enzyme or by stimulating its activity: these two mechanisms are not mutually exclusive and might operate simultaneously in a complementary fashion. Whether and to what extent either of them operate in the liver of rodents will be determined by immunochemical studies along the lines of Whiting and Granick's (1976) experiments and also by extending and clarifying the observations of Irving and Elliot (1969) and of Patton and Beattie (1973).

Abbreviations

AIA	2-Allyl-2-isopropylacetamide
ALA	5-Aminolevulinate
ALA-S	5-Aminolevulinate synthetase
DC	3,5-Diethoxycarbonylcollidine
DDC	3,5-Diethoxycarbonyl-1,4-dihydrocollidine
HET-griseofulvin	2'-β-Hydroxyethyl thioether analog of griseofulvin
PBG	Porphobilinogen
PIA	2-Propyl-2-isopropylacetamide
SKF 525-A	2-Diethylamino-3,3-diphenylpropylacetate

References

Abbritti, G., De Matteis, F.: Decreased levels of cytochrome P-450 and catalase in hepatic porphyria caused by substituted acetamides and barbiturates. Importance of the allyl group in the molecule of the active drugs. Chem. biol. Interact. **4**, 281 – 286 (1971)
Abbritti, G., De Matteis, F.: Effect of 3,5-diethoxycarbonyl-1,4-dihydrocollidine on degradation of liver heme. Enzyme **16**, 196 – 202 (1973)

Abou-El-Makarem, M.M., Bock, K.W.: UDP-glucuronyl transferase in perfused rat liver and in microsomes. Europ. J. Biochem. **62**, 411 – 416 (1976)

Badawy, A.A.-B., Evans, M.: The effects of chemical porphyrogens and drugs on the activity of rat liver tryptophan pyrrolase. Biochem. J. **136**, 885 – 892 (1973 a)

Badawy, A.A.-B., Evans, M.: The effects of chronic phenobarbitone administration and subsequent withdrawal on the activity of rat liver tryptophan pyrrolase and their resemblance to those of ethanol. Biochem. J. **135**, 555 – 557 (1973 b)

Badawy, A.A.-B., Evans, M.: Regulation of rat liver tryptophan pyrrolase activity. Biochem. J. **150**, 511 – 520 (1975)

Baird, M.B., Samis, H.V., Massie, H.R., Zimmerman, J.A., Sfeir, G.A.: Evidence for altered hepatic catalase molecules in allylisopropylacetamide-treated mice. Biochem. Pharmacol. **25**, 1101 – 1105 (1976)

Bissell, D.M., Hammaker, L.E.: Cytochrome P-450 heme and the regulation of δ-aminolevulinic acid synthetase in the liver. Arch. Biochem. Biophys. **176**, 103 – 112 (1976)

Bock, K.W., Weiner, R., Fröhling, W.: Regulation of δ-aminolevulinic acid synthetase by drugs and steroids in isolated perfused rat liver. Enzyme **16**, 295 – 301 (1973)

Burnham, B.F., Lascelles, J.: Control of porphyrin biosynthesis through a negative-feedback mechanism. Biochem. J. **87**, 462 – 472 (1963)

Correia, M.A., Meyer, U.A.: Apo-cytochrome P-450: Reconstitution of functional cytochrome with hemin in vitro. Proc. nat Acad. Sci. (Wash.) **72**, 400 – 404 (1975)

Creighton, J.M., Racz, W.J., Tyrrell, D.L.J., Schneck, D.W., Marks, G.S.: Drug-induced porphyrin biosynthesis, S. Afr. J. Lab. clin. Med. **17**, 79 – 81 (1971)

Del Favero, A., Gamulin, S., Gray, C.H., Norman, M.R.: Ribosome function in livers of porphyric mice. Biochem. J. **150**, 573 – 576 (1975)

De Matteis, F.: Hypercholesterolaemia and liver enlargement in experimental hepatic porphyria. Biochem. J. **98**, 23 C – 25 C (1966)

De Matteis, F.: Toxic hepatic porphyrias. Semin. Hematol. **5**, 409 – 423 (1968)

De Matteis, F.: Rapid loss of cytochrome P-450 and heme caused in the liver microsomes by the porphyrogenic agent 2-allyl-2-isopropylacetamide. Febs Lett. **6**, 343 – 345 (1970)

De Matteis, F.: Loss of heme in rat liver caused by the porphyrogenic agent 2-allyl-2-isopropylacetamide. Biochem. J. **124**, 767 – 777 (1971 a)

De Matteis, F.: Drugs and porphyria. S. Afr. J. Lab. clin. Med. **17**, 126 – 133 (1971 b)

De Matteis, F.: Drug-induced destruction of cytochrome P-450. Drug Metab. Dispos. **1**, 267 – 272 (1973 a)

De Matteis, F.: Drug interactions in experimental hepatic porphyria. A model for the exacerbation by drugs of human variegate porphyria. Enzyme **16**, 266 – 275 (1973 b)

De Matteis, F.: The effect of drugs on 5-aminolaevulinate synthetase and other enzymes in the pathway of liver heme biosynthesis. In: Enzyme Induction. Parke, D.V. (ed.), pp. 185 – 205. London – New York: Plenum Press 1975

De Matteis, F., Abbritti, G., Gibbs, A.H.: Decreased liver activity of porphyrin metal chelatase in hepatic porphyria caused by 3,5-diethoxycarbonyl-1,4-dihydrocollidine. Studies in rats and mice. Biochem. J. **134**, 717 – 727 (1973)

De Matteis, F., Gibbs, A.: Stimulation of liver 5-aminolevulinate synthetase by drugs and its relevance to drug-induced accumulation of cytochrome P-450. Biochem. J. **126**, 1149 – 1160 (1972)

De Matteis, F., Gibbs, A.H.: Stimulation of the pathway of porphyrin synthesis in the liver of rats and mice by griseofulvin, 3,5-diethoxycarbonyl-1,4-dihydrocollidine and related drugs: evidence for two basically different mechanisms. Biochem. J. **146**, 285 – 287 (1975)

De Matteis, F., Gibbs, A.H.: Inhibition of heme synthesis caused by cobalt in rat liver. Evidence for two different sites of action. Biochem. J. **162**, 213 – 216 (1977)

De Matteis, F., Rimington, C.: Disturbances of porphyrin metabolism caused by griseofulvin in mice. Brit. J. Derm. **75**, 91 – 104 (1963)

Doss, M.: Über die Porphyrinsynthese in der Leberzellkultur unter der Einwirkung von Pharmaka und Steroiden. Z. klin. Chem. u. klin. Biochem. **2**, 133 – 147 (1969)

Druyan, R., Kelly, A.: The effect of exogenous δ-aminolaevulinate on rat liver heme and cytochromes. Biochem. J. **129**, 1095 – 1099 (1972)

Gayathri, A.K., Rao, M.R.S., Padmanaban, G.: Studies on the induction of δ-aminolevulinic acid synthetase in mouse liver. Arch. Biochem. Biophys. **155**, 299 – 306 (1973)

Gelboin, H.V., Wortham, J.S., Wilson, R.G.: 3-Methylcholanthrene and phenobarbital. Stimulation of rat liver RNA polymerase. Nature (Lond.) **214**, 281—283 (1967)

Ginsburg, A.D., Dowdle, E.B.: Biochemical changes in dicarbethoxy dihydrocollidine-induced porphyria in the rat. S. Afr. J. Lab. clin. Med. **9**, 206—211 (1963)

Goldberg, A., Rimington, C.: Experimentally produced porphyria in animals. Proc. roy. Soc. B **143**, 257—280 (1955)

Granick, S.: The induction in vitro of the synthesis of δ-aminolevulinic acid synthetase in chemical porphyria: A response to certain drugs, sex hormones, and foreign chemicals. J. biol. Chem. **241**, 1359—1375 (1966)

Granick, S., Sassa, S.: δ-aminolevulinic acid synthetase and the control of heme and chlorophyll synthesis. Metab. Regulation **5**, 77—141 (1971)

Granick, S., Sinclair, P., Sassa, S., Grieninger, G.: Effects by heme, insulin, and serum albumin on heme and protein synthesis in chick embryo liver cells cultured in a chemically defined medium, and a spectrofluorometric assay for porphyrin composition. J. biol. Chem. **250**, 9215—9225 (1975)

Granick, S., Urata, G.: Increase in activity of δ-aminolevulinic acid synthetase in liver mitochondria induced by feeding of 3,5-dicarbethoxy-1,4-dihydrocollidine. J. biol. Chem. **238**, 821—827 (1963)

Haeger-Aronsen, B.: Porphyria induced in the rabbit by diethyl-1,4-dihydro-2,4,6-trimethylpyridine-3,5-dicarboxylate. II. Catalase activity and concentration of green porphyrins in the liver and a comparison with apronal-induced porphyria. Acta pharmacol. (Kbh.) **19**, 156—164 (1962)

Irving, E.A., Elliott, W.H.: A sensitive radiochemical assay method for δ-aminolevulinic acid synthetase. J. biol. Chem. **244**, 60—67 (1969)

Jacob, S.T., Scharf, M.B., Vessel, E.S.: Role of RNA in Induction of hepatic microsomal mixed function oxidases. Proc. nat. Acad. Sci. (Wash.) **71**, 704—707 (1974)

Jones, M.S., Jones, O.T.G.: The structural organization of heme synthesis in rat liver mitochondria. Biochem. J. **113**, 507—514 (1969)

Kaplan, B.H.: δ-Aminolevulinic acid synthetase from the particulate fraction of liver of porphyric rats. Biochim. biophys. Acta (Amst.) **235**, 381—388 (1971)

Kato, R., Vassanelli, P., Frontino, G., Chiesara, E.: Variation in the activity of liver microsomal drug-metabolizing enzymes in rats in relation to the age. Biochem. Pharmacol. **13**, 1037—1051 (1964)

Kaufman, L., Swanson, A.L., Marver, H.S.: Chemically induced porphyria: Prevention by prior treatment with phenobarbital. Science **170**, 320—322 (1970)

Kawamata, F., Sakurai, T., Higashi, T.: Biosynthesis of liver catalase in rats treated with allylisopropylacetylcarbamide. J. Biochem. (Japan) **78**, 969—974 (1975a)

Kawamata, F., Sakurai, T., Higashi, T.: Biosynthesis of liver catalase in rats treated with allylisopropylacetylcarbamide. J. Biochem. (Japan) **78**, 975—980 (1975b)

Labbe, R.F., Hanawa, Y., Lottsfeldt, F.I.: Heme and fatty acid biosynthesis in experimental porphyria. Arch. Biochem. Biophys. **92**, 373—374 (1961)

Landaw, S.A., Callahan, E.W. Jr., Schmid, R.: Catabolism of heme in vivo: comparison of the simultaneous production of bilirubin and carbon monoxide. J. clin. Invest. **49**, 914—925 (1970)

Lazarow, P.B., De Duve, C.: The synthesis and turnover of rat liver peroxisomes. IV. Biochemical pathway of catalase synthesis. J. Cell Biol. **59**, 491—506 (1973)

Levin, W., Jacobson, M., Sernatinger, E., Kuntzman, R.: Breakdown of cytochrome P-450 heme by secobarbital and other allyl-containing barbiturates. Drug Metab. Dispos. **1**, 275—284 (1973)

Liem, H.H., Muller-Eberhard, U.: Effect of allylisopropylacetamide on the conversion of heme (Ferriprotoporphyrin IX) to bilirubin in rat liver perfusion in vitro. In: Porphyrins in Human Diseases. Doss, M. (ed.), pp. 80—85. Basel: S. Karger 1976

Lockhead, A.C., Dagg, J.H., Goldberg, A.: Experimental griseofulvin porphyria in adult and foetal mice. Brit. J. Derm. **79**, 96—102, (1967)

Maines, M.D., Janousek, V., Tomio, J.M., Kappas, A.: Cobalt inhibition of synthesis and induction of δ-aminolevulinate synthase in liver. Proc. nat. Acad. Sci. (Wash.) **73**, 1499—1503 (1976)

Maines, M.D., Kappas, A.: Cobalt stimulation of heme degradation in the liver. Dissociation of microsomal oxidation of heme from cytochrome P-450. J. biol. Chem. **250**, 4171 – 4177 (1975)

Marks, G.S., Hunter, E.G. Terner, U.K., Schneck, D.: Studies of the relationship between chemical structure and porphyria-inducing activity. Biochem. Pharmacol. **14**, 1077 – 1084 (1965)

Marks, G.S., Krupa, V., Creighton, J.C., Roomi, M.W.: Investigation of the role of an allyl group in substituted acetamides in porphyrin-inducing activity. Hoppe-Seylers Z. physiol. Chem. **354**, 856 – 857 (1973)

Marver, H.S.: The role of heme in the synthesis and repression of microsomal protein. In: Microsomes and Drug Oxidation. Gillette, J.R., Conney, A.H., Cosmides, G.J., Estabrook, R.W., Fouts, J.R., Mannering, G.J. (eds.), pp. 495 – 511. New York: Academic Press 1969

Marver, H.S., Collins, A., Tschudy, D.P., Rechcigl, M.: δ-Aminolevulinic acid synthetase. II. Induction in rat liver. J. biol. Chem. **241**, 4323 – 4329 (1966)

Maxwell, J.D., Meyer, U.A.: Effect of lead on hepatic δ-aminolaevulinic acid synthetase activity in the rat: A model for drug sensitivity in intermittent acute porphyria. Europ. J. clin. Invest. **6**, 373 – 379 (1976 a)

Maxwell, J.D., Meyer, U.A.: Drug sensitivity in hereditary hepatic porphyria. In: Proceedings of the International Porphyrin Meeting, Freiburg, May 1 – 4, 1975. Doss, M. (ed.), pp. 1 – 9. Basel: S. Karger 1976 b

McKay, R., Druyan, R., Getz, G.S., Rabinowitz, M.: Intramitochondrial localization of δ-aminolaevulate synthetase and ferrochelatase in rat liver. Biochem. J. **114**, 455 – 461 (1969)

Meyer, U.A., Schmid, R.: The porphyrias. In: The Metabolic Basis of Inherited Disease, Stanburg, J.B., Wyngaarden, J.B., Frederickson, D.S. (eds.), 4th ed. Chapter 50. New York: McGraw-Hill 1977

Moses, H.L., Spelsberg, T.C., Korinek, J., Chytil, F.: Porphyria-inducing drugs: Comparative effects on nuclear ribonucleic acid polymerases in rat liver. Molec. Pharmacol. **12**, 731 – 737 (1976)

Murphy, F.R., Krupa, V., Marks, G.S.: Drug-induced porphyrin synthesis. XIII. Role of lipophilicity in determining porphyrin-inducing activity of aliphatic amides after blockade of their hydrolysis by bis-[*p*-nitrophenyl]phosphate. Biochem. Pharmacol. **24**, 883 – 889 (1975)

Nakao, K., Wada, O., Takaku, F., Sassa, S., Yano, Y., Urata, G.: The origin of the increased protoporphyrin in erythrocytes of mice with experimentally induced porphyria. J. Lab. clin. Med. **70**, 923 – 932 (1967)

Nawata, H., Kato, K.: Ribonucleic acid synthesis in porphyric rat liver induced by 3,5-dicarbethoxy-1,4-dihydrocollidine. Biochem. J. **136**, 209 – 215 (1973)

Onisawa, J., Labbe, R.F.: Effects of diethyl-1,4-dihydro-2,6-trimethylpyridine-3,5-dicarboxylate on the metabolism of porphyrins and iron. J. biol. Chem. **238**, 724 – 727 (1963)

Padmanaban, G., Satyanarayana Rao, M.R., Malathi, K.: A model for the regulation of δ-aminolaevulinate synthetase induction in rat liver. Biochem. J. **134**, 847 – 857 (1973)

Patton, G.M., Beattie, D.S.: Studies on hepatic δ-aminolevulinic acid synthetase. J. biol. Chem. **248**, 4467 – 4474 (1973)

Piper, W.N., Bousquet, W.F.: Phenobarbital and methylcholanthrene stimulation of rat liver chromatin template activity. Biochem. biophys. Res. Commun. **33**, 602 – 609 (1968)

Powell, K.A., Cox, R., McConville, M., Charles, H.P.: Mutations effecting porphyrin bio yn-thesis in *Escherichia coli*. Enzymes **16**, 65 – 73 (1973)

Price, V.E., Sterling, W.R., Tarantola, V.A., Hartley, R.W. Jr., Rechcigl, M. Jr.: The kinetics of catalase synthesis and destruction in vivo. J. biol. Chem. **237**, 3468 – 3475 (1962)

Racz, W.J., Marks, G.S.: Drug-induced porphyrin biosynthesis II. Simple procedure for screening drugs for porphyria-inducing activity. Biochem. Pharmacol. **18**, 2009 – 2018 (1969)

Racz, W.J., Marks, G.S.: Drug-induced porphyrin biosynthesis. IV. Investigation of the differences in response of isolated liver cells and the liver of the intact chick embryo to porphyria-inducing drugs. Biochem. Pharmacol. **21**, 143 – 151 (1972)

Rajamanickam, C., Satyanarayana Rao, R., Padmanaban, G.: On the sequence of reactions leading to cytochrome P-450 synthesis. Effect of drugs. J. biol. Chem. **250**, 2305 – 2310 (1975)

Rein, H., Maricic, S., Jänig, G.-R., Vuk-Pavlovic, S., Benko, B., Ristau, O., Ruckpaul, K.:
    Heme accessibility in cytochrome P-450 from rabbit liver. A proton magnetic relaxation
    study by stereochemical probes. Biochim. biophys. Acta (Amst.) **446**, 325 – 330 (1976)
Rothwell, J.D., Lacroix, S., Sweeney, G.D.: Evidence against a regulatory role for heme
    oxygenase in hepatic synthesis. Biochim biophys. Acta (Amst.) **304**, 871 – 874 (1973)
Sardana, M.K., Rajamanickam, C., Padmanaban, G.: Differential role of heme in the syn-
    thesis of mitochondrial and microsomal hemoproteins. In: Porphyrins in Human Diseases.
    Doss, M. (ed.), pp. 62 – 70. Basel: S. Karger 1976
Sardana, M.K., Satyanarayana Rao, M.R., Padmanaban, G.: Effect of allylisopropylacetamide
    on nuclear ribonucleic acid synthesis in rat liver. Biochem. J. **147**, 185 – 186 (1975)
Sassa, S., Granick, S.: Induction of δ-aminolevulinic acid synthetase in chick embryo liver
    cells in culture. Proc. nat. Acad. Sci. (Wash.) **67**, 517 – 522 (1970)
Satyanarayana Rao, M.R., Malathi, K., Padmanaban, G.: The relationship between δ-amino-
    laevulinate synthetase induction and the concentrations of cytochrome P-450 and catalase
    in rat liver. Biochem. J. **127**, 553 – 559 (1972)
Schimke, R.T., Sweeney, E.W., Berlin, C.M.: The role of synthesis and degradation in the
    control of rat liver tryptophan pyrrolase. J. biol. Chem. **240**, 322 – 331 (1965)
Schmid, R., Figen, J.F., Schwartz, S.: Experimental porphyria. IV. Studies of liver catalase
    and other heme enzymes in Sedormid porphyria. J. biol. Chem. **217**, 263 – 274 (1955)
Schmid, R., McDonagh, A.F.: The enzymatic formation of bilirubin. Ann. N.Y. Acad. Sci.
    244, 533 – 552 (1975)
Scholnick, P.L., Hammaker, L.E., Marver, H.S.: Soluble δ-aminolevulinic acid synthetase of
    rat liver. II. Studies related to the mechanism of enzyme action and hemin inhibition. J. biol.
    Chem. **247**, 4132 – 4137 (1972)
Scott, J.J.: The metabolism of δ-aminolaevulic acid. In: Ciba Foundation Symposium on
    Porphyrin Biosynthesis and Metabolism. Wolstenholme, G.E.W., Millar, E.C.P. (eds.),
    pp. 43 – 58. London: J. and A. Churchill 1955
Sinclair, P.R., Granick, S.: Heme control on the synthesis of δ-aminolevulinic acid synthetase
    in cultured chick embryo liver cells. Ann. N.Y. Acad. Sci. **244**, 509 – 518 (1975)
Snyder, A., Schmid, R.: The conversion of hematin to bile pigment in the rat. J. Lab. clin. Med.
    65, 817 – 824 (1965)
Stich, W., Decker, P.: Studies on the mechanism of porphyrin biosynthesis with the aid of
    inhibitors. In: Ciba Foundation Symposium on Porphyrin Biosynthesis and Metabolism.
    Wolstenholme, G.E.W., Millar, E.C.P. (eds.), pp. 254 – 260. London: J. and A. Churchill
    1955
Strand, L.J., Manning, J., Marver, H.S.: The induction of δ-aminolevulinic acid synthetase
    in cultured liver cells. The effect of end product and inhibitors of heme synthesis. J. biol. Chem.
    247, 2820 – 2827 (1972)
Sweeney, G.D.: Hepatic catalase activity during states of altered heme synthesis. In: Proceed-
    ings of the International Porphyrin Meeting. Freiburg, May 1 – 4, 1975. Doss, M. (ed.),
    pp. 53 – 61. Basel: S. Karger 1976
Sweeney, G.D., Janigan, D., Mayaman, D., Lai, H.: The experimental porphyrias. A group of
    distinctive metabolic lesions. S. Afr. J. Lab. clin. Med. **17**, 68 – 72 (1971)
Tomita, Y., Ohashi, A., Kikuchi, G.: Induction of δ-aminolevulinate synthetase in organ
    culture of chick embryo liver by allylisopropylacetamide and 3,5-dicarbethoxy-1,4-dihydro-
    collidine. J. Biochem. **75**, 1007 – 1015 (1974)
Tschudy, D.P., Bonkowsky, H.L.: Experimental porphyria. Fed. Proc. **31**, 147 – 159 (1972)
Tyrrell, D.L.J., Marks, G.S.: Drug-induced porphyrin biosynthesis. V. Effect of protohemin
    on the transcriptional and post-transcriptional phases of δ-aminolevulinic acid synthetase
    induction. Biochem. Pharmacol. **21**, 2077 – 2093 (1972)
Wada, O., Yano, Y., Urata, G., Nakao, K.: Behaviour of hepatic microsomal cytochromes
    after treatment of mice with drugs known to disturb porphyrin metabolism in liver. Bio-
    chem. Pharmacol. **17**, 595 – 603 (1968)
Waterfield, M.D., Del Favero, A., Gray, C.H.: Effect of 1,4-dihydro-3,5-dicarbethoxycollidine
    on hepatic microsomal heme, cytochrome b_5 and cytochrome P-450 in rabbits and mice.
    Biochim. biophys. Acta (Amst.) **184**, 470 – 473 (1969)

Wetterberg, L.: Report on an international survey of safe and unsafe drugs in acute intermittent porphyria. In: Proceedings of International Porphyrin Meeting—Porphyrins in
Human Diseases. Doss, M., Nawrocki, P. (eds.), Vol. 2, pp. 191–202. Freiburg im
Breisgau: Falk 1976
Whiting, M.J., Elliott, W.H.: Purification and properties of solubilized mitochondrial δ-aminolevulinic acid synthetase and comparison with the cytosol enzyme. J. biol. Chem. **247,**
6818–6826 (1972)
Whiting, M.J., Granick, S.: δ-Aminolevulinic acid synthase from chick embryo liver mitochondria. II. Immunochemical correlation between synthesis and activity in induction and
repression. J. biol. Chem. **251,** 1347–1353 (1976)
Woods, J.S., Dixon, R.L.: Studies of the perinatal differences in the activity of hepatic δ-aminolevulinic acid synthetase. Biochem. Pharmacol. **21,** 1735–1744 (1972)
Zuyderhoudt, F.M.J., Borst, P., Huijng, F.: Intramitochondrial localization of 5-aminolaevuli-
nate synthase induced in rat liver with allylisopropylacetamide. Biochim. biophys. Acta
(Amst.) **178,** 408–411 (1969)

Porphyria Caused by Hexachlorobenzene and Other Polyhalogenated Aromatic Hydrocarbons

G. H. ELDER

A. Introduction

The polyhalogenated aromatic hydrocarbons which cause the specific form of hepatic porphyria described in this Chapter are shown in Figure 1. Prolonged administration of these compounds to susceptible mammals and birds leads to the development, after a delay which varies between species but is usually at least a week, of massive overproduction of uroporphyrin and heptacarboxylic porphyrin and, to a lesser extent, porphyrins with 6, 5 and 4 carboxyl groups.

The member of this group of chemicals that has been most extensively studied as a cause of porphyria is hexachlorobenzene (HCB), which is used as a seed dressing to control fungi (TILLETIA spp.) that destroy cereal crops and also in the manufacture of some chlorophenols. Its porphyrogenic action was discovered when consumption of seed wheat treated with HCB was shown to be the cause of an outbreak of cutaneous porphyria which occurred in south-east TURKEY between 1955 and 1959. This was confirmed by epidemiological investigations and by the demonstration that HCB feeding produced porphyria in animals (SCHMID, 1960), and has been reviewed by DE MATTEIS (1967, 1968) and TSCHUDY and BONKOWSKY (1972). 2,3,7,8-Tetrachlorodibenzo-p-dioxin (TCDD) was shown to be the most potent inducer of 5-aminolaevulinate synthetase (ALA-S) in chick-embryos yet discovered (POLAND and GLOVER, 1973a) and to cause porphyria in mice (GOLDSTEIN et al., 1973) as the result of investigations into the cause of the high incidence of porphyria in a factory producing the herbicides 2,4-D and 2,4,5-T (2,4-dichloro- and 2,4,5-trichloro-phenoxyacetic acids) (BLEIBERG et al., 1964; POLAND et al., 1971a). In 1970, VOS and KOEMAN found that a commercial polychlorinated biphenyl (PCB) mixture produced porphyrin accumulation in chickens, Japanese quail and rats. Later VOS and NOTENBOOM-RAM (1972) showed that pure 2,4,5,2',4',5'-hexachlorobiphenyl was porphyrogenic, as is hexabromobiphenyl (STRIK, 1973a). PCB porphyria has not been reported in man, although wide-scale poisoning due to the use of cooking oil containing a PCB mixture occurred in Japan in 1968 (KIMBROUGH, 1974). Recently STRIK and KOEMAN (1976) have shown that octachlorostyrene causes porphyria in the rat.

In man, HCB is one of the causes of the syndrome known as porphyria cutanea tarda symptomatica (PCTS) (synonyms in current use: porphyria cutanea tarda; symptomatic porphyria). PCTS is a syndrome in which skin lesions due to the photosensitising action of porphyrins are associated with a characteristic pattern of porphyrin excretion, the most important feature of which is marked uroporphyrinuria, with massive accumulation of uroporphyrin in the liver (MARVER and SCHMID, 1972; ELDER et al., 1972). Attacks of abdominal pain and neuropsychiat-

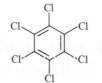

Hexachlorobenzene

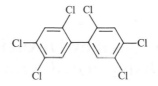

2, 4, 5, 2', 4', 5'–Hexachlorobiphenyl

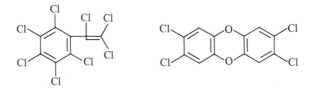

Octachlorostyrene   2, 3, 7, 8–Tetrachlorodibenzo–p–dioxin

Fig. 1. Chlorinated aromatic hydrocarbons that produce porphyria in mammals and birds

ric manifestations do not occur, and porphobilinogen excretion is always normal. The syndrome is seen most commonly as a sporadic disorder of insidious onset in middle-aged men with liver-cell damage due to alcohol, although it may complicate other types of chronic liver disease or be precipitated by oestrogens. PCTS in more than one member of a family is rare. The condition is particularly common in areas with a high incidence of iron-overload and alcoholism, as among the Bantu people of South Africa. Total body iron stores are moderately increased in about two-thirds of European patients with PCTS (LUNDVALL, 1971a; TURNBULL et al., 1973). Depletion of body iron stores by repeated venesection leads to clinical and biochemical remission, even in patients with normal iron stores (RAMSAY et al., 1974).

The increased loss of heme precursors in the urine and faeces is less marked in PCTS than in other forms of hepatic porphyria. In keeping with this, the activity of the rate-limiting enzyme of heme biosynthesis in the liver, 5-aminolaevulinate synthetase (ALA-S) is not raised to the same extent and may even be normal (MARVER and SCHMID, 1972). ALA-S activity decreases as porphyrin excretion declines in remission (MOORE et al., 1972). As in the other hepatic porphyrias, it is probable that both the increase in ALA-S activity and the specific pattern of porphyrin excretion are secondary to a decrease in the activity of one of the intermediate enzymes of heme biosynthesis. KUSHNER and co-workers have recently shown that in at least some patients with PCTS the activity of uroporphyrinogen decarboxylase (UROG-D) is decreased both in the liver and in red blood cells (KUSHNER and BARBUTO, 1974, 1975a). The concentration of cytochrome P-450 may be increased in the liver of alcoholic subjects with PCTS (PIMSTONE et al., 1973). Many of the features of PCTS described above are also present in the experimental porphyria that is produced in animals by prolonged administration of the compounds listed in Figure 1.

The type of porphyria produced by polyhalogenated aromatic hydrocarbons is of interest for a number of reasons. First, its discovery showed that porphyria in man could be toxic in origin. Second, it provides an experimental model for PCTS which has the closest resemblance to a human disease of any experimental porphyria. Third, and perhaps most important, elucidation of the mechanism of the porphyria may provide an insight into the mechanism of the hepatotoxicity of these compounds.

B. Properties and Metabolism of Porphyrogenic Polyhalogenated Aromatic Hydrocarbons

In this section only those aspects of the chemistry, toxicology and metabolism of these compounds that appear relevant to their porphyrogenic action are described. As far as possible the discussion is restricted to the effect of porphyrogenic doses in species which are susceptible to this action of these compounds.

The porphyrogenic polyhalogenated aromatic hydrocarbons all have important toxic actions in addition to their ability to cause porphyria. These have recently been reviewed for the polyhalogenated biphenyls (KIMBROUGH, 1974; FISHBEIN, 1974) and TCDD (KIMBROUGH, 1974). In contrast, toxicological investigation of HCB has largely been restricted to its porphyrogenic action, but its very low acute toxicity (CAMERON et al., 1937; STRIK, 1973c) has been documented. Its chronic toxic actions are described in Section C.

I. Chemistry and Nomenclature

HCB, TCDD and the polyhalogenated biphenyls are white, crystalline solids which are insoluble in water but soluble to varying degrees in organic solvents, fats and vegetable oils.

The PCBs are marketed as viscous liquids under trade names, e.g. Aroclor, Clophen, Phenoclor and Kanechlor. These contain mixtures of biphenyls which differ both in the number and position of chlorine subtituents. The Aroclors are differentiated by numbers, (e.g. Aroclor 1254). The first two digits indicate the molecular type (12 for biphenyls; 25 and 44 for biphenyl—terphenyl mixtures, containing 75% and 60% biphenyl respectively; and 54 for terphenyls); the last two digits indicate the weight % of chlorine. Hexachlorobiphenyls are major components of Aroclors with greater than 50% chlorine by weight (54% chlorine corresponds to an average of five chlorine substituents per molecule). Experiments in which commercial PCB preparations, such as Aroclors, have been used are difficult to interpret because it is never certain which component of the mixture is responsible for the observed effect, since each component may be absorbed, retained within the body and metabolised differently (HUTZINGER et al., 1972).

Chlorinated dibenzodioxins and the related chlorinated dibenzofurans are potential contaminants of a wide range of products manufactured from chlorophenols and chlorobenzenes, notably herbicides, pentachlorophenol, polychlorinated biphenyls and hexachlorobenzene. Their formation has been reviewed by KIMBROUGH (1974). These and other potentially porphyrogenic contaminants are often present in samples of chlorinated hydrocarbons and it is important to ensure that the compound under investigation does not contain significant amounts of such materials. Thus Vos et al. (1970) found that two commercial PCB mixtures contained tetra- and penta-chlorodibenzofuran and chlorinated naphthalenes and ascribed the differences in toxicity between these and another commercial sample to their presence. Some commercial samples of hexachlorobenzene contain not only pentachlorobenzene as a major impurity (200 – 81,000 ppm) but also traces of hepta- and octa-chlorinated dibenzodioxins and dibenzofurans and other chlorinated compounds (VILLENEUVA et al., 1974).

II. Absorption, Distribution in the Body, Metabolism and Excretion

1. Hexachlorobenzene

a) *Absorption and Distribution*

In order to produce porphyria in small mammals or birds, HCB is usually administered by allowing free access to a standard powdered diet containing crystalline HCB (20 – 5000 ppm, according to the species). Crystalline hexachlorobenzene suspended in water is poorly adsorbed from a single dose (PARKE and WILLIAMS, 1960; KOSS, 1976) and it is probable that absorption of crystals mixed with the diet is also poor and variable, particularly if the die is not homogeneous. With continuous feeding of diets containing 10 – 160 ppm HCB, steady incorporation into tissue stores occurs so that the net amount accumulated in adipose tissue, liver and other tissues after 9 months is directly related to the dose (GRANT et al., 1974; VILLENEUVE et al., 1974). More efficient absorption of HCB from an oral dose is obtained by administering it as a solution in vegetable oil. With this method as much as 80% of doses in the range 20 – 180 mg/kg body weight may be absorbed (KOSS, 1976; VILLENEUVE, 1975). It is probable that the absorption of HCB is also enhanced by increasing the fat content and decreasing the fibre content of the diet. For acute experiments, HCB suspended in olive oil has been given i.p. (SWEENEY et al., 1971).

   After absorption from the gut, HCB is distributed to most body tissues in rats of both sexes but, like other fat-soluble compounds, it is stored mainly in adipose tissue where the concentration (expressed per g wet weight of tissue) may be at least ten times that in the next most important storage site, the liver (VILLENEUVE et al., 1974; VILLENEUVE, 1975). Redistribution of HCB between tissues follows food restriction (VILLENEUVE, 1975) which in the rat causes rapid depletion of body fat depots and consequent release of stored HCB, and exposure to hepatotoxins, such as carbon tetrachloride (VILLENEUVE et al., 1974), an effect which may be secondary to the production of a fatty liver. Large amounts of HCB can be stored in adipose tissue. When HCB concentrations were measured in fat after rats had been given doses of HCB in corn oil varying from 1 – 100 mg/kg body weight daily for 14 days, there was no evidence that storage capacity was becoming saturated at concentrations in fat of about 4000 ppm, and concentrations greater than 10,000 ppm have been reported (VILLENEUVE, 1975). However, in rats accumulation in the liver begins to fall off once a concentration of about 850 μg/total liver of 100 g body weight has been reached (STONARD, 1974; VILLENEUVE, 1975).

HCB, like other fat-soluble hydrocarbons that are resistant to metabolic degradation, is extremely persistent in body fat and is probably widely distributed
in the ecosystem. Trace amounts have been identified in the tissues of fish, shell-
fish and birds in the Netherlands (KOEMAN et al., 1969) and in samples of human
fat in the United Kingdom (ABBOTT et al., 1972), Australia, Papua and New Guinea
(BRADY and SIYALI, 1972).

b) *Metabolism and Excretion*

HCB is slowly eliminated from the body, mainly as unchanged HCB in the faeces
(PARKE and WILLIAMS, 1960; VILLENEUVE, 1975; KOSS, 1976). For rats, the bio-
logical half-life of ^{14}C-labelled HCB within the body appears to be about 10 days
(KOSS, 1976).

   In the 1950's WILLIAMS and his co-workers showed that, in general, the more
chlorine a halogenated benzene contained, the less readily was it metabolised. The
position of the chlorine substituents was also important, with *ortho*-unsubstituted
positions favouring metabolism. PARKE and WILLIAMS (1960) studied the fate of
HCB (0.4–0.5 g/kg suspended in water) given as a single oral dose to rabbits.
After 5 days only 6% had appeared in the faeces, the bulk of the dose being still
in the gastro-intestinal tract. Examination of the urine by absorption spectroscopy
of steam distillates revealed no significant urinary excretion of phenolic metabolites and there was no increase in the output of conjugated glucuronic acids,
ethereal sulphates or mercapturic acid. In addition, no metabolites were detected
in expired air. Steam distillates of the gut contents contained hexachlorobenzene
and, possibly, traces of 1,2,4,5-tetrachlorobenzene which may have been formed
by bacterial dechlorination in the gut. On the basis of these studies in rabbits it is
usually considered that HCB is not metabolised within the body. However, recent
studies of the fate of HCB administered to rats have shown conclusively that, in
this species at least, HCB is converted to polar metabolites. After i.p. administration of ^{14}C-labelled HCB (total dose 390 mg/kg), 8% of the total dose was excreted
in the urine, and 22% in the faeces, within 4 weeks (KOSS, 1976). About half the total
radioactivity excreted was in the form of metabolites which were mainly present in
the urine, unchanged HCB being the major component in the faeces. The major
metabolite was identified as pentachlorophenol, which accounted for 41% of the
radioactivity in the urine and 22% in the faeces. Tetrachloroquinone and pentachlorothiophenol were also present. These metabolites, as well as tetrachlorocatechol, have also been identified in the urine of rats chronically poisoned with
HCB (LUI and SWEENEY, 1975; LUI et al., 1976).

2. Other Porphyrogenic Polychlorinated Aromatic Hydrocarbons

The storage, distribution, metabolism and excretion of PCBs and TCDD has recently been reviewed (KIMBROUGH, 1974). Like HCB they are fat-soluble, resistant
to metabolism and persist within the body in adipose tissue and the liver.

   There have been few studies of the metabolism of pure porphyrogenic PCBs in
susceptible species. HUTZINGER et al. (1972) demonstrated that, as with the chlorinated benzenes, resistance to metabolism increases with degree of chlorination.
They were unable to detect any metabolites of 2,4,5,2',4',5'-hexachlorobiphenyl in

the urine or faeces of rats and pigeons, but subsequently JENSEN and SUNDSTROM (1974) showed conclusively that rats excrete a small amount of a monohydroxy derivative in their faeces. Study of the metabolism of TCDD is difficult due to its very high acute toxicity (oral LD_{50} values for rats: females 44.7 µg/kg, males 22.5 µg/kg; KIMBROUGH, 1974). PIPER et al. (1973) studied the fate of a single oral dose of ^{14}C-labelled TCDD in the rat. About 65 – 70% of the radioactivity was eliminated from the body within 21 days, mostly in the faeces, although 13% appeared in the urine and 3% in expired air, but the radioactive compounds were not identified. VINOPAL and CASIDA (1973) using ^{3}H-labelled TCDD were unable to detect any significant formation of metabolites in mice.

C. Porphyria Caused by Hexachlorobenzene and Other Halogenated Aromatic Hydrocarbons

In this section the effect of hexachlorobenzene and other halogenated aromatic hydrocarbons on the excretion and accumulation of heme precursors by mammals and birds is described. For any type of porphyria, a precise description of the pattern of overproduction of heme precursors is an essential preliminary, for it defines the condition, indicates the nature of the underlying disturbance of heme metabolism and must be fully explained by any proposed biochemical mechanism. For the compounds discussed here, the complexity of the excretion pattern and the great variation in response between species and, within species, between different strains and sexes presents special problems of interpretation.

I. Hexachlorobenzene

1. HCB Porphyria in Man

In man, HCB is one of the causes of the syndrome of PCTS (SCHMID, 1960). An outbreak of porphyria due to poisoning by HCB occurred in south-eastern Turkey between 1955 and 1960. The first patients presented in the spring and summer of 1955 (WRAY et al., 1962) and by 1960 at least 3000 (PETERS et al., 1966) and possibly as many as 5000 (SCHMID, 1960) people had developed porphyria. CAM (1958, 1959) was the first to suspect that the outbreak was due to the consumption of seed wheat treated with HCB to control wheat smut due to the fungus *Tilletia tritici*. In 1954 seed wheat mixed with either Chlorable or Surmesan (0.2% by weight) was distributed for the first time in the provinces of Urfa, Mardin, Diyarbakir, Elazig, Siirt, Bitlis and Mus, where cases of porphyria were later reported (CAM, 1958; WRAY et al., 1962). Both these seed dressings contain HCB (10% by weight) mixed with mercury salts. All the patients with porphyria had eaten treated wheat intended for sowing, probably due to the local economic factors described by WRAY et al. (1962). The aetiology of the porphyria was confirmed when HCB was shown to be porphyrogenic in rabbits and rats (KANTEMIR, 1960; SCHMID, 1960; OCKNER and SCHMID, 1961; DE MATTEIS et al., 1961; GAJDOS and GAJDOS-TÖRÖK, 1961) and by the disappearance of new cases within 2 years of withdrawal of these seed dressings by the Turkish Government in 1959 (WRAY et al., 1962; PETERS et al., 1966). Although one of the patients reported by CETINGIL and ÖZEN (1960) developed porphyria after only one month on an HCB-contaminated diet, most had had a continuous intake of HCB for one to three years before the onset of skin lesions, and CAM and NIGOGOSYAN (1963) estimated that such patients had consumed about 0.05 – 2.0 g HCB/day. Considerable variation in response between individual members of families eating the same food was noted (DOGRAMACI et al., 1962a). No measurements of HCB levels in blood or body fat have been reported for any of the Turkish patients.

a) *Clinical Features*

The majority of the patients were children and most of these were boys (DOGRAMACI et al., 1962a). Of 348 patients studied by CAM and NIGOGOSYAN (1963), 76% were male and about 80% were between 4 and 14 years old. When porphyria occurred in adults, the same sex difference was noted (CETINGIL and ÖZEN, 1960). A mortality rate of 10% has been reported (PETERS et al., 1966). The most striking clinical features were skin lesions on sun-exposed areas, similar to those of congenital erythropoietic porphyria and the cutaneous hepatic porphyrias, which consisted of bullae, fragility, hypertrichosis and hyperpigmentation. The hypertrichosis and pigmentation were sufficiently marked for many of the affected children to be named "monkey children". Secondary infections of the skin lesions and sclerodermatous changes were common. Extensive scarring from healed skin lesions and atrophic changes, especially of the nails, which often fell off, were frequent and in some patients there was partial resorption of the distal phalanges. An unexplained, painless arthritis of the interphalangeal joints with swelling and spindling of the fingers, which persisted after the porphyrinuria and other clinical features had disappeared, was present in about half the children (DOGRAMACI et al., 1962b). Most patients had active lesions during the summer months and there was often some healing of skin lesions during the winter. Asymptomatic enlargement of the thyroid was present in over 30% of the patients (CAM and NIGOGOSAN, 1963).

The attacks of acute abdominal pain and neurological and psychiatric symptoms which are characteristic of the genetic hepatic porphyrias (MARVER and SCHMID, 1972) did not occur in any of the patients (SCHMID, 1960; DOGRAMACI et al., 1962a; PETERS et al., 1966; DEAN, 1971). A few patients had marked limb weakness initially but no sensory changes were reported (PETERS et al., 1966).

Many of the patients, especially the children, were malnourished and cachectic and about a third had hepatomegaly (CETINGIL and ÖZEN, 1960; SCHMID, 1960; DOGRAMACI et al., 1962a; CAM and NIGOGOSYAN, 1963; PETERS et al., 1966; DEAN, 1971). Abnormal turbidity tests and reversal of the albumin/globulin ratio were present in some patients (PETERS et al., 1966; CETINGIL and ÖZEN, 1960) but hyperbilirubinaemia was not reported. There are few reports of the histology of the liver: two patients had cirrhosis (PETERS et al., 1966), two others had "advanced hydropic and granular degeneration of the parenchyma with yellow pigment in some parenchymal cells" (CETINGIL and ÖZEN, 1960) while one had chronic hepatitis (DOGRAMACI et al., 1962c). Measurements of liver porphyrin concentration were not made, but needle biopsy samples showed intense red fluorescence due to porphyrin when examined in ultraviolet light (DOGRAMACI et al., 1962c).

The only hematological abnormalities described in patients with HCB porphyria were those of chronic infection (PETERS et al., 1966). There was no accumulation of porphyrin within the bone marrow and no red-fluorescent cells were seen
when bone-marrow smears were examined by ultraviolet microscopy (CETINGIL and
ÖZEN, 1960).

The acute skin manifestations usually disappeared 20 – 30 days after discontinu-
ing the ingestion of HCB and this was accompanied by a decrease in urine porphyrin excretion (CAM and NIGOGOSYAN, 1963). Many patients appeared clinically
to be cured, but in others the condition persisted, with occasional periodic exacerbation of the skin lesions, especially during the summer, being present even ten
years later (DEAN, 1971). Seven patients were treated with year-long courses of
ethylenediaminetetraacetic acid (EDTA) (PETERS et al., 1966). An initial increase
in porphyrin excretion was followed by a progressive decline to near normal levels
which was accompanied by healing of the skin lesions and an improvement in the
general clinical condition of all seven patients. One patient later relapsed but a
further course of EDTA was successful.

Children under the age of 4 rarely developed porphyria but in this age group,
and particularly in breast-fed infants, a condition known as pembe yara or "pink
sore" with a mortality rate greater than 95%, was common (CAM, 1960). The
mother of the infants either had porphyria or had eaten HCB-treated wheat
and samples of breast milk were shown to contain HCB (PETERS et al., 1966).
Pembe yara was not confined to children and PETERS et al. (1966) reported that an
adult with the condition later developed porphyria. Although the epidemic of this
condition paralleled that of the porphyria it has not been experimentally reproduced
in animals and it is not clear whether it was purely a manifestation of poisoning
by HCB or whether mercury compounds in the seed dressing were involved (DEAN,
1971).

b) *Biochemical Features*

All the patients had marked porphyrinuria, often sufficient to colour the urine
reddish-brown, but qualitative tests for porphobilinogen were consistently negative
(SCHMID, 1960) and the few quantitative estimations reported were within the normal range (WATSON, quoted by CAM and NIGOGOSYAN, 1963). The increase in
urinary porphyrin excretion was mainly due to uroporphyrin and heptacarboxylate porphyrin, but coproporphyrin and porphyrins with 5 and 6 carboxyl groups
were also present (Table 1) (CETINGIL and ÖZEN, 1960; CAM and NIGOGOSYAN,
1963; PETERS et al., 1966; CHU and CHU, 1967). There was a moderate increase in
the concentration of porphyrin in the faeces of some patients (CETINGIL and ÖZEN,
1960; BARNES, quoted by CAM and NIGOGOSYAN, 1963; WATSON, 1960) with increases in the coproporphyrin and uroporphyrin fractions as the most consistent
abnormalities (Table 2). Investigation of the composition of these fractions has not
been reported. CETINGIL and ÖZEN (1960) determined the melting points of the
methyl ester derivatives of uroporphyrin and coproporphyrin, isolated from faeces
and urine, and concluded that the former was a series I isomer and the latter,
series III. CHU and CHU (1967), using a chromatographic method of isomer determination, which is more suitable for the analysis of mixtures, found that uroporphyrin from the urine of four patients was 45 – 60% isomer I, while coproporphyrin-

Table 1. Heme precursors in urine in HCB-porphyria and PCTS

	Porphyrin precursors µmol/24 h		Porphyrin fraction nmol/24 h		% Total porphyrin				
	ALA	PBG	COPRO	URO	URO	7-CO$_2$H	6-CO$_2$H	5-CO$_2$H	COPRO
PCTS									
(1) Sporadic									
Dowdle et al. (1970) (12 pts.)			200–1746	1934–12333	51–76 (24–40)	18–32 (82–97)	1–4 (74–96)	1–3 (37–66)	2–12 (26–72)
Doss et al. (1971)					46–78	17–30	1–9	1–9	1–14
(2) Due to HCB									
Watson (1960) (4 pts.)			65–519	4154–9332					
Chu and Chu (1967) (4 pts.)					52–62 (40–55)	29–37 (>90)	1–4 (>90)	1–5 (>90)	1–5 (70–75)
HCB porphyria (rat)									
Ockner and Schmid (1961)	11	75	322	433					
San Martin de Viale et al. (1970)					50 (>90)	16 (100)	5 (100)	7 (>90)	22 (100)
Taljaard et al. (1971)									
HCB			49	110	28	19	9	24	20
HCB + iron			113	331	52	14	10	9	16

Values in parentheses give the isomer III composition expressed as % of total. Ranges are given for patients; means (2–5 animals) or single estimations for rats.

Table 2. Faecal porphyrins in HCB porphyria and PCTS

	Porphyrin fraction (nmol/g dry wt.)				% 4–8 CO$_2$H porphyrin				
	COPRO	PROTO	Ether-insol "URO"	URO	7-CO$_2$H	6-CO$_2$H	5-CO$_2$H	Isocopro	Copro
PCTS									
(1) *Sporadic*									
ELDER (1973) (20 pts.)	21–395 (156)	30–498 (153)	7–431 (140)						
ELDER (1973) (4 pts.)				6	24	14	20	21	15
(2) *Due to HCB*									
WATSON (1960)	1360[1] 7390[1]	96[1] 570[1]	309[1]				not investigated		
CAM and NIGOGOSYAN (1963)	104 28	68 81							
Normal values	<32	<133	<24						
HCB porphyria (rat)									
ELDER (1973)	Total porphyrin 1113 nmol/24 h			21	32	24	12	7	4

Ranges (with means in parentheses), means or single estimations are given for patients; and means for 4 animals are given for rats.
[1] nmol/100 g faeces.

phyrin was 70 – 75% isomer III and penta-, hexa- and heptacarboxylate porphyrins were all about 90% isomer III. Increased excretion of isomer I series porphyrins is not seen in HCB porphyria in other mammals and is of particular interest since a similar overproduction of type I porphyrins is seen in PCTS of non-toxic origin. The pattern of porphyrin excretion found in the Turkish cases is compared with that found in sporadic cases of the syndrome of PCTS in Tables 1 and 2.

c) Porphyria due to Occupational Exposure to HCB

The risk of developing porphyria due to occupational exposure to HCB appears to be low. MORLEY et al. (1973) screened 54 male workers, who prepared and distributed HCB-treated grain, for increased urine porphyrin excretion. Only one subject was abnormal with small increases in uroporphyrin and coproporphyrin excretion (170 and 255 µg/24 h respectively). He had been exposed to HCB for longer than the others, 25 years, but his alcohol intake is described as moderate and the finding of latent porphyria may have been coincidental (MORLEY et al., 1973). Blood levels of HCB are only marginally higher in people using and preparing HCB-treated products for agricultural use than in the general population (SIYALI, 1972).

Measurements of HCB levels in the blood of workers manufacturing the compound do not appear to have been reported, but one worker in a factory producing various cyclic chlorinated hydrocarbons, but who was in contact with HCB, developed chloracne and PCTS (GOMBOS et al., 1969).

2. HCB Porphyria in the Rat

a) General Features

The response of rats to the prolonged administration of a diet containing 0.2 – 0.5% (w/w) HCB shows marked variation between individuals, strains and sexes with respect to the length of time taken for porphyria to develop, the extent of the increase in porphyrin excretion and the pattern of heme precursor excretion. A large single dose of HCB does not cause porphyria (SWEENEY et al., 1971). The effect of HCB on urinary porphyrin excretion by female Wistar rats is shown in Figure 2. The response can be divided into three phases. After a period of some 4 weeks during which there is relatively litte change in porphyrin excretion, the onset of porphyria is indicated by a rapid increase in porphyrin excretion which then levels off as porphyria becomes well-established by about 10 weeks. During the final phase porphyrin excretion continues to increase, but at a slower rate, until the animal dies. The changes in faecal porphyrin excretion parallel those in the urine (Fig. 2). The original reports of the porphyrogenic action of HCB in rats stressed that the excretion of 5-aminolaevulinate and, especially, porphobilinogen becomes greatly increased as porphyria develops (Table 1) (OCKNER and SCHMID, 1961; DE MATTEIS et al., 1961) but this aspect of the porphyria has subsequently been largely ignored, possibly because it is not seen in man and some other animals.

OCKNER and SCHMID (1961) found that when HCB is removed from the diet at the end of the onset phase porphyrin excretion returns to normal within a week but that if feeding is continued for a further 2 – 3 weeks before HCB is withdrawn,

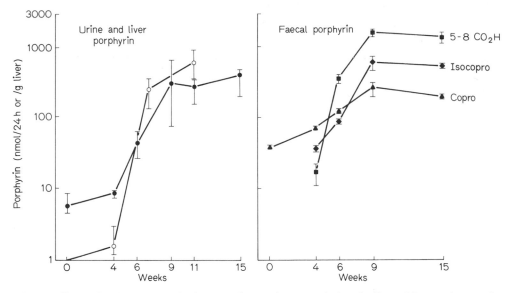

Fig. 2. Effect of HCB on porphyrin excretion and accumulation in liver. Mean values and ranges are shown for 4 female Wistar rats receiving HCB (0.3%, w/w). ● : urinary porphyrin excretion; ○ : porphyrin concentration in liver. Urinary porphyrin was >90% copropor-phyrin at 4 weeks, 60% coproporphyrin and 25% uroporphyrin at 7 weeks, 31% coropor-phyrin and 51% uroporphyrin at 11 weeks, with the remainder being 5−7 carboxyl por-phyrins. Faeces did not contain measurable amounts of isocoproporphyrin or porphyrins with 5−8 carboxyl groups at start of experiment

porphyrin excretion does not fall during the subsequent ten days. A less rapid decrease in porphyrin excretion towards normal on withdrawal of HCB has been described by PEARSON and MALKINSON (1965).

HCB causes cutaneous and neurological lesions in rats (DE MATTEIS et al., 1961; GAJDOS and GAJDOS-TÖRÖK, 1961). The cutaneous lesions are seen most com-monly when high doses (0.5−2% w/w) are administered and may appear before the onset of porphyrinuria. They consist of changes in the hair, which becomes discoloured and of poor quality, and depilated sores with hemorrhagic crusts, often symmetrically placed near the shoulders but also seen elsewhere on the back and on the head and feet. Doses in the range 0.2−2% (w/w) prevent all animals from gaining weight normally and kill some animals before porphyria develops. Those animals which die in the early stages of poisoning show generalised tremors, weakness and immobility progressing to paresis and death. Similar but more chronic neurotoxic manifestations are seen, especially pre-terminally, in animals which survive long enough to develop porphyria. Newborn and very young rats are particularly susceptible to the neurotoxic effects of HCB (DE MATTEIS et al., 1961). The number of rats that die from this cause before developing porphyria can be decreased by not giving HCB until they are at least 6 weeks old. It is of interest that limb weakness was noted in some patients by PETERS et al. (1966) during the early stages of HCB poisoning. The neurotoxicity does not appear to be related to the porphyria since it may occur in the absence of any change in the excretion of heme precursors both in rats and other species (DE MATTEIS et al., 1961). The mechanism of the neurotoxic effect is unknown. Morphological lesions have not been found in the central nervous system (CAMPBELL, 1963). VILLENEUVE (1975) has shown that adult male Sprague-Dawley rats die when the concentration of HCB in the brain exceeds 300 ppm, but the reason for the marked susceptibility of some rats to this action of HCB, which presumably underlies the death of some animals early in the course of poisoning, is unknown.

Although neither of the toxic effects described above provides an experimental model for the clinical features of human porphyria, cutaneous lesions due to the photosensitising action of porphyria in the skin have been produced in rats with HCB porphyria. Thus PEARSON and MALKINSON (1965) showed that chronic exposure of plucked or shaved rats to longwave ultraviolet light led to delayed hair regrowth and that gentle rubbing of the exposed skin produced erosions and subepidermal blisters identical to those of PCTS. Fluorescence microscopy of sections of the skin showed that porphyrin was selectively concentrated in the epidermis and follicular epithelium. Skin lesions do not appear to be produced by short-term exposure to ultraviolet light (DE MATTEIS et al., 1961; BURNETT and PATHAK, 1964).

b) *Porphyrins in Urine, Faeces and Tissues*

The composition of the mixture of porphyrins excreted in the urine in HCB porphyria in the rat has been investigated by solvent partition (OCKNER and SCHMID, 1961; DE MATTEIS et al., 1961; SIMON et al., 1970; TALJAARD et al., 1971, 1972a; STONARD, 1974) and chromatographic techniques (Table 1) (SAN MARTIN DE VIALE et al., 1970; ELDER, 1972; TALJAARD et al., 1971, 1972a). The porphyrin excretion pattern changes as HCB administration proceeds and varies according to the strain of rat studied. Thus differences in the descriptions of the porphyrin excretion patterns given by these workers are to be expected. However, there is a reasonable agreement on the main features. The earliest change, which occurs before the onset of porphyria, is a slight increase in coproporphyrin excretion. The phase of onset of porphyria is marked by a progressive increase in the excretion of uroporphyrin and, to a lesser extent, porphyrins with 5, 6 and 7 carboxyl groups, but coproporphyrin also continues to increase during this phase (OCKNER and SCHMID, 1961; DE MATTEIS et al., 1961; TALJAARD et al., 1971, 1972a; STONARD, 1974; DOSS et al., 1976; ELDER et al., 1976a). Most workers have reported that uroporphyrin eventually becomes the main urinary porphyrin (Table 1) (OCKNER and SCHMID, 1961; GAJDOS and GAJDOS-TÖRÖK, 1961; PEARSON and MALKINSON, 1965; KALIVAS et al., 1969; SAN MARTIN DE VIALE et al., 1970; TALJAARD et al., 1971, 1972a; ELDER et al., 1976a; DOSS et al., 1976). Those who have reported persistent coproporphyrinuria either carried out short-term experiments or used resistant strains of rats (DE MATTEIS et al., 1961; ELDER, 1972; STONARD, 1974). SAN MARTIN DE VIALE et al. (1970) have pointed out that the porphyrin excretion pattern of female Wistar rats (also used by TALJAARD et al., 1971; 1972a and b; ELDER et al., 1976a) resembles the pattern described by DE MATTEIS et al. (1961) for the rabbit more closely than that reported by the latter authors for male rats. In most strains of rats, uroporphyrinuria does appear to be the hallmark of established HCB porphyria, as it is in other susceptible species, but, since porphobilinogen is also present in the urine, care has to be taken to ensure that uroporphyrin measurements

accurately reflect uroporphyrin excretion and are not increased by the inclusion of
uroporphyrin formed by in vitro condensation of porphobilinogen.

The excretion of porphyrins in the faeces is increased (OCKNER and SCHMID,
1961; GAJDOS and GAJDOS-TÖRÖK, 1961; ELDER, 1972; STONARD, 1974; ELDER
et al., 1976a) to a greater extent than urinary porphyrin excretion (Fig. 2) (ELDER,
1972; STONARD, 1974; ELDER et al., 1976a). The increase is mainly due to porphyrins with 4—8 carboxyl groups, with relatively larger amounts of the more
hydrophobic porphyrins being present than in the urine (Table 2). The faeces contain large amounts of porphyrins of the isocoproporphyrin series, which are metabolites of pentacarboxylate porphyrinogen III (ELDER, 1972; ELDER, 1974; ELDER
et al., 1976a). Reports of increases (OCKNER and SCHMID, 1961) or decreases
(STONARD, 1974) in the protoporphyrin fraction of the faeces are difficult to
evaluate due to technical problems in the analysis of this fraction by solvent-partition methods and due to uncertainty about the origin of this fraction in rat faeces.
However, the protoporphyrin concentration of the bile is increased about 5-fold
in HCB porphyria (ELDER, 1973).

There is general agreement that the porphyrins excreted in the urine and in the
faeces belong to the type III isomer series (DE MATTEIS et al., 1961; SAN MARTIN
DE VIALE et al., 1970; JACKSON et al., 1976). Recent studies in which porphyrins
prepared by unambiguous synthesis have been compared with natural material by
physico-chemical methods have shown that hepta-, hexa- and penta-carboxylate
porphyrins and isocoproporphyrin are single isomers derived from the III series
(STOLL et al., 1973; JACKSON et al., 1976; BAPTISTA DE ALMEIDA et al., 1975).

As porphyria develops, heme precursors accumulate progressively within the
liver and, to a lesser extent, the kidney (OCKNER and SCHMID, 1961; GAJDOS and
GAJDOS-TÖRÖK, 1961; STONARD, 1974) and are incorporated into growing bones
(OCKNER and SCHMID, 1961), including the incisors (PEARSON and MALKINSON,
1965), but do not accumulate in bone marrow or red cells. The increase in liver
porphyrin, which is mainly uroporphyrin III (about 70—90% of the total) and
heptacarboxylic porphyrin with traces of lower carboxylated porphyrins (SIMON
et al., 1970; TALJAARD et al., 1972a; STONARD, 1974), parallels the increase in porphyrin excretion (Fig. 2) and similarly tends to level-off once porphyria is established (STONARD, 1974). Porphobilinogen also accumulates in the liver (OCKNER
and SCHMID, 1961) but to a lesser extent than uroporphyrin (RAJAMANICKAM et al.,
1972).

c) Factors Influencing the Porphyrogenic Action of HCB in rats

A number of factors influence the response of rats of the same strain to HCB or
alter the course of the porphyria. Female rats develop porphyria more rapidly
than males (SAN MARTIN DE VIALE et al., 1970; GRANT et al., 1974; STONARD,
1974). This difference is seen even when the rate of accumulation of HCB within
the liver and other tissues is the same in the two sexes (GRANT et al., 1974). The
resistance of male rats to the porphyrogenic action of HCB can be overcome by
administering oestradiol, either alone or in combination with 17 α-hydroxypro-
gesterone or testosterone (IPPEN et al., 1972a). In female rats, the response to HCB
is diminished by ovariectomy and enhanced by high doses of oestrogen (SAN MARTIN
DE VIALE et al., 1976a).

Alterations in body iron stores are known to influence the course of PCTS in man and the possibility that a similar effect operates in HCB porphyria in the rat has been investigated. KALIVAS et al. (1969) were unable to demonstrate an effect of iron loading on HCB-induced changes in urinary porphyrin excretion by giving iron-dextran i.p. at the start of HCB feeding or after the onset of porphyria. Subsequently JOUBERT and his co-workers showed that the onset of porphyria could be accelerated if rats were made siderotic before feeding HCB and that porphyrin concentrations in the urine and liver then reached higher levels than in control rats treated with HCB alone. In addition, the final preponderance of uroporphyrin was more marked and the urine porphyrin pattern more closely resembled that of PCTS (BACH et al., 1971; TALJAARD et al., 1971, 1972 a). Recently STONARD (1976) has shown that the administration of iron during the course of feeding HCB to a strain of rat that is particularly sensitive to the porphyrogenic action of this compound markedly enhances the accumulation of porphyrin in the liver.

Alcohol, which is another factor that has been implicated in the pathogenesis of PCTS, has little influence on the course (PEARSON and MALKINSON, 1965) or development of HCB porphyria (IPPEN et al., 1972 b) in rats.

3. HCB Porphyria in Other Species

The response of several species of mammals and birds to the porphyrogenic, hepatotoxic and neurotoxic actions of HCB has been compared by DE MATTEIS et al. (1961), STRIK and WIT (1972) and STRIK (1973 a).

a) *Mammals*

Of all the species studied, the disturbance of porphyrin metabolism in the female rabbit (males do not appear to have been studied) most closely resembles that seen in the Turkish epidemic (DE MATTEIS et al., 1961). After six weeks on a diet containing 0.5% HCB (w/w), urinary porphyrin excretion increases progressively, without any change in porphobilinogen or 5-aminolaevulinate excretion, until the animals die after 8 – 12 weeks. When analysed by solvent-partition methods most of the urinary porphyrin was found to be ether-insoluble, although there was also some increase in the ether-soluble fraction. The former was predominantly heptacarboxylate porphyrin, while coproporphyrin III and hepta-, hexa- and pentacarboxylate porphyrins were present in the ether-soluble fraction. Uroporphyrin III, with some heptacarboxylate porphyrin, accumulated in the liver. Faecal porphyrin excretion was not investigated.

Mice and guinea pigs are unsuitable species for the study of the chronic toxic effects of HCB since they are very susceptible to its neurotoxic action and die within 10 days without developing porphyria (DE MATTEIS et al., 1961; IPPEN and AUST, 1972). The effect of HCB on heme metabolism in mice has been investigated in short-term experiments (NAKAO et al., 1967; WADA et al., 1968).

b) *Birds*

Chicken and Japanese quail are more sensitive than mammals to the porphyrogenic action of HCB (STRIK and WIT, 1972; STRIK, 1973 c). In these species the incidence and severity of porphyria at a particular level of HCB in the diet appears to be

related to the severity of other toxic actions—weight loss, tremor and liver damage—
and to the number of animals that die during long-term feeding experiments (Vos
et al., 1971; Vos et al., 1972). Two indices of porphyria have been used in birds;
an increase in the concentration of the coproporphyrin fraction in faeces, which
is the more sensitive (Vos et al., 1971), and macro- and microscopic examination of internal organs in ultraviolet light for red fluorescence due to porphyrins.
Vos et al. (1971) fed diets containing 5, 20 and 80 ppm HCB to Japanese quail for
90 days, and found a dose-related increase in the faecal coproporphyrin fraction
that was first observed after 10 days. Changes in faecal protoporphyrin levels were
difficult to assess since values for control birds fluctuated markedly. Five out of
15 birds in the group fed 80 ppm HCB died and these showed macroscopic fluorescence of liver, bile, small intestine, kidney and bones, but the remaining birds
which were killed after 90 days only showed weak fluorescence in the bones. Fewer
birds died in the 20 ppm group and the incidence of red fluorescence was lower.
Red fluorescence of the bile due to an increased concentration of porphyrin has
been observed as soon as 17 h after a single large oral dose of HCB (1000 mg/kg)
(STRIK, 1973b) but it is not clear whether this indicates the very early onset of a
porphyria of the HCB-type or reflects an increase in porphyrin excretion during
microsomal enzyme induction, a response that has been reported in some mammals
(MOORE et al., 1970).

Analyses of the composition of the increased faecal porphyrin fractions have
not been reported for HCB porphyria in the Japanese quail but it is probable that
porphyrins with 4−8 carboxyl groups would be found as in mammals, since STRIK
(1973b) has shown that the bile contains increased amounts of porphyrins with
5−8 carboxyl groups. The pattern of porphyrin accumulation in the liver is the
same as in other species, while porphyrins with 6, 7 and 8 carboxyl groups are
present in the kidney.

The greater sensitivity of Japanese quail, compared with rats, to the porphyrogenic action of HCB which is indicated by the earlier onset (within 10−90 days)
of porphyria at lower dietary levels (5−80 ppm), may be partly due to a more
rapid accumulation of HCB in the liver. Thus comparison of the concentrations
of HCB in the livers of female Sprague-Dawley rats reported by GRANT et al. (1974)
with those given for quail by Vos et al. (1972) suggests that there may be no great
difference between the concentrations at which porphyria (as judged by liver porphyrin concentrations or red fluorescence of liver) develops in the two species.

Carnivorous birds are resistant to the porphyrogenic, but not to the other toxic
actions of HCB (Vos et al., 1971; Vos et al., 1972).

II. Other Polyhalogenated Aromatic Hydrocarbons

1. Polyhalogenated Biphenyls

The prolonged administration of polyhalogenated biphenyls, either mixed with the
diet or by absorption through the skin (Vos and BEEMS, 1971), produces a porphyria in rabbits, rats and birds which is very similar to HCB porphyria. However,
clinical porphyria was not a feature of the outbreak of PCB poisoning that occurred
in Japan in 1968 (KIMBROUGH, 1974) due to contamination of rice oil with Kane-

chlor-400, a commercial mixture containing about 48% chlorine. Although some of the commercial PCB mixtures used in most investigations may contain other chlorinated hydrocarbons (Vos et al., 1970), PCBs themselves are undoubtedly porphyrogenic since Vos and NOTENBOOM-RAM (1972) have shown that pure 2,4,5,2',4',5'-hexachlorobiphenyl causes porphyria. Of the commercial mixtures tested, Phenoclor DP6, Clophen A60 and Aroclors 1242, 1254 and 1260 are porphyrogenic (Vos and KOEMAN, 1970; Vos and NOTENBOOM-RAM, 1972; BRUCKNER et al., 1974; GOLDSTEIN et al., 1974). Hexabrominated biphenyls also cause porphyria (STRIK, 1973a).

GOLDSTEIN et al. (1974) fed female Sherman rats with a diet containing Aroclor 1254 (100 ppm) for 13 months. During this time the animals gained weight normally, no skin lesions or neurotoxicity were seen and no deaths occurred. Slight coproporphyrinuria was present from the first week of feeding but porphyria did not develop for $2-7$ months. The first and most consistent sign of porphyria was a rapid increase in the urinary uroporphyrin fraction which continued over 4 6 weeks and then levelled-off at a value some 500-fold that of controls. This was accompanied by porphobilinogenuria (maximum increase: 50-fold) and later by a less marked increase in the excretion of coproporphyrin (27-fold) and 5-aminolaevulinate (18-fold). Most of the urine porphyrin was shown to be uroporphyrin (73%) and heptacarboxylic porphyrin (16%) by thin-layer chromatography but increased quantities of coproporphyrin and hexa- and pentacarboxylic porphyrins were also present. The porphyrin concentration in the liver (uroporphyrin and heptacarboxylic porphyrin, 75% and 25% of the total respectively) increased progressively as porphyria developed. No red fluorescence was seen when the bone marrow was examined in ultraviolet light. A single large oral dose (1000 mg/kg) of Aroclor 1254 did not produce porphyria in these animals.

Other studies of the porphyrogenic action of polyhalogenated biphenyls have been less detailed. Vos and NOTENBOOM-RAM (1972) showed that the dermal application of both Aroclor 1260 and 2,4,5,2',4',5'-hexachlorobiphenyl (120 mg in isopropanol/day, 5 times/week for 4 weeks) to rabbits led to accumulation of porphyrin in the liver, kidney and small intestine and to an increase in the faecal coproporphyrin fraction. STRIK (1973c) compared the porphyria produced by polyhalogenated biphenyls and by HCB in Japanese quail and found no essential difference between them.

2. Porphyria Associated with the Manufacture of Chlorinated Phenols: TCDD

a) Porphyria in Herbicide Factories

A form of porphyria, indistinguishable from PCTS, has been reported in association with outbreaks of chloracne among workers in two factories producing the herbicides 2,4-D(2,4-dichlorophenoxyacetic acid) and 2,4,5-T(2,4,5-trichlorophenoxyacetic acid) and related compounds (BLEIBERG et al., 1964; JIRÁSEK et al., 1973). In both outbreaks uroporphyrinuria was commoner than overt porphyria with skin lesions. BLEIBERG et al. (1964) studied 29 patients with chloracne. Two of these had active porphyric skin lesions which in one patient were exacerbated when a fungus infection was treated with griseofulvin. Both patients had uroporphyrinuria with a smaller increase in coproporphyrin excretion, and one of them was reported to have had an increased urinary porphobilinogen concentration. A third patient gave a history of severe chloracne and bullous eruptions but had not been in contact with chlorinated hydrocarbons for two years and had no uroporphyrinuria when examined. Eight of the remaining 26 patients had uroporphyrinuria without clinical porphyria; three of these had no chloracne at the time of examination. Of the 76 patients with chloracne studied by JIRÁSEK et al. (1973, 1974), 11 had a persistent increase in uroporphyrin excretion ranging from 172 – 2230 µg/24 h and 10 of these had porphyric skin lesions. A further 12 patients had intermittent increases in uroporphyrin excretion which never exceeded 100 µg/24 h (normal < 35 µg/24 h). Although clinical porphyria and chloracne occurred together in the same patients in both outbreaks, in neither was there any correlation between the severity of chloracne and the presence of chemical or clinical evidence of porphyria. In many workers with chloracne urinary porphyrin excretion was normal, while in others uroporphyrinuria persisted after the chloracne had healed.

Clinical and biochemical evidence of liver dysfunction was present in some of the patients with porphyria and histological examination of needle biopsy samples showed "parenchymal cell regeneration and hemofuscin deposition" (BLEIBERG et al., 1964) or "mild steatosis or mild periportal fibrosis" (JIRÁSEK et al., 1974). Samples of liver from patients with porphyria showed intense red fluorescence in ultraviolet light, as did liver tissue from one patient without uroporphyrinuria who died (JIRÁSEK et al., 1974). The latter finding suggests that the true incidence of abnormal porphyrin metabolism in such outbreaks is probably greater than that revealed by urine screening procedures which are known to be less sensitive for the detection of latent PCTS than direct examination of liver tissue for porphyrin (LUNDVALL and ENERBACK, 1969). JIRÁSEK et al. (1974) found that the bonemarrow of some of their patients with increased hepatic porphyrin concentrations also showed red fluorescence, but the precise localisation of this fluorescence is not reported.

b) *TCDD*

In recent years evidence has accumulated that porphyria in workers manufacturing herbicides may be due to exposure to TCDD rather than to chlorophenols or chlorobenzenes as previously suggested (POLAND et al., 1971a; CROW, 1970). TCDD is a potent chloracneigenic agent (CROW, 1970) which may be formed during the manufacture of 2,4,5-T as one of the side products of the alkaline hydrolysis of 1,2,4,5-tetrachlorobenzene to 2,4,5-trichlorophenate, especially if the reaction is carried out at too high a temperature (MILNES, 1971; MAY, 1973) as happened in the Czechoslovakian outbreak (JIRÁSEK, 1974). POLAND et al. (1971a), on re-investigating the workers in the factory that BLEIBERG et al. (1964) had studied 6 years before, found uroporphyrinuria in only one of the 73 employees, a man who had had clinical porphyria at the time of the first investigation, although the incidence of chloracne was still high. They suggested that a recent change in the manufacturing process, so as to decrease the level of TCDD in the 2,4,5-trichlorophenate from 10 – 25 ppm to less than 1 ppm, may have been related to the decreased incidence of uroporphyrinuria. Subsequently POLAND and GLOVER (1973a; 1973b) showed that a number of chlorinated dibenzo-*p*-dioxins increase the activity of

ALA-S in the chick embryo and that TCDD, which doubles ALA-S activity at a dose of 1.5 ng/egg, is the most potent inducer of this enzyme yet discovered.

Studies in mammals are made difficult by the very high acute toxicity of TCDD. WOODS (1973) found no alteration in the activity of ALA-S during a period of 28 days after giving a single dose of TCDD (25 – 100 µg/kg) to male and female rats and to mice. Although not all compounds which induce ALA-S in chick embryo systems are porphyrogenic in mammals (DE MATTEIS, 1967), this does not seem to be the case with TCDD since GOLDSTEIN et al. (1973) have since produced porphyria in male C 57/BL 6 mice by giving either four weekly doses of 25 µg/kg (in corn oil : acetone, 6 : 1 v/v) or a single dose of 150 µg/kg orally. Mice that were killed or died 21 – 28 days after the first or only dose showed massive increases in liver porphyrin concentration (2000 – 4000-fold: uroporphyrin 90%, hepta-carboxylic porphyrin, 10%). The time course of porphyrin accumulation was not studied. These investigations show that, although there may be considerable strain and species variation in susceptibility to the porphyrogenic action of TCDD, in susceptible animals exposure to little more than trace amounts, as in the manu-facture of herbicides, may be sufficient to provoke porphyria. Further investigations of the porphyrogenic action of TCDD in mammals are clearly required. Mean-while, in view of the dissociation between chloracne and porphyria in some patients, it is worth recalling that the patients described by BLEIBERG et al. (1964) and JIRÁSEK et al. (1974) had been exposed to chlorinated hydrocarbons other than TCDD, and that reports of industrial accidents in which chloracne and exposure to TCDD are well-documented make no mention of porphyria (CROW, 1970; MAY, 1973).

3. Other Halogenated Aromatic Compounds

The compounds described in this section can be divided into two groups. In the first group are compounds, such as octachlorostyrene, tetrachlorodibenzofuran and hexachloronaphthalene, that share many of the properties of the porphyrogens described above. Of these, only octachlorostyrene, has been shown to be por-phyrogenic causing a porphyria in the rat identical to that produced by HCB (STRIK and KOEMAN, 1976); however the others compounds have not been rigor-ously tested.

The second group of compounds contains the lower chlorinated benzenes in-vestigated by RIMINGTON and ZIEGLER (1963). These compounds were given orally to male rats in amounts (250 – 800 mg/kg/day, about 0.5 – 1.6%, w/w) close to the lethal dose for periods of 30 – 40 days. With the exception of 1,2,4,5-tetrachloro-benzene, which may have been poorly absorbed, all produced a similar disturbance of porphyrin metabolism, which was most marked with those compounds with chlorine substituents *para* to each other; 1,4-, 1,2,4- and 1,2,3,4-chlorobenzene (pentachlorobenzene was not investigated). There was an immediate increase in the urinary excretion of coproporphyrin III which rose steadily until it reached a plateau (7 – 15 times control) at around 30 days when the animals were killed. The concentration of uroporphyrin in the urine, although increased some 10 – 50-fold, never exceeded more than 10% of the coproporphyrin concentration. At the higher doses there was a late increase in the excretion of porphyrin precursors.

Both porphyrin and porphobilinogen accumulated in the livers of markedly porphyric animals. In contrast to the findings with HCB, the liver porphyrin was uroporphyrin, protoporphyrin and coproporphyrin in approximately equal amounts,
much of it appeared to be stored as porphyrinogen, and the total concentration
was increased no more than 10-fold. The disturbance of porphyrin metabolism
described in these experiments clearly shows some differences from that produced
both by HCB and by porphyrogens such as AIA (RIMINGTON and ZIEGLER, 1963).
It can be distinguished from HCB porphyria by the lack of a delayed onset, the
low uroporphyrin excretion, and the pattern of porphyrin(ogen) accumulation in
the liver. The last of these is not an early feature of HCB porphyria and thus it is
unlikely that the differences are due to failure to continue the experiments for long
enough or to the use of a resistant strain of male rat. POLAND et al. (1971b) were
also unable to produce a porphyria of the HCB-type in short-term experiments
with 1,3-dichlorobenzene and its major metabolite, 2,4-dichlorophenol. The porphyrogenic action of the lower chlorinated benzenes needs further investigation,
but at present there is no evidence that they produce a porphyria of the HCB-type
in animals, and therefore they may not cause PCTS in man—a point of some
practical relevance since some of them are used in the manufacture of herbicides.

III. Conclusion

In susceptible strains and species, HCB, hexabromobiphenyl, octachlorostyrene
and a component(s) of the higher chlorinated commercial PCB mixtures produce
a specific disturbance of porphyrin metabolism in the liver, which is characterised
by overproduction of isomer series III porphyrins with acetate substituents, notably
uroporphyrin III. Although the pattern of heme precursor excretion varies between
strains and species, the overproduction of these porphyrins is a constant feature
that defines this type of chemically induced porphyria. Compounds that produce
this response are potential causes of the syndrome of PCTS in man. The response
to these porphyrogens in animals and the course of PCTS in man is influenced by
alterations in body iron stores and by oestrogens.

D. The Effect of Polyhalogenated Aromatic Hydrocarbons on Heme Metabolism in the Liver

The administration of porphyrogenic polyhalogenated hydrocarbons to animals
produces an increase in the concentration of microsomal hemoproteins in the liver
and alterations in the activity of some of the enzymes of the heme biosynthetic pathway. The increase in microsomal hemoprotein concentration is an early response
to exposure to the chemical, whereas the changes in enzyme activity are delayed
and occur in parallel with the development of porphyria. The actions of these
compounds on hepatic heme metabolism thus differ from those of other porphyrogenic chemicals in two respects: they cause an increase, rather than a decrease, in hemoprotein concentration and there is no close relationship between
the time of onset of the changes in hemoprotein concentration and the alterations
in enzyme activity.

I. Effect on Hemoproteins in the Liver

1. Microsomal Hemoproteins

HCB and polyhalogenated biphenyls, like many other xenobiotics (CONNEY, 1967), increase the concentration of microsomal protein and cytochromes P-450 and b_5, and the activity of associated drug-metabolising enzymes, in the liver of mammals and birds (Table 3) (WADA et al., 1968; SWEENEY et al., 1971; ALVARES et al., 1973; RAJAMANICKAM et al., 1972; STRIK, 1973c; FARBER and BAKER, 1974; GOLDSTEIN et al., 1974; GRANT et al., 1974; STONARD, 1974; STONARD and NENOV, 1974; TURNER and GREEN, 1974; STONARD, 1975). These changes are paralleled morphologically by proliferation of the smooth endoplasmic reticulum (SWEENEY et al., 1971; KIMBROUGH et al., 1972; MEDLINE et al., 1973) especially in centrilobular cells which appear hypertrophied when examined by light microscopy (CAMPBELL, 1963; SWEENEY et al., 1971; KIMBROUGH et al., 1972; TIMME et al., 1974).

When porphyrogenic doses of HCB are fed to rats hepatomegaly develops within a week (MEDLINE et al., 1973, STONARD, 1974) and is largely due to the increase in smooth endoplasmic reticulum (KUIPER-GOODMAN et al., 1974). It is probable that the hepatomegaly produced by PCBs (KIMBROUGH et al., 1972; GOLDSTEIN et al., 1974) is due to the same cause. With both HCB and PCBs hepatomegaly and induction of microsomal hemoproteins and drug-metabolising enzymes is more marked in male rats, which are more resistant to the porphyrogenic and lethal effects of these compounds, than in female rats (KIMBROUGH

Table 3. The effect of porphyrogenic halogenated aromatic hydrocarbons on microsomal drug metabolising enzymes

Reaction and substrate	Effect of: —	HCB	PCB	TCDD	
Aliphatic hydroxylation					
pento- or hexobarbitol		$+$ [1,4]	$+$ [5,6,7]	8,4	*[9]
Aromatic hydroxylation					
zoxazolamine		$+$ [1,4]	$+$ [5]	$+$ [9,10]	$+$ *[9]
3,4-benzopyrene			$+$ [5]	$+$ [10]	
biphenyl		$+$ [2]			
N-Hydroxylation					
aniline		$+$ [1,2,4]	$+$ [6]	$+$ [10]	
N-Dealkylation					
ethylmorphine		$-$ [3]	$+$ [5]	$-$ [10]	
aminopyrine		$+$ [1,4]	$+$ [6,7]	$-$ [10]	
O-Dealkylation					
4-nitroanisole		$+$ [2]	$+$ [6]		
Nitro-reduction					
p-nitrobenzoate			$+$ [6,7]		

Enzyme systems in italics are not induced by 3-methylcholanthrene. Data for rats or * mice (C 57 BL/6) from [1] STONARD and NENOV (1974), [2] TURNER and GREEN (1974), [3] SWEENEY et al. (1971), [4] GRANT et al. (1974), [5] ALVARES et al. (1973), [6] JOHNSTONE et al. (1974), [7] FARBER and BAKER (1974), [8] GREIG (1972), [9] GREIG and DE MATTEIS (1973), [10] LUCIER et al. (1973).

et al., 1972; KUIPER-GOODMAN et al., 1974; STONARD and NENOV, 1974; STONARD, 1974; GRANT et al., 1974).

The time course of the induction of microsomal hemoproteins by HCB and PCB has been studied in several investigations of the porphyrogenic actions of these compounds. With HCB an increase in microsomal cytochrome P-450 is apparent within 24 h (RAJAMANICKAM et al., 1972), a maximum of $3-5$ times the control values is reached after $7-13$ days (RAJAMANICKAM et al., 1972; STONARD, 1974) and the cytochrome subsequently remains elevated at $2-3$ times control values without any detectable change when porphyria develops (STONARD, 1974). Proliferation of the smooth endoplasmic reticulum and increases in the activity of drug-metabolising enzymes persist for at least eight weeks after withdrawal of HCB from the diet (KUIPER-GOODMAN et al., 1974). Similar changes are seen when female rats receive a diet containing Aroclor 1254 (100 ppm) over a period of 13 months (GOLDSTEIN et al., 1974). Aroclor 1254 is a mixture of chlorinated biphenyls, and it is therefore possible that separate components may be responsible for the induction of microsomal hemoprotein and the porphyria. However, 2,4,5,2',4',5'-hexachlorobiphenyl possesses both actions (VOS and NOTENBOOM-RAM, 1972; JOHNSTONE et al., 1974). Short-term studies have shown that the initial increase in cytochrome P-450 is accompanied by an increase in the activity of drug-metabolising enzymes which is probably greatest when hemoprotein levels are at their maximum (ALVARES et al., 1973; STONARD and NENOV, 1974; KUIPER-GOODMAN et al., 1974). Few investigations of the functional state of the smooth endoplasmic reticulum during the later stages of HCB poisoning have been reported. SWEENEY et al. (1971) found that ethylmorphine N-demethylase activity was decreased in HCB porphyria, and it is possible that the hypertrophied smooth endoplasmic reticulum eventually becomes hypoactive. This aspect of the changes in the microsomal drug-metabolising system requires further investigation, particularly since the ultrastructural changes in the hepatocyte after prolonged HCB feeding resemble those seen after similar exposure to dieldrin and other compounds which are known to produce a hypertrophic hypoactive smooth endoplasmic reticulum (HUTTERER et al., 1968; PEREZ et al., 1972; MEDLINE et al., 1973).

Compounds that induce microsomal drug-metabolising enzymes in the liver can be divided into two groups (CONNEY, 1967; ALVARES et al., 1973). One group contains compounds that, like phenobarbitone, increase the concentration of cytochrome P-450 and the activity of a wide range of drug-metabolising enzymes. The second group of compounds—typified by 3-methylcholanthrene—induce the synthesis of cytochrome P-448 and increase the activity of fewer drug-metabolising enzymes (CONNEY, 1967). Although most reports refer to the major microsomal hemoprotein induced by HCB and PCB as cytochrome P-450 it is probable that these compounds represent a third class of inducers which promote the formation of a hemoprotein, or group of hemoproteins, which share the properties of both main types of inducer (ALVARES et al., 1973; STONARD, 1975). Thus, although the carbon monoxide difference spectrum of microsomes from rats treated with Aroclor 1254 (ALVARES et al., 1973) or HCB (STONARD, 1975) has a peak at 448 nm, as is found after 3-methylcholanthrene treatment, the pattern of induction of microsomal enzyme activities resembles that found after phenobarbitone administration (Table 3). Reduced microsomes from treated rats bind ligands, such as ethylisocyanide or pyridine, to give pH-dependent difference spectra which, with Aroclor 1254 (ALVARES et al., 1973) resemble those obtained with microsomes from 3-methylcholanthrene treated rats but, with HCB (STONARD, 1975) are intermediate between those from 3-methylcholanthrene and phenobarbitone-treated animals. Binding of hexobarbitone or aniline to oxidised microsomes from rats treated with either compound gives both type I (hexobarbitone) and type II (aniline) difference spectra, as would be obtained with microsomes from rats treated with phenobarbitone and 3-methylchloranthrene together (ALVARES et al., 1973; STONARD, 1975). In view of the known heterogeneity of microsomal hemoproteins (RYAN et al., 1975) and the observation that simultaneous administration of 3-methylcholanthrene and phenobarbitone produces a pattern of enzyme induction similar to that described above (CONNEY, 1967), it seems likely that HCB combines in one molecule structural features that are capable of inducing both types of response. It is probable that the same is true for PCB since, although ALVARES et al. (1973) used a commercial mixture, a number of pure chlorinated biphenyls have now been shown to induce a similar wide range of microsomal enzyme activities (JOHNSTONE et al, 1974), even though the spectral properties of the induced hemoproteins have not been studied.

There are a number of reasons for believing that the changes in the concentration and properties of hepatic microsomal cytochromes that follow exposure to polyhalogenated aromatic hydrocarbons may not be directly related to the porphyrogenic action of these compounds. Thus, the effect on microsomal hemoproteins can be dissociated from the porphyria, since the former precedes the latter by several weeks, occurs with doses which are lower than those required to produce porphyria (GRANT et al., 1974) and is more marked in the sex which is less susceptible to the porphyrogenic action. Similarly, the relevance of the specific pattern of microsomal hemoprotein and enzyme induction is difficult to assess since the apparent restriction of this type of response to PCB and HCB may be due solely to the lack of detailed investigation of the spectral properties of the hemoproteins induced by other lipophilic compounds that similarly accumulate within the body but do not cause porphyria. Certainly this pattern of response is not found with all porphyrogenic polychlorinated aromatic hydrocarbons since TCDD is a potent inducer of changes in liver microsomes in rats and mice—including the strain that is susceptible to its porphyrogenic action—that are identical to those caused by 3-methylcholanthrene (GREIG, 1972; GREIG and DE MATTEIS, 1973) (Table 3).

2. Other Hemoproteins

In contrast to other types of experimental porphyria, the concentration of catalase in the liver remains normal in HCB porphyria (OCKNER and SCHMID, 1961; DE MATTEIS et al., 1961), a finding which may indicate that the supply of protoheme for hemoprotein synthesis is adequate in this condition (SWEENEY, 1976). Other heme-enzymes and mitochondrial hemoproteins have not been studied in HCB porphyria in mammals. In Japanese quail the concentration of both mitochondrial hemoproteins and soluble heme-enzymes in the liver is unaffected by HCB (STRIK, 1973 b).

II. Effect on Enzymes of the Heme Biosynthetic Pathway

Measurements of the activity of enzymes of the heme biosynthetic pathway in HCB porphyria are summarised in Table 4.

Table 4. Enzyme activities in the liver of rats with HCB porphyria

Enzyme	HCB porphyria	HCB porphyria + iron overload	Control	References
ALA-S	146		42	Sweeney et al. (1971)
	27.2 ± 2.1		16.1 ± 2.1	Rajamanickam et al. (1972)
	81.5 ± 16.7	79.2 ± 23.9		Taljaard et al. (1972a)
ALA-de-hydratase	360		700	Rajamanickam et al. (1972)
UROG-D	64.2 ± 16.3	Not detectable	52.3 ± 24.9	Taljaard et al. (1971)
	136 − 248 (184)		896 − 1472 (1240)	Elder et al. (1975a)
CPG-OX	900 − 1269 (1056)		1008 − 1216 (1120)	Elder et al. (1975a)

Activities, expressed as nmoles of 5-ALA equivalents produced/g liver/h, are given as means ± S.D. or as ranges with means in parentheses.

1. 5-Aminolaevulinate Synthetase (ALA-S)

The activity of the rate-limiting enzyme of protoheme synthesis, ALA-S, is increased in the liver in HCB porphyria in the rat (Simon et al., 1970; Sweeney et al., 1971; Taljaard et al., 1971, 1972a; Rajamanickam et al., 1972; Strik, 1973c; Stonard, 1974) and other species (Strik, 1973a and c), and in porphyria caused by polyhalogenated biphenyls (Strik, 1973a; Goldstein et al., 1974) and by TCDD (Goldstein et al., 1973). The increase is less than in other types of experimental porphyria and is rarely greater than 2 − 3-fold.

Large single doses of HCB (Wada et al., 1968; Sweeney et al., 1971) and PCB (Goldstein et al., 1974) cause an immediate increase in hepatic ALA-S activity which is probably related to the induction of microsomal hemoproteins in the liver. Prolonged administration of the smaller doses of these compounds that are used to produce porphyria does not increase ALA-S activity until the onset of porphyria (Simon et al., 1970; Rajamanickam et al., 1972; Goldstein et al., 1974). At these lower doses, the initial increase in microsomal hemoprotein concentration is not accompanied by a measurable increase in ALA-S activity, although a small increase in the rate of total heme synthesis to a maximum of one-and-a-half times the basal rate at 72 h can be detected (Rajamanickam et al., 1972). Thus the increase in hepatic ALA-S activity is a delayed effect which is related to the manifestation of porphyria, rather than to the increase in microsomal hemoprotein concentration.

The onset of porphyria in the rat is, therefore, marked by two events: an increase in the excretion and accumulation of porphyrins and an increase in the activity of hepatic ALA-S. In other types of experimental porphyria, where similar changes develop over a shorter period of time, it has been shown that they indicate compensatory increases designed to maintain the required rate of protoheme synthesis when the activity of one of the enzymes of the pathway is decreased (see Chapt. 5). The excess excretion of heme precursors reflects the accumulation of the substrates of the defective enzyme, and, often, of the enzymes preceding it, brought about by the increase in ALA-S activity which operates to keep the rate of formation of product constant in spite of a decrease in the level of active enzyme. Thus, the pattern of heme precursor excretion should indicate the site of the enzyme defect.

2. Uroporphyrinogen Decarboxylase (UROG-D)

In 1961, DE MATTEIS et al. noted that massive excretion of porphyrins with acetate side chains characterises HCB porphyria and suggested that the porphyria might be due to "interference to the uroporphyrinogen decarboxylating mechanism" in the liver. The sequential decarboxylation of the four acetate side chains of uroporphyrinogen III to form coproporphyrinogen III is catalysed by an enzyme system, uroporphyrinogen decarboxylase (UROG-D), which is located in the cytosol in mammalian and avian erythroid tissue (MAUZERALL and GRANICK, 1958; TOMIO et al., 1970; ROMEO and LEVIN, 1971) and in rat liver (ELDER et al., 1976b). No detailed investigations of the properties of the enzyme system from mammalian liver have been reported, but UROG-D from avian and mammalian erythroid tissue appears to be a single enzyme (TOMIO et al., 1970; ROMEO and LEVIN, 1971), which can utilise hepta-, hexa-, and pentacarboxylate porphyrinogens of the isomer III series as well as uroporphyrinogen I and III as substrates (BATLLE and GRINSTEIN, 1964; SAN MARTIN DE VIALE and GRINSTEIN, 1968; GARCIA et al., 1973). Studies of the pattern of accumulation of intermediates during the course of the reaction and comparison of the rates of decarboxylation of uroporphyrinogen III and heptacarboxylate porphyrinogen III suggest that in avian erythrocytes, but not in mammalian erythroid tissue (ROMEO and LEVIN, 1971), elimination of the first carboxyl group from uroporphyrinogen III is more rapid than the subsequent decarboxylations. The same may also be true of the enzyme system from mammalian liver (SAN MARTIN DE VIALE et al., 1976b). In both avian erythrocytes and rat liver the acetate substituents of uroporphyrinogen III are decarboxylated in order around the ring starting with that at position 8 and ending at position 5 (JACKSON et al., 1976).

The first measurements of UROG-D in HCB porphyria were reported by TALJAARD et al. (1971), who found that the enzyme was readily demonstrable in the livers of normal animals but could not be detected in the livers of rats with iron-overload made porphyric by HCB. However, the activity of UROG-D in the livers of rats with HCB porphyria alone was the same as in control animals. Subsequently SAN MARTIN DE VIALE et al. 1972, 1976b) showed that the activity of UROG-D was decreased by 76%, with uroporphyrinogen III as substrate, and by 95%, with heptacarboxylate porphyrinogen as substrate, in liver fractions from rats with HCB porphyria without iron overload. The activity of UROG-D was normal in the spleen and red cells from these animals. SAN MARTIN DE VIALE et al. (1976b) excluded the possibility that the large amounts of porphyrin present

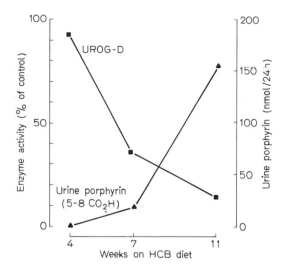

Fig. 3. Effect of HCB on the activity of UROG-D in liver. Mean values for 4 female Wistar rats receiving HCB (0.3%, w/w) are shown

in the liver extracts may have directly inhibited the enzyme, or enhanced the aut-oxidation of the substrate (MAUZERALL and GRANICK, 1958), by removing the porphyrin by Sephadex G-25 chromatography before assaying the enzyme. How-ever, it is unlikely that uroporphyrin, even in the concentrations that may be reached in the liver in HCB porphyria, produces significant inhibition of the en-zyme in vitro, provided that sufficient glutathione or thioglycollate is present in the assay system (MAUZERALL and GRANICK, 1958; TALJAARD et al., 1971; ELDER et al., 1976b).

ELDER et al. (1976a and b) have followed the changes in UROG-D activity that occur during the course of feeding HCB to rats. Using pentacarboxylate porphyrinogen III as substrate, they showed that the activity of the enzyme in rat liver homogenates falls progressively as porphyria develops (Fig. 3). The rate of decarboxylation of two other substrates of UROG-D, uroporphyrinogen III and isocoproporphyrinogen, was also found to be markedly decreased when measured after 13 weeks on a diet containing HCB. The correlation between the changes in the rates of decarboxylation of pentacarboxylate porphyrinogen III and excretion of porphyrins with $8-5$ carboxyl groups during the onset of HCB porphyria (Fig. 3), considered together with the low activity of UROG-D, measured with uroporphyrinogen III as substrate, in the liver once porphyria is established, stongly suggests that HCB porphyria is due to the decreased activity of UROG-D in liver. A precise description of the relationship between the pattern of porphyrin excretion and accumulation and the level of activity of UROG-D in the liver requires more knowledge of the kinetics of the interaction of rat liver UROG-D with its substrates than is available at present.

JOUBERT and co-workers (TALJAARD et al., 1972b; JOUBERT et al., 1973) have emphasised that, since initially accumulation of porphyrin is restricted to the

centrilobular zones of the liver (CAMPBELL, 1963; SWEENEY et al., 1971), the enzyme defect may be similarly localised in the early stages of the porphyria. If this
is so, measurements of enzyme activities in whole liver homogenates may show
little change from control values at a time when both accumulation of porphyrins
in affected cells and excretion of porphyrins from these cells are readily detectable.
Thus ELDER et al. (1976a) found that the concentration of isocoproporphyrin and
pentacarboxylate porphyrin in the faeces, and of uroporphyrin in the liver, was
increased at a time when there was no statistically significant decrease in the
activity of UROG-D, and GOLDSTEIN et al. (1974) reported that liver porphyrin
levels increase before ALA-S activity in PCB porphyria. JOUBERT et al. (1973)

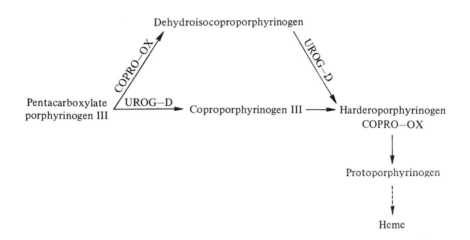

Fig. 4. Metabolism of pentacarboxylate porphyrinogen III in liver

suggested that their finding of normal UROG-D activities in the liver of porphyric rats without iron overload might also be explained in this way, particularly
if there is a compensatory increase in enzyme activity in unaffected hepatocytes.
However, it is likely that the discrepancy between their findings and those of other
workers, as well as the low activity they report for control rats (Table 3), is due

to their use of an assay method in which only the formation of porphyrinogens corresponding to ether-soluble porphyrins is measured, since subsequent work has shown that heptacarboxylate porphyrinogen (i.e. the porphyrinogen of an ether-in soluble porphyrin) may be a major product of decarboxylation of uroporphyrinogen III under similar assay conditions (San Martin De Viale et al., 1975b; Kushner et al., 1975a; Elder et al., 1976b).

The increased excretion of porphyrins of the isocoproporphyrin series that occurs in HCB porphyria in the rat is a direct consequence of the decrease in the activity of UROG-D. Dehydroisocoproporphyrinogen, the precursor of these porphyrins (Elder, 1974), is produced when the 2-propionate group of pentacarboxylate porphyrinogen III is converted to a vinyl group by coproporphyrinogen oxidase (CPG-OX) (Fig. 4). It is probable that under normal circumstances little dehydroisocoproporphyrinogen is formed because pentacarboxylate porphyrinogen III is rapidly converted to coproporphyrinogen III by UROG-D and because the affinity of CPG-OX for coproporphyrinogen III is greater than for pentacarboxylate porphyrinogen III. Furthermore, the 5-acetate group of any dehydroisocoproporphyronigen formed will be decarboxylated by UROG-D to form harderoporporphyrinogen (Fig. 4). In HCB porphyria, the low activity of UROG-D leads to an increase in the amount of pentacarboxylate porphyrinogen III formed relative to coproporphyrinogen III and to a decrease in the rate of decarboxylation of dehydroisocoproporphyrinogen (Fig. 4). Consequently, dehydroisocoproporphyrinogen and the porphyrins derived from it (Elder, 1972) are formed and excreted in excess. It seems likely that increased excretion of these porphyrins relative to coproporphyrin, which is also seen in PCTS (Elder, 1975), may prove to be a reliable indicator of the presence of a UROG-D defect.

3. Coproporphyrinogen Oxidase (CPG-OX)

The increase in coproporphyrin III excretion, which is a feature of HCB porphyria (Ockner and Schmid, 1961; De Matteis et al., 1961; San Martin De Viale et al., 1970; Taljaard et al., 1972a) is, at first sight, incompatible with the concept that a UROG-D defect underlies the overproduction of porphyrins in this condition. Taljaard et al. (1972b) have suggested that the coproporphyrin may come from hepatocytes unaffected by the porphyric process and would thus be another manifestation of compensatory changes in heme biosynthesis in non-porphyric cells. Alternatively, coproporphyrinogen III accumulation, and coproporphyrinuria, may be a direct consequence of the decreased activity of UROG-D. Thus, although the activity of coproporphyrinogen oxidase is normal in HCB porphyria (Elder et al., 1976a), the production of dehydroisocoproporphyrinogen in this condition indicates that pentacarboxylate porphyrinogen III is competing with coproporphyrinogen III as a substrate for this enzyme. Since the conversion of dehydroisocoproporphyrinogen via harderoporphyrinogen to protoheme is impaired by the UROG-D defect, pentacarboxylate porphyrinogen III acts effectively as a competitive inhibitor of heme synthesis. Under these circumstances, maintenance of the rate of heme synthesis would require an increase in coproporphyrinogen concentration and would be expected to produce coproporphyrinuria.

The slight coproporphyrinuria, which precedes the onset of porphyria (OCKNER and SCHMID, 1961; TALJAARD et al., 1972a; STONARD, 1974), cannot be explained by the above mechanism. It may be similar in origin to the accumulation of co-proporphyrin that accompanies induction of microsomal hemoproteins by other compounds (MOORE et al., 1972).

4. Other Enzymes

Few measurements of other enzymes of the heme biosynthetic pathway in porphyria caused by polyhalogenated aromatic hydrocarbons have been reported. RAJAMANICKAM et al. (1972) reported that the activity of hepatic 5-aminolaevulinate dehydratase is decreased in rats with HCB porphyria, although the activity remains well in excess of that of ALA-S and formation of porphobilinogen does not become rate-limiting. In contrast, HCB increased the activity of 5-aminolaevulinate de-hydratase and porphobilinogen deaminase in the liver in female rats of a different strain, an effect that is oestrogen-dependent (SAN MARTIN DE VIALE et al., 1976c). Differences in the relative activities of enzymes of heme biosynthesis may underlie some of the variations in the pattern of heme-precursor excretion seen between different strains and species.

5. Conclusion

The evidence described above indicates that HCB causes porphyria by decreasing the activity of UROG-D in the liver. The same is probably true for the other porphyrogenic polyhalogenated compounds, since they produce an identical pattern of porphyrin overproduction. Initially the defect is most marked in the centri-lobular hepatocytes but eventually all parenchymal cells become involved. The rate of protoheme synthesis or hemoprotein turnover in HCB porphyria has not been investigated. Early in the course of HCB feeding, when induction of micro-somal hemoproteins is at a maximum, there is a small increase in the rate of proto-heme synthesis (RAJAMANICKAM et al., 1972). It is probable that, once the new steady-state level of increased microsomal hemoprotein concentration is reached, the rate declines towards normal, since the activity of ALA-S remains indistin-guishable from that of control animals until porphyria develops. The sustained increase in ALA-S activity which accompanies the porphyria is presumably suf-ficient to maintain this rate of protoheme synthesis in the face of the combined effects of the decrease in UROG-D activity and the consequent competitive inhibi-tion of CPG-OX by pentacarboxylate porphyrinogen III, since microsomal cyto-chrome levels do not change as porphyria develops. Figure 5 shows that the amount of ALA produced in the liver, determined by in vitro measurements of ALA-S activity, is in reasonable agreement with the amount utilized for porphyrin overproduction and protoheme synthesis. The accumulation of intermediates of the heme biosynthetic pathway which accompanies these changes in enzyme activ-ity is reflected in the pattern of heme-precursor accumulation and excretion which defines this type of porphyria.

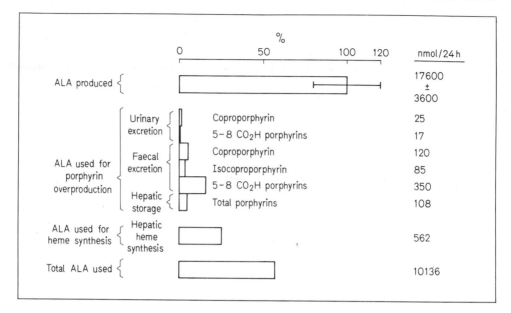

Fig. 5. Production and utilisation of ALA in experimental HCB porphyria. ALA production (mean ±S.D.) was calculated from ALA-S measurements given by TALJAARD et al. (1972a), porphyrin overproduction from data in Fig. 2, and rate of hepatic heme synthesis from figures given by MEYER and MARVER (1971) for normal rats. In the bar diagram, amounts are expressed as a percentage of mean ALA production; rates used to construct the diagram are also shown (8 moles ALA are equivalent to one mole of porphyrin or heme). Figures are for female Wistar rats (liver wt. 9.0 g) after 6 weeks on a diet containing 0.3% (w/w) HCB

E. The Mechanism of the Porphyrogenic Action of Polyhalogenated Aromatic Hydrocarbons

The mechanism of the porphyrogenic action of HCB and other polyhalogenated aromatic hydrocarbons is obscure. They are all water-insoluble, lipophilic, planar or near-planar molecules which produce similar effects on the liver. Thus, in addition to causing porphyria, they induce microsomal drug-metabolising enzymes in the liver, yet are themselves resistant to metabolism and persist to produce liver cell damage. The theories that have been proposed to explain their porphyrogenic action have centred on the relationship between morphological changes in the liver and the porphyria, the possibility of a direct inhibitory action of the compound or a metabolite on an enzyme of the biosynthetic pathway, and the role of abnormalities of iron metabolism within the liver. Before these theories are examined in relation to the recent finding that the activity of hepatic UROG-D is decreased in HCB porphyria, some possible explanations for the delayed onset of this type of porphyria will be discussed.

I. The Mechanism of the Delayed Response to the Porphyrogenic Action of Polyhalogenated Aromatic Hydrocarbons

There is some evidence that the delay in the onset of HCB porphyria may be due, at least in part, to the time taken to accumulate a critical porphyrogenic concentration of HCB in the liver. GRANT et al. (1974) have shown that porphyria does not develop in female rats until liver HCB concentrations exceed about 30 µg/g wet weight, and a similar relationship has been demonstrated for Japanese quail (Vos et al., 1972) in which porphyria develops very rapidly after large doses (STRIK, 1973b). A similar threshold effect, but in respect of dose given, is found when mice are fed the very potent porphyrogen, TCDD. In this case the total amount required to produce porphyria is so small that it can be administered in a single dose (GOLDSTEIN et al., 1973). It is not known whether there is a delay in the onset of porphyria after administering this compound. Differences between species, strains, sexes and individuals in the concentration of HCB in the liver that must be reached before porphyria will develop, as well as in the rate of accumulation in the liver, may partly explain the variability between different animals with respect to the length of time before porphyria develops, as well as the failure to define a dose—response relationship in individual rats (STONARD, 1974). Male rats do not develop porphyria at HCB levels which are associated with porphyria in females (GRANT et al., 1974), a finding that is probably due to a combination of factors: the lack of oestrogens (SAN MARTIN DE VIALE et al., 1976a), the more marked adaptive response in the males and, possibly, differences in iron metabolism between the sexes (HERSHKO and EILON, 1974).

Although it seems likely that at least part of the delay in the onset of porphyria is due to the time taken to achieve a critical level of the porphyrogenic compound in the liver, it is not clear whether porphyria develops as soon as this level is reached, or whether some other change is initiated, e.g. damage to intracellular organelles, which itself leads to porphyria. The first possibility would be supported if a positive correlation between the concentration of HCB in the liver and the severity of the porphyria could be demonstrated.

II. The Relationship Between Porphyria and Morphological Changes in the Liver

Various morphological abnormalities are prominent in the liver by the time porphyria develops in response to HCB, PCB and, especially, TCDD; and some evidence of liver cell damage is usually present in patients with PCTS. Thus several theories of the pathogenesis of both the experimental and human porphyrias have attempted to link the ultrastructural alterations within the hepatocyte to the disorder of heme biosynthesis.

Prolonged administration of porphyrogenic doses of HCB and Aroclors 1254 and 1260 to rats produces similar changes in the liver (OCKNER and SCHMID, 1961; CAMPBELL, 1963; SWEENEY et al., 1971; KIMBROUGH et al., 1972; MEDLINE et al., 1973; BURSE et al., 1974; HANSELL and ECOBICHON, 1974; TIMME et al., 1974). The liver cells are enlarged, especially in the centre of the lobule, with foamy or vacuolated cytoplasm, often containing eosinophilic inclusions. Examination of these cells with the electron microscope reveals massive hypertrophy of the smooth endoplasmic reticulum with displacement of the rough endoplasmic reticulum and mitochondria into scattered clumps, especially around the nucleus. Most mitochondria are of normal appearance. The cytoplasm contains lipid vacuoles and large lipid droplets and localised concentric or laminated membrane arrays—the eosinophilic inclusions of light microscopy—which are probably derived from smooth endoplasmic reticulum. Slender tubular inclusions may represent precipitated porphyrin (TIMME et al., 1974). Occasional necrotic cells and small foci of necrosis, with some evidence of liver cell regeneration, are usually present by the time porphyria develops. The presence of liver cell damage is also indicated by the increased levels of liver enzymes in the serum (SIMON et al., 1970; STRIK, 1973b). Liver cell damage is also present in HCB porphyria in humans, rabbits (DE MATTEIS et al., 1961), Japanese quail (VOS et al., 1971) and in PCB porphyria in rabbits (VOS and NOTENBOOM-RAM, 1972) and quail (STRIK, 1973b). Apart from porphyrin accumulation, the morphological changes produced by these compounds are not specific but are seen with other toxic chemicals (KIMBROUGH et al., 1972; MEDLINE et al., 1973; PEREZ et al., 1972). TCDD is a potent hepatotoxin (JONES and BUTLER, 1974), and porphyrogenic doses of TCDD cause severe liver damage in mice with centrilobular necrosis and inflammation (GOLDSTEIN et al., 1973). Proliferation of smooth endoplasmic reticulum is less marked than with HCB and PCB. The hepatotoxic effect of these compounds is not restricted to animals which are susceptible to the porphyrogenic action.

In general, two theories that link these changes in hepatocytes to the development of porphyria have been proposed. In one, intracellular disorganisation is considered to disrupt the compartmentation of protoheme biosynthesis so that intermediate porphyrinogens accumulate in the cytosol due to a decrease in the uptake, and further metabolism, of coproporphyrinogen III by the mitochondrion (SWEENEY et al., 1971; ELDER, 1972). This theory, which implies that these compounds produce a specific (porphyrogenic) disorganisation of intracellular structure, is not supported by the finding that the intracellular distribution of the mitochondrial enzyme, CPG-OX, is unaltered in HCB porphyria (ELDER and EVANS, unpublished work). The suggestion that dehydroisocoproporphyrinogen is formed in the cytosol by CPG-OX that has leaked from the mitochondrion (ELDER, 1972) now seems less likely than the alternative explanation that its formation is the consequence of entry of accumulated pentacarboxylate porphyrinogen III into the mitochondrion. At present nothing is known of the process of uptake of porphyrinogens by mitochondria, but it is unlikely that an anion of the size of coproporphyrinogen III enters passively. A decreased rate of entry of coproporphyrinogen III into the mitochondrion could explain the coproporphyrinuria of HCB porphyria (STONARD, 1974) but a complete explanation of the porphyria on this basis is not compatible with the decrease in the activity of UROG-D. HCB may exert at least part of its toxic action by altering membrane permeability (SIMON et al., 1976), perhaps by becoming incorporated into membrane lipid, and the possibility of an effect on the mitochondrial membrane requires further investigation. Although at present it is difficult to relate the ultrastructural changes in the liver to the decreased activity of UROG-D, it is of interest that in some patients with PCTS, who may have an inherited defect in UROG-D (KUSHNER and BARBUTO, 1975a), the onset of clinical porphyria appears to be related to non-specific liver cell damage.

The other main theory proposes that the increased excretion of those porphyrins which are utilised as porphyrinogens for heme synthesis may be due to "escape" of porphyrinogens from the pathway due to enhanced intracellular oxidation to porphyrins (HEIKEL et al., 1958; RIMINGTON, 1963; SWEENEY et al., 1971; TALJAARD et al., 1972b), perhaps due to an alteration in the redox state of the cytosol associated with liver damage. In HCB porphyria, the NAD: NADH ratio is increased in liver cytosol (TALJAARD et al., 1972b), but it is not clear whether this is a specific feature of HCB liver damage (SLATER and ZIEGLER, 1966) or whether it is likely to increase the oxidation of porphyrinogens, since the mechanism that maintains porphyrinogens in the reduced state is not understood. In porphyria due to polyhalogenated aromatic hydrocarbons and in PCTS, the liver contains predominantly porphyrin, rather than porphyrinogen, since fresh tissue shows an intense red fluorescence in ultraviolet light, which is not intensified by oxidants. However, comparison of the pattern of porphyrin accumulation in the liver with that of porphyrin excretion indicates that the retention of uroporphyrin and, to a lesser extent, other hydrophilic porphyrins within the hepatocyte represents selective storage of these porphyrins (TALJAARD et al., 1973). The mechanism of this process and its relation to the intracellular oxidation of porphyrinogens is not understood. It is clear that storage as porphyrin does not imply loss from the pathway as porphyrin, but may be the end-result of a primary accumulation of porphyrinogen with later oxidation and storage. Evidence for the accumulation of porphyrinogens is provided by the increased formation of dehydroisocoproporphyrinogen, since this is a consequence of an increase in the intracellular concentration of pentacarboxylate porphyrinogen III, and by the report that up to 24% of the uroporphyrin in the urine in PCTS may be excreted as uroporphyrinogen (KALIVAS, 1969). Similar studies of the excretion of porphyrinogens are required in HCB porphyria.

III. Inhibition of UROG-D by Porphyrogenic Compounds or Their Metabolites

If the porphyria caused by polyhalogenated aromatic hydrocarbons is due to a direct effect of the compound or a metabolite on UROG-D, it should be possible to demonstrate inhibition of UROG-D by these compounds. HCB produces accumulation of porphyrin in chick-embryo liver cell cultures (GRANICK, 1966), but identification of the porphyrin has not been reported. Recently, SINCLAIR and GRANICK (1974) have shown that Aroclor 1254, 2,4,5,2',4',5'-hexachlorobiphenyl, TCDD and γ-hexachlorocyclohexane induce rapid accumulation of uroporphyrin III by chick-embryo liver cell cultures. In this system chlorinated hydrocarbons both induce ALA-S and cause accumulation of uroporphyrin. These two effects are independent of each other, since the conversion of added ALA to uroporphyrin rather than to protoporphyrin, as in cultures without a chlorinated hydrocarbon present, continues when ALA-S is inhibited by heme. Production of uroporphyrin was prevented by iron-chelators, by inhibition of protein synthesis and by two inhibitors of drug metabolism, SKF 525-A and piperonyl butoxide. Uroporphyrin was also formed when liver homogenates from chick embryos previously injected with Aroclor 1254 were incubated with ALA, whereas homogenates from un- treated embryos formed protoporphyrin. This effect appeared to be due to a meta- bolite of Aroclor 1254, since direct addition of this compound to homogenates from untreated embryos did not lead to formation of uroporphyrin on incubation with ALA. Incubation of liver homogenates from Aroclor-treated embryos for 1 h at 37°C before addition of ALA prevented the formation of uroporphyrin. The metabolite was not identified, but incubation of pentachlorophenol, a metabolite of HCB (Lui and Sweeney, 1975; Koss, 1976), 2,4-dinitrophenol or tetrachlorophenol with chick-embryo liver homogenates and ALA caused an accumulation of uro- porphyrin, which was not prevented by iron-chelators. Sinclair and Granick (1974) concluded that the accumulation of uroporphyrin in chick-embryo liver cell cultures treated with chlorinated hydrocarbons is probably due to the inhibition of UROG-D by an unstable metabolite of the hydrocarbon, possibly an hydroxylated derivative, the formation of which requires iron. Direct measurements of the activ- ity of UROG-D in this system are clearly required.

These experiments, by providing indirect evidence that some chlorinated hydro- carbons may decrease the activity of UROG-D in chick-embryo liver cell cultures within a short time of addition, support the hypothesis that polyhalogenated aro- matic hydrocarbons or their metabolites cause porphyria by a direct action on this enzyme. However, results obtained with the chick-embryo liver must be extra- polated to the mammalian liver with caution, for the two systems respond differently to various porphyrogens, and at least some of these differences depend on differences in the rates of metabolism of the compounds. Neither γ-hexachlorocyclohexane (Simon and Siklosi, 1974) nor pentachlorophenol, the major metabolite of HCB, causes porphyria in rats (Lui et al., 1976). There is, as yet, no evidence that a metabolite of HCB inhibits UROG-D in mam- malian liver. UROG-D in mammalian erythropoietic tissue, and therefore, prob- ably in the liver, contains sulphydryl groups which are essential for activity (Romeo and Levin, 1971). The isolation of pentachlorothiophenol from the urine of rats treated with HCB suggests that a metabolite of HCB may react with thiol groups (Koss, 1976; Lui et al., 1976). However, Wolf et al. (1962) found no change in hepatic glutathione levels in HCB porphyria in rats. If a metabolite of HCB in- hibits UROG-D in mammals and adult birds, the delay in onset of the porphyria has to be explained, possibly either by progressive accumulation of the metabolite until it reaches porphyrogenic levels or by a change in the pattern of metabolism of HCB as it accumulates.

IV. The Role of Iron in the Production of Porphyria

The frequent association of hepatic siderosis with PCTS has prompted investiga- tion of the role of iron in the pathogenesis of HCB porphyria. Although adminis- tration of HCB to rats has been reported to increase the total iron concentration of the liver (Saunders et al., 1963), HCB porphyria can develop without any increase in the non-heme iron concentration of the liver (Elder et al., 1976a). Similarly, total body iron stores and liver non-heme iron concentrations are normal in about one-third of European patients with PCTS (LUNDVALL, 1971a; TURNBULL et al., 1973). Thus, in neither condition is decreased activity of UROG-D dependent on an increase in liver iron stores. However, there is ample evidence that a change in the level of the body iron stores influences the severity of both experimental HCB porphyria and PCTS. Thus iron overload accelerates the development of HCB porphyria in rats (Section C.I.2.c) while, in PCTS, depletion of iron stores by repeated venesection returns porphyrin excretion towards normal (RAMSAY et al., 1974), a response that is reversed by administration of iron (LUNDVALL, 1971b). Patients with normal iron stores respond as well to venesection as those with increased stores.

In both experimental HCB porphyria and PCTS the major effect of any change in the iron stores is to alter the amount of porphyrin produced and excreted. If the action of iron was related to inhibition of an enzyme other than UROG-D one would expect a major change in porphyrin excretion pattern. This is not observed, even in PCTS where it has been suggested that iron may inhibit uroporphyrinogen co-synthetase (KUSHNER et al., 1972). Thus, in order to explain the effect of iron, only the two interacting factors that determine the degree of porphyrin excretion need to be considered: the activity of the enzyme UROG-D and the rate of ALA production.

Iron overload could decrease the activity of UROG-D either directly, through an effect of iron on the enzyme, or indirectly by potentiating the action of HCB, or a metabolite of HCB, on the enzyme. The first mechanism should be demonstrable by investigating the effect of iron on UROG-D in normal liver, the second would only operate in the presence of HCB. The UROG-D activity of pig liver extracts is decreased by up to 40% by incubation with ferrous iron (0.7 mM) for 2 h at 37°C (KUSHNER et al., 1973; 1975b), but inhibition of this enzyme by ferrous iron without prior incubation has not been reported. Although this concentration of ferrous iron is unlikely to be reached in vivo in iron overload, the possibility that the effect observed was due to ferritin, which is likely to have been formed from pre-existing apoferritin during the incubation, cannot be excluded. These experiments suggest that iron in some form may influence the stability of UROG-D in vitro. At present there is no evidence that iron overload decreases the activity of UROG-D in vivo. Rats with hepatic siderosis have slight uroporphyrinuria but do not show porphyrin fluorescence in their livers (SHANLEY et al., 1970). Since in HCB porphyria accumulation of porphyrin in the liver is as early an indicator of a decrease in UROG-D activity as uroporphyrinuria, hepatic fluorescence would have been expected if the increased uroporphyrin excretion was due to a defect in this enzyme. Moreover, abnormalities of porphyrin excretion are not a feature of severe iron overload in man. Clearly measurements of UROG-D activity in iron overload are required.

At present, a more likely alternative explanation for the effect of iron overload in HCB porphyria is that iron potentiates the action of HCB, or a metabolite of HCB on UROG-D. TALJAARD et al. (1971) have shown that the increased severity of HCB porphyria in siderotic rats is associated with levels of UROG-D that are lower than in porphyric rats with normal iron stores, suggesting that iron overload and HCB feeding together produce lower levels of UROG-D than HCB alone. This potentiation could be brought about through an effect of iron overload on the pattern of metabolism or distribution of HCB within the liver so that a given dose produces a greater decrease in UROG-D activity. In chick-embryo liver, endogenous iron may be involved in the conversion of polychlorinated hydrocarbons to active inhibitors of UROG-D (SINCLAIR and GRANICK, 1974).

A problem with the mechanisms discussed above is that they do not readily explain the effect of venesection in PCTS of non-toxic origin, especially in those patients with normal iron stores. If the effects of iron-overload and venesection are different aspects of the same phenomenon, the correct mechanism for the role of iron should explain both. At present there is no direct evidence that the two effects are related. In this respect, investigation of the effect of iron depletion in experimental HCB porphyria would be of interest.

Finally, there is evidence that iron overload increases the rate of heme synthesis by stimulating heme catabolism both in the presence (TALJAARD et al., 1972b) and absence of HCB (DE MATTEIS and SPARKS, 1973; DE MATTEIS, 1976). This action, by indirectly increasing the substrate concentration for UROG-D, almost certainly contributes to the greater production of porphyrin by siderotic porphyric rats.

F. General Conclusions

The porphyrinogenic polyhalogenated aromatic hydrocarbons described in this Chapter have two separate actions on heme biosynthesis in the liver: they cause an early sustained increase in the level of microsomal cytochromes and later produce porphyria by decreasing the activity of UROG-D. The first of these properties is possessed by a variety of lipophilic molecules that are resistant to metabolism, but the second appears to be restricted to a small group of halogenated aromatic compounds. Furthermore, the porphyrogenic action of these compounds is restricted to certain species and strains of animal whereas the induction of hemoproteins appears to be a much more widespread response. Production of porphyria requires the administration of larger doses than are necessary to increase hemoprotein levels. The delay in onset, and the failure to produce porphyria with single large doses, which is a feature of both HCB and PCB porphyria (SWEENEY et al., 1971; GOLDSTEIN et al., 1974), may reflect the difficulty of achieving porphyrogenic concentrations of these compounds in the liver by any way other than prolonged oral administration. Experiments with the potent porphyrogen, TCDD, which produces porphyria in mice after a single dose, may clarify this problem.

A decrease in the activity of UROG-D in laboratory animals is readily detected by the specific pattern of porphyrin overproduction, which is remarkably constant for different porphyrogens and different strains and species. However, the testing of compounds for their ability to produce this type of porphyria in mammals is difficult due to the long period of administration required and the species selectivity shown. A similar pattern of porphyrin overproduction characterises the syndrome of PCTS in man, in which the underlying UROG-D defect is only rarely due to exposure to polychlorinated hydrocarbons. The features that are shared by this type of experimental porphyria and by PCTS are summarised in Table 5.

Table 5. Features common to those porphyrias in which there is a decrease in the activity of UROG-D in the liver

	Experimental porphyria in animals (HCB, PCB, TCDD, octachlorostyrene)	due to HCB (? TCDD)	PCTS sporadic (alcoholic liver damage, etc.)
ALA-S activity	Increased up to 3-fold		Normal to increased 6-fold
Cytochrome P-450 concentration	Increased		(?) Increased
Liver cell damage	Usually (? always) present	Common	Usually present
Effect of oestrogens	Enhances response to HCB in rats		May be precipitated by oestrogens
Effect of alterations in iron stores	Increased iron stores enhances response to HCB in rats	Porphyrin excretion decreased by treatment with EDTA	Porphyrin excretion decreased by depletion of iron stores

The pathogenesis of this homogeneous group of human and experimental porphyrias is obscure. Both the mechanism of the decrease in the activity of UROG-D and the role of factors such as iron, oestrogens and, possibly, liver damage, which apparently modify the expression of the defect, whatever its origin, are poorly understood. Identification of a decrease in the activity of UROG-D as the enzyme defect that underlies this group of conditions provides a starting point for an approach to these problems.

Abbreviations

HCB	Hexachlorobenzene
TCDD	Tetrachloro-p-dioxin
ALA-S	5-Aminolaevulinate synthetase
PCB	Polychlorinated biphenyl
PCTS	Porphyria cutanea tarda symptomatica
UROG-D	Uroporphyrinogen decarboxylase

References

Abbott, D.C., Collins, G.B., Goulding, R.: Organochlorine pesticide residues in human fat in the United Kingdom 1969−1971. Brit. med. J. **1972 II,** 553−556

Alvares, A.P., Bickers, D.R., Kappas, A.: Polychlorinated biphenyls: a new type of inducer of cytochrome P-448 in the liver. Proc. nat. Acad. Sci. (Wash.) **70,** 1321−1325 (1973)

Bach, P.H., Taljaard, J.J.F., Joubert, S.M., Shanley, B.C.: The effect of iron overload on the development of hexachlorobenzene (HCB) porphyria. S. Afr. J. Lab. clin. Med. **17,** 75−76 (1971)

Baptista de Almeida, J.A.P., Kenner, G.W., Smith, K.M., Sutton, M.J.: A stepwise synthesis of unsymmetrically substituted porphyrins: isocoproporphyrin. J. C. S. Chem. Commun., 111−112 (1975)

Batlle, A.M. del C., Grinstein, M.: Porphyrin biosynthesis.II Phyriaporphyrinogen III, a normal intermediate in the biosynthesis of protoporphyrin IX. Biochim. biophys. Acta (Amst.) **82,** 13 – 20 (1964)

Bleiberg, J., Wallen, M., Brodkin, R., Applebaum, I.L.: Industrially-acquired porphyria. Arch. Derm. (Chic.) **89,** 793 – 797 (1964)

Brady, M.N., Siyali, D.S.: Hexachlorobenzene in human body fat. Med. J. Aust. **1,** 158 – 161 (1972)

Bruckner, J.V., Khanna, K.L., Cornish, H.H.: Effect of chronic ingestion of polychlorinated biphenyls on the rat. Toxicol. appl. Pharmacol. **29,** 103 (1974)

Burnett, J., Pathak, M.: Effect of light upon porphyrin metabolism of rats. Arch. Derm. (Chic.) **89,** 257 – 266 (1964)

Burse, V.M., Kimbrough, R.D., Villeneuva, E.C., Jennins, R.W., Linder, R.E., Sovocool, G.W.: Polychlorinated biphenyls. Arch. environm. Hlth. **29,** 301 – 307 (1974)

Cam, C.: Hexachlorobenzen ile muzmin zehirlenmeye bagli deri porfirisi vakalari. Sağl. Derg. **32,** 215 – 216 (1958)

Cam, C.: Intoksikasyona bagli deri porfirilevi. Dirim **34,** 11 (1959)

Cam, C.: A new epidemic dermatosis of children. Ann. Derm. Syph. (Paris) **87,** 393 – 397 (1960)

Cam, C., Nigogosyan, G.: Acquired toxic porphyria cutanea tarda due to hexachlorobenzene. J. Amer. med. Ass. **183,** 88 – 91 (1963)

Cameron, G.R., Thomas, J.C., Ashmore, S.A., Buchan, J.L., Warren, E.H., Hughes, A.W.McK.: The toxicity of certain chlorine derivatives of benzene, with special reference to O-dichlorobenzene. J. Path. Bact. **44,** 281 – 296 (1937)

Campbell, J.A.H.: Pathological aspects of hexachlorobenzene feeding in rats. S. Afr. J. Lab. clin. Med. **9,** 203 – 206 (1963)

Cetingil, A.I., Özen, M.A.: Toxic porphyria. Blood **16,** 1002 – 1011 (1960)

Chu, T.C., Chu, E.J.-H.: Porphyrin patterns in different types of porphyria. Clin. Chem. **13,** 371 – 387 (1967)

Conney, A.H.: Pharmacological implications of microsomal enzyme induction. Pharmacol. Rev. **19,** 317 – 366 (1967)

Crow, K.D.: Chloracne. Trans. St. John's Hosp. derm. Soc. (Lond.) **56,** 79 – 99 (1970)

Dean, G.: The Porphyrias: A Story of Inheritance and Environment, 2nd ed. London: Pitman Medical Publishing 1971

De Matteis, F.: Disturbances of liver porphyrin metabolism caused by drugs. Pharmacol. Rev. **19,** 523 – 557 (1967)

De Matteis, F.: Toxic hepatic porphyrias. Sem. Haematol. **5,** 409 – 423 (1968)

De Matteis, F.: Iron-dependent degradation of liver heme in vivo. In: Porphyrins in Human Diseases. Doss, M. (ed.), pp. 37 – 42. Basel: Karger 1976

De Matteis, F., Prior, B.E., Rimington, C.: Nervous and biochemical disturbances following hexachlorobenzene intoxication. Nature (Lond.) **191,** 363 – 366 (1961)

De Matteis, F., Sparks, R.G.: Iron-dependent loss of liver cytochrome P-450 heme in vivo and in vitro. FEBS Lett. 141 – 143 (1973)

Dogramaci, I., Kenanoglu, A., Muftu, Y., Ergene, T., Wray, J.D.: Bone and joint changes in patients with porphyria turcica. Turk. J. Pediat. **4,** 149 – 156 (1962 b)

Dogramaci, I., Tinaztepe, B., Gunalp, A.: Condition of the liver in patients with toxic cutaneous porphyria. Turk. J. Pediat. **4,** 103 – 106 (1962 c)

Dogramaci, I., Wray, J.D., Ergene, T., Sezer, V., Muftu, Y.: Porphyria turcica, a survey of 592 cases of cutaneous porphyria seen in southeastern Turkey. Turk. J. Pediat. **4,** 138 – 147 (1962 a)

Doss, M., Meinhof, W., Look, D., Henning, H., Nawrocki, P., Dolle, W., Strohmeyer, G., Filippini, L.: Porphyrins in liver and urine in acute intermittent and chronic hepatic porphyrias. S. Afr. J. Lab. clin. Med. **17,** 50 – 54 (1971)

Doss, M., Schermuly, E., Koss, G.: Hexachlorobenzene porphyria in rats as a model for human chronic hepatic porphyrias. Ann. Clin. Res. **8,** Suppl. **17,** 171 – 181 (1976)

Dowdle, E., Goldswain, P., Spong, N., Eales, L.: The pattern of porphyrin isomer accumulation and excretion in symptomatic porphyria. Clin. Sci. **39,** 147 – 158 (1970)

Elder, G.H.: Identification of a group of tetracarboxylate porphyrins, containing one acetate and three propionate β-substituents, in faeces from patients with symptomatic cutaneous hepatic porphyria and from rats with porphyria due to hexachlorobenzene. Biochem. J. **126**, 877–891 (1972)

Elder, G.H.: The porphyrin excretion pattern of symptomatic cutaneous hepatic porphyria. M.D. Thesis, University of Cambridge, 1973

Elder, G.H.: The metabolism of porphyrins of the isocoproporphyrin series. Enzyme **17**, 61–68 (1974)

Elder, G.H.: The differentiation of porphyria cutanea tarda symptomatica from other types of porphyria by the measurement of isocoproporphyrin in faeces. J. clin. Path. **28**, 601–607 (1975)

Elder, G.H., Evans, J.O., Matlin, S.: The porphyrogenic action of polychlorinated hydrocarbons. In: Porphyrins in Human Diseases. Doss, M. (ed.), pp. 424–431. Basel: Karger 1976a

Elder, G.H., Evans, J. O., Matlin, S.: The effect of the porphyrogenic compound, hexachlorobenzene, on the activity of uroporphyrinogen decarboxylase in rat liver. Clin. Sci. molec. Med. **51**, 71–80 (1976b)

Elder, G.H., Nicholson, D.C., Gray, C.H.: The porphyrias: a review. J. clin. Path. **25**, 1013–1033 (1972)

Farber, T.M., Baker, A.: Microsomal enzyme induction by hexabromobiphenyl. Toxicol. appl. Pharmacol. **29**, 102 Abstr. No. 68 (1974)

Fishbein, L.: Toxicity of chlorinated biphenyls. Ann. Rev. Pharmacol. **14**, 139–156 (1974)

Gajdos, A., Gajdos-Török, M.: The therapeutic effect of adenosine-5-monophosphoric acid in porphyria. Lancet **1961 II**, 175–177

Garcia, D.C., San Martin de Viale, L.L., Tomio, J.M., Grinstein, M.: Porphyrin biosynthesis. X. Porphyrinogen carboxy-lyase from avian erythrocytes: further properties. Biochim. biophys. Acta (Amst.) **309**, 203–210 (1973)

Goldstein, J.A., Hickman, P., Bergman, H., Vos, J.G.: Hepatic porphyria induced by 2,3,7,8-tetrachlorodibenzo-*p*-dioxin in the mouse. Res. Commun. chem. Path. Pharmacol. **6**, 919–928 (1973)

Goldstein, J.A., Hickman, P., Jue, D.L.: Experimental hepatic porphyria induced by polychlorinated biphenyls. Toxicol. appl. Pharmacol. **27**, 437–448 (1974)

Gombos, B., Pechanova, A., Koziak, B., Moscovicova, E.: Porphyria cutanea tarda and *acne chlorina* at the production of cyclic chlorinated hydrocarbons. Bratisl. lek. Listy **51**, 640 (1969)

Granick, S.: The induction in vitro of the synthesis of δ ALA synthetase in chemical porphyria: a response to certain drugs, sex hormones and foreign chemicals. J. biol. Chem. **24**, 1359–1375 (1966)

Grant, D.L., Iverson, F., Hatina, G.V., Villeneuve, D.C.: Effects of hexachlorobenzene on liver porphyrin levels and microsomal enzymes in the rat. Environ. Physiol. Biochem. **4**, 159–165 (1974)

Greig, J.B.: Effect of 2,3,7,8-tetrachlorodibenzo-1,4-dioxin on drug metabolism in the rat. Biochem. Pharmacol. **21**, 3196–3198 (1972)

Greig, J.B., De Matteis, F.: Effects of 2,3,7,8-tetrachlorodibenzo-*p*-dioxin on drug metabolism and hepatic microsomes of rats and mice. Environ. Hlth. Perspect. **5**, 211–219 (1973)

Hansell, M.M., Ecobichon, D.J.: Effects of chemically pure biphenyls on the morphology of rat liver. Toxicol. appl. Pharmacol. **28**, 418–427 (1974)

Heikel, T., Lockwood, W.H., Rimington, C.: Formation of non-enzymic heme. Nature (Lond.) **182**, 313 (1958)

Hershko, Ch., Eilon, L.: The effect of sex difference on iron exchange in the rat. Brit. J. Haemat. **28**, 471–482 (1974)

Hutterer, F., Schaffner, F., Klion, F.M., Popper, H.: Hypertrophic, hypoactive smooth endoplasmic reticulum: A sensitive indicator of hepatotoxicity exemplified by dieldrin. Science **161**, 1017–1019 (1968).

Hutzinger, O., Nash, D.M., Safe, S., Defreitas, A.S.W., Norstrom, R.J., Wildish, D.J., Zitko, V.: Polychlorinated biphenyls: metabolic behaviour of pure isomers in pigeons, rats and brook trout. Science **178**, 312–314 (1972)

Ippen, H., Aust, D.: Klinisch-experimentelle Untersuchungen zur Entstehung der Porphyrien. I. Allgemeine und tierexperimentelle Modellversuche. Arch. Derm. Forsch. **245**, 110–124 (1972)

Ippen, H., Aust, D., Goerz, G.: Klinisch-experimentelle Untersuchungen zur Entstehung der Porphyrien. III. Wirkung einiger Steroid-Hormone auf die "latente Hexachlorobenzol-Porphyrie" der Ratte. Arch. Derm. Forsch. **245**, 305–317 (1972a)

Ippen, H., Hüttenhain, S., Aust, D.: Klinisch-experimentelle Untersuchungen zur Entstehung der Porphyrien. II. Wirkung von Äthylalkohol auf die Hexachlorobenzol-Porphyrie der Ratte. Arch. Derm. Forsch. **245**, 191–202 (1972b)

Jackson, A.H., Sancovich, H.A., Ferramola, A.M., Evans, N., Games, D.E., Matlin, S.A., Elder, G.H., Smith, S.G.: Macrocyclic intermediates in the biosynthesis of porphyrins. Phil. Trans. B **273**, 191–206 (1976)

Jensen, S., Sundstrom, G.: Metabolic hydroxylation of a chlorobiphenyl containing only isolated unsubstituted positions – 2,2′,4,4′,5,5′-hexachlorobiphenyl. Nature (Lond.) **251**, 219–220 (1974)

Jirásek, L., Kalensky, J., Kubec, K.: Acne chlorina, porphyria cutanea tarda pri výrobě herbicid. Čsl. Derm. **48**, 306–317 (1973)

Jirásek, L., Kalenský, J., Kubec, K., Pazderová, J., Lukáš. E.: Acne chlorina, porphyria cutanea tarda a jiné projevy celkové intoxikace pri výrobě herbicid. II. Čsl. Derm. **49**, 145–157 (1974)

Johnstone, G.J., Ecobichon, D.J., Hutzinger, O.: The influence of pure polychlorinated biphenyl compounds on hepatic function in the rat. Toxicol. appl. Pharmacol. **28**, 66–81 (1974)

Jones, G., Butler, W.H.: A morphological study of the liver lesion induced by 2,3,7,8-tetra-chlorodibenzo-*p*-dioxin in rats. J. Path. **112**, 93–98 (1974)

Joubert, S.M., Taljaard, J.J.F., Shanley, B.C.: Aetiological relationship between hepatic siderosis and symptomatic porphyria cutanea tarda. Enzyme **16**, 305–313 (1973)

Kalivas, J.: Urinary clues to the pathogenesis of porphyria cutanea tarda. Clin. Biochem. **2**, 417–421 (1969)

Kalivas, J.T., Pathak, M.A., Fitzpatrick, T.B.: Phlebotomy and iron overload in porphyria cutanea tarda. Lancet **1969 I**, 1184–1187

Kantemir, I.: Porphyrin kimyasi ve analiz metodlari. Türk Ij. tecr. Biyol. Derg. **20**, 1 (1960)

Kimbrough, R.D.: The toxicity of polychlorinated polycyclic compounds and related chemicals. CRC Crit. Rev. Toxicol. **2**, 445–498 (1974)

Kimbrough, R.D., Linder, R.E., Gaines, T.B.: Morphological changes in livers of rats fed polychlorinated biphenyls. Arch. environm. Hlth. **25**, 354–365 (1972)

Koeman, J.H., Noever de Brauw, M.C., Vos, R.H.: Chlorinated biphenyls in fish, mussels and birds from the river Rhine and the Netherlands coastal area. Nature (Lond.) **221**, 1126–1128 (1969)

Koss, G.: Studies on the pharmacokinetics of hexachlorobenzene in rats. In: Porphyrins in Human Diseases. Doss, M. (ed.), pp. 414–417. Basel: Karger 1976

Kuiper-Goodman, T., Grant, D., Korsrod, G., Moodie, C.A., Munro, I.C.: Toxic effects of hexachlorobenzene in the rat: correlations of electron microscopy with other toxic parameters. Toxicol. appl. Pharmacol. **29**, 101 Abstr. 67 (1974)

Kushner, J.P., Barbuto, A.J.: Decreased activity of hepatic uroporphyrinogen decarboxylase (urodecarb) in porphyria cutanea tarda (PCT). Clin. Res. **22**, 178 (1974)

Kushner, J.P., Barbuto, A.J.: An inherited defect in porphyria cutanea tarda (PCT): decreased uroporphyrinogen decarboxylase. Clin. Res. **23**, 403 (1975a)

Kushner, J.P., Lee, G.R., Nacht, S.: The role of iron in the pathogenesis of porphyria cutanea tarda: an in vitro model. J. clin. Invest. **51**, 3044–3051 (1972)

Kushner, J.P., Steinmuller, D.P., Lee, G.R.: Inhibition of uroporphyrinogen decarboxylase activity by iron. Clin. Res. **21**, 266 (1973)

Kushner, J.P., Steinmuller, D.P., Lee, G.R.: The role of iron in the pathogenesis of porphyria cutanea tarda. II. Inhibition of uroporphyrinogen decarboxylase. J. clin. Invest. **56**, 661–667 (1975b)

Lucier, G.W., McDaniel, O.S., Hook, G.E.R., Fowler, B.A., Sonawane, B.R., Faeder, E.: TCDD-induced changes in rat liver microsomal enzymes. Environ. Hlth. Perspect. **5**, 199–209 (1973)

Lui, H., Sweeney, G.D.: Hepatic metabolism of hexachlorobenzene in rats. Febs Lett. **51,** 225–226 (1975)

Lui, H., Sampson, R., Sweeney, G.D.: Hexachlorobenzene porphyria: purity and metabolic fate of hexachlorobenzene. In: Porphyrins in Human Diseases. Doss, M. (ed.), pp. 405–413. Basel: Karger 1976

Lundvall, O.: The effect of phlebotomy therapy in porphyria cutanea tarda. Its relation to the phlebotomy induced reduction of iron stores. Acta. med. scard. **189,** 33–50 (1971a)

Lundvall, O.: The effect of replenishment of iron stores after phlebotomy therapy in porphyria cutanea tarda. Acta med. scand. **189,** 51–63 (1971b)

Lundvall, O., Enerback, L.: Hepatic fluorescence in porphyria cutanea tarda studied in fine needle aspiration biopsy smears. J. clin. Path. **22,** 704–709 (1969)

Marver, H.S., Schmid, R.: The porphyrias. In: The Metabolic Basis of Inherited Disease. 3rd ed. New York: McGraw-Hill 1972

Mauzerall, D., Granick, S.: Porphyrin biosynthesis in erythrocytes. II. Uroporphyrinogen and its decarboxylase. J. biol. Chem. **232,** 1141–1161 (1958)

May, G.: Chloracne from the accidental production of tetrachlorodibenzodioxin. Brit. J. Industr. Med. **30,** 276–283 (1973)

Medline, A., Bain, E., Menon, A.I., Haberman, H.F.: Hexachlorobenzene and rat liver. Arch. Path. (Chic.) **96,** 61–65 (1973)

Meyer, U.A., Marver, H.S.: Enhancement of the fractional catabolic rate of microsomal heme in chemically induced porphyria. S. Afr. J. Lab. clin. Med. **17,** 175–177 (1971)

Milnes, M.H.: Formation of 2,3,7,8-tetrachlorodibenzodioxin by thermal decomposition of 2,4,5-trichlorophenate. Nature (Lond.) **232,** 395–396 (1971)

Moore, M.R., Battistini, V., Beattie, A.D., Goldberg, A.: The effect of certain barbiturates on the hepatic porphyrin metabolism of rats. Biochem. Pharmacol. **19,** 751–757 (1970)

Moore, M.R., Turnbull, A.L., Barnado, D., Beattie, A.D., Magnus, I.A., Goldberg, A.: Hepatic δ-aminolaevulinic acid synthetase activity in porphyria cutanea tarda. Lancet **1972 II,** 97–100

Morley, A., Geary, D., Harben, F.: Hexachlorobenzene pesticides and porphyria. Med. J. Aust. **1,** 565 (1973)

Nakao, K., Wada, O., Takaku, F., Sassa, S., Yano, Y., Urata, G.: The origin of the increased protoporphyrin in erythrocytes of mice with experimentally induced porphyria. J. Lab. clin. Med. **70,** 923–932 (1967)

Ockner, R.K., Schmid, R.: Acquired porphyria in man and rat due to hexachlorobenzene intoxication. Nature (Lond.) **189,** 499 (1961)

Parke, D.V., Williams, R.T.: Studies in detoxication. 81. The metabolism of halogenobenzenes: (a) Penta- and hexa-chlorobenzenes (b) Further observations on 1:3:5-trichlorobenzene. Biochem. J. **74,** 5–9 (1960)

Pearson, R.W., Malkinson, F.D.: Some observations on hexachlorobenzene induced experimental porphyria. J. invest. Derm. **44,** 420–432 (1965)

Perez, V., Schaffner, F., Popper, H.: Hepatic drug reactions. In: Progress in Liver Diseases, Vol. 4. London–New York: Grune and Stratton 1972

Peters, H.A., Johnson, S.A.M., Cam, S., Oral, S., Müftü, Y., Ergene, T.: Hexachlorobenzene-induced porphyria: effect of chelation of the disease, porphyrin and metal metabolism. Amer. J. med. Sci. **251,** 314–322 (1966)

Pimstone, N.R., Blekkenhorst, G., Eales, L.: Enzymatic defects in hepatic porphyria: preliminary observations in patients with porphyria cutanea tarda and variegate porphyria. Enzyme **16,** 354–366 (1973)

Piper, W.N., Rose, J.Q., Gehring, P.J.: Excretion and tissue distribution of 2,3,7,8-tetrachloro-dibenzo-*p*-dioxin in the rat. Environ. Hlth. Perspect. **5,** 241–244 (1973)

Poland, A., Glover, E.: 2,3,7,8-tetrachlorodibenzo-*p*-dioxin: a potent inducer of δ-amino-levulinic acid synthetase. Science **179,** 476–477 (1973a)

Poland, A., Glover, E.: Studies on the mechanism of toxicity of the chlorinated dibenzo-*p*-dioxins. Environ. Hlth. Perspect. **5,** 245–251 (1973b)

Poland, A., Goldstein, J., Hickman, P., Burse, V.W.: A reciprocal relationship between the induction of δ-aminolevulinic acid synthetase and drug metabolism produced by m-dichlorobenzene. Biochem. Pharmacol. **20,** 1281–1290 (1971b)

Poland, A.P., Smith, D., Metter, G., Possick, P.: A health survey of workers in a 2,4-D and 2,4,5-T plant. Arch. environm. Hlth. **22**, 316 – 327 (1971a)

Rajamanickam, C., Amrutavalli, J., Rao, M.R.S., Padmanaban, G.: Effect of hexachloro-benzene on heme synthesis. Biochem. J. **129**, 381 – 387 (1972)

Ramsay, C.A., Magnus, I.A., Turnbull, A., Baker, H.: The treatment of porphyria cutanea tarda by venesection. Quart. J. med. N.S. **43**, 1 – 24 (1974)

Rimington, C.: Patterns of porphyrin excretion and their interpretation. S. Afr. J. Lab. clin. Med. **9**, 255 – 261 (1963)

Rimington, C., Ziegler, G.: Experimental porphyria in rats induced by chlorinated benzenes. Biochem. Pharmacol. **12**, 1387 – 1397 (1963)

Romeo, G., Levin, E.Y.: Uroporphyrinogen decarboxylase from mouse spleen. Biochim. bio-phys. Acta (Amst.) **230**, 330 – 341 (1971)

Ryan, D., Lu, A.Y.H., West, S., Levin, W.: Multiple forms of cytochrome P-450 in pheno-barbital and 3-methylcholanthrene-treated rats. Separation and spectral properties. J. biol. Chem. **250**, 2157 – 2163 (1975)

San Martin de Viale, L.C., Grinstein, M.: Porphyrin biosynthesis. IV. 5- and 6-COOH por-phyrinogens (type III) as normal intermediates in heme biosynthesis. Biochim. biophys. Acta (Amst.) **158**, 79 – 91 (1968)

San Martin de Viale, L.C., Rios de Molina, M. del C., Wainstock de Calmanovici, R., Tomio, J.M.: Experimental porphyria produced in rats by hexachlorobenzene IV. Studies on the stepwise decarboxylation of uroporphyrinogen and phyriaporphyrinogen 'in vivo' and 'in vitro' in several tissues. In: Porphyrins in Human Diseases. Doss, M. (ed.), pp. 445 – 452. Basel: Karger 1976b

San Martin de Viale, L.C., Russo, M.C., Rios de Molina, M. del C., Grinstein, M.: Experi-mental porphyria induced in rats by hexachlorobenzene II. The effect of oestradiol-17β. Abstracts of 1st International Porphyrin Meeting, Freiburg, (1976a)

San Martin de Viale, L.C., Tomio, J.M., Ferramola, A.M., Sancovich, H.A., Tigier, H.A.: Nat. Meeting Arg. Soc. biochem. Invest. Abstr. 8 (1972)

San Martin de Viale, L.C., Tomio, J.M., Ferramola, A.M., Sancovich, H.A., Tigier, H.A.: Experimental porphyria induced in rats by hexachlorobenzene III. Studies on enzymes associated with heme pathway—the effect of oestradiol-17β. In: Porphyrins in Human Diseases. Doss, M. (ed.), pp. 453 – 458. Basel: Karger 1976c

San Martin de Viale, L.C., Viale, A.A., Nacht, S., Grinstein, M.: Experimental porphyria induced in rats by hexachlorobenzene. A study of the porphyrins excreted by urine. Clin. chim. Acta **28**, 13 – 25 (1970)

Saunders, S.J., Williams, J., Levey, M.: Iron metabolism in symptomatic porphyria. S. Afr. J. Lab. clin. Med. **9**, 277 – 282 (1963)

Schmid, R.: Cutaneous porphyria in Turkey. New Engl. J. Med. **263**, 397 – 398 (1960)

Shanley, B.C., Zail, S.S., Joubert, S.M.: Porphyrin metabolism in experimental hepatic siderosis in the rat. Brit. J. Haemat. **18**, 79 – 87 (1970)

Simon, N., Dobozy, A., Berko, G.: Porphyrinstoffwechsel und klinisch-laboratorium-mäßige Untersuchungen in Modellversuchen und an Patienten mit Porphyria cutanea tarda. Arch. klin. exp. Derm. **238**, 38 – 43 (1970)

Simon, N., Siklosi, C.: Experimentelles Porphyrie-Modell mit Hexachlor-Cyclohexan. Z. Hautkr. **49**, 497 – 504 (1974)

Simon, N., Siklosi, C., Koszo, F.: The role of damages in cellular membrane structures in the development of phorphyria cutanea tarda. In: Porphyrins in Human Diseases. Doss, M. (ed.), pp. 432 – 437. Basel: Karger 1976

Sinclair, P.R., Granick, S.: Uroporphyrin formation induced by chlorinated hydrocarbons (lindane, polychlorinated biphenyls, tetrachlorodibenzo-p-dioxin): requirements for en-dogenous iron, protein synthesis and drug-metabolising activity. Biochem. biophys. Res. Commun. **61**, 124 – 133 (1974)

Siyali, D.S.: Hexachlorobenzene and other organochlorine pesticides in human blood. Med. J. Aust. **2**, 1063 – 1066 (1972)

Slater, T.F., Ziegler, G.: Nicotinamide adenine dinucleotides in the liver in experimentally induced porphyrias. Biochem. Pharmacol. **15**, 1279 – 1285 (1966)

Stoll, M., Elder, G.H., Games, D.E., O'Hanlon, P., Millington, D.S., Jackson, A.H.: Isocoproporphyrin: Nuclear-magnetic-resonance and mass-spectral methods for the determination of porphyrin structure. Biochem. J. **131**, 429 – 432 (1973)

Stonard, M.D.: Experimental hepatic porphyria induced by hexachlorobenzene as a model for human symptomatic porphyria. Brit. J. Haemat. **27**, 617 – 125 (1974)

Stonard, M.D.: Mixed type hepatic microsomal enzyme induction by hexachlorobenzene. Biochem. Pharmacol. **24**, 1959 – 1963 (1975)

Stonard, M.D.: Abstracts of 1st International Porphyrin Meeting, Freiburg 1976

Stonard, M.D., Nenov, P.Z.: Effect of HCB on hepatic microsomal enzymes in the rat. Biochem. Pharmacol. **23**, 2175 – 2184 (1974)

Strik, J.J.T.W.A.: Toxicity of hexachlorobenzene (HCB) and hexabromobiphenyl (HBB). Meded. Fak. Landbouwweten-Schappen, Gent, **38**, 709 – 716 (1973 a)

Strik, J.J.T.W.A.: Chemical porphyria in Japanese Quail (Coturnix c. Japonica). Enzyme **16**, 211 – 223 (1973 b)

Strik, J.J.T.W.A.: Species differences in experimental porphyria caused by polyhalogenated aromatic compounds. Enzyme **16**, 224 – 228 (1973 c)

Strik, J.J.T.W.A., Koeman, J.H.: Porphyrinogenic action of hexachlorobenzene and octachlorostyrene. In: Porphyrins in Human Diseases. Doss, M. (ed.), pp. 418 – 423. Basel: Karger 1976

Strik, J.J.T.W.A., Wit, J.G.: Hepatic porphyria in birds and mammals. TNO-nieuws **27**, 604 – 610 (1972)

Sweeney, G.D.: Hepatic catalase activity during states of altered heme synthesis. In: Porphyrins in Human Diseases. Doss, M. (ed.), pp. 53 – 61. Basel: Karger 1976

Sweeney, G.D., Janigan, D., Mayman, D., Lai, H.: The experimental prophyrias—a group of distinctive metabolic lesions. S. Afr. J. Lab. clin. Med. **17**, 68 – 72 (1971)

Taljaard, J.J.F., Shanley, B.C., Deppe, W.M., Joubert, S.M.: Porphyrin metabolism in experimental hepatic siderosis in the rat. II. Combined effect of iron overload and hexachlorobenzene. Brit. J. Haemat. **23**, 513 – 519 (1972 a)

Taljaard, J.J.F., Shanley, B.C., Deppe, W.M., Joubert, S.M.: Porphyrin metabolism in experimental hepatic siderosis in the rat. III. Effect of iron overload and hexachlorobenzene on liver heme biosynthesis. Brit. J. Haemat. **23**, 587 – 593 (1972 b)

Taljaard, J.J.F., Shanley, B.C., Joubert, S.M.: Decreased uroporphyrinogen decarboxylase activity in "experimental symptomatic porphyria". Life Sci. **10**, 887 – 893 (1971)

Taljaard, J.J.F., Shanley, B.C., Joubert, S.M., Deppe, W.M.: Incorporation of (4-^{14}C) δ-aminolaevulinate into urinary porphyrins in porphyria cutanea tarda: effect of chloroquine therapy. Clin. Sci. **44**, 571 – 581 (1973)

Timme, A.H., Taljaard, J.J.F., Shanley, B.C., Joubert, S.M.: Symptomatic porphyria. II. Hepatic changes with hexachlorobenzene. S. Afr. med. J. **48**, 1833 – 1836 (1974)

Tomio, J.M., Garcia, R.C., San Martin de Viale, L.C., Grinstein, M.: Porphyrin biosynthesis. VII. Porphyrinogen carboxy-lyase from avian erythrocytes. Purification and properties. Biochim. biophys. Acta (Amst.) **198**, 353 – 363 (1970)

Tschudy, D.P., Bonkowsky, H.L.: Experimental porphyria. Fed. Proc. **31**, 147 – 159 (1972)

Turnbull, A., Baker, H., Vernon-Roberts, B., Magnus, I.A.: Iron metabolism in porphyria cutanea tarda and erythropoietic protoporphyria. Quart. J. Med., New Series **42**, 341 – 355 (1973)

Turner, J.C., Green, R.S.: Effect of hexachlorobenzene on microsomal enzyme systems. Biochem. Pharmacol. **23**, 2387 – 2390 (1974)

Villeneuva, E.C., Jennings, R.W., Burse, V.M., Kimbrough, R.D.: Evidence of chlorodibenzo-p-dioxin and chlorodibenzofuran in hexachlorobenzene. J. agric. Food Chem. **22**, 916 – 917 (1974)

Villeneuve, D.C.: The effect of food restriction on the redistribution of hexachlorobenzene in the rat. Toxicol. app. Pharmacol. **31**, 313 – 319 (1975)

Villeneuve, D.C., Phillips, W.E.J., Panopio, L.G., Mendoza, C.E., Hatina, G.V., Grant, D.L.: The effects of phenobarbital and carbon tetrachloride on the rate of decline of body burdens of hexachlorobenzene in the rat. Arch. environ. Contam. Toxicol. **2**, 243 – 252 (1974)

Vinopal, J.N., Casida, J.E.: Metabolic stability of 2,3,7,8-tetrachlorodibenzo-p-dioxin in mammalian liver microsomal systems and in living mice. Arch. environ. Contam. Toxicol. **1**, 122 – 132 (1973)

Vos, J.G., Beems, R.B.: Dermal toxicity studies of technical polychlorinated biphenyls and fractions there of in rabbits. Toxicol. appl. Pharmacol. **19**, 617 – 633 (1971)

Vos, J.G., Botterweg, P.F., Strik, J.J.T.W.A., Koeman, J.H.: Experimental studies with HCB in birds. TNO-nieuws **27**, 599 – 603 (1972)

Vos, J.G., Koeman, J.H.: Comparative toxicologic study with polychlorinated biphenyls in chickens with special reference to porphyria, edema formation, liver necrosis, and tissue residues. Toxicol. appl. Pharmacol. **17**, 656 – 668 (1970)

Vos, J.G., Koeman, J.H., Van der Maas, H.L., Ten Noever de Brauw, M.C., De Vos, R.H.: Identification and toxicological evaluation of chlorinated dibenzofurans and chlorinated naphthalene in two commercial polychlorinated biphenyls. Food Cosmet. Toxicol. **8**, 625 – 633 (1970)

Vos, J.G., Notenboom-Ram, E.: Comparative toxicity study of 2,4,5,2',4',5'-hexachlorobiphenyl and a polychlorinated biphenyl mixture in rabbits. Toxicol. appl. Pharmacol. **23**, 563 – 578 (1972)

Vos, J.G., Van der Maas, H.L., Musch, A., Ram, E.: Toxicity of hexachlorobenzene in Japanese Quail with special reference to porphyria, liver damage, reproduction and tissue residues. Toxicol. appl. Pharmacol. **18**, 944 – 957 (1971)

Wada, O., Yano, Y., Urata, G., Nakao, K.: Behaviour of hepatic microsomal cytochromes after treatment of mice with drugs known to disturb porphyrin metabolism in liver. Biochem. Pharmacol. **17**, 595 – 603 (1968)

Watson, C.J.: The problem of porphyria—some facts and questions. New Engl. J. Med. **263**, 1205 – 1215 (1960)

Wolf, M., Lester, R., Schmid, R.: Hepatic GSH in hexachlorobenzene induced porphyria. Biochem. biophys, Res. Commun. **8**, 278 – 279 (1962)

Woods, J.S.: Studies of the effects of 2,3,7,8-tetrachlorodibenzo-p-dioxin on mammalian hepatic δ-aminolaevulinic acid synthetase. Environ. Hlth. Perspect. **5**, 221 – 225 (1973)

Wray, J.D., Müftü, Y., Dogramaci, I.: Hexachlorobenzene as a cause of porphyria turcica. Turk. J. Pediat. **4**, 132 – 137 (1962)

CHAPTER 7

The Effect of Chemicals on Hepatic Heme Biosynthesis*

Differences in Response to Porphyrin-Inducing Chemicals Between Chick Embryo Liver Cells, the 17-Day-Old Chick Embryo and Other Species

GERALD S. MARKS

A. Introduction

The administration of Sedormid (2-isopropylpent-4-enoylurea) to rabbits resulted in an experimental porphyria (SCHMID und SCHWARTZ, 1952) and the liver which was shown to be the major site of the metabolic disturbance contained large amounts of uro-, copro-, and proto-porphyrin. Sedormid (Fig. 1a) has a structure closely similar to the barbiturate group of drugs (Fig. 1b). Investigation of the relationship between structure and porphyrin inducing activity revealed the following requirements for activity: an allyl group together with either a cyclic ureide (as in the barbiturates), a ureide (as in Sedormid), or an acid amide [as in allylisopropylacetamide (AIA, Fig. 1c)].

B. Porphyrin Induction in Chick Embryo Liver Cells

1. Structure-Activity Relationships

TALMAN et al. (1957) compared the porphyrin inducing activity of Sedormid analogues by injecting them into the yolk sac of 8-day-old chick embryos, and measuring the porphyrin concentration in the allantoic fluid. GRANICK (1966) developed a procedure for maintaining liver cells of 16- to 17-day-old chick embryos on glass cover slips and showed that these cells would accumulate porphyrins several hours after exposure to chemicals such as AIA (Fig. 1c). The ability to accumulate porphyrins was apparent early in the development of the chick embryo and could be detected in the 9-day-old embryo. Further study revealed that the ability to accumulate porphyrins in response to AIA and other porphyrin inducing drugs was restricted to the liver cell—cells cultured in vitro from kidney, spleen and brain tissue of the 16-day-old chick embryo were unresponsive (GRANICK, 1966). With this technique GRANICK (1966) showed that many drugs possessed the potential to induce porphyrin accumulation and were contraindicated in patients with inherited hepatic porphyria. GRANICK (1966) suggested that five specific chemical groups were capable of inducing porphyrin biosynthesis.

* This work was supported by a grant from the Medical Research Council, Canada.

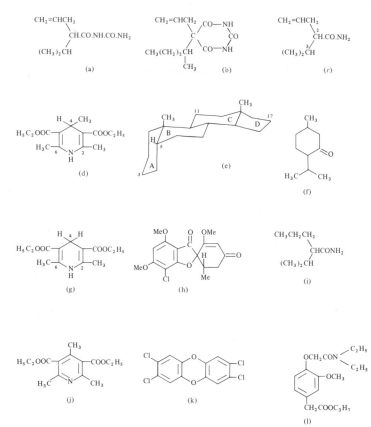

Fig. 1. (a) 2-Isopropylpent-4-enoylurea (Sedormid); (b) secobarbital; (c) allylisopropylacetamide (AIA); (d) 3,5-diethoxycarbonyl-1,4-dihydro-2,4,6-trimethylpyridine (DDC); (e) basic nuclear structure of a 5β-H steroid (A:B cis); (f) menthone; (g) 3,5-diethoxycarbonyl-1,4-dihydro-2,6-dimethylpyridine; (h) griseofulvin; (i) propylisopropylacetamide (PIA); (j) 3,5-diethoxy-carbonyl-2,4,6-trimethylpyridine (Ox-DDC); (k) 2,3,7,8-tetrachlorodibenzo-p-dioxin (TCDD); (l) propanidid

The finding that steroidal sex hormones induced porphyrin biosynthesis in chick embryo liver cells in culture (GRANICK, 1966) led to an extensive investigation of the relationship between structure and activity in this group of compounds. A number of steroid metabolites derived from the biotransformation of testosterone and progesterone were found to be highly active inducers (GRANICK and KAPPAS, 1967a, b; KAPPAS and GRANICK, 1968). Steric factors were found to be of importance for activity. A hydrocarbon nucleus of the 5β-androstane or 5β-pregnane type, in which the A:B ring junction was highly angular (Fig. 1e) rather than planar, was required. Other features which contributed to optimal activity were alcohol or ketone substituents at C-3, C-17, C-20 and possibly C-11. Of interest was the finding that several steroid components of contraceptive pills had weak inducing activity in chick embryo liver cell culture. A group of terpene compounds were investigated for porphyrin inducing activity (GRANICK and SASSA, 1971).

Menthone (Fig. 1f) α- or β-Thujone, and β-ionone were found to be potent porphyrin inducing compounds while d,1-menthol, camphor and camphenol had
moderate porphyrin inducing activity. Cyclopentadecanone (exaltone), a per-
fumery fixative, was found to be more potent than AIA. It was concluded that
the basic structural requirement in the terpene group of compounds was a bulky
hydrophobic group containing a carbonyl as a polar group.

DE MATTEIS (1971) studied the porphyrin-inducing activity of a series of compounds in chick embryo liver cells maintained in culture. He demonstrated that
the potency of a series of substituted acetamides and barbiturates depended upon
their lipophilicity. HIRSCH et al. (1967) and SCHNECK et al. (1968) studied the relationship between chemical structure and porphyrin-inducing activity in a series of
esters and amides. They concluded that in this class of compounds, the essential
feature for activity was an ester or amide group which was hindered from hydrolysis. 3,5-Diethoxycarbonyl-1,4-dihydro-2,4,6-trimethylpyridine (DDC, Fig. 1d),
for example, is an ester whose hydrolysis is sterically hindered by three methyl
groups in the 2-, 4- and 6-position of the dihydropyridine ring. Its inactive analogue, on the other hand, 3,5-diethoxycarbonyl-1,4-dihydro-2,6-dimethylpyridine
(Fig. 1g) is not sterically hindered from hydrolysis. AIA (Fig. 1c), an active inducer,
is an aliphatic amide which is branched at the 2- and 3-carbon atoms. This endows
the structure with considerable steric hindrance to chemical and enzymic hydrolysis. On the other hand, the inactive straight-chain amide, valeramide, is not
sterically hindered from hydrolysis. The studies of RACZ and MARKS (1972) indicated that for a chemical to induce hepatic porphyrin accumulation, it had to remain in contact with liver cells in active form for a period of at least several hours
in order to induce and maintain high levels of ALA-synthetase. Chemicals containing readily hydrolysable ester or amide groups would be inactivated rapidly
and therefore not persist in active form in contact with liver cells. On the other
hand, chemicals containing ester or amide groups which were resistant to hydrolysis would presumably persist in an active form to maintain high levels of ALA-
synthetase for an adequate period of time. The requirement for sterically hindered
ester or amide groups could thereby be explained. Since chemicals lacking ester
or amide groups such as menthone (Fig. 1f) and griseofulvin (Fig. 1h) are active
it is clear that ester or amide groups are not essential for porphyrin-inducing activity. However, if they are present in a molecule, they must be resistant to enzymic
hydrolysis; otherwise they will be hydrolyzed and the molecules will lose their
essential lipophilicity. An opportunity to test this hypothesis became available
through the work of KRISCH (1972) and HEYMANN et al. (1969). These workers
showed that bis-[p-nitrophenyl] phosphate (BNPP) is a specific, relatively non-
toxic, inhibitor of liver carboxylesterase (carboxylic-ester hydrolase, E.C. 3.1.1.1.).
The liver carboxylesterase also possesses amidase activity and the hydrolysis of
several amides can be inhibited by BNPP. The amides, phenacetin and acetanilide,
are substrates of the liver carboxylesterase, which are hydrolyzed to aromatic
amines with potent methemoglobin-forming properties. Following blockade of
liver carboxylesterase with BNPP the hydrolysis of the amides and the consequent
production of methemoglobin is inhibited. If the ideas of HIRSCH et al. (1967),
SCHNECK et al. (1968), and RACZ and MARKS (1972) were correct, then inhibition
of chick embryo liver carboxylesterase by BNPP should: 1) slow the rate of meta-

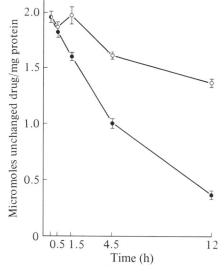

Fig. 2. Amount of unchanged decanamide-1-^{14}C found in the media after different periods of incubation of decanamide-1-^{14}C (30 μg/ml) with a monolayer of chick embryo liver cells without BNPP pretreatment (●———●) and with BNPP pretreatment (○———○) (From Murphy, F.R. et al.,Biochem. Pharmac. **24**, 883 [1975], with permission)

bolism of inactive, sterically unhindered esters and amides and 2) allow the sterically unhindered esters and amides to exert porphyrin-inducing activity comparable to that exhibited by sterically hindered esters and amides in the absence of BNPP. This was in general found to be the case. Decanamide presents an illustrative example (Murphy et al., 1975); inhibition of hydrolysis by BNPP results in significantly higher levels of unchanged drug in contact with the liver cell at all periods of time studied (Fig. 2). Inhibition of hydrolysis is accompanied by a large increase in porphyrin-inducing activity (Fig. 3a). The activity of the sterically hindered 2-ethylbutyramide was the same in the presence and absence of BNPP (Fig. 3b). Similarly (Marks et al., 1975) the activity of the sterically hindered aromatic ester diethyl 2,3,5,6-tetramethyl-terephthalate was not significantly changed by BNPP pretreatment of the cells (Fig. 3c), while the activity of the sterically unhindered ester, ethyl benzoate, was markedly potentiated (Fig. 3d).

It is worthwhile at this stage to recapitulate the different requirements for porphyrin-inducing activity stressed by different groups of workers:

1. An allyl group in barbiturates and substituted acetamides
2. Specific chemical groupings
3. Lipophilicity
4. Bulky hydrophobic group containing a carbonyl group
5. Steric factors inhibiting hydrolysis in esters and amides

The question that arises is whether it might be possible to construct a uniform hypothesis embracing all the above requirements. The importance of an allyl group in substituted acetamides and barbiturates for porphyrin-inducing activity has been reinvestigated in recent years and confirmed in studies using the 17-day-old chick embryo, chicken, mice (Marks et al., 1973), and rats (De Matteis, 1971; Abbritti

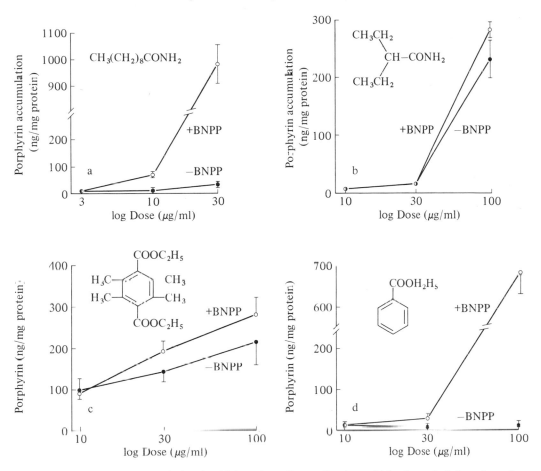

Fig. 3. Porphyrin accumulation in chick embryo liver cell culture 24 h after administration of a) decanamide (●———●) and BNPP (10 µg/ml medium) followed by decanamide (○———○); b) 2-ethylbutyramide (●———●) and BNPP (10 µg/ml medium) followed by 2-ethylbutyramide (○———○); c) diethyl 2,3,5,6-tetramethylterephthalate (●———●) and BNPP (10 µg/ml medium) followed by diethyl 2,3,5,6-tetramethylterephthalate (○———○); d) ethyl benzoate (●———●) and BNPP (10 µg/ml medium) followed by ethyl benzoate (○———○). Each point represents the mean of four determinations ±SEM

and DE MATTEIS, 1971). However in chick embryo liver cells in culture the allyl group is not required for activity (HIRSCH et al., 1966; DE MATTEIS, 1971; MARKS et al., 1973). In fact the saturated analogue of AIA viz., propyl-isopropylacetamide (PIA, Fig. 1i) is more potent than AIA in this test system (MURPHY et al., 1975). Recently lipophilicity alone has been shown to be insufficient to account for the porphyrin-inducing activity of chemicals in chick embryo liver cells (MURPHY et al., 1975, 1976). For example, decanamide, which has higher lipophilicity than AIA, is considerably less potent as a porphyrin-inducing drug. Moreover, resistance to hydrolysis of amides has been shown to be insufficient to account for the activity of all aliphatic amides. For example, 2-methylbutyramide, which is a poor substrate of chick embryo liver amidase and therefore expected to be active, was found to be devoid of porphyrin-inducing activity (MURPHY et al., 1975). Subsequent detailed studies of aliphatic and aromatic amides, aromatic esters, and aliphatic di esters in the presence and absence of BNPP showed that activity in these compounds depended upon two properties viz., lipophilicity and resistance to rapid hydrolysis to compounds of lower lipophilicity (MURPHY et al., 1975, 1976; MARKS et al., 1975). Thus, decanamide, although a highly lipophilic compound, is of low potency because it has little resistance to hydrolysis to the acid, a compound of low lipophilicity. The low potency of 2-methylbutyramide, a compound resistant to hydrolysis, could be attributed to its low lipophilicity. The high potency of AIA could be attributed to the fact that it is lipophilic and resistant to hydrolysis to the acid, a compound of markedly lower lipophilicity (MURPHY et al., 1975).

HANSCH and co-workers (HANSCH and DUNN, 1972; HANSCH and CLAYTON, 1973; HANSCH, 1972) have been able to correlate the relative biological activity of many different series of drugs with their lipophilicity. They have shown that the relationship between relative activity and lipophilicity can be either linear (HANSCH and DUNN, 1972) or parabolic (HANSCH and CLAYTON, 1973). MURPHY et al. (1975) utilized the procedures of HANSCH and DUNN (1972) and HANSCH and CLAYTON (1973) to explore the relationship between lipophilicity and porphyrin-inducing activity in a series of aliphatic amides. As a measure of lipophilicity, HANSCH has used $\log P$, where P is defined as the octanol-water partition coefficient of a drug. The $\log P$ values (Table 2) of AIA and PIA were obtained experimentally. The $\log P$ values of pentanamide and hexanamide (Table 1) were available (HANSCH and DUNN, 1972; HANSCH and CLAYTON, 1973) and the $\log P$ values of other amides (Tables 1 and 2) were calculated by adding a value of 0.5 for each additional CH_2 group added to hexanamide (LEO et al., 1971). In the case of branched-chain compounds, a value of 0.2 was subtracted from the calculated $\log P$ to compensate for branching (LEO et al., 1971). HANSCH has defined the relative biological activity of a drug in terms of $\log 1/C$ were C is the molar concentration of a drug producing a standard biological response. MURPHY et al. (1975) defined the standard biological response as the porphyrin-inducing activity observed 24 h after the addition of AIA (10 µg/ml) to chick embryo liver cells. Dose response

Table 1. Observed and calculated concentrations of straight-chain aliphatic amides which give the same porphyrin-inducing activity as AIA (10 µg/ml)

Amide	$\log P$	$\log 1/C$		$\lvert \Delta \log 1/C \rvert$
		Obs'd	Calc'd	
Pentanamide	0.29	2.00	2.07	0.07
Hexanamide	0.79	2.89	2.72	0.17
Heptanamide	1.29	3.06	3.25	0.19
Octanamide	1.79	3.74	3.65	0.09
Nonanamide	2.29	4.04	3.93	0.11
Decanamide	2.79	3.93	4.07	0.14
Dodecanamide	3.79	4.02	3.99	0.03

The "observed" and "calculated" values of $\log 1/C$ were obtained as indicated in the text.

curves were constructed for the straight-chain amides in the presence of BNPP and for the branched-chain amides alone, and the molar concentration (C) was determined which gave the same response as AIA (10 µg/ml) in the same experiment. From this information the observed log $1/C$ values (Tables 1 and 2) were derived. The degree of correlation between log P and observed log $1/C$ was determined for the straight-chain amides in the presence of BNPP and for the branched-chain amides in the absence of BNPP. This procedure was adopted since BNPP was found to inhibit hydrolysis of straight-chain but not of branched-chain amides (MURPHY et al., 1975). Regression analysis by the method of least squares was used to determine equations defining the "best" fit straight line (Eq. 1) and the "best" fit parabola (Eq. 2) through the data. For the straight-chain amides in the presence of BNPP, the equations derived were:

	n	r	SD	
log $1/C =$ 0.560 log $P + 2.341$	7	0.732	0.396	(1)
log $1/C = -0.255$ (log $P)^2 + 1.589$ log $P + 1.626$	7	0.954	0.164	(2)

where n is the number of data points, r is the correlation coefficient and SD is the standard deviation (HANSCH and DUNN, 1972; HANSCH and CLAYTON, 1973).

The log P value, the observed log $1/C$ value, the log $1/C$ value calculated from the parabolic equation (2), and the difference between log $1/C$ (observed) and log $1/C$ (calculated) for each amide are shown in Table 1. The log P values were plotted against the observed log $1/C$ values in Figure 4 and the parabola defined by Equation (2) was drawn through the data points. These results demonstrate that the porphyrin-inducing activity of the straight-chain amides after BNPP pretreatment can be correlated with lipophilicity and that the correlation is highest ($r - 0.954$) for the parabolic case (Eq. 2).

In the case of the branched-chain amides, the equations derived were:

	n	r	SD	
log $1/C =$ 0.171 log $P + 1.972$	5	0.970	0.189	(3)
log $1/C - -0.640$ (log $P)^2 + 2.805$ log $P + 1.712$	5	0.996	0.070	(4)

Table 2. Observed and calculated concentrations of branched-chain aliphatic amides which give the same porphyrin-inducing activity as AIA (10 µg ml)

Amide	log P	log $1/C$		$\|\Delta$ log $1/C\|$
		Obs'd	Calc'd	
2-Methylbutyramide	0.1	2.00	1.99	0.01
2-Ethylbutyramide	0.6	3.11	3.16	0.05
Allylisopropyl-acetamide	1.14	4.15	4.08	0.07
Propylisopropyl-acetamide	1.48	4.43	4.46	0.03
Dipropylacetamide	1.59	4.55	4.56	0.01

See footnote, Table 1.

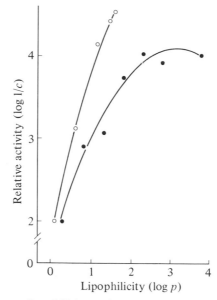

Fig. 4. Relationship between lipophilicity and porphyrin-inducing activity of straight-chain amides in the presence of BNPP (●) and of branched-chain amides alone (○). (From MURPHY, F.R. et al.: Biochem. Pharmac. **24**, 883 [1975] with permission)

The log P value, the experimentally observed log $1/C$ value, the log $1/C$ value calculated from the parabolic equation (4), and the difference between log $1/C$ (observed) and log $1/C$ (calculated) for each amide are shown in Table 2. The log P values are plotted against the observed log $1/C$ values in Figure 4 and the parabola defined by Equation (4) is drawn through the data points. The results demonstrate that the porphyrin-inducing activity of the branched-chain amides can also be correlated with lipophilicity; however, one is unable to determine from the limited data whether the correlation is linear ($r=0.970$) or parabolic ($r-0.996$).

A similar study, carried out with aromatic esters in the presence of BNPP and aromatic amides alone (MURPHY et al., 1976), revealed a correlation between porphyrin-inducing activity and lipophilicity. Since the above correlations could not be achieved if the activity of aromatic esters or aliphatic straight-chain amides was determined in the absence of BNPP pretreatment, it is clear that lipophilicity can explain the porphyrin-inducing activity of these compounds provided that hydrolysis to compounds of lower lipophilicity is inhibited by BNPP.

The next question that requires to be answered is the following: will any compound that is lipophilic and resistant to metabolism to compounds of lower lipophilicity induce porphyrin biosynthesis in chick embryo liver cells in culture? The compounds studied by MURPHY et al. (1975, 1976) and MARKS et al. (1975) all contained ester or amide groups and it is possible that the electronic properties of these or similar groups are required for optimal activity. GRANICK and SASSA (1971), who examined the porphyrin-inducing activity of terpenes and related compounds, suggested that the basic structural requirement for activity was a bulky hydrophobic non-planar structure containing a carbonyl as a polar group. A compound of minimal structural complexity shown to have marked porphyrin-inducing activity when tested in the presence of BNPP was ethyl benzoate (MARKS et al., 1975). Ethyl benzoate possesses a hydrophobic group (the benzene ring) and a carbonyl function in the ester group. A survey of the structures of porphyrin-inducing compounds (GRANICK, 1966; GRANICK and SASSA, 1971; SCHNECK et al., 1968; DE MATTEIS, 1971) shows that with the exception of the halogenated hydrocarbons and collidine almost all porphyrin-inducing compounds surveyed contain at least one carbonyl group or a hydroxy group which could be oxidized to a carbonyl group. A carbonyl group might function as the electron-donor group in the formation of a hydrogen bond and the nitrogen atom in collidine could perform the same function. On the basis of these considerations we would like to suggest the following working hypothesis to explain the porphyrin-inducing activity of chemicals in chick embryo liver cells: In order for a drug to induce, it must be —

1. lipophilic;
2. resistant to metabolism to compounds of lower lipophilicity;
3. a compound containing a group capable of participating as an electron-donor in hydrogen bond formation or capable of being converted to such a group in the cell.

It is possible that the underlying feature in the five chemical groupings suggested by GRANICK (1966) to induce porphyrin biosynthesis is a carbonyl group or N atom able to participate as electron-donor groups in hydrogen bond formation. The halogenated hydrocarbons do not apparently fit into this hypothesis. There are two possible reasons for this: These drugs may induce porphyrin accumulation by a different mechanism to those of the more common carbonyl containing compounds (SINCLAIR and GRANICK, 1974). Alternatively they may be converted to metabolites prior to exerting porphyrin-inducing activity (GRANICK and SASSA, 1971). While the allyl group is not required for activity in chick embryo liver cells, it is an important chemical group when drugs are tested in other test systems. Apparently the allyl group confers resistance to metabolism. This factor will be considered later in this review.

2. Pattern of Porphyrin Accumulation

Since porphyrin-inducing chemicals induce a rapid increase in ALA-synthetase activity in chick embryo liver cells in culture (GRANICK, 1966), it has been assumed that porphyrins accumulate as a result of the overproduction of ALA and the inability of the enzymes of the heme biosynthetic pathway to cope with an increased flux of intermediates through the pathway (GRANICK, 1966). If this is the correct explanation, one would expect (1) that the same porphyrins should accumulate in response to all porphyrin-inducing chemicals, and (2) that the pattern of porphyrin accumulation in response to drugs should be the same as that observed when exogenous ALA is added to the chick embryo liver cell culture medium. Following the addition of a porphyrin-inducing drug (presumably AIA)

GRANICK (1966) showed that the porphyrin which accumulated consisted of over 80% coproporphyrin and small amounts of di- and tri-carboxylic acid porphyrin. DOSS and KALTEPOTH (1971) compared the porphyrins accumulating in response to two porphyrin-inducing drugs (meprobamate and etiocholanolone) and to exogenous ALA in chick embryo liver cells. The pattern of accumulation, proto->copro->uro-porphyrin was found to be the same whether porphyrin-inducing drugs or ALA was added. Protoporphyrin accumulated first, followed by coproporphyrin and finally by uroporphyrin. GRANICK and SASSA (1971) suggested that differences in the pattern of porphyrin accumulation might depend on the conditions of culture since older cultures were observed to contain greater quantities of copro- and uro-porphyrin. SINCLAIR and GRANICK (1974) cultured chick embryo liver cells in a serum-free Ham medium containing insulin and showed that uroporphyrin accumulated in response to several chlorinated hydrocarbons while protoporphyrin was the major porphyrin which accumulated in response to AIA. These workers suggested that a metabolite of the chlorinated hydrocarbons inhibited uroporphyrinogen decarboxylase, thus causing uroporphyrin to accumulate. When exogenous ALA was added to control cells, protoporphyrin accumulated. These observations indicate that some porphyrin-inducing agents are acting in ways other than by overproduction of ALA. This conclusion is supported by results obtained by FISCHER et al. (1976). Thus, in serum-free medium, coproporphyrin accumulated in response to AIA and PIA (Fig. 5), while uroporphyrin was the major porphyrin to accumulate in response to 3,5-diethoxycarbonyl-2,4,6-trimethyl-pyridine (Ox-DDC, Fig. 1j) and a mixture of proto-, copro- and uro-porphyrin in response to DDC (Fig. 5). These results suggest that Ox-DDC inhibits uroporphyrinogen decarboxylase and that AIA and PIA inhibit coproporphyrinogen oxidase. It would appear that one of the mechanisms by which porphyrin-inducing drugs act is by inhibiting a step in the porphyrin biosynthetic pathway (STRAND et al., 1972). This would result in decreased levels of protoheme which in turn would release ALA-synthetase from feedback repression. It would appear that determination of the pattern of porphyrin accumulation in chick embryo liver cells may be a useful tool in elucidating the mechanism of action of porphyrin-inducing drugs. How can one reconcile the possibility that different porphyrin-inducing drugs act at a variety of sites with the previously considered structure-activity relationship? If one assumes that all the possible sites of action are intracellular sites and that these sites must be occupied for a considerable period of time, then the requirements for lipophilicity and resistance to metabolism to compounds of lower lipophilicity are understandable. Moreover, the third structural requirement, viz., a group capable of participating as an electron-donor in hydrogen bond formation or capable of being converted to such a group, is sufficiently general to accommodate several classes of compounds acting at a variety of sites.

The pattern of porphyrin accumulation response to Ox-DDC was similar in serum-free and serum-containing medium (Fig. 5). With DDC the pattern of porphyrin accumulation was similar qualitatively but not quantitatively (Fig. 5). In the case of AIA and PIA the pattern of porphyrin accumulation was markedly different in serum-containing and serum-free medium (Fig. 5). Thus while coproporphyrin was the principle porphyrin in serum-free medium, a mixture of uro-, proto-, and copro-porphyrins accumulated in serum-containing medium. This ex-

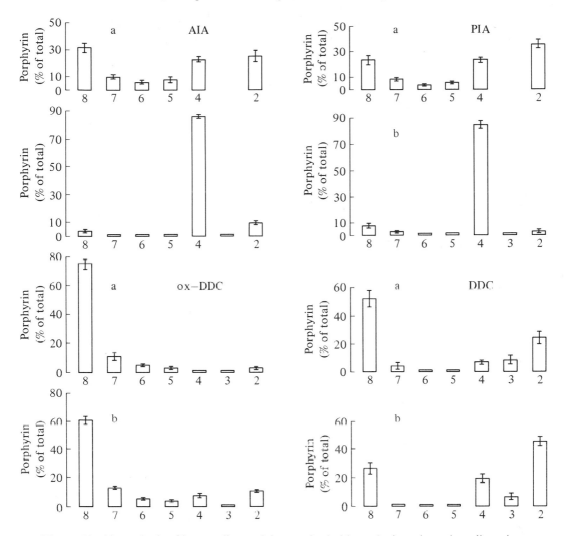

Fig. 5. The biosynthesis of intermediates of the porphyrin biosynthetic pathway by cells maintained in serum-containing Eagle's basal medium (A) and serum-free Waymouth MD 705/1
medium (B) in response to AIA and PIA (100 µg/ml), Ox-DDC (50 µg/ml) and DDC (1.5 µg/ml).
The accumulation of the intermediates is expressed as the percentage of total porphyrins
formed ±SEM. The intermediates are: 8, uro-; 7, heptacarboxylic; 6, hexacarboxylic; 5, pentacarboxylic; 4, copro-; 3, tricarboxylic; 2, proto-porphyrin. (From FISCHER, P.W.F. et al.: Biochem. Pharmac. [1976] with permission)

periment suggests that factors in serum markedly effect porphyrin biosynthesis.
There are at least three factors in serum that exert an effect on porphyrin bio-
synthesis-heme, albumin, and hormones. GRANICK et al. (1975) showed that when
serum albumin was added to chick embryo liver cells, cultured in serum-free
medium it enhanced the synthesis of protoporphyrin and the transfer of protoporphyrin from cells to medium. Recently MORGAN et al. (1975, 1976) have shown

that thyroid hormone, hydrocortisone, and other hormones markedly enhance drug-induced porphyrin biosynthesis when added to chick embryo liver cells cultured in serum-free Waymouth medium. It is thus likely that the differences observed by previous investigators in the pattern of porphyrin accumulation might be explained by differences in the levels of hormones, albumin, and heme in the serum-containing and serum-free media used. We are currently investigating the effects of hormones such as thyroxine on the patterns of drug-induced porphyrin accumulation in serum-free Waymouth medium. It is worth pointing out that chick embryo liver cells cultured in serum-free Waymouth medium are ideal for studying hormonal effects on porphyrin biosynthesis and hormonal effects on other aspects of liver metabolism.

3. Mechanism of Action of Porphyrin-Inducing Drugs

GRANICK (1966) showed that the accumulation of porphyrins in chick embryo liver cell culture in response to a variety of chemicals resulted from an increase in the activity of ALA-synthetase, the rate-limiting enzyme in the protoheme biosynthetic pathway. The increased activity of the enzyme was considered to result from an increase in the amount of the enzyme rather than from activation of the inactive enzyme. The drug-induced synthesis of the enzyme was inhibited by protoheme. On the basis of this observation and the ideas of JACOB and MONOD (1961), GRANICK (1966) suggested that the repressor for ALA-synthetase consisted of a protein aporepressor combined with protoheme which functioned as a corepressor. The porphyrin-inducing chemicals were suggested to displace protoheme from the aporepressor so that the mRNA for ALA-synthetase was formed. This would be followed by increased synthesis of ALA-synthetase, and porphyrins and protoheme would be produced as a consequence. It was suggested that the protoheme produced was used for the formation of protoheme enzymes in the endoplasmic reticulum that act as mixed function oxidases to hydroxylate and inactivate the porphyrin-inducing chemical (GRANICK, 1966). If the above hypothesis of GRANICK (1966) was correct, then there are two consequences that follow: (1) porphyrin-inducing compounds induce ALA-synthetase activity by increasing the amount of the mRNA for the enzyme; (2) protoheme prevents the induction of ALA-synthetase by repression of transcription. The studies reported below were designed to test the validity of the first consequence of Granick's hypothesis. TYRRELL and MARKS (1972) incubated chick embryo liver cells in a medium containing DDC; ALA-synthetase activity increased during the 8-h measurement period (*curve a*, Fig. 6). When cycloheximide was added with DDC, the enzyme induction was suppressed. When the cells were pretreated with a combination of DDC and cycloheximide for 5 h, washed and reincubated in fresh medium (FM), ALA-synthetase activity increased markedly without a lag period (*curve b*, Fig. 6). This increase was not prevented by the addition of actinomycin D to the fresh medium (*curve c*, Fig. 6) but instead was augmented. On the other hand, cycloheximide added to fresh medium completely blocked the increase in ALA-synthetase activity normally seen on reincubation (*curve d*, Fig. 6). Similar results were obtained when AIA was used as the porphyrin-inducing drug instead of DDC. The results were interpreted (NEBERT and GELBOIN, 1970; PETERKOFSKY and TOMKINS, 1968) by

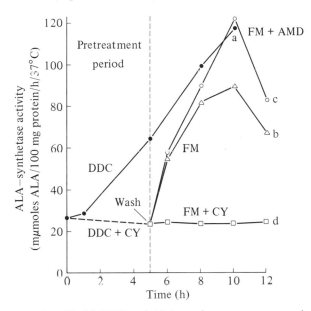

Fig. 6. Cells were exposed to 37 μM DDC and ALA-synthetase was measured over 8 h (*curve a*, ●———●). Cells were exposed to 37 μM DDC and 20 μM cycloheximide (CY) for 5 h (●----- □), washed and reincubated in fresh medium (*curve b*, △———△), or fresh medium and 0.8 μM actinomycin D (AMD; *curve c*, ○———○), or fresh medium and 20 μM cycloheximide (*curve d*, □———□) (From TYRRELL, D.L.J. and MARKS, G.S.: Biochem. Pharmac. **21**, 2077 [1972] with permission)

assuming that RNA had accumulated prior to washing in cells treated with AIA or DDC and cycloheximide. The induction-specific RNA which had accumulated while the translation step of protein synthesis was inhibited was thought to mediate increased ALA-synthetase activity after washing, by translation into either this enzyme or into some other protein responsible for ALA-synthetase activation. Since the addition of actinomycin D to the medium after washing cells pretreated with AIA or DDC and cycloheximide did not prevent the increase in ALA-syn-thetase activity normally observed after washing, this second phase of induction is independent of transcription. The second phase of induction was inhibited by cycloheximide and therefore was dependent on translation. These observations were in accordance with the hypothesis of GRANICK (1966) which suggested that porphyrin-inducing compounds induce ALA-synthetase activity by increasing the amount of the mRNA for the enzyme. TOMITA et al. (1974) studied the induction of ALA-synthetase by AIA and DDC in organ culture of 18-day-old chick embryo liver. These workers showed that both AIA and DDC stimulated an increased synthesis of mRNA for ALA-synthetase. Thus the results obtained in the organ culture of chick embryo liver were in essential agreement with those obtained in the chick embryo liver cell culture system (TYRRELL and MARKS, 1972). SASSA and GRANICK (1970) obtained results compatible with the view that DDC (and etio-cholanolone) stimulated an increased synthesis of mRNA for ALA-synthetase in chick embryo liver cells. However, both these authors and STRAND et al. (1972)

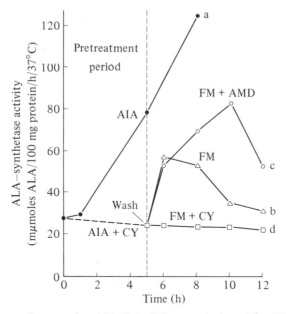

Fig. 7. Same as Figure 6 except that AIA (2.1 mM) was substituted for DDC (37 µM). (From TYRRELL, D.L.J. and MARKS, G.S., Biochem. Pharmac. **21**, 2077 [1972] with permission)

reported only small or negligible effects with AIA. In addition, SASSA and GRANICK (1970) found the porphyrin-inducing chemical γ-hexachlorocyclohexane (Lindane) to be ineffective in stimulating an increased synthesis of the mRNA for ALA-synthetase. The inability of STRAND et al. (1972) to observe significant effects with AIA may be explained by comparing their experimental technique with that of TYRRELL and MARKS (1972). After preincubation of chick embryo liver cells in culture with AIA and cycloheximide, TYRRELL and MARKS (1972) measured the ALA-synthetase activity 1, 3, 5, and 7 h after washing to remove AIA and cycloheximide (Fig. 7). Activity was maximal after 1 h and dropped thereafter reaching levels closely similar to control after 7 h. TOMITA et al. (1974), who demonstrated an effect with AIA, measured ALA-synthetase activity $1^1/_2$, 3, and 5 h after washing to remove AIA and cycloheximide. On the other hand, STRAND et al. (1972) measured ALA-synthetase activity 8 h after washing out the AIA and cycloheximide, by which time they would have missed measuring the effect. It is possible that the inability of SASSA and GRANICK (1970) to record a significant effect with AIA may be due to the fact that they used a concentration of 60 µg/ml of AIA in their experiments compared to 300 µg/ml used by TYRRELL and MARKS (1972).

SASSA and GRANICK (1970) have, on the basis of the following experiments, subdivided porphyrin-inducing drugs into those acting on translation and those acting on transcription. After the addition of acetoxycycloheximide to the cells, ALA-synthetase decayed at a first order rate with a half-life of 3 h. When porphyrin-inducing drugs were added with acetoxycycloheximide the half-life of the enzyme remained unchanged showing that these drugs do not affect the rate of degradation of ALA-synthetase. After the addition of actinomycin D to the cells the apparent half-life of the enzyme was 5.2 h. When AIA or Lindane was added with actinomycin D the apparent half-life of the enzyme was markedly increased. On the other hand, when either of the two porphyrin-inducing drugs, etiocholanolone or DDC, was added with actinomycin D the half-life of the enzyme was unchanged. This result was interpreted as indicating that AIA and Lindane acted at the translational level-bringing about a marked increase in synthesis of the enzyme from preformed mRNA by either increasing the lifetime of the mRNA for ALA-synthetase or its activity for translation. Etiocholanolone and DDC were suggested to act primarily at the transcriptional level. If the above experiments can be confirmed the techniques used should allow one to distinguish between porphyrin-inducing drugs acting at a transcriptional and translational level. It would be useful to examine other porphyrin-inducing chemicals by these techniques in order to gain further information on their mechanism of action. Moreover, from the point of view of studying the relationship between structure and activity it is of importance to obtain information on the mechanisms of action of these drugs.

TOMITA et al. (1974) using chick embryo liver organ culture showed that the half-life of ALA-synthetase, after the addition of actinomycin D, was the same whether the incubation medium contained AIA or not. These results are in apparent conflict with those of SASSA and GRANICK (1970) but might be due to the difference between organ and cell culture of chick embryo liver. In summary, the combined evidence indicates that AIA and DDC both act at the transcriptional level by stimulating an increased synthesis of mRNA for ALA-synthetase in chick embryo liver cells. It is possible that AIA has an additional effect at the translational stage, but this claim (SASSA and GRANICK, 1970) requires confirmation.

The second consequence of GRANICK's hypothesis (1966) was that protoheme prevents the induction of ALA-synthetase by repression of transcription. The experiments reported below were directed to investigating this question. Protohemin is used in experimental work instead of protoheme because of the difficulty of maintaining protoheme in the reduced state. The normal induction of ALA-synthetase activity by DDC is shown in Figure 8 (*curve a*). When cells pretreated with a porphyrin-inducing compound and cycloheximide for 5 h were washed and reincubated in fresh medium, ALA-synthetase activity increased (*curve b*, Fig. 8). On the other hand, when cells pretreated with DDC and cycloheximide for 5 h were washed and reincubated with fresh medium and protohemin (PH), no increase in ALA-synthetase activity was observed (*curve c*, Fig. 8). These results were not anticipated on the basis of the model for the control of protoheme biosynthesis suggested by GRANICK (1966), since the model limits the ability of protoheme to prevent ALA-synthetase induction to repression of transcription. The ability of protoheme to repress the transcriptional phase of ALA-synthetase induction was examined (Fig. 9). The normal induction of ALA-synthetase activity by porphyrin-inducing compounds is shown in Figure 9 (*curve a*). When cells pretreated with a porphyrin-inducing compound and cycloheximide for 5 h were washed and reincubated in fresh medium, ALA-synthetase activity increased (*curve b*, Fig. 9). When cells pretreated for 5 h with medium containing DDC, cycloheximide, and protoheme were washed and reincubated in fresh medium, ALA-synthetase activity increased (*curve c*, Fig. 9). The dose of protoheme used in this study was twice the

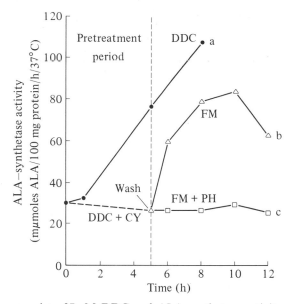

Fig. 8. Cells were exposed to 37 µM DDC and ALA-synthetase activity was measured over 8 h (*curve a*, ●——●). Cells were exposed to 37 µM DDC and 20 µM cycloheximide (CY) for 5 h, washed and reincubated in fresh medium (*curve b*, △————△), or in fresh medium containing 10 µM protohemin (PH; *curve c*, □————□). (From TYRRELL, D.L.J., and MARKS, G.S.: Biochem. Pharmac. **21**, 2077 [1972] with permission)

dose required to inhibit completely the rise in ALA-synthetase activity when added in the post-wash phase. Thus transcription of mRNA occurs in the presence of concentrations of protohemin which completely inhibited the post-transcriptional process.

SASSA and GRANICK (1970) studied the effect of protoheme on ALA-synthetase induction as follows: The chick embryo liver cells were treated with AIA to increase the level of ALA-synthetase. The cells were washed and reincubated in fresh medium containing actinomycin D. The apparent half-life of ALA-synthetase was found to be 5.2 h. When protohemin was added together with actinomycin D the apparent half-life of the enzyme decreased to 3.6 h. On the basis of this experiment it was suggested that protoheme inhibited the synthesis of ALA-synthetase at the translational level. TOMITA et al. (1974) came to the same conclusion after carrying out similar experiments. The effect of protoheme on porphyrin accumulation (SCHNECK and MARKS, 1969) and ALA-synthetase induction (STRAND et al., 1972) was found to resemble that of cycloheximide rather than that of actinomycin D. It was therefore suggested that protoheme exerts its effect at a translational rather than at a transcriptional level.

In rats and in adult chickens AIA induces ALA-synthetase both in liver mitochondria and in the cytosol (HAYASHI et al., 1972; OHASHI and KIKUCHI, 1972). It appears that ALA-synthetase is synthesized in the endoplasmic reticulum and after undergoing some change in structure enters and is incorporated into mito-

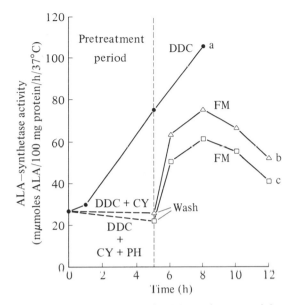

Fig. 9. Cells were exposed to 37 μM DDC and ALA-synthetase activity was measured over 8 h (*curve a*, ●———●). Cells were exposed to 37 μM DDC and 20 μM cycloheximide for 5 h, washed and reincubated in fresh medium (*curve b*, △———△). Cells were exposed to 37 μM DDC, 20 μM cycloheximide and 20 μM protohemin (PH) for 5 h, washed and reincubated in fresh medium (*curve c*, □———□). (From TYRRELL, D.L.J. and MARKS, G.S.: Biochem. Pharmac. **21**, 2077 [1972] with permission)

chondria. Protohemin was shown to inhibit the conversion of the "soluble" form of ALA-synthetase into the mitochondrial ALA-synthetase. It was possible that the effects of protoheme on translation observed by TYRRELL and MARKS (1972) and SASSA and GRANICK (1970) might at least in part have been due to protoheme preventing the conversion of "soluble" into mitochondrial ALA-synthetase. This possibility has been tested by TOMITA et al. (1974). These workers treated chick embryo liver in organ culture or in ovo with AIA or DDC and showed that the accumulation of ALA-synthetase in the cytosol was minor. Moreover, protohemin did not cause an appreciable accumulation of ALA-synthetase in the liver cytosol. It was concluded (TOMITA et al., 1974) that in chick embryo liver protohemin did not prevent the conversion of "soluble" into mitochondrial ALA-synthetase as it did in adult chicken or rat liver (HAYASHI et al., 1972; OHASHI and KIKUCHI, 1972).

C. Porphyrin Induction in 17-Day-Old-Chick Embryos

TALMAN et al. (1957) injected drugs into the yolk sac of 8-day-old chick embryos and measured the porphyrin concentration in the allantoic fluid. These workers noted that the kidneys fluoresced intensely while the livers rarely fluoresced. GRANICK (1966) extended this technique by inoculating 17-day-old chick embryos with AIA, onto the air sac, through a pinhole made in the shell. The hole was covered and the egg reincubated. Fluorescing porphyrins were detected $2^1/_2$ h later in the kidney tubules while 4 to 24 h later fluorescing porphyrins were detected in the liver localized to bile canaliculi. Since induction of ALA synthetase was a specific property of chick embryo liver parenchymal cells, GRANICK (1966) concluded that the liver excreted ALA or other porphyrin precursors into the blood stream from which they were concentrated by the kidney tubules and converted to porphyrins.

On the basis of results obtained with chick embryo liver cells in culture, GRANICK (1964) cautioned against the use of glutethimide, methsuximide, barbiturates, mephenytoin, griseofulvin, and other drugs in patients and relatives of patients with porphyria. WATSON (1966) suggested that many pharmaceuticals, especially sedatives and analgesics should be screened by the Granick procedure as latent cases of acute intermittent *porphyria* are apparently more prevalent than generally realized. Since several drugs which are highly active in the liver cell culture system are inactive when given orally to guinea pigs (MARKS et al., 1965) it appeared possible that on the basis of the test in vitro, several drugs might be unnecessarily excluded from clinical use. It was thus of interest to determine whether liver cells grown as a monolayer culture responded in the same way to porphyrin-inducing drugs as the liver of the intact 17-day-old chick embryo. RACZ and MARKS (1969) described a simplified procedure for determining porphyrin-inducing activity. Drugs, usually dissolved in dimethylsulfoxide (0.1 ml), were injected into the fluids surrounding the 17-day-old chick embryo; after re-incubation for 24 h, the liver was removed and porphyrins estimated quantitatively. Twenty-one compounds previously shown to be active in chick embryo liver cell culture (GRANICK, 1966) were tested in the 17-day-old chick embryo (RACZ and MARKS, 1969). Fifteen of the 21 compounds were found to be active and 6 inactive. Thus in the case of the majority of drugs tested, those that caused porphyrin accumulation in chick embryo liver cells in culture also caused porphyrin accumulation in the 17-day-old chick embryo liver. Some of the important exceptions were hexachlorobenzene, griseofulvin, bemegride, 3,5-diethoxycarbonyl-2,4,6-trimethylpyridine and 1,4-diethoxycarbonyl-2,3,5,6-tetramethylbenzene. In laboratories which are not equipped for cell culture studies the intact chick embryo is a useful practical means for screening drugs prior to administration to porphyria patients.

RIFKIND et al. (1973) examined 51 drugs, most of which are in common clinical use, for their effects on chick embryo hepatic ALA-synthetase. Eleven of these drugs had previously been tested by RACZ and MARKS (1969) for their in vivo porphyrin-stimulating activity in chick embryo livers. Ten of the 11 drugs stimulated both porphyrin formation and ALA-synthetase in vivo and the remaining drug, bemegride, stimulated neither. The chick embryo liver was shown to undergo drug-induced ALA-synthetase stimulation when as young as 13 days and to increase markedly in drug-inducibility during the few days prior to hatching. RIFKIND et al. (1973) compared the ability of 27 drugs to induce ALA-synthetase activity in chick embryo liver in vivo with their ability to induce porphyrin accumulation in chick embryo liver cells in culture. With 23 out of the 27 drugs there was a correlation between ALA-synthetase stimulation in vivo and porphyrin accumulation in vitro. These studies suggested a direct correlation between the induction of porphyrin accumulation and the ability to synthesize ALA. However, the latter does not necessarily lead to porphyria as discussed below.

Studies of CREIGHTON and MARKS (1971), and TAUB (1973) did not support the correlation between ALA-synthetase activity and porphyrin accumulation in chick embryo liver. Thus the 5β-H steroids caused a marked elevation of hepatic ALA-synthetase levels in chick embryos which was not accompanied by a parallel porphyrin accumulation (CREIGHTON and MARKS, 1972). Pentobarbital sodium and phenobarbital sodium caused marked elevations of hepatic ALA-synthetase activity while porphyrin levels remained low. Thalidomide caused a marked elevation of ALA-synthetase activity without effecting porphyrin levels (TAUB, 1973). On the basis of these results it appears that a new drug should be screened for its ability to induce ALA-synthetase as well as porphyrin accumulation in the 17-day-old chick embryo.

The hypnotic-sedatives constitute the group of drugs most frequently implicated in the precipitation of hepatic porphyria (EALES, 1971). Some patients with hepatic porphyria experience difficulty in sleeping and the question arises whether there are any sedative-hypnotic drugs which may be safely administered to these patients. In an attempt to answer this question, TAUB (1973) screened a large number of sedative-hypnotics in vivo in the chick embryo liver. In view of the poor relationship observed in some cases between ALA-synthetase activity and porphyrin levels both ALA-synthetase activity and porphyrin accumulation was measured. All the barbiturates tested were found to induce elevated levels of ALA-synthetase. The barbiturates which were most active in inducing porphyrin accumulation, viz., methohexital, secobarbital, hexobarbital, and aprobarbital contained an unsaturated side chain. This observation is in accord with previous reports (RACZ and MARKS, 1969; TALMAN et al., 1957).

Since all the barbiturate drugs are contraindicated in porphyric patients, the benzodiazepine group of sedative-hypnotics, which has achieved popularity in recent years, was investigated. The order of potency in causing hepatic ALA-synthetase elevation was found to be flurazepam > diazepam > oxazepam > nitrazepam > chlordiazepoxide. A significant elevation of hepatic porphyrin levels was observed after 12 h with flurazepam and after 24 h with diazepam. In agreement with these findings is the report of RIFKIND et al. (1973) that diazepam was a potent inducer of ALA-synthetase while chlordiazepoxide was an inducer of low potency in 17-day-old chick embryos.

The following non-barbiturate hypnotics were screened (TAUB, 1973): glutethimide, ethinamate, ethchlorvynol, methaqualone, chloral hydrate, paraldehyde, and thalidomide. All the drugs tested with the exception of chloral hydrate produced a dose-dependent increase in ALA-synthetase activity. Glutethimide, ethinamate, ethchlorvynol and methaqualone caused a marked porphyrin accumulation; the remaining drugs did not alter porphyrin levels significantly. RIFKIND et al. (1973), who measured hepatic ALA-synthetase activity but not porphyrin levels, obtained similar results with chloral hydrate, paraldehyde, and glutethimide. Thus the only hypnotic-sedative totally devoid of activity in the 17-day-old chick embryo was chloral hydrate. It is of interest that chloral hydrate appears to be unique amongst sedative-hypnotics in that it is metabolized by a reductive rather than by an oxidative mechanism.

KOSKELO et al. (1966) reported that some apparently normal women, taking oral contraceptive pills, excrete elevated levels of ALA in the urine. For this reason, RIFKIND et al. (1970) examined the ability of oral contraceptive steroids to induce hepatic ALA-synthetase in vivo in 15- to 16-day-old chick embryo. All the pro-gestational components of the contraceptive mixtures induced elevated levels of ALA-synthetase with the exception of chlormadinone acetate. Neither of the estrogenic components of the oral contraceptives, mestranol or ethinyl estradiol, were active alone, nor did they effect the results obtained with the progestational compounds alone. KAPPAS et al. (1968) examined the ability of a series of natural steroids to induce hepatic ALA-synthetase in vivo in the 16-day-old chick embryo. The following steroids exhibited marked potency: 5β-pregnane-3α,17α-diol, 11,20-dione, etiocholanolone, etiocholanedione, pregnanedione, 11-ketopregnano-lone. Progesterone, testosterone, estradiol, and cortisol exhibited weak activity or no activity.

The herbicide 2,4,5-trichlorophenoxyacetic acid (2,4,5-T) is contaminated with an extremely toxic substance 2,3,7,8-tetrachlorodibenzo-p-dioxin (TCDD, Fig. 1k). This contaminant is believed to be responsible for an outbreak of acne and por-phyria cutanea tarda in workers engaged in the manufacture of 2,4,5-T. POLAND and GLOVER (1973a, b) showed that TCDD was an extremely potent inducer of hepatic ALA-synthetase in vivo in the 15- to 20-day-old chick embryo. After a single dose of TCDD ALA-synthetase levels remained elevated for 5 days; this prolonged elevation was attributed to the resistance of TCDD to metabolic degrada-tion. Fifteen analogues of TCDD were screened for their ability to induce ALA-synthetase and it was shown that for activity halogen atoms were required at a minimum of three of the four lateral ring positions. Moreover, at least one ring position was required to be non-halogenated. POLAND and GLOVER (1973b) have indicated that several important questions remain to be answered viz., "would the 2,3,7,8-tetrachloro derivatives of other tricyclic planar ring systems be active? And does the interaction of the TCDD molecule with the hypothetical induction receptor depend on the steric configuration of the molecule or primarily on the electron distribution?" To the reviewer it appears that an additional question requires answering, viz., both the active and inactive congeners are lipophilic compounds and differences in activity can therefore not be attributed to differences in lipo-philicity alone. However, in addition to being lipophilic, TCDD is resistant to metabolic degradation. Could differences in activity observed between congeners be explained, at least in part, by differences in rates of metabolism from com-pounds of high to compounds of low lipophilicity?

A point of interest which emerges from the work of POLAND and GLOVER (1973b) is that cycloheximide and actinomycin D produced more pronounced effects when administered intravenously (FINKELSTEIN, 1964) than when adminis-tered into the air sac or yolk sac. In the author's laboratory some drugs have been observed to be active in chick embryo liver cells in culture but inactive when administered in vivo into the fluids surrounding the 17-day-old chick embryo (RACZ and MARKS, 1969). It is possible that the inactivity in vivo of some drugs which are active in vitro might be attributed, at least in part, to the route of administration. It would be worth comparing the activity of a series of drugs administered by the I-V. route into the 17-day-old chick embryo with their activ-ity when injected into the fluids surrounding the embryo.

HANSCH et al. (1968) presented evidence that the hypnotic activity of groups of barbiturates depends largely upon their relative lipophilic character as defined by their octanol/water partition coefficient P. DE MATTEIS (1971) noted that the porphyrin-inducing activity of barbiturates in chick embryo liver cells in culture could be correlated with their lipophilicity. TAUB (1973) examined the relationship between lipophilicity and the ALA-synthetase inducing activity of barbiturate and non-barbiturate sedative-hypnotics including thalidomide in vivo in the 17-day-old chick embryo liver. In the barbiturate and non-barbiturate series (Table 3) a correlation was noted between lipophilicity and activity. When propanidid (log P, 1.97) an ultra short-acting non-barbiturate anesthetic, was first tested in this system the level of hepatic ALA-synthetase was found to be unaltered 12 h after injection of the drug. Propanidid is an ester (Fig. 1*l*) which is rapidly hydrolyzed in vivo by esterases and its activity was therefore re-determined in a chick embryo whose liver carboxylesterase (carboxylic-ester hydrolase, E.C. 3.1.1.1) was blocked with BNPP (TAUB and MARKS, 1973). In the BNPP-treated embryo propanidid exhibited marked activity in accordance with that anticipated from its lipophilicity (Table 3). This study indicated that in this in vivo test system as in chick embryo liver cells in culture at least two properties are required for activity: a) lipophilicity and b) resistance to metabolism to compounds of lower lipophilicity.

The presence of cytochrome P-450 in chick embryo liver was demonstrated by STRITTMATTER and UMBERGER (1969). Phenobarbital treatment resulted in marked

Table 3. The relationship between lipophilicity and hepatic ALA-synthetase activity of sedative-hypnotics in the 17-day-old chick embryo

Drug	Lipophilicity (log P)[a]	Dose causing 10-fold elevation of ALA-synthetase activity	
		(mg/egg)	(μmol/egg)
Aprobarbital	1.15	2.4	11.4
Diallylbarbiturate	1.19	7	33.6
Phenobarbital	1.42	3.9	15.4
Hexobarbital	1.68	1.15	4.87
Amobarbital	1.95	1.50	6.05
Pentobarbital	2.05	1.46	5.87
Secobarbital	2.34	1.07	4.11
Thiopental	3.00	0.44	1.66
Methohexital	2.84	0.50	1.75
Thalidomide	0.33	4.1	15.9
Paraldehyde	0.70	6.8	51.5
Glutethimide	1.90	0.89	4.1
Propanidid (after BNPP pretreatment)	1.97	0.4	1.2
Ethchlorvynol	2.00	0.65	4.5
Chloral hydrate	0.67	Cannot induce at any dose	

[a] log P values of pentobarbital, hexobarbital and propanidid were determined in our laboratory using [3]H- or ^{14}C-labeled compounds. The other log P values were obtained from the following two sources: HANSCH et al. (1968) and LEO et al. (1971).

increases in cytochrome P-450. RIFKIND et al. (1973) reported that all drugs that were potent stimulators of ALA-synthetase in chick embryo liver also increased the cytochrome P-450 content of the liver measured 30 h after drug administration. KRUPA et al. (1974) showed that the porphyrin-inducing drugs, AIA, PIA and DDC, produced an elevation of cytochrome P-450 in the 17-day-old chick embryo liver. DDC and its analogues have been shown to inhibit aminopyrine N-demethylase activity of the 17-day-old chick embryo (CREIGHTON and MARKS, 1969). A possible explanation of this result is that DDC and its analogues are competitive substrates of aminopyrine (CREIGHTON and MARKS, 1969).

D. Porphyrin Induction in Chickens and Japanese Quail

GOLDBERG and RIMINGTON (1955) administered AIA (200 mg/kg) in gelatin capsules to two Rhode Island Red chickens. A rapid rise in copro- and proto-porphyrin content of the excreta was observed while porphobilinogen and uroporphyrin were detected on the fourth and seventh day, respectively. CREIGHTON and MARKS (1972) investigated the activity of a series of compounds in 5- to 7-week-old chickens and the following compounds were shown to induce hepatic porphyrin accumulation: glutethimide, methsuximide, secobarbital, methyprylon and mephenytoin. The 5β-H steroids, 5β-pregnan-3α, 17α-diol-11,20-dione and 5β-androstan-3,17-dione, produced little or no increase in hepatic porphyrins. TAUB (1973) tested a series of barbiturates for their activity in 6-week-old chickens. Phenobarbital and thiopental caused slight but significant elevations of ALA-synthetase after 12 h. Low but significant hepatic porphyrin accumulation was observed 12 h after administration of phenobarbital and hexobarbital. Methohexital was found to be inactive. In 1967 the porphyrin-inducing chemical hexachlorobenzene was detected in the tissues of wild birds (Vos et al., 1972). This led to a study of the porphyrin-inducing effects of halogenated hydrocarbons in the Japanese quail (Vos et al., 1972; STRIK and WIT, 1972; STRIK, 1973). In this species hexachlorobenzene and the halogenated biphenyls produced a disturbance of porphyrin metabolism with different features to that observed with AIA and DDC. Uroporphyrin accumulates in response to hexachlorobenzene while protoporphyrin accumulates in response to AIA and DDC. The effect appeared more slowly with hexachlorobenzene than with AIA and DDC. With the chlorinated hydrocarbons no correlation could be found between hepatic porphyrin accumulation and ALA-synthetase activity. The accumulation of porphyrins after administration of polyhalogenated aromatic compounds was related to liver mitochondrial damage. It was of interest that the administration of protoheme did not result in any inhibition of porphyrin accumulation in this type of experimental *porphyria*.

E. Differences in Response to Porphyrin Inducing Drugs in Different Species and Model Test Systems

1. Comparison of Response in Chick Embryo and Rat Liver Cells in Culture

EDWARDS and ELLIOTT (1974) developed an in vitro experimental system where regulation of ALA-synthetase could be studied in a suspension of isolated, normal adult rat liver cells. In order to obtain reproducible induction of the enzyme the rat liver cells required supplementation with dibutyryl cyclic AMP. In chick embryo liver cells in culture dibutyryl cyclic AMP is not essential for drug-induced porphyrin biosynthesis but it does enhance drug-induced porphyrin biosynthesis when added to the cells (MORGAN et al., 1976). Of great interest was the finding in rat liver cells that for a variety of androstane and pregnane derivatives, induction by 5α-H steroids was as great or greater than that by 5β-H steroids (EDWARDS and ELLIOTT, 1975). This finding contrasts markedly with results in the chick embryo liver cells in culture where 5β-H steroids are reported to be markedly more potent than 5α-H steroids.

2. Comparison of Response in Chick Embryo Liver Cells in Culture with the Response of the 17-Day-Old Chick Embryo

In the studies of RACZ and MARKS (1969) and RIFKIND et al. (1973) several compounds were found to induce porphyrin accumulation in chick embryo liver cells in culture but to be inactive when injected into the fluids surrounding the 17-day-old chick embryo, e.g., bemegride, griseofulvin, hexachlorobenzene, chloramphenicol, pyrazinamide and 3,5-diethoxycarbonyl-2,4,6-trimethylpyridine (Ox-DDC, Fig. 1 j). To investigate the reason for the difference in responsiveness of isolated liver cells and the liver of the intact chick embryo the following studies were performed (RACZ and MARKS, 1972): Ox-DDC-^{14}C and DDC-^{14}C were injected into 17-day-old chick embryos and the total amount of drug and metabolite(s) in the livers measured at different time intervals. Ox-DDC was found to undergo a more rapid metabolic degradation in liver than DDC and its low potency in the chick embryo was attributed to its rapid metabolic degradation. The fact that Ox-DDC causes porphyrin accumulation in chick embryo liver cells in culture is due to the inability of the cells to rapidly metabolize the drug (RACZ and MOFFAT, 1974).

3. Comparison of Responsiveness of the 17-Day-Old Chick Embryo and the Chicken

Hexobarbital induces a marked increase in ALA-synthetase activity and porphyrin levels in chick embryo liver (Fig. 10) but is inactive in the 18-day-old chicken (Fig. 11). Following pretreatment of chickens with SKF 525-A, hexobarbital exhibits marked activity (Fig. 11). PIA elevates hepatic ALA-synthetase activity in the 17-day-old chick embryo and produces a small increase in porphyrin levels (MARKS et al., 1973). In contrast to this result, PIA produced a small elevation of ALA-synthetase activity in the 18-day-old chicken accompanied by a small increase in porphyrin levels (Fig. 11). Following pretreatment of chickens with SKF 525-A, PIA exhibits marked activity (Fig. 11). Apparently SKF 525-A blocks metabolism of PIA and hexobarbital in the chicken liver resulting in higher levels of unchanged drug in the livers and therefore greater activity (Fig. 11).

4. Comparison of Responsiveness of Avian and Mammalian Species

STRIK (1973) reported differences in drug-induced porphyrin biosynthesis in various species of birds. Thus the Japanese quail was sensitive to the porphyrinogenic action

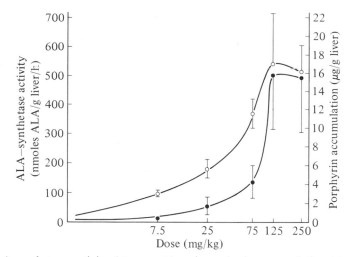

Fig. 10. ALA-synthetase activity (○———○) and porphyrin accumulation (●———●) in the livers of chick embryos 12 h following administration of increasing doses of hexobarbital. Each point represents the mean of 5−6 determinations (±SEM). (From TAUB, H. et al.: Biochem. Pharmac. **25**, 511 [1976] with permission)

of hexachlorobenzene and hexabromobiphenyl whereas carniverous birds were not susceptible to these compounds. STRIK and WIT (1972) suggested that species differences might be attributable to differences in diet. STRIK (1973) reported that the Japanese quail appeared to be more sensitive to the porphyrinogenic action of hexachlorobenzene and hexabromobiphenyl than the rat.

RACZ and MARKS (1969) and CREIGHTON and MARKS (1972) tested a series of compounds for their ability to induce porphyrin accumulation in the 17-day-old chick embryo, 5- to 7-week-old chickens and mice. Glutethimide, methsuximide, secobarbital, methyprylon and mephenytoin induced hepatic porphyrin accumulation in chick embryos and chickens but not in mice. Mice have been shown to be more sensitive than rats to DDC but less sensitive than rats to AIA (DE MATTEIS et al., 1973). The marked sensitivity of mice to DDC-induced porphyrin accumulation has been attributed by the above workers to the sensitivity of mouse hepatic ferrochelatase to inhibition by this chemical. It is of considerable interest that differences exist in the inducibility of hepatic ALA-synthetase in selected inbred strains of mice (HUTTON and GROSS, 1970; GROSS and HUTTON, 1971).

KAPPAS et al. (1968) were unable to induce hepatic ALA-synthetase activity with 5β-H steroids in guinea pigs or rats despite the fact that these compounds were highly active in chick embryo liver cells in culture. The 5β-H steroids induce ALA-synthetase activity in suspensions of rat liver cells (EDWARDS and ELLIOTT, 1975); it is possible that differences between the results in the rat and in isolated rat liver cells are due to differences between the concentration of drug in contact with rat liver cells in vitro and in vivo, and to the period of time that the cells are exposed to an effective concentration of drug.

MOORE et al. (1970) examined the ability of a series of barbiturates to induce hepatic ALA-synthetase and porphyrin accumulation in rats; the order of activity

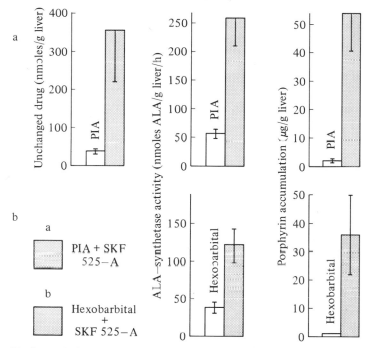

Fig. 11. A. Unchanged drug, ALA-synthetase activity and porphyrin accumulation in the livers of 18-day-old chickens 12 h after administration of PIA (100 mg/kg), without SKF 525-A pretreatment (*open bars*); with SKF 525-A (25 mg/kg) pretreatment (*hatched bars*). B. ALA-synthetase activity and porphyrin accumulation in the livers of 18-day-old chickens 12 h after administration of hexobarbital (100 mg/kg), without SKF 525-A pretreatment (*open bars*); with SKF 525 A (25 mg/kg) pretreatment (*hatched bars*). The results in A and B represent the mean of four determinations for unchanged drug and the mean of six determinations for ALA-synthetase activity and porphyrin accumulation (±SEM). The asterisk denotes significance at the 0.05 level. SKF 525-A does not exert any significant effect alone. (From TAUB, H. et al.: Biochem. Pharmac. **25**, 511 (1976) with permission)

was diallylbarbituric acid > aprobarbital > secobarbital > pentobarbital > phenobarbital > thiopental > amobarbital. In rabbits GOLDBERG (1954) and STICH and DECKER (1955) demonstrated porphyrin-inducing activity with aprobarbital, diallylbarbituric acid, pentobarbital, phenobarbital and secobarbital; amobarbital and thiopental were inactive. These results contrast markedly with results obtained in the 17-day-old chick embryo (TAUB, 1973) and chick embryo liver cells in culture (DE MATTEIS, 1971). Thus diallylbarbituric acid, which is the most active drug in rats, is least active in chick embryo, and thiopental, which is weakly active in the rat, is highly active in the chick embryo. No difference has been found between male and female chickens in their response to DDC (CREIGHTON and MARKS, 1972).

Control levels of ALA-synthetase in 17-day-old chick embryos are only one-third those of adult chickens while levels in newborn chicks are intermediate between adult and embryonic levels (CREIGHTON and MARKS, 1972). In contrast to these results the levels of hepatic ALA-synthetase are greater in the embryos than in

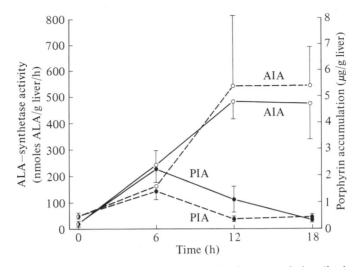

Fig. 12. ALA-synthetase activity (*solid lines*) and porphyrin accumulation (*broken lines*) in the livers of chick embryos following administration of AIA (1 mg) and PIA (1 mg). Each point represents the mean of five determinations (±SEM). (From MARKS, G.S. et al.: Canad. J. Physiol. and Pharmacol. **51**, 863 [1973] with permission)

adults of rats, rabbits and guinea pigs (WOODS and DIXON, 1970a, b). DDC induces large increases in ALA-synthetase activity in both newborn and adult chickens (CREIGHTON and MARKS, 1972). In contrast, newborn rabbits are much less responsive than adult rabbits to induction with this drug (WOODS and DIXON, 1970a, b) and newborn rats are completely refractory to induction by AIA and DDC (SONG et al., 1968). The properties of ALA-synthetase from fetal rat liver differ from those of the adult enzyme. For example, unlike the enzyme from adult rat liver, the fetal enzyme is not inhibited by protohemin (MURTHY and WOODS, 1974).

   An illustrative example of differences in porphyrin-inducing activity in different test systems is available from studies with AIA and PIA. AIA was found to be considerably more potent than PIA in inducing hepatic ALA-synthetase activity and hepatic porphyrin accumulation in the 17-day-old chick embryo (Fig. 12), chickens, mice of the CBA/J strain (MARKS et al., 1973), and rats (ABBRITTI and DE MATTEIS, 1971; STICH and DECKER, 1955). On the other hand in chick embryo liver cell culture (Fig. 13) PIA was found to be either equipotent with AIA (HIRSCH et al., 1966; MARKS et al., 1973; DE MATTEIS, 1971) or to be of greater potency (MURPHY et al., 1975). In order to attempt to understand these findings the metabolism of AIA-^{14}C and PIA-^{14}C was studied in the 17-day-old chick embryo, chicken, CBA/J mice and chick embryo liver cells in culture (KRUPA et al., 1973; MURPHY et al., 1975; TAUB et al., 1976). In the 17-day-old chick embryo liver the levels of ALA-synthetase and porphyrins were shown (MARKS et al., 1973) to be similar (Fig. 12) 6 h after administration of AIA and PIA (1 mg/egg). However, after this time period the levels of ALA-synthetase and porphyrins fell in the PIA-treated embryos but continued to rise in the AIA-treated

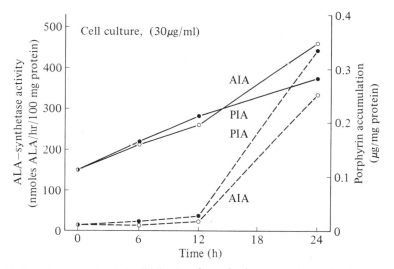

Fig. 13. ALA-synthetase activity (*solid lines*) and porphyrin accumulation (*broken lines*) in chick embryo liver cell culture following administration of AIA and PIA (30 µg/ml). Each point is the mean of three separate determinations. (From MARKS, G.S. et al.: Canad. J. Physiol. Pharmacol. **51**, 863 [1973] with permission)

embryos. Examination of the results shown in Figure 14 (KRUPA et al., 1973) provides a possible explanation for these results: 6 h after drug administration the amount of unchanged PIA in the liver drops rapidly and 24 h after drug administration there is no unchanged drug remaining in the liver. The drop in ALA-synthetase and porphyrin levels after 6 h (Fig. 12) correlates with a reduction of PIA levels in the liver (Fig. 14). Despite the disappearance of PIA from the liver, a large amount of metabolite(s) derived from PIA remains in the liver. It may therefore be concluded that the metabolite(s) is inactive in inducing ALA-synthetase or porphyrin accumulation. The rise in ALA-synthetase and porphyrin levels 6 h after the administration of AIA (Fig. 12) correlates with a large amount of unchanged AIA in the liver between 6 and 24 h (Fig. 14). The amount of unchanged AIA remaining in the liver, 24 h after drug injection, is equal to or greater than the maximum observed level of unchanged PIA. The lowered potency of PIA relative to AIA in the chick embryo liver at periods of time longer than 6 h may be attributed, at least in part, to the rapid exhaustion of hepatic PIA. The lowered potency of PIA relative to AIA in chickens and in CBA/J mice was similarly attributed, at least in part, to the more rapid disappearance of unchanged PIA than of AIA from chickens and from mouse liver. An additional effect may be exerted by the allyl group. In rats, and possibly in other species, the allyl group appears to cause a rapid loss of rat liver microsomal cytochrome P-450 accompanied by a loss of microsomal heme (DE MATTEIS, 1971). The drop in heme levels would in turn result in enhanced ALA-synthetase levels.

AIA-^{14}C and PIA-^{14}C were added to chick embryo liver cell cultures (Fig. 15) and the percentage of unchanged drug measured after several time periods (MURPHY et al., 1975). After 24 h 86% of AIA-2-^{14}C and 62% of PIA-2-^{14}C was recovered

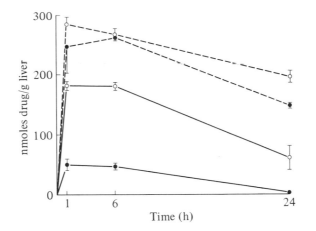

Fig. 14. The amount of total drug and unchanged drug in livers of 17-day-old chick embryos at different times after injection of AIA-^{14}C (7125 nmol) and PIA-^{14}C (6993 nmol). ○-----○ = Total drug AIA-^{14}C; ●------● = total drug PIA-^{14}C; ○————○ = unchanged drug AIA-^{14}C; ●————● = unchanged drug PIA-^{14}C. Each point represents the mean of four determinations ±SEM. (From Krupa et al.: Enzyme, **16**, 276 [1973] with permission)

in the unchanged form. Thus, as in the in vivo studies, PIA appears to be more rapidly metabolized than AIA. However, in contrast to the in vivo studies (Fig. 14), where PIA has disappeared after 24 h, in the cells in culture the amount of PIA available to the cells, over the 24 h study period, is sufficient to ensure an effective concentration to stimulate ALA-synthetase and cause porphyrin accumulation. The remarkable sensitivity of the chick embryo liver cells in culture can therefore be attributed, at least in part, to the unique pharmacokinetics of the system; unlike the intact animal, the cell culture cannot terminate the action of a drug by redistribution to other organs or by excretion. Moreover, sufficient drug may be added in the cell culture to effectively overwhelm the capacity of the liver cells to metabolize and inactivate the drug over a 24 h period.

Our results (Creighton and Marks, 1972; Marks et al., 1973; Krupa et al., 1973; Taub et al., 1976) indicate the following order of sensitivity to porphyrin-inducing drugs: chick embryo liver cells in culture > 17-day-old chick embryo > chickens (and other avian species) > mammals (e.g. mice, rats, rabbits and guinea pigs). The exquisite sensitivity of chick embryo liver cells in culture can be explained, at least in part, by the unique pharmacokinetic properties of this system. How do we explain the differing sensitivity of chicken, chick embryo, mice (and other mammals)? Brodie et al. (1965) have suggested two possible reasons for species variation in response to a drug: (1) variation in drug metabolism resulting in differences in the amount of drug at the site of action, and (2) variation in sensitivity of receptor sites. Let us consider the possibility that the greater responsiveness of the 17-day-old chick embryo compared to the chicken or the mouse was due to slower drug metabolism in the chick embryo than in the chicken or mouse. Data assembled in Table 4 (Marks et al., 1973; Krupa et al., 1973; Taub et al., 1976) do not support this idea for it is clear that in these three systems there is no correlation between ALA-synthetase activity at 6 h and concentration

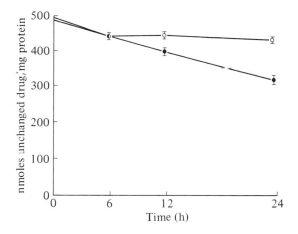

Fig. 15. Amount of unchanged AIA-2-^{14}C ($\circ$———$\circ$) and unchanged PIA-2-^{14}C ($\bullet$———$\bullet$) found in the media after different periods of incubation of AIA-2-^{14}C (7 µg/ml) and PIA-2-^{14}C (7 µg/ml) with a monolayer of chick embryo liver cells. (From MURPHY, F R et al.: Biochem. Pharmac. **24**, 883 [1975] with permission)

Table 4. ALA-synthetase activity and amount of unchanged AIA in the livers of 18-day-old chickens, mice of the CBA/J strain and 17-day-old chick embryos 6 h after administration of AIA

Time after drug adminis- tration	18-Day-old chicken		17-Day-old chick embryo		CBA/J mice	
	ALA-syn- thetase activity (% of control)	Unchanged drug (nmol/g liver)	ALA-syn- thetase activity (% of control)	Unchanged drug (nmol/g liver)	ALA-syn- thetase activity (% of control)	Unchanged drug (nmol/g liver)
6	600	1550	1100	178	400	1700

of AIA. It is therefore probable that differences in response between the chick embryo, chicken and mouse, must be explained by differences in the sensitivity of receptor sites in the liver cell to the porphyrin-inducing drugs. Since hormones greatly influence the sensitivity of chick embryo liver cells to drug-induced por- phyrin biosynthesis (MORGAN et al., 1975, 1976) it is possible that differences in species response may be attributed at least in part to different hormonal influences on the liver.

5. Extrapolation of Results from Animals and Model Test Systems to Man

An important question that remains to be answered concerns the relevance of results obtained in chick embryo liver cells in culture and in avian and mammalian tests in vivo to patients with hereditary hepatic porphyria. Since a drug may induce ALA-synthetase activity and porphyrin accumulation in one test system but not in another, the problem arises in deciding which test system allows the best prediction to be made of the results to be expected in the porphyric patient. The correct choice of a test system is crucial in deciding which drugs may be safely administered to patients with hereditary hepatic porphyria. It is therefore worth comparing results observed in a variety of test systems with experience in patients with porphyria. Results have been tabulated (Table 5) to facilitate the comparison. We have selected for inclusion in this table only those drugs which have been both tested in one or other of the test systems and administered to patients with porphyria.

The positive results of the chick embryo tests (in vitro and in vivo) are in accord with the ability of the following drugs to induce attacks in porphyric patients: phenobarbital, secobarbital, pentobarbital, amobarbital, glutethimide, methyprylon, meprobamate, thiopental, diphenylhydantoin, methsuximide and tolbutamide. Moreover the inactivity of the following drugs in chick embryo tests accord with their evaluation as safe or probably safe drugs in porphyric patients by EALES (1971) and others (WATSON, 1974): diphenhydramine, guanethidine, morphine, codeine, meperidine, penicillins, streptomycin, chloral hydrate, neostigmine, chlorpromazine and melphalan.

Griseofulvin, which induced attacks of porphyria in porphyric patients is highly active in chick embryo liver cells in culture but does not cause porphyrin accumulation in the chick embryo. Chloramphenicol, which has been reported to be safe by EALES (1971), is active in chick embryo liver cells in culture but inactive in the chick embryo. Drugs of the sulfonamide group have been reported to induce attacks of porphyria in man, although the particular compounds involved have not been specified (EALES, 1971). The parent drug in this group, sulfanilamide, was inactive in chick embryo liver cell culture (DE MATTEIS, 1971). Propanidid

Table 5. A comparison of the ability of drugs to induce attacks of porphyria in man with their ability to effect porphyrin biosynthesis in animals and liver cell cultures[a]

Drug	Man	Chick embryo liver cell culture (porphyrins)	17-Day-old chick embryo Porphyrins	17-Day-old chick embryo ALA-synthetase	Mice	Rabbits	Rats
Sedative-hypnotics							
A. Barbiturate type							
Phenobarbital	+	+	+	+			+
Secobarbital	+	+	+	+	−	+	+
Pentobarbital	+	+	+	+		+	+
Amobarbital	+	+	+	+			+
B. Non-barbiturate type							
Glutethimide	+	+	+	+	−		
Methyprylon	+(?)	+	+	+	−		
Meprobamate	+	+	+	+	−		
Chloral hydrate	−		−	−			
Diazepam	−(?)	+	+	+			
Chlordiazepoxide	−(?)	−(?)	−	+			

Table 5 (continued)

Drug	Man	Chick embryo liver cell culture (porphyrins)	17-Day-old chick embryo		Mice	Rabbits	Rats
			Porphyrins	ALA-synthetase			
Ultra-short-acting Anesthetics							
Thiopental	+	+	+	+			+
Propanidid	−	+	+	+			
Anticonvulsants							
Diphenylhydantoin	+	+	+	+	−		
Methsuximide	+	+	+	+	−		
Hypoglycemic agents							
Tolbutamide	+	+		+			
Antihistamines							
Diphenhydramine	−			−			
Antipsychotic agents							
Chlorpromazine	−			−			
Antihypertensive agents							
Guanethidine	−	−					
Propranolol	−	−					
Narcotic analgesics							
Morphine	−			−			
Codeine	−			−			
Meperidine	−						
Anticholinestease agents							
Neostigmine	−	−					
Antibacterial agents							
Chloramphenicol	−	+		−			
Penicillins	−	−					
Streptomycin	−						
Sulfonamides	+	−					
Antifungal agents							
Griseofulvin	+	+	−		+		+
Anticancer agents							
Melphalan	−	−	−	−			

[a] The human data was obtained from the following: EALES, 1971; SCHLESINGER and GASTEL, 1961; COWGER and LABBE, 1965; WATSON, 1974. The chick embryo liver cell culture data was obtained from the work of GRANICK, 1966; DE MATTEIS, 1971; HIRSCH et al., 1966; and MARKS, 1975. The chick embryo data were obtained from the work of RACZ and MARKS (1969); RIFKIND et al. (1973) and TAUB (1973). The mice data are from the work of RACZ and MARKS (1969); rabbit data are from the work of STICH and DECKER (1955) and GOLDBERG (1954) and rat data are from the work of MOORE et al. (1970). The propranolol data were obtained from the following: BLUM et al., 1973; ATSMON and BLUM, 1970, and ATSMON, 1975. Additional information on man and animals was derived from DE MATTEIS (1967).

has been reported to be safe for use in porphyria patients (DEAN, 1969; DEAN, 1971) despite the report that it was active in liver cell culture (DEAN, 1969). In our studies it was shown to be markedly active in chick embryo liver cells in culture but weakly active in the chick embryo in vivo (TAUB and MARKS, 1973). However, its activity in the chick embryo test in vivo was markedly increased when hepatic carboxylesterase was inhibited by BNPP. Clearly, propanidid should be used with care, particularly in patients receiving other drugs with a possible potential to inhibit hepatic carboxylesterase. The situation regarding diazepam and chlordiazepoxide is controversial. EALES (1971) reported that in his experience these drugs are safe to use when given alone. Other workers have implicated these drugs as precipitants of attacks of porphyria. In chick embryo liver cell culture chlordiazepoxide was found to be inactive and diazepam slightly active by MARKS (1975) but DE MATTEIS (1971) reported that chlordiazepoxide is active. Both diazepam and chlordiazepoxide induce ALA-synthetase activity in the 17-day-old chick embryo, diazepam displaying considerably greater potency than chlordiazepoxide (RIFKIND et al., 1973; TAUB, 1973). Both drugs however displayed less potency than secobarbital (TAUB, 1973).

Thus of 29 drugs listed in the table the chick embryo data was in complete accord with clinical experience in 23 cases. In the remaining 6 cases the results were not clear-cut although they were indicative. The tests in the chick embryo thus appear to have considerable predictive value for hereditary hepatic porphyria. If a drug induces porphyrin accumulation in chick embryo liver cell culture and in the 17-day-old chick embryo and is of a potency similar to that of secobarbital, it is probable that it will have the capacity to induce an attack of porphyria in patients with the inherited trait. The results to date indicate that if one desires to administer a drug of unknown porphyrin-inducing potential to a patient with porphyria it should be screened (for porphyrin accumulation) in chick embryo liver cell culture and for porphyrin accumulation and ALA-synthetase activity in the intact chick embryo. The potency of the drug should be compared in these systems with a drug known to induce acute attacks, such as secobarbital.

While a variety of drugs will, in small doses, cause a derangement of hepatic porphyrin biosynthesis accompanied by clinical symptoms in patients with hereditary hepatic porphyria, normal man will be relatively insensitive to these agents. Similarly normal rats and mice are relatively insensitive to drugs known to induce porphyria in patients with hereditary hepatic porphyria.

Several drugs which were active in the chick embryo test systems viz., secobarbital, glutethimide, methyprylon, meprobamate, diphenylhydantoin and methsuximide failed to cause hepatic porphyrin accumulation after prolonged administration to mice (RACZ and MARKS, 1969). Since these drugs have been shown to produce a clinical relapse in porphyric patients (COWGER and LABBE, 1965; EALES, 1971) it appears that the results obtained using the chick embryo test systems allow a more accurate prediction of the results to be expected in the porphyric patient than the results in mice. DE MATTEIS (1971) has similarly concluded that the results in chick embryo liver cells in culture allow better prediction of results to be expected in porphyric patients than results in rats and rabbits. Possible reasons for this phenomenon are the following: There is evidence for a partial block in heme biosynthesis in avian (DE MATTEIS, 1973) and human porphyric liver cells (MEYER et al., 1972), leading to increased sensitivity to the action of porphyrin-inducing drugs when compared to rat and mouse liver cells. Moreover, slow metabolism of drugs in chick embryo liver cells in culture (Fig. 15) and in patients with acute intermittent porphyria (SONG et al., 1974) might in part explain increased sensitivity to these drugs.

Abbreviations

AIA	Allylisopropylacetamide
ALA	δ-Aminolevulinic acid
BNPP	Bis-[p-nitrophenyl]phosphate
DDC	3,5-Diethoxycarbonyl-1,4-dihydro-2,4,6-trimethylpyridine
Ox-DDC	3,5-Diethoxycarbonyl-2,4,6-trimethylpyridine
PIA	Propylisopropylacetamide
SKF-525-A	2-Diethylaminoethyl-3,3-diphenylpropylacetate
TCDD	2,3,7,8-Tetrachlorodibenzo-p-dioxin

References

Abbritti, G., De Matteis, F.: Decreased levels of cytochrome P-450 and catalase in hepatic porphyria caused by substituted acetamides and barbiturates. Importance of the allyl group in the molecule of the active drugs. Chem. biol. Interact. **4**, 281 − 286 (1971)

Atsmon, A.: Personal communication (1975)

Atsmon, A., Blum, I.: Treatment of acute porphyria variegata with propranolol. Lancet **1970 I**, 196 − 197

Blum, I., Schoenfeld, N., Atsmon, A.: The effect of DL-propranolol on δ-aminolevulinic acid synthetase activity and urinary excretion of porphyrins in allylisopropylacetamide-induced experimental porphyria. Biochim. biophys. Acta (Amst.) **320**, 242 − 248 (1973)

Brodie, B.B., Cosmides, G.J., Rall, D.P.: Toxicology and the biomedical sciences. Science **148**, 1547 − 1554 (1965)

Cowger, M.L., Labbe, R.F.: Contraindications of biological oxidation inhibitors in the treatment of porphyria. Lancet **1965 I**, 88 − 89

Creighton, J.M., Marks, G.S.: Drug-induced porphyrin biosynthesis—I. The effect of porphyria-inducing drugs on N-demethylase activity of chick embryo liver. Biochem. Pharmacol. **18**, 2040 − 2045 (1969)

Creighton, J.M., Marks, G.S.: Drug-induced porphyrin biosynthesis—VII. Species, sex, and developmental differences in the generation of experimental porphyria. Canad. J. Physiol. Pharmacol. **50**, 485 − 489 (1972)

Dean, G.: A report on propanidid, an intravenous anaesthetic in Porphyria variegata. S. Afr. med. J. **43**, 227 − 229 (1969)

Dean, G.: The Porphyrins. 2nd ed., p. 132. Philadelphia − Montreal: J.B. Lippincott Co. 1971

De Matteis, F.: Drugs and porphyria, S. Afr. J. Lab. clin. Med. **17**, 126 − 133 (1971)

De Matteis, F.: Disturbances of liver porphyrin metabolism caused by drugs. Pharmacol. Rev. **19**, 523 − 557 (1967)

De Matteis, F.: Drug interactions in experimental hepatic porphyria. A model for the exacerbation by drugs of human variegate porphyria. Enzyme **16**, 266 − 275 (1973)

De Matteis, F., Abbritti, G., Gibbs, A.H.: Decreased liver activity of porphyrin-metal chelatase in hepatic porphyria caused by 3,5-diethoxycarbonyl-1,4-dihydrocollidine. Biochem. J. **134**, 717 − 727 (1973)

Doss, M., Kaltepoth, B.: Porphyrin biosynthesis in liver cell cultures. S. Afr. J. Lab. clin. Med. **17**, 73 − 75 (1971)

Eales, L.: Acute porphyria: The precipitating and aggravating factors. S. Afr. J. Lab. clin. Med. **17**, 120 − 125 (1971)

Edwards, A.M., Elliott, W.H.: Induction of δ-aminolevulinic acid synthetase in isolated rat liver cell suspensions. Adenosine 3':5'-monophosphate dependence of induction by drugs. J. biol. Chem. **249**, 851 – 855 (1974)

Edwards, A.M., Elliott, W.H.: Induction of δ-aminolevulinic acid synthetase in isolated rat liver cells by steroids. J. biol. Chem. **250**, 2750 – 2755 (1975)

Finkelstein, R.A.: Observations on mode of action of endotoxin in chick embryos. Proc. Soc. exp. Biol. (N.Y.) **115**, 702 – 707 (1964)

Fischer, P.W.F., Morgan, R.O., Krupa, V., Marks, G.S.: Drug-induced porphyrin biosynthesis—XV. Induction of porphyrin biosynthesis in chick embryo liver cells maintained in serum-free Waymouth medium. Biochem. Pharmacol. **25**, 687 – 693 (1976)

Goldberg, A.: The effects of certain barbiturates on the porphyrin metabolism of rabbits. Biochem. J. **57**, 55 – 61 (1954)

Goldberg, A., Rimington, C.: Experimentally produced porphyria in animals. Proc. roy. Soc. B **143**, 257 – 280 (1955)

Granick, S.: A test for detection of porphyria-inducing drugs. J. Amer. med. Ass. **190**, 475 (1964)

Granick, S.: The induction in vitro of the synthesis of δ-aminolevulinic acid synthetase in chemical porphyria: A response to certain drugs, sex hormones and foreign chemicals. J. biol. Chem. **241**, 1359 – 1375 (1966)

Granick, S., Kappas, A.: Steroid control of porphyrin and heme biosynthesis: A new biological function of steroid hormone metabolites. Proc. nat. Acad. Sci. (Wash.) **57**, 1463 – 1467 (1967a)

Granick, S., Kappas, A.: Steroid induction of porphyrin synthesis in liver cell culture. I. Structural basis and possible physiological role in the control of heme formation. J. biol. Chem. **24**, 4587 – 4593 (1967b)

Granick, S., Sassa, S.: δ-Aminolevulinic acid synthetase and the control of heme and chlorophyll synthesis. In: Metabolic Regulation. Vogel H.J. (ed.), Vol. 5 of Metabolic Pathways, pp. 77 – 141. New York – London: Academic Press 1971

Granick, S., Sinclair, P., Sassa, S., Grieninger, G.: Effects by heme, insulin, and serum albumin on heme and protein synthesis in chick embryo liver cells cultured in a chemically defined medium, and a spectrofluorometric assay for porphyrin composition. J. biol. Chem. **250**, 9215 – 9225 (1975)

Gross, S.R., Hutton, J.J.: Induction of hepatic δ-aminolevulinic acid synthetase activity in strains of inbred mice. J. biol. Chem. **246**, 606 – 614 (1971)

Hansch, C.: Quantitative relationships between lipophilic character and drug metabolism. Drug Metab. Rev. **1**, 1 – 14 (1972)

Hansch, C., Clayton, J.M.: Lipophilic character and biological activity of drugs II: The parabolic case. J. pharm. Sci. **62**, 1 – 21 (1973)

Hansch, C., Dunn, W.J.: Linear relationship between lipophilic character and biological activity of drugs. J. pharm. Sci. **61**, 1 – 19 (1972)

Hansch, C., Steward, A.R., Anderson, S.M., Bentley, D.: The parabolic dependence of drug action upon lipophilic character as revealed by a study of hypnotics. J. med. Chem. **11**, 1 – 11 (1968)

Hayashi, N., Kurashima, Y., Kikuchi, G.: Mechanism of allylisopropylacetamide-induced increase of δ-aminolevulinate synthetase in liver mitochondria. V. Mechanism of regulation by hemin of the level of δ-aminolevulinate synthetase in rat liver mitochondria. Arch. Biochem. Biophys. **148**, 10 – 21 (1972).

Heymann, E., Krisch, K., Büch, H., Buzello, W.: Inhibition of phenacetin- and acetanilide-induced methemoglobinemia in the rat by the carboxylesterase inhibitor bis-[p-nitrophenyl] phosphate. Biochem. Pharmacol. **18**, 801 – 811 (1969)

Hirsch, G.H., Bubbar, G.L., Marks, G.S.: Studies of the relationship between chemical structure and porphyria-inducing activity—III. Biochem. Pharmacol. **16**, 1455 – 1462 (1967)

Hirsch, G.H., Gillis, J.D., Marks, G.S.: Studies of the relationship between chemical structure and porphyria-inducing activity—II. Biochem. Pharmacol. **15**, 1006 – 1008 (1966)

Hutton, J.J., Gross, S.R.: Chemical induction of hepatic porphyria in inbred strains of mice. Arch. Biochem. Biophys. **141**, 284 – 292 (1970)

Jacob, F., Monod, J.: Genetic regulatory mechanisms in the synthesis of proteins. J. molec. Biol. **3**, 318 – 356 (1961)

Kappas, A., Granick, S.: Steroid induction of porphyrin synthesis in liver cell culture II. The effects of heme, uridine diphosphate glucuronic acid, and inhibitors of nucleic acid and protein synthesis on the induction process. J. biol. Chem. **243**, 346 – 351 (1968)

Kappas, A., Song, C.S., Levere, R.D., Sachson, R.A., Granick, S.: The induction of δ-amino-levulinic acid synthetase in vivo in chick embryo liver by natural steroids. Proc. nat. Acad. Sci. (Wash.) **61**, 509 – 513 (1968)

Koskelo, P., Eisalo, A., Toivonen, I.: Urinary excretion of porphyrin precursors and copro-porphyrin in healthy females on oral contraceptives. Brit. med. J. **1966 I**, 652 – 654

Krisch, K.: Carboxylic ester hydrolases. In: The Enzymes 3rd ed., Vol. 5, edit. by P.D. Boyer, pp. 43 – 69. New York – London: Academic Press 1972

Krupa, V., Blattel, R.A., Marks, G.S.: Drug-induced porphyrin biosynthesis IX. Levels of ^{14}C-allylisopropylacetamide, ^{14}C-propylisopropylacetamide and metabolite(s) in the livers of chick embryos and mice. Enzyme **16**, 276 – 285 (1973)

Krupa, V., Creighton, J.C., Freeman, M., Marks, G.S.: Drug-induced porphyrin biosynthesis—XII. Levels of cytochrome P-450 in chick embryo liver following administration of allylisopropylacetamide and propylisopropylacetamide. Canad. J. Physiol. Pharmacol. **52**, 891 – 895 (1974)

Leo, A., Hansch, C., Elkins, D.: Partition coefficients and their uses. Chem. Rev. **71**, 525 – 616 (1971)

Marks, G.S.: Unpublished observations (1975)

Marks, G.S., Hunter, E.G., Terner, U.K., Schneck, D.: Studies of the relationship between chemical structure and porphyria-inducing activity. Biochem. Pharmacol. **14**, 1077 – 1084 (1965)

Marks, G.S., Krupa, V., Murphy, F., Taub, H., Blattel, R.A.: Mechanisms of drug-induced porphyrin biosynthesis. Ann. N.Y. Acad. Sci. **244**, 472 – 480 (1975)

Marks, G.S., Krupa, V., Roomi, M.W.: Drug-induced porphyrin biosynthesis—VIII. Investigation of the importance of an allyl group for activity in substituted acetamides. Canad. J. Physiol. Pharmacol. **51**, 863 – 868 (1973)

Meyer, U.A., Strand, L.J., Doss, M., Rees, A.C., Marver, H.S.: Intermittent acute porphyria-demonstration of a genetic defect in porphobilinogen metabolism. New Engl. J. Med. **286**, 1277 – 1282 (1972)

Moore, M.R., Battistini, V., Beattie, A.D., Goldberg, A.: The effects of certain barbiturates on the hepatic porphyrin metabolism of rats. Biochem. Pharmacol. **19**, 751 – 757 (1970)

Morgan, R.O., Fischer, P.W.F., Marks, G.S.: Unpublished observations (1976)

Morgan, R.O., Fischer, P.W.F., Stephens, J.K., Marks, G.S.: Thyroid hormone enhancement of drug-induced porphyrin biosynthesis in chick embryo liver cells maintained in serum-free Waymouth medium. Biochem. Pharmacol. **25**, 2609 – 2612 (1976)

Murphy, F.R., Krupa, V., Marks, G.S.: Drug-induced porphyrin biosynthesis—XIII. Role of lipophilicity in determining porphyrin-inducing activity of aliphatic amides after blockade of their hydrolysis by bis-[p-nitrophenyl] phosphate. Biochem. Pharmacol. **24**, 883 – 889 (1975)

Murphy, F.R., Krupa, V., Marks, G.S.: Drug-induced porphyrin biosynthesis—XIV. Role of lipophilicity in determining porphyrin-inducing activity of esters and amides following blockade of their hydrolysis by bis-[p-nitrophenyl) phosphate. Biochem. Pharmacol. **25**, 1351 – 1354 (1976)

Murthy, V.V., Woods, J.S.: Solubilization and partial purification of mitochondrial δ-amino-levulinate synthase from fetal rat liver. Biochim. biophys. Acta (Amst.) **350**, 240 – 246 (1974)

Nebert, D.W., Gelboin, H.V.: The role of ribonucleic acid and protein synthesis in micro-somal aryl hydrocarbon hydroxylase induction in cell cultures: The independence of transcription and translation. J. biol. Chem. **245**, 160 – 168 (1970)

Ohashi, A., Kikuchi, G.: Mechanism of allylisopropylacetamide-induced increase of δ-amino-levulinate synthetase in liver mitochondria. VI. Multiple molecular forms of δ-amino-levulinate synthetase in the cytosol and mitochondria of induced cock liver. Arch. Biochem. Biophys. **153**, 34 – 46 (1972)

Peterkofsky, B., Tomkins, G.M.: Evidence for the steroid-induced accumulation of tyrosine aminotransferase messenger RNA in the absence of protein synthesis. Proc. nat. Acad. Sci. (Wash.) **60**, 222 – 228 (1968)

Poland, A., Glover, E.: 2,3,7,8-Tetrachlorodibenzo-*p*-dioxin: A potent inducer of δ-amino-levulinic acid synthetase. Science **179**, 476 – 477 (1973 a)

Poland, A., Glover, E.: Chlorinated dibenzo-*p*-dioxins: Potent inducers of δ-aminolevulinic acid synthetase and aryl hydrocarbon hydroxylase. II. A study of the structure-activity relationship. Molec. Pharmacol. **9**, 736 – 747 (1973 b)

Racz, W.J., Marks, G.S.: Drug-induced porphyrin biosynthesis—II. Simple procedure for screening drugs for porphyria-inducing activity. Biochem. Pharmacol. **18**, 2009 – 2018 (1969)

Racz, W.J., Marks, G.S.: Drug-induced porphyrin biosynthesis—IV. Investigation of the differences in response of isolated liver cells and the liver of the intact chick embryo to porphyria-inducing drugs. Biochem. Pharmacol. **21**, 143 – 151 (1972)

Racz, W.J. Moffat, J.A.: Drug metabolism in cell culture—I. Importance of steric factors for activity in porphyrin-inducing drugs. Biochem. Pharmacol. **23**, 215 – 221 (1974)

Rifkind, A.B., Gillette, P.N. Song, C.S., Kappas, A.: Induction of hepatic δ-aminolevulinic acid synthetase by oral contraceptive steroids. J. clin. Endocr. **30**, 330 – 335 (1970)

Rifkind, A.B., Gillette, P.N., Song, C.S., Kappas, A.: Drug stimulation of δ-aminolevulinic acid synthetase and cytochrome P-450 in vivo in chick embryo liver. J. Pharmacol. exp. Ther. **185**, 214 – 225 (1973)

Sassa, S., Granick, S.: Induction of δ-aminolevulinic acid synthetase in chick embryo liver cells in culture. Proc. nat. Acad. Sci. (Wash.) **67**, 517 – 522 (1970)

Schlesinger, F.G., Gastel (van), C.: Possible aggravation of abdominal symptoms by tolbutamide in a patient with diabetes and hepatic porphyria. Acta med. scand. **169**, 433 – 435 (1961)

Schmid, R., Schwartz, S.: Experimental porphyria III. Hepatic type produced by Sedormid. Proc. Soc. exp. Biol. (N.Y.) **81**, 685 – 689 (1952)

Schneck, D.W., Marks, G.S.: The inhibition of drug-induced porphyria by hemin. Pharmacologist **11**, 285 (1969)

Schneck, D.W., Racz, W.J., Hirsch, G.H., Bubbar, G.L., Marks, G.S.: Studies of the relationship between chemical structure and porphyria-inducing activity—IV. Investigations in a cell culture system. Biochem. Pharmacol. **17**, 1385 – 1399 (1968)

Sinclair, P.R., Granick, S.: Uroporphyrin formation induced by chlorinated hydrocarbons (lindane, polychlorinated biphenyls, tetrachlorodibenzo-*p*-dioxin). Requirements for endogenous iron, protein synthesis and drug-metabolizing activity. Biochem. biophys. Res. Commun. **61**, 124 – 133 (1974)

Song, C.S., Bonkowsky, H.L., Tschudy, D.P.: Salicylamide metabolism in acute intermittent porphyria. Clin. Pharmacol. Ther. **15**, 431 – 435 (1974)

Song, C.S., Singer, J.W., Levere, R.D., Harris, D.F., Kappas, A.: Developmental and gestational influences on drug induction of δ-aminolevulinic acid (ALA) synthetase in rat liver. J. Lab. clin. Med. **72**, 1019 – 1020 (1968)

Stich, W., Decker, P.: Studies on the mechanism of porphyrin biosynthesis with the aid of inhibitors. In: Ciba Foundation Symposium on Porphyrin Biosynthesis and Metabolism. Wolstenholme, G.E.W. and Miller, E.C.P. (eds.), pp. 254 – 260. London: J. and A. Churchill 1955

Strand, L.J., Manning, J., Marver, H.S.: The induction of δ-aminolevulinic acid synthetase in cultured liver cells. The effects of end product and inhibitors of heme synthesis. J. biol. Chem. **247**, 2820 – 2827 (1972)

Strik, J.J.T.W.A.: Chemical porphyria in Japanese quail (*Coturnix c. Japonica*). Enzyme **16**, 211 – 223 (1973)

Strik, J.J.T.W.A., Wit, J.G.: Hepatic porphyria in birds and mammals. TNO-nieuws **27**, 604 – 610 (1972)

Strittmatter, C.F., Umberger, F.T.: Oxidative enzyme components of avian liver microsomes. Changes during embryonic development and the effects of phenobarbital administration. Biochim. biophys. Acta (Amst.) **180**, 18 – 27 (1969)

Talman, E.L., Labbe, R.F., Aldrich, R.A.: Porphyrin metabolism. IV. Molecular structure of acetamide derivatives affecting porphyrin metabolism. Arch. Biochem. Biophys. **66,** 289 – 300 (1957)

Taub, H.: Drug-induced porphyrin biosynthesis. Effects of lipophilicity and hepatic metabolism on the porphyria-inducing activity of sedative-hypnotic drugs. M. Sc. Thesis, Queen's University, Kingston, Canada (1973)

Taub, H., Krupa, V., Marks, G.S.: Drug-induced porphyrin biosynthesis—XI. Effect of SKF 525-A on the activity of porphyrin-inducing drugs in chick embryos, chickens and rats. Biochem. Pharmacol. **25,** 511 – 516 (1976)

Taub, H., Marks, G.S.: Drug-induced porphyrin biosynthesis—X. Potentiation of propanidid-induced elevation of δ aminolevulinic acid synthetase and porphyrins in chick embryo liver by the carboxylesterase inhibitor bis-[*p*-nitrophenyl] phosphate. Canad. J. Physiol. Pharmacol. **51,** 700 – 704 (1973)

Tomita, Y., Ohashi, A., Kikuchi, G.: Induction of δ-aminolevulinate synthetase in organ culture of chick embryo liver by allylisopropylacetamide and 3,5-dicarbethoxy-1,4-dihydrocollidine. J. Biochem. **75,** 1007 – 1015 (1974)

Tyrrell, D.L.J., Marks, G.S.: Drug-induced porphyrin biosynthesis—V. Effect of protohemin on the transcriptional and post-transcriptional phases of δ-aminolevulinic acid synthetase induction. Biochem. Pharmacol. **21,** 2077 – 2093 (1972)

Vos, J.G., Botterweg, P.F., Strik, J.J.T.W.A., Koeman, J.H.: Experimental studies with HCB in birds. TNO-news, **27,** 599 – 603 (1972)

Watson, C.J.: Pursuit of the purple. J. Amer. med. Ass. **197,** 1074 – 1080 (1966)

Watson, C.J.: Private communication (1974)

Woods, J.S., Dixon, R.L.: Neonatal differences in the induction of hepatic aminolevulinic acid synthetase. Biochem. Pharmacol. **19,** 1951 – 1954 (1970a)

Woods, J.S., Dixon, R.L.: Perinatal differences in delta-aminolevulinic acid synthetase activity. Life Sci. **9,** 711 – 719 (1970b)

Pharmacogenetics in the Field of Heme Metabolism: Drug Sensitivity in Hereditary Hepatic Porphyria

J. Douglas Maxwell and Urs A. Meyer

Sir Archibald Garrod (1902), who pioneered the study of inborn errors of metabolism, was the first to suggest that unusual reactions to drugs might be caused by genetically determined aberrations in metabolic pathways. This far-sighted observation was neglected for many years. However, with the recognition in the 1950's that several "idiosyncratic" drug reactions, such as primaquine-induced hemolytic anemia and suxamethonium-induced prolonged apnoea, could be explained on the basis of genetically determined enzyme deficiencies, pharmacogenetics was established. Initially, the term referred only to hereditary disorders involving adverse reactions to drugs that were uncovered by administration of the particular agents. This definition seemed too restrictive, as it excluded from consideration genetically determined differences in drug metabolism or disposition (pharmacokinetics) and drug response (pharmacodynamics) between healthy non-medicated subjects (Vesell, 1975). When it became apparent that the interplay between genetics and pharmacology influenced the action of many drugs, the scope of pharmacogenetics was extended to include all studies at the interface of these two sciences. Pharmacogenetics now incorporates all clinically important hereditary variations in drug metabolism and response.

This paper is devoted to a consideration of a group of classical pharmaco-genetic disorders—the hereditary hepatic porphyrias. Recent clinical and laboratory studies will be presented which suggest that many of the previously unexplained features of this group of disorders can be understood on a mechanistic basis, and that the "idiosyncratic" reaction to many common drugs, which is such a characteristic feature of the hereditary hepatic porphyrias, is a direct consequence of the primary genetic defect in porphyrin and heme biosynthesis.

A. Hereditary Hepatic Porphyrias

The hepatic porphyrias are a group of disorders whose principal clinical manifestations are intermittent attacks of neuropsychiatric dysfunction and/or photosensitivity. They include intermittent acute porphyria (IAP), hereditary coproporphyria (HCP), variegate porphyria (VP), and porphyria cutanea tarda (PCT). All four are biochemically characterized by increased formation, accumulation, and excretion of porphyrin precursors and/or porphyrins in the liver, reflecting dysfunction of hepatic heme biosynthesis (Meyer and Schmid, 1977).

IAP, HCP, and VP constitute the three classical hereditary hepatic porphyrias. In these three disorders acute, often life-threatening attacks of an identical neuropsychiatric syndrome are commonly precipitated by normal therapeutic doses of

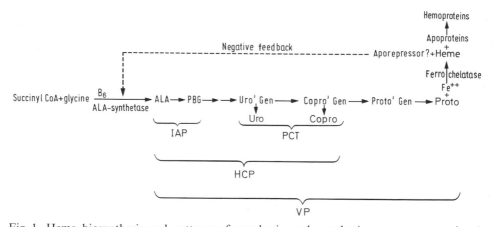

Fig. 1. Heme biosynthesis and patterns of porphyrin and porphyrin precursor excretion in the hepatic porphyrias. Intermediates of the pathway excessively excreted during the acute phase of each of the hepatic porphyrias are within the respective brackets. (ALA, δ-amino-levulinic acid; PBG, porphobilinogen; URO'GEN, uroporphyrinogen; COPRO'GEN, copro-porphyrinogen; PROTO'GEN, protoporphyrinogen; URO, uroporphyrin; COPRO, copro-porphyrin; PROTO, protoporphyrin; IAP, intermittent acute porphyria; PCT, porphyria cutanea tarda; HCP, hereditary coproporphyria; VP, variegate porphyria)

a variety of drugs. These three forms of hepatic porphyria can be distinguished, however, on the basis of additional clinical manifestations (such as the presence or absence of skin photosensitivity) and a unique pattern of porphyrin precursor and/or porphyrin excretion.

In PCT, less defined genetic and acquired abnormalities of hepatic heme bio-synthesis interact in causing hepatic accumulation of porphyrins. In contrast to IAP, HCP, and VP, the major clinical manifestations of PCT are limited to the skin, and the disease frequently is associated with evidence of hepatic dysfunc-tion. Acute attacks of neuropsychiatric disturbance and the associated massive excretion of porphyrin precursors do not occur in PCT; moreover, drugs that aggravate or precipitate symptoms in IAP, HCP, and VP in general have no adverse effect in PCT. In regard to the sensitivity to drugs, PCT is therefore clearly different from the classical hereditary hepatic porphyrias.

I. Enzyme Defects in the Hepatic Porphyrias

In all the hepatic porphyrias, the liver appears to be the major site where the inborn enzymatic error manifests itself metabolically by accumulation and, con-sequently, by excretion of porphyrins and porphyrin precursors. This does not mean that the genetic defect is limited to the liver; in IAP for example, cha-racteristic enzymatic abnormalities have been demonstrated in other tissues (MEYER, 1973). It is now established that increased activity of hepatic δ-amino-levulinic acid synthetase (ALA-synthetase), the first and rate-limiting enzyme in heme synthesis, is an enzymatic abnormality common to the three classical heredi-tary hepatic porphyrias (ELDER et al., 1972; MEYER and SCHMID, 1973; Fig. 1).

Furthermore, there is some evidence that during acute attacks, the activity of this enzyme is enhanced still further (TADDEINI and WATSON, 1968; STRAND et al., 1970; MCINTYRE et al., 1971), apparently contributing to the accumulation of porphyrin precursors characteristically seen at this time. However, although strikingly increased activity of hepatic ALA-synthetase is a constant feature of IAP, HCP, and VP, this is not seen in PCT, even in severe cases (MEYER and SCHMID, 1977). Furthermore, it has to be realized that increased activity of ALA-synthetase could not by itself account for the distinct patterns of porphyrin or porphyrin precursor excretion that typifies each of the hepatic porphyrias (Fig. 1).

Recent studies indicate that in IAP reduced activity of uroporphyrinogen I synthetase (which catalyses the condensation of 4 moles of PBG to 1 mol of uroporphyrinogen) represents the primary genetic defect in heme synthesis (MEYER et al., 1972). A partial block at this site conveniently explains both the specific pattern of porphyrin precursor excretion in IAP, and suggests that increased hepatic ALA-synthetase activity is a secondary phenomenon, possibly the result of a decreased negative feedback regulation by heme (SASSA and GRANICK, 1970; STRAND et al., 1972). The demonstration of a primary partial defect in heme synthesis in IAP supports the concept that the other forms of hereditary hepatic porphyria may be explained by analogous enzymatic defects at more distant sites in the pathway of heme biosynthesis.

1. Intermittent Acute Porphyria (IAP)

IAP is characterised by acute attacks of neuropsychiatric manifestations, including abdominal colic, hypertension, peripheral and central neuropathies and mental disturbance. Photosensitivity does not occur. Acute attacks are frequently precipitated by drugs as well as by hormonal, nutritional and other metabolic factors. Like the other hereditary hepatic porphyrias, it is inherited as an autosomal dominant disorder. The primary genetic defect in IAP is a generalized deficiency of uroporphyrinogen I synthetase. In the liver, this defect results in a secondary rise and apparently in enhanced "inducibility" of ALA-synthetase. As a consequence, urinary excretion of the porphyrin precursors δ-aminolevulinic acid (ALA) and porphobilinogen (PBG) is increased, without a proportional increase in porphyrin excretion (Fig. 1).

2. Hereditary Coproporphyria (HCP)

HCP resembles IAP both in its drug sensitivity and the occurrence of acute attacks with neuropsychiatric manifestations. In addition, photosensitivity may occur. HCP is inherited as an autosomal dominant disorder with variable clinical expression. The suspected defect is a deficiency of coproporphyrinogen oxidase, which secondarily affects the regulation of hepatic ALA-synthetase. The characteristic chemical finding is the unremitting excretion of large amounts of coproporphyrin in the feces and, to a lesser extent, in the urine. During acute attacks, urinary excretion of the porphyrin precursors ALA and PBG is increased.

3. Variegate Porphyria (VP)

VP is also inherited as an autosomal dominant disorder; it is characterized by drug sensitivity, and may exhibit neuropsychiatric manifestations. However, in addition, chronic skin sensitivity to light and to mechanical trauma is a prominent feature. Biochemically, VP is characterized by greatly enhanced excretion of faecal protoporphyrin and, to a lesser degree, of coproporphyrin. The suspected primary defect is a deficiency of an enzyme between protoporphyrinogen and heme. As in HCP, the urinary excretion of ALA and PBG is increased during acute attacks.

4. Porphyria Cutanea Tarda (PCT)

Photosensitivity is the only noteworthy clinical manifestation of this form of hepatic porphyria. Biochemically, it is characterized by excessive urinary excretion of uroporphyrins, together with smaller amounts of copro- and other porphyrins. Recent research suggests that, at least in some patients, PCT may be related to a dominantly inherited defect in uroporphyrinogen decarboxylase, but the metabolic expression of this genetic anomaly appears to require additional acquired factors, such as hepatic iron overload, alcohol, and estrogens. In PCT, the underlying primary genetic defect (in contrast to the classical hereditary hepatic porphyrias) does not appear to result in significantly altered regulation of the heme pathway, as ALA-synthetase activity remains normal or only minimally increased, even in overt cases. This observation probably accounts for the critical clinical and biochemical difference between PCT and the classical hereditary hepatic porphyrias— namely the absence of acute neuropsychiatric attacks, normal urinary excretion of porphyrin precursors ALA and PBG, and the lack of sensitivity to drugs such as barbiturates.

II. Biochemical Basis for Clinical Features in the Hepatic Porphyrias

It has been difficult to establish a causal relationship between the metabolic defects in porphyrin and heme biosynthesis and the various clinical abnormalities in the hereditary hepatic porphyrias, because little is known of the pharmacological effects of porphyrins and porphyrin precursors. However, it is most likely that *porphyrin* accumulation in plasma or skin is responsible for photosensitivity in VP, HCP, and PCT (RIMINGTON et al., 1967). The other noncutaneous features characteristic of an acute attack of hereditary hepatic porphyria can all be explained by disturbances of central or peripheral nervous system functions (RIDLEY, 1969), but the pathogenetic link between the biochemical abnormality in heme synthesis and these clinical manifestations remains obscure. Numerous hypotheses have been advanced to explain the neuropsychiatric manifestations, but none is supported by convincing experimental evidence. The neurologic dysfunction cannot yet be defined in biochemical terms, but a partial enzymatic block in heme synthesis has a number of possible theoretical implications for the pathogenesis of neurotoxicity. If it is assumed that enzyme activity is also deficient in cells of the nervous system, this could lead to intraneuronal accumulation of porphyrin precursors and possibly result in neurocytotoxicity. Alternatively, if heme synthesis in the nervous system were regulated in a different manner from that in the liver, the enzymatic defect could result in impaired availability of heme for hemoproteins, which might in turn result in metabolic impairment. It is also conceivable that the neuropsychiatric manifestations might be caused by depletion of critical metabolites or by accumulation of neurotoxic substances which, while not directly related to heme synthesis, may be a consequence of the inherited defect (MEYER and SCHMID, 1974). However, the most attractive explanation at present for the neuropsychiatric phenomena is that excess *porphyrin precursors* (ALA and/or PBG) formed in the liver may gain access to the nervous system and there exert a toxic effect. This hypothesis is supported by the observation that the neurologic manifestations occur only in those hepatic porphyrias in which there is excessive hepatic accumulation and urinary excretion of porphyrin precursors (IAP, VP, and HCP). Moreover, in patients with IAP, a rough correlation has been found between the concentration of ALA and PBG in serum and the extent of neuropsychiatric manifestations (DHAR et al., 1975). Furthermore, the recently demonstrated effectiveness of hematin infusion in patients with acute attacks of hepatic porphyria (WATSON, 1975) is also consistent with the concept that elevated plasma levels of ALA and/or PBG may be causally related to the pathogenesis of the neurologic lesion. Because of the similarities between some clinical features of lead poisoning and acute porphyria (DAGG et al., 1965), ALA is a prime suspect as a mediator of the neurologic lesion. Although various studies have shown ALA and PBG to affect nerve function in vitro, the significance of these effects for the pathogenesis of acute porphyria remains controversial. The neurotoxicity of the porphyrin precursors has not been conclusively demonstrated in vivo, but no studies have yet been carried out in animal models of hepatic porphyria with generalized partial blocks in heme synthesis mimicking the genetic defect in man.

B. Precipitation of Hereditary Hepatic Porphyria by Drugs

In his classical monograph on intermittent acute porphyria published in 1937, WALDENSTROM drew attention to the role of barbiturates in precipitating acute porphyria, an association which had first been reported some 30 years earlier by DOBRSCHANSKY (1906). Further evidence of a relationship between drug administration and acute attacks of hepatic porphyria has come from South Africa, where a large genetic reservoir of one form of inherited porphyria—variegate porphyria— has existed for over two centuries. Interestingly, the clinical expression of this genetic disorder was virtually unrecognized until the therapeutic revolution of the past three to four decades, resulting in the widespread use of drugs, such as the barbiturates. Since that time, acute attacks of variegate porphyria have become a substantial problem in South Africa (DEAN, 1963).

In all forms of the hereditary hepatic porphyrias, both the intermittent nature of the clinical disorder and the existence of latent cases (WITH, 1963; MEYER, 1973) provide evidence that the primary genetic defect is frequently not expressed and point to the importance of additional endogenous or environmental factors in initiating acute attacks. Imprudent drug administration appears to be particularly important in this respect and has been implicated as a precipitating factor in between 50% and 75% of acute attacks (STEIN and TSCHUDY, 1970; EALES, 1971). Moreover, it has been claimed that drug-related attacks are associated with a more severe neurologic disturbance than spontaneous episodes of acute porphyria (GOLDBERG, 1959). Barbiturates remain the drugs most commonly associated with acute attacks of hepatic porphyria, and in one report they featured in over 50% of acute attacks (EALES, 1971). A heterogeneous group of nonbarbiturate sedatives and other structurally dissimilar drugs have also been implicated as possible precipitating factors of the acute attack. The association of drugs and acute attacks may have been under-estimated, as cases of deliberate suppression of a history of prior drug ingestion have been recognized (Table 1). The natural course of the disease is variable and unpredictable, and because of this the evidence associating any given drug with an acute attack is open to question. Many patients had been taking several drugs at the time of an acute attack, and under these circumstances it was difficult to implicate one drug rather than another. Furthermore, the primary indication for drug treatment (e.g., infection), rather than the drug itself (e.g., sulphonamide), may have been the major factor responsible for precipitating an acute attack (STEIN and TSCHUDY, 1970; EALES, 1971). However, for the barbiturates at least, the evidence for a causal relationship between drug intake and an acute attack seems undeniable. There are many well-documented reports of previously healthy individuals who developed acute attacks following thiopentone anesthesia for minor extraabdominal surgery. On the other hand, the susceptibility of porphyric subjects to barbiturates seems to be unpredictable, as there are many patients who have undergone drug administration or thiopentone anesthesia without ill effect.

Recent clinical and laboratory studies have provided information that now allows a better understanding of the possible mode of action of drugs in precipitating acute attacks of human hepatic porphyria. The key to this progress has been a better understanding of factors regulating heme biosynthesis, particularly the negative feedback control of ALA-synthetase by the end product of the pathway, heme (for review see MEYER and SCHMID, 1977; and the chapter by TAIT in this volume). Moreover, the elucidation of the mechanism of action of certain chemicals that cause experimental porphyria in rodents and cell culture has contributed to this progress (TSCHUDY and BONKOWSKY, 1972; and see chapters by DE MATTEIS and MARKS in this volume).

Table 1. Some drugs known or reported to precipitate acute attacks of porphyria

Alcohol	Ethylalcohol
Anticonvulsants	Hydantoins; Succinimides
Barbiturates	All varieties, including thiopentone
Chemotherapeutics	Griseofulvin; Sulphonamides
Hypoglycaemics	Tolbutamide
Hypotensives	Methyl dopa
Nonbarbiturate hypnotics	Dichloralphenazone; Glutethimide
Tranquillizers	Meprobamate
Steroids	Estrogens; Progestagens

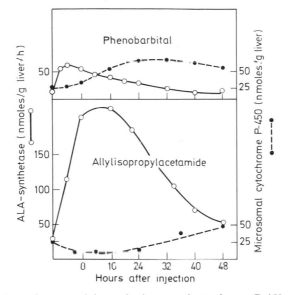

Fig. 2. Hepatic ALA-synthetase activity and microsomal cytochrome P-450 concentration after a single injection of phenobarbital or allylisopropylacetamide in rats (from MEYER and MARVER, 1971, copyright 1971 by the American Association for the Advancement of Science)

C. Experimental Models for the Exacerbation of Hereditary Hepatic Porphyria by Drugs

Drugs implicated in precipitating acute attacks in patients with inherited porphyria are structurally diverse. However, this varied group of drugs shares with the experimental porphyrinogenic compounds the property of lipid solubility. Indeed, many of these drugs are recognised as potent inducers of cytochrome P-450 and the hepatic microsomal mixed-function oxidase system (CONNEY, 1967). Normally, induction of cytochrome P-450 by such drugs in laboratory animals is preceded by a slight rise in hepatic ALA-synthetase activity. This response has been interpreted as providing the additional heme required for increased synthesis of hemoproteins and contrasts strikingly with the divergent effect of porphyrinogenic compounds, such as allylisopropylacetamide (AIA), which stimulate markedly hepatic ALA-synthetase activity but cause an initial loss, not an increase of cytochrome P-450 concentration (Fig. 2 and see chapter by DE MATTEIS in this volume).

Barbiturates do not cause clinical attacks of porphyria in normal subjects, nor do they increase porphyrin or porphyrin precursor excretion in laboratory rodents. These and other common drugs, which are innocuous in normal individuals but which provoke acute attacks in subjects with inherited hepatic porphyria, are thought to do so by eliciting a sustained increase in ALA-synthetase activity. Why they should cause this idiosyncratic reaction in patients with a genetically determined abnormality in heme synthesis has until recently been unexplained.

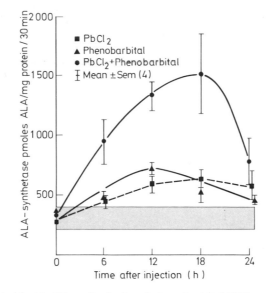

Fig. 3. Effect of lead chloride (10 mg/kg i.v.) and phenobarbital (100 mg/kg i.p.), alone and in combination, on hepatic ALA-synthetase in rats (from MAXWELL and MEYER, 1976, reproduced with permission of the Europ. J. Clin. Invest.)

Studies from our own and other laboratories have indicated that a similar basic regulatory mechanism may account for massive induction of hepatic ALA-synthetase in both experimental porphyria and the human pharmacogenetic disorder. These studies will be briefly outlined, and a hypothesis presented which may explain the idiosyncrasy to common drugs shown by susceptible patients. Experiments in cultures of chick embryo liver (STRAND et al., 1972; SINCLAIR and GRANICK, 1975) and in rodents (DE MATTEIS and GIBBS, 1972; DE MATTEIS, 1973b; MAXWELL and MEYER, 1976) have suggested that the extreme sensitivity to drugs of patients with hepatic porphyria may be a consequence of increased sensitivity of hepatic ALA-synthetase to induction by these drugs. Evidence in favour of this hypothesis is provided by the studies considered in detail below.

Partial inhibition of heme biosynthesis was produced in rats by lead, which inhibits several enzymes of the pathway (GOLDBERG, 1972). Following such experimentally acquired partial blocks in heme synthesis (mimicking the genetic partial block in heme synthesis in IAP), a modest rise in ALA-synthetase activity occurs, possibly due to negative feedback derepression. However, when phenobarbital is given in combination with lead, induction of ALA-synthetase is greatly enhanced (MAXWELL and MEYER, 1974, 1976; Fig. 3).

A similar synergistic effect of lead was observed with various other barbiturates, chloral hydrate, antipyrine, progesterone, and small doses of the porphyrinogenic compound AIA. Cycloheximide administered before the injection of lead, phenobarbital, or of the combination of lead and phenobarbital, completely abolished the rise in ALA-synthetase activity. Additional studies revealed that the potentiation of the effect of lead on drug-mediated induction of ALA-synthetase

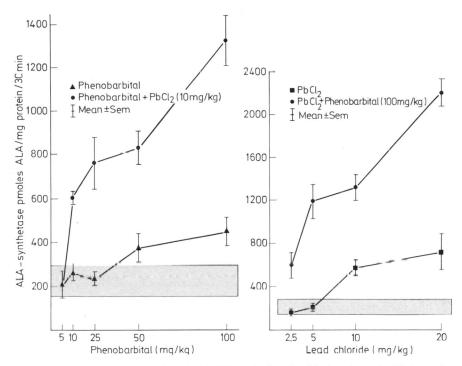

Fig. 4. Effects of varying doses of lead chloride and phenobarbital on hepatic ALA-synthetase activity in rats (from MAXWELL and MEYER, 1976, reproduced with permission of the Europ. J. Clin. Invest.)

was related to both the dose of lead and the dose of the inducing agent (Fig. 4). Moreover, the effects of lead and phenobarbital on ALA-synthetase were paralleled by similar striking changes in the urinary excretion of ALA. Lead alone predictably caused an increase in the excretion of the porphyrin precursor ALA, which was dose related, but this effect was greatly enhanced by the addition of phenobarbital (Fig. 5).

A similar potentiation of ALA-synthetase activity was observed when phenobarbital, phenylbutazone, or many other lipid-soluble drugs were administered together with small doses of 3,5-diethoxycarbonyl-1,4-dihydro-2,4,6-trimethyl-pyridine (DDC) or AIA (DE MATTEIS, 1973b; BOCK et al., 1973; PADMANABAN et al., 1973). Thus, partial blocks in heme synthesis appear to greatly increase the sensitivity of ALA-synthetase to induction.

Since partial blocks in heme synthesis may also interfere with hemoprotein formation, the effects of lead on cytochrome P-450 and drug metabolism were studied. Lead administration resulted in a significant fall in microsomal cytochrome P-450 concentration, and the combination of lead and phenobarbital delayed and impaired the normal adaptive rise in cytochrome P-450 concentration observed after phenobarbital alone (Fig. 6). This effect was paralleled by reduced drug metabolism in hepatic microsomes in vitro (demethylation of paranitroanisole) (MAXWELL and MEYER, 1974, 1976).

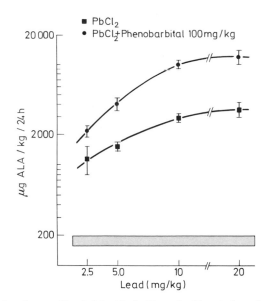

Fig. 5. Effect of varying doses of lead chloride (with and without phenobarbital) on the urinary excretion of ALA in the rat (from MAXWELL and MEYER, 1976, reproduced with permission of the Europ. J. Clin. Invest.)

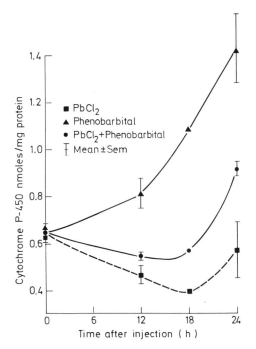

Fig. 6. Effect of lead chloride (10 mg/kg i.v.) and phenobarbital, alone and in combination, on hepatic microsomal cytochrome P-450 concentration (from MAXWELL and MEYER, 1976, reproduced with permission of the Europ. J. Clin. Invest.)

The idiosyncratic reaction to many common drugs in patients with the hereditary hepatic porphyrias has naturally inhibited clinical studies of drug metabolism in this group of disorders. However, two recent clinical studies indicated definite impairment of the metabolism of salicylamide and antipyrine in patients with overt IAP, while glucuronidation of the drug was unaffected (SONG et al., 1974; ANDERSON et al., 1976).

As explained above, barbiturates and other drugs have by themselves little effect on ALA-synthetase activity in laboratory animals with unimpaired heme biosynthesis and do not cause a marked increase in porphyrin or porphyrin precursor excretion in these animals. Curiously, however, they are capable of causing striking induction of ALA-synthetase and porphyrin accumulation in cultured chick embryo liver cells (GRANICK, 1966). This system thus appears to be a model for human-inherited hepatic porphyria and has been used to screen for drugs potentially dangerous to porphyric subjects (RIFKIND et al., 1973). In the chick embryo liver system, the stimulatory effect on ALA-synthetase activity appears to be related both to the lipid solubility of the test drug (DE MATTEIS, 1971 a) and possibly also its low rate of metabolism (see chapter by MARKS in this volume).

D. Common Basis for Induction of Hepatic ALA-Synthetase in Clinical and Experimental Porphyria

Recognition of a common underlying basis for both the drug idiosyncrasy characteristic of the hereditary hepatic porphyrias and for experimental porphyrogenesis has emerged from the laboratory studies outlined above. Increased activity of hepatic ALA-synthetase with consequent overproduction of porphyrins and/or porphyrin precursors (features common to both the acute attacks of hereditary hepatic porphyria and experimental chemical porphyria) appears to result from the coexistence of two separate requirements, each of which alone may have only moderate or no effect on the enzyme. These are 1. an affect on heme synthesis or degradation, and 2. exposure to lipid-soluble inducers of hemoprotein synthesis, such as certain drugs and possibly endogenous substances (Fig. 7). Thus, experi-

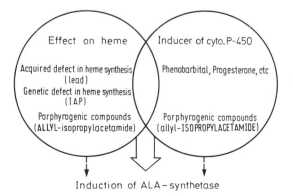

Fig. 7. Dual requirements for potentiation of the induction of hepatic ALA-synthetase

mental reduction of a certain pool of intracellular heme, for example, when heme synthesis is partially blocked by lead, may moderately induce ALA-synthetase. Likewise, phenobarbital and other inducers of hemoprotein cytochrome P-450 may also moderately stimulate the activity of this enzyme but without affecting porphyrin or porphyrin precursor excretion. However, when both factors are present together, a synergistic effect is seen, with massive induction of ALA-synthetase (depicted by the broad arrow in Fig. 7), which is accompanied by greatly enhanced excretion of precursors (Maxwell and Meyer, 1974, 1976).

The analogy with IAP is clear, since in this clinical setting, defective adaptation of heme synthesis is a consequence of the intrinsic genetic disorder. It has been proposed that the partial defect in heme synthesis in IAP may result in derepression of ALA-synthetase through negative feedback regulation, and that because of the kinetic properties of the enzymatic steps following ALA-synthetase, the increase in PBG production may be sufficient to partially overcome the defect in heme synthesis (Meyer and Schmid, 1973). Thus, despite the partial block, the "effective" heme concentration and heme available for basal hemoprotein synthesis may approach normal levels, provided ALA-synthetase and, therefore, heme synthesis remains induced. Such a "compensated" block may reflect the situation in a patient with "latent" porphyria where clinical symptoms are absent and precursor excretion in the urine may be negligible. However, this precarious equilibrium is readily disturbed by any of a large number of drugs (and possibly naturally occurring endogenous inducers) which have little or no effect on ALA-synthetase in the normal hepatocyte but may precipitate "acute porphyria" in individuals with a genetic defect in heme synthesis.

The exact mechanism of increased sensitivity of ALA-synthetase to induction in the presence of partial inhibition of heme synthesis remains to be determined, but it appears to be related to the negative feedback regulation of heme synthesis. Thus, the inability of an hepatocyte with compromised heme synthesis to respond appropriately to a sudden demand for increased synthesis of heme (such as is created by inducers of hemoprotein cytochrome P-450) would result in persistence of the regulatory feedback signal and hence exaggerated stimulation of ALA-synthetase activity. Recent studies by Correia and Meyer (1975) and Meyer et al. (1976) have shown that partial enzymatic blocks in heme synthesis disturb the normally closely coordinated synthesis of mitochondrial heme and microsomal apoprotein during induction of cytochrome P-450 and result in a relative excess of free apocytochrome P-450 in the liver. Further studies have suggested that increased synthesis of apocytochrome P-450 is the primary event in drug-mediated induction of holocytochrome P-450 (Correia and Meyer, 1975; Rajamanickam et al., 1975). This has provided support to the speculation that free apocytochrome P-450 may quantitatively reflect the regulatory signal for induction of ALA-synthetase by drugs. Massive induction of ALA-synthetase by inducers of cytochrome P-450 in the presence of partial blocks in heme synthesis may represent an attempt to overcome the block and provide the heme required for combination with free apocytochrome P-450. Whether the regulatory signal for synthesis of ALA-synthetase is mediated directly via free apoprotein concentration ("positive feedback") (Padmanaban et al., 1973) or in response to the prevailing deficiency of a certain heme pool ("negative feedback") (DE MATTEIS and GIBBS, 1972), or by some other mechanism remains to be determined.

The recent clinical studies indicating impaired hepatic biotransformation of salicylamide and antipyrine in patients with IAP (SONG et al., 1974; ANDERSON et al., 1976) raise the possibility that impaired hepatic biotransformation may contribute to the drug idiosyncrasy in hepatic porphyria. One consequence of impaired metabolism of an inducing agent is that its stimulatory effect on ALA-synthetase activity will be enhanced, as enzyme induction is a dose-dependent phenomenon and may be influenced by the rate of biotransformation of the inducer in the target organ (see chapter by MARKS in this volume). Slowing the metabolism of an inducing drug would increase its effectiveness as an inducer and thus may contribute to the massive induction of ALA-synthetase. The in vitro studies in lead-treated rats indeed showed impaired demethylation of paranitroanisole (MAXWELL and MEYER, 1976). A necessary corollary to this definition of the hereditary hepatic porphyrias as a group of pharmacogenetic disorders of heme synthesis characterized by a unique sensitivity to enzyme inducing agents is the recognition that those drugs which may be safely used in these patients are relatively weak or ineffective inducers of microsomal hemoproteins (Table 2). A further consequence of the dual requirements underlying massive induction of hepatic ALA-synthetase is the recognition that it is inappropriate to screen drugs as safe for use in patients with inherited hepatic porphyria simply on the basis of their failure to affect ALA-synthetase activity in laboratory animals with an intact heme pathway, as for example in the report of BEATTIE et al. (1973).

The scheme depicted in Fig. 7 may also be relevant to an understanding of the mechanism of action of potent experimental porphyrinogenic compounds, such as AIA, DDC, and griseofulvin. These compounds may functionally be analogous to the experimental combination of lead and phenobarbital in that each possesses in a single molecule the dual properties for massive induction of ALA-synthetase. This duality is most readily apparent with allyl-substituted compounds, where the allyl group is responsible for the effect on heme, while the remainder of the lipid-soluble molecule may provide the inducing moiety.

The paradoxic effect of prior exposure of an experimental animal to enzyme-inducing drugs in enhancing heme degradation but at the same time diminishing the porphyrinogenic effect of subsequently administered AIA (KAUFMAN et al., 1970; DE MATTEIS, 1973a; SCHMID, 1973) can now be understood on a rational basis. Thus, while microsomal enzyme induction will enhance the effect of AIA on

Table 2. Some drugs considered to be safe (or probably safe) in the hereditary hepatic porphyrias

Analgesics	Aspirin; morphine and related opiates; paracetamol
Antibiotics	Penicillin
Psychoactive drugs	Amitriptyline; chlorpromazine
Antihistamines	Diphenhydramine; mepyramine
Hypotensives	Bethanidine; guanethidine
Miscellaneous	Atropine; digoxin; neostigmine/prostigmine; propranolol; vitamins B, C, E

heme degradation by accelerating the biotransformation of the allyl moiety to the active metabolite responsible for this effect (De Matteis, 1971b), it also accelerates the metabolism of the remainder of the molecule (the inducing moiety) (Kaufman et al., 1970), reducing its availability and thus its inducing potential. This latter effect apparently negates the former and could account for the net reduction in ALA-synthetase activity observed.

While these recent studies have given some insight into the basis of these pharmacogenetic disorders of heme synthesis, the concept of dual requirements for massive induction of ALA-synthetase in IAP, HCP, and VP is necessarily an oversimplification. In an individual with the underlying genetic disorder, response to drug administration is unpredictable, and it is likely that a number of factors will determine whether or not an acute attack will be precipitated. These include the genetically determined activity of the defective enzyme in heme biosynthesis, together with the individual dose of drug absorbed and its inducing potential. A variety of other factors, such as the hormonal environment and nutritional state ("glucose effect") have been shown to influence the inducibility of mitochondrial ALA-synthetase (see chapter by Tschudy in this volume), and there is considerable evidence that the inducibility of the microsomal P-450 system is to a large extent genetically determined (Vesell, 1975). Moreover, the apparent insensitivity of patients with PCT to the effects of enzyme-inducing drugs is puzzling. However, the explanation for this discrepancy, as suggested earlier, seems to lie in the fact that in this form of hereditary hepatic porphyria, the partial enzymatic defect is insufficient to affect the feedback-regulation of ALA-synthetase by heme. Hence, ALA-synthetase activity and its inducibility remain unaffected. Finally, our explanation for the pathogenesis of this group of pharmacogenetic disorders requires that the development of the neurologic syndrome is directly related to massive induction of ALA-synthetase and consequent accumulation of porphyrin precursors, for which there is as yet only indirect evidence (Meyer and Schmid, 1974).

Acknowledgements: Original studies reported in this chapter were supported in part by Grants GM 16496 and AM 11275 from the National Institutes of Health, Grant ASC 48 from the Academic Senate, University of California, San Francisco, Grant 3.9140.72 from the Schweizerische Nationalfonds zur Förderung der wissenschaftlichen Forschung, and by a Bay Area Heart Association Fellowship awarded to J.D.M.

References

Anderson, K.E., Alvarez, A.P., Sassa, S., Kappas, A.: Studies in porphyria. V. Drug oxidation rates in hereditary hepatic porphyria. Clin. Pharmacol. Ther. **19**, 47−54 (1976)

Beattie, A.D., Moore, M.R., Goldberg, A., Ward, R.L.: Acute intermittent porphyria: Response of tachycardia and hypertension to propranolol. Brit. med. J. **1973 III**, 257−260

Bock, K.W., Weiner, R., Frohling, W.: Regulation of δ-aminolevulinate synthetase by steroids and drugs in isolated perfused rat liver. Enzyme **16**, 295−301 (1973)

Conney, A.H.: Pharmacological implications of microsomal enzyme induction. Pharmacol. Rev. **19**, 317−366 (1967)

Correia, M.A., Meyer, U.A.: Apocytochrome P-450: Reconstitution of functional cytochrome with hemin in vitro. Proc. nat. Acad. Sci. (Wash.) **72**, 400−404 (1975)

Dagg, J.H., Goldberg, A., Lochhead, A., Smith, J.A.: The relationship of lead poisoning to acute intermittent porphyria. Quart. J. Med. **34**, 163 – 175 (1965)

Dean, G.: The prevalence of the porphyrias. S. Afr. J. Lab. clin. Med. **9**, 145 – 151 (1963)

De Matteis, F.: Drugs and porphyria. S. Afr. med. J. **45**, 126 – 133 (1971 a)

De Matteis, F.: Loss of heme in rat liver caused by the porphyrogenic agent 2-allyl-2-isopropylacetamide. Biochem. J. **124**, 767 – 777 (1971 b)

De Matteis, F.: Drug-induced destruction of cytochrome P-450. Drug Metab. Dispos. **1**, 267 – 272 (1973 a)

De Matteis, F.: Drug interactions in experimental hepatic porphyria: A model for the exacerbation by drugs of human variegate porphyria. Enzyme **16**, 266 – 275 (1973 b)

De Matteis, F., Gibbs, A.H.: Stimulation of liver δ-aminolaevulinate synthetase by drugs and its relevance to drug-induced accumulation of cytochrome P-450. Biochem. J. **126**, 1149 – 1160 (1972)

Dhar, G.J., Bossenmaier, I., Petryka, Z.J., Cardinal, R., Watson, C.J.: Effects of hematin in hepatic porphyria. Further studies. Ann. intern. Med. **83**, 20 – 30 (1975)

Dobrschansky, M.: Einiges über Malonal. Wien med. Presse **47**, 2145 – 2151 (1906)

Eales, L.: Acute porphyria: The precipitating and aggravating factors. S. Afr. med. J. **45**, 120 – 125 (1971)

Elder, G.H., Gray, C.H., Nicholson, D.C.: The porphyrias: a review. J. clin. Path. **25**, 1013 – 1033 (1972)

Garrod, A.E.: The incidence of alkaptonuria: A study in chemical individuality. Lancet **1902 II**, 1616 – 1620

Goldberg, A.: Acute intermittent porphyria. Quart. J. Med. **28**, 183 – 209 (1959)

Goldberg, A.: Lead poisoning and heme biosynthesis. Brit. J. Haemat. **23**, 521 – 524 (1972)

Granick, S.: The induction in vitro of the synthesis of δ-aminolaevulinic acid synthetase in chemical porphyria. A response to certain drugs, sex hormones, and foreign chemicals. J. biol. Chem. **241**, 1359 – 1375 (1966)

Kaufman, L., Swanson, A.L., Marver, H.S.: Chemically induced porphyria: Prevention by prior treatment with phenobarbital. Science **170**, 320 – 322 (1970)

Maxwell, J.D., Meyer, U.A.: Drug sensitivity in hepatic porphyria: Relationship to defect in heme synthesis. J. clin. Invest. **53**, 51 A (1974)

Maxwell, J.D., Meyer, U.A.: Effect of lead on hepatic δ-aminolaevulinic acid synthetase activity in the rat: A model for drug sensitivity in intermittent acute porphyria. Europ. J. clin. Invest. **6**, 373 – 379 (1976)

McIntyre, N., Pearson, A.J.G., Allan, D.J., Craske, S., West, G.M.L., Moore, M.R., Paxton, J., Beattie, A.D., Goldberg, A.: Hepatic δ-aminolaevulinic acid synthetase in an attack of hereditary coproporphyria and during remission. Lancet **1971 I**, 560 – 564

Meyer, U.A.: Intermittent acute porphyria: Clinical and biochemical studies of disordered heme biosynthesis. Enzyme **16**, 334 – 342 (1973)

Meyer, U.A., Marver, H.S.: Chemically induced porphyria: increased microsomal heme turnover after treatment with allyl isopropylacetamide. Science **171**, 64 – 66 (1971)

Meyer, U.A., Meier, P.J., Correia, A.M.: Interaction between mitochondria and rough endoplasmic reticulum during induction of cytochrome P-450. In: The Liver. Quantitative Aspects of Structure and Function. Preisig, R., Bircher, J., Paumgartner, G. (eds.), pp. 172 – 178. Aulendorf, Germany: Editio Cantor 1976

Meyer, U.A., Schmid, R.: Hereditary hepatic porphyrias. Fed. Proc. **32**, 1649 – 1655 (1973)

Meyer, U.A., Schmid, R.: Intermittent acute porphyria. Res. Publ. Ass. nerv. ment. Dis. **33**, 211 – 223 (1974)

Meyer, U.A., Schmid, R.: The porphyrias. In: The Metabolic Basis of Inherited Disease. Stanbury, J.B., Wyngaarden, J.B., Frederickson, D.S. (eds.), 4th edit. New York: McGraw-Hill 1977

Meyer, U.A., Strand, L.T., Doss, M., Rees, A.C., Marver, H.S.: Intermittent acute porphyria: Demonstration of a genetic defect in porphobilinogen metabolism. New Engl. J. Med. **286**, 1277 – 1282 (1972)

Padmanaban, G., Rao, M.R.S., Malathi, K.: A model for the regulation of δ-aminolevulinate synthetase induction in rat liver. Biochem. J. **134**, 847 – 857 (1973)

Rajamanickam, C., Rao, M.R.S., Padmanaban, G.: On the sequence of reactions leading to cytochrome P-450 synthesis. Effect of drugs. J. biol. Chem. **250**, 2305 – 2310 (1975)

Ridley, A.: The neuropathology of acute intermittent porphyria. Quart. J. Med. **38**, 307 – 333 (1969)

Rifkind, A.B., Gillette, P.N., Song, C.S., Kappas, A.: Drug stimulation of δ-aminolevulinic acid synthetase and cytochrome P-450 in vivo in chick embryo liver. J. Pharmacol. exp. Ther. **185**, 214 – 225 (1973)

Rimington, C., Magnus, I.A., Ryan, E.A., Cripps, D.J.: Porphyria and photosensitivity. Quart. J. Med. **36**, 29 – 57 (1967)

Sassa, S., Granick, S.: Induction of δ-aminolevulinic acid synthetase in chick embryo liver cells in culture. Proc. nat. Acad. Sci. (Wash.) **67**, 517 – 522 (1970)

Schmid, R.: Discussion of paper by De Matteis, F. Drug Metab. Dispos. **1**, 273 (1973)

Sinclair, P.R., Granick, S.: Heme control of the synthesis of δ-aminolevulinic acid synthetase in cultured chick embryo liver cells. Ann. N.Y. Acad. Sci. **244**, 509 – 520 (1975)

Song, C.S., Bonkowsky, H.L., Tschudy, D.P.: Salicylamide metabolism in acute intermittent porphyria. Clin. Pharmacol. Ther. **15**, 431 – 435 (1974)

Stein, J.A., Tschudy, D.P.: Acute intermittent porphyria: A clinical and biochemical study of 46 patients. Medicine (Baltimore) **49**, 1 – 16 (1970)

Strand, J.L., Felsher, B.F., Redeker, A.G., Marver, H.S.: Heme biosynthesis in intermittent acute porphyria: decreased hepatic conversion of porphobilinogen to porphyrins and increased δ-aminolevulinic acid synthetase activity. Proc. nat. Acad. Sci. (Wash.) **67**, 1315 – 1320 (1970)

Strand, J.L., Manning, J., Marver, H.S.: The induction of δ-aminolevulinic acid synthetase in cultured liver cells. J. biol. Chem. **247**, 2820 – 2827 (1972)

Taddeini, L., Watson, C.J.: The clinical porphyrias. Sem. Hemat. **5**, 335 – 369 (1968)

Tschudy, D.P., Bonkowsky, H.L.: Experimental porphyria. Fed. Proc. **31**, 147 – 159 (1972)

Vesell, E.S.: Pharmacogenetics. Biochem. Pharmacol. **24**, 445 – 450 (1975)

Waldenstrom, J.: Studien über Porphyrie. Acta med. scand. Suppl. **82** (1937)

Watson, C.T.: Haematin and porphyria. New Engl. J. Med. **293**, 605 – 607 (1975)

With, T.K.: Acute intermittent porphyria: Family studies on the excretion of PBG and delta-ALA with ion exchange chromatography. Z. klin. Chem. **1**, 134 – 143 (1963)

CHAPTER 9

The Influence of Hormonal and Nutritional Factors on the Regulation of Liver Heme Biosynthesis

D. P. TSCHUDY

A. Introduction

The liver plays a major role in maintaining the chemical homeostasis of the organism. It does this by a variety of mechanisms. Some compounds of both endogenous and exogenous origin are chemically modified for eventual excretion in the urine and others are excreted into the gut before or after modification by the liver. In addition to its excretory functions the liver also serves as a sort of "chemical valve" between materials ingested from the environment and the "internal milieu." In this capacity it handles the standard components of the diet, adjusting their composition to the needs of the body as well as modifying other foreign compounds for excretion. Some of the reactions involved in these processes are catalyzed by heme-containing enzymes. Since the demands for these reactions vary with changing conditions of diet, drug intake, and hormonal changes, it would seem that the most efficient way for the liver to adjust to these changing needs would be through the development of control mechanisms which can appropriately alter the activities of the enzymes involved. Such changes in carbohydrate-metabolizing enzymes have been studied extensively and for the most part the changes fit rather nicely into a logical or readily understood pattern. The heme biosynthetic pathway would also be expected to respond to various demands, which it clearly does. The changes, however, do not always fit into simple logical patterns, as will be shown by the subsequent discussion, which will be mainly restricted to the effect of hormonal and nutritional factors in the liver.

B. The Influence of Nutritional Factors

I. Carbohydrates and Protein

1. The "Glucose Effect" in Experimental Porphyria

The sequence of studies in experimental porphyria is an excellent example of how basic research in an experimental disease in animals led to discoveries which had considerable value in the understanding and treatment of the human porphyrias. While attempting to elucidate the basic enzyme changes which explain the excessive porphyrin precursor excretion in allylisopropylacetamide (AIA)-induced porphyria, it was found that the porphyria could be prevented by sufficient intake of diet (ROSE et al., 1961). The active components of the diet were found to be carbohydrate and protein. Other types of experimental porphyria were also shown to be inhibited by increasing diet intake (De Matteis, 1964). Increasing food intake decreased the excretion of δ-aminolevulinic acid (ALA), porphobilinogen (PBG), and porphyrins. Sufficient amounts of glucose could completely prevent the porphyria. At the time the initial discovery of the effect of diet was made, there was no reasonable explanation which could account for this phenomenon. In fact, the effect of protein in inhibiting the development of experimental porphyria seemed somewhat paradoxical, since the increased intake of a porphyrin precursor in the form of glycine in protein might be expected to augment, rather than diminish, porphyrin and porphyrin-precursor production.

The key discovery that hepatic ALA-synthetase is an inducible enzyme (Granick and Urata, 1963) provided the basis for an explanation. After the initial finding that hepatic ALA-synthetase is induced in 3,5-dicarbethoxy-1,4-dihydrocollidine (DDC) porphyria, a similar induction was demonstrated in AIA-induced porphyria (Tschudy et al., 1964; Marver et al., 1966a). These findings indicated that over-production of porphyrin precursors resulting from hepatic ALA-synthetase induction might be a mechanism common to various experimental porphyrias. The fact that glucose can block the induction of certain enzymes in microorganisms (Epps and Gale, 1942; Monod, 1947; Neidhardt and Magasanik, 1956; Nakada and Magasanik, 1964; Clarke and Brammar, 1964) had been known for some time. Later work extended this phenomenon to mammalian liver when it was shown that the induction of two liver enzymes in the rat, threonine dehydrase and ornithine δ-transaminase, could be repressed by carbohydrate feeding (Pitot and Peraino, 1963; Peraino and Pitot, 1964). The ability of carbohydrate to block the induction of certain enzymes was named the "glucose effect" and "catabolite repression." Analysis of the above facts suggested that the mechanism by which diet suppressed the production of experimental porphyria was via a "glucose effect" on the induction of hepatic ALA-synthetase. This was shown to be the correct explanation (Tschudy et al., 1964; Marver et al., 1966a).

2. The "Glucose Effect" in Human Hepatic Porphyria

Since diet could prevent experimental porphyria, it was only a short time after the experimental findings that the effect of diet on porphyrin-precursor excretion in human hepatic porphyria was investigated. It was shown that porphyrin-precursor excretion was reciprocally related to carbohydrate and/or protein intake in acute intermittent porphyria (Welland et al., 1964; Felsher and Redeker, 1967) and that a high carbohydrate intake lowers porphyrin and porphyrin-precursor excretion in variegate porphyria (Perlroth et al., 1968). At the time of the initial demonstration of the effect of high carbohydrate intake on lowering porphyrin-precursor excretion in acute intermittent porphyria, there was no explanation for the effect. The finding of the genetically mediated induction of hepatic ALA-synthetase in this disease (Tschudy et al., 1965; Nakao et al., 1966; Dowdle et al., 1967) indicated that the "glucose effect" was operating in the human disease as well as the experimental porphyrias.

Subsequent experience in the study of the effects of diet in acute intermittent porphyria has shown great variation in the response of different patients to a high carbohydrate intake (Stein and Tschudy, 1970). The biochemical response, lowering of porphyrin-precursor excretion, usually mirrors the clinical response. In some patients, an intake of 450 g/day or more of carbohydrate can cause a profound decline in porphyrin-precursor excretion, sometimes to approximately normal levels, accompanied by spectacular clinical improvement. There are some patients in whom this therapeutic approach has been a life-saving procedure. The paradox relating to the "glucose effect" in the disease is the wide spectrum of responsiveness of patients. The range appears to extend from little or no effect to the striking effect described above. There is no explanation at present for this heterogeneity of response, although several possibilities require further investigation. Patients with acute intermittent porphyria often have abnomalities of carbohydrate metabolism as manifested by a tendency toward adult onset type diabetic glucose tolerance tests and insulin secretion patterns (WAXMAN et al., 1967; TSCHUDY, 1968). Their growth-hormone response to a glucose load is often abnormal, sometimes manifested as an inappropriate release of growth hormone (PERLROTH et al., 1967). It might be suspected, therefore, that the spectrum of responsiveness to the "glucose effect" might relate to the varying ability of these patients to utilize glucose. Preliminary data did not suggest that inappropriate release of growth-hormone explained the failure of some patients to experience a significant "glucose effect," although this requires further study.

The above discussion illustrates how the complex interplay between diet and hormones is involved in the manifestations of a human disease and relates to its treatment. The significance of the "glucose effect" in mammals extends well beyond porphyrin metabolism and porphyria, since other liver enzymes in the rat also appear to be effected. These include phosphoenolpyruvate carboxykinase (YOUNG et al., 1964), cytochrome P-450 (REMMER, 1964), dimethylazobenzene reductase (JERVELL et al., 1965), other drug metabolizing enzymes (McLEAN and McLEAN, 1966), histidase, serine dehydratase, homoserine dehydratase, mitochondrial aspartate transaminase, cytoplasmic alanine transaminase (PESTAÑA, 1969), and tyrosine aminotransferase (YUWILER et al., 1970; SUDILOVSKY et al., 1971).

3. Possible Mechanisms Underlying the "Glucose Effect"

The mechanism by which glucose blocks the induction of certain enzymes has been the subject of considerable study, but the effect of protein in blocking the induction of hepatic ALA-synthetase has not been investigated in detail. It is possible that this may in principle be the same process and merely reflect the activity of the gluconeogenic amino acids present in protein.

Specific mention of one particular amino acid is warranted. Tryptophane is an inducer of hepatic ALA-synthetase (MARVER et al., 1966b) presumably through the following sequence of events: (1) increased binding of dissociable heme to the apoenzyme of tryptophane pyrrolase which causes, (2) increased levels of tryptophane pyrrolase resulting from its decreased rate of degradation, (3) decreased availability of heme for repression of ALA-synthetase resulting in, (4) induction of ALA-synthetase. This amino acid, therefore, acts antagonistically to the "glucose effect" mediated by carbohydrate and protein. It is interesting that tryptophane can induce certain other hepatic enzymes such as serine dehydratase, alanine transaminase, tyrosine transaminase, and aspartate transaminase (Pestaña, 1969).

Early work on the mechanism of the "glucose effect" led to the concept of "catabolite repression" (Neidhardt and Magasanik, 1956; Magasanik, 1961) which is as follows: all glucose-sensitive enzymes are capable of converting their substrates to metabolites which the cell can also obtain independently and more readily by the metabolism of glucose; conversely the ultimate products of the action of glucose-insensitive enzymes cannot be produced independently by separate pathways from glucose. It was thought that catabolites formed rapidly from glucose accumulate in the cell and repress the formation of enzymes whose activity would augment the already large intracellular pools of these compounds. In applying this theory to the "glucose effect" on hepatic ALA-synthetase, it would be necessary to postulate that metabolites of glucose could be converted to heme by reactions which bypass ALA-synthetase. This possibility does exist in the form of reversal of the so-called succinate−glycine cycle originally postulated by Shemin et al. (1955). In this pathway ALA is converted to α-ketoglutaraldehyde by transamination, the latter then being converted to ketoglutarate or succinate by the appropriate reactions. If this pathway were reversible, then ALA and ultimately heme could be produced by a second mechanism which bypasses the well-known ALA-synthetase catalyzed condensation of glycine and succinyl CoA. The enzymatic conversion of α-ketoglutaraldehyde to ALA has been demonstrated and the equilibrium in some systems favors ALA (Gibson et al., 1961; Neuberger and Turner, 1963). However, although enzymatic conversion of α-ketoglutarate to α-ketoglutaraldehyde has not been shown in animal tissues, synthesis of ALA from ketoglutarate and glutamate have been demonstrated in greening plants (Beale et al., 1975). It is possible that a reverse succinate−glycine cycle is the primary mechanism of ALA synthesis in these organisms. The more recent work on cyclic AMP and its relationship to the "glucose effect" as discussed below may appear to make a discussion of "catabolite repression" irrelevant. It is presented for two reasons. First is the fact that it now appears almost certain that the cyclic AMP mechanism may not apply to all glucose-sensitive enzymes. Second, it emphasizes the question of whether it is metabolites of glucose which are the ultimate mediators of the "glucose effect" in some systems.

The mechanism by which glucose blocks the induction of enzymes controlled by the lac and gal operons in *Escherichia coli* has been elucidated by outstanding work in several laboratories (De Crombrugghe et al., 1969; Varmus et al., 1970; Zubay et al., 1970; Arditti et al., 1970; Nissley et al., 1971; Anderson et al., 1971). In *E. coli* cyclic AMP leaks out of the cells into the medium when glucose is added to the medium, thus lowering the intracellular concentration of cyclic AMP. Cyclic AMP was shown to react with a protein which has been called CAP (catabolite-gene activating protein) and CRP (cyclic AMP receptor protein). This cyclic AMP protein complex attaches to DNA at the promoter locus (the site at which RNA polymerase is thought to attach to DNA) and augments transcription of the genes of these operons. It is in this manner that cyclic AMP stimulates the synthesis of certain proteins. These data raise the question of whether a glucose load in mammalian organisms causes its inhibition of induction of certain hepatic enzymes by similarly affecting a cyclic-AMP-dependent mechanism. At present the question cannot be answered with certainty, since there are findings which suggest conflicting conclusions. The relationship of cyclic AMP to induction of certain hepatic enzymes is highly relevant to the present discussion since this compound may lie at the crossroads of dietary and hormonal effects for some enzymes.

Early studies of the glucose effect on hepatic ALA-synthetase suggested that it was mediated at the level of transcription (HICKMAN et al., 1968), a finding which has not yet been confirmed. This locus corresponds to that for the cyclic AMP mechanism in microorganisms. Furthermore, it has been established that cyclic AMP plays a role in supporting the synthesis of certain enzymes in mammalian liver which are subject to the glucose effect. This compound induces phosphoenolpyruvate carboxykinase (WICKS et al., 1969), serine dehydrase (WICKS et al., 1969), and tyrosine aminotransferase (WICKS, 1968) (WICKS et al., 1969). In a study attempting to examine the role of cyclic AMP in the glucose effect in rat liver it was found that intragastric glucose inhibits the induction of tyrosine aminotransferase and serine dehydratase by glucagon, but has no effect on the increase of hepatic cyclic AMP resulting from administration of glucagon (SUDILOVSKY et al., 1971). Although hepatic tyrosine aminotransferase can be induced by cyclic AMP, it can also undergo a cyclic-AMP-independent induction mediated by hydrocortisone, as can tryptophane pyrrolase. Since glucose can block these cyclic-AMP-independent inductions (PESTAÑA, 1969; YUWILER et al., 1970), the mechanism of the glucose effect on these enzymes, as well as on the cyclic-AMP-dependent induction of tyrosine aminotransferase and serine dehydratase cited above, is clearly different from that described in *E. coli* where glucose acts by lowering intracellular cyclic AMP levels. It is clear, therefore, that there are heterogeneous mechanisms involved in the "glucose effect" in various organisms.

With regard to the relationship of cyclic AMP to hepatic ALA-synthetase, the findings are complex and somewhat conflicting but much of the evidence does not support a role of this compound in stimulating ALA-synthetase production. Although glucagon administration (known to increase hepatic cyclic AMP) produced slight hepatic ALA-synthetase induction in 18-day-old chick embryo liver, there was no induction when cyclic AMP was given (SIMONS, 1970). Furthermore, glucagon did not induce the enzyme in rat liver and slightly lowered the induced activity produced by AIA (MARVER et al., 1966a), a finding which has been confirmed and studied in further detail (KIM and KIKUCHI, 1974), as discussed later.

Studies in chick embryos, however, suggest that cyclic AMP may play some role in enhancing hepatic ALA-synthetase production. Dibutyryl cyclic AMP enhanced AIA-mediated induction by $10-15\%$ and at 10^{-4} M completely blocked the glucose effect ($25-30\%$ lowering of induction) in 17-day-old chick embryo liver (KORINEK and MOSES, 1973a).

In isolated rat liver cell suspensions AIA alone (1.2 mM) or dibutyryl cyclic AMP alone (50 µM) produced no induction of ALA-synthetase. In combination, however, a $4-5$ fold increase of ALA-synthetase was seen over a 6-h period (EDWARDS and ELLIOT, 1974). The same phenomenon was seen with dicarbethoxy-dihydrocollidine. This finding suggests a "permissive effect" of cyclic AMP on the induction, a phenomenon which has been shown previously in vivo for hydrocortisone (MARVER et al., 1966c). Significant induction cannot be produced in adrenalectomized animals by either hydrocortisone or known inducers administered separately, but occurs normally when they are administered together. In isolated rat liver cell suspensions neither hydrocortisone succinate (in concentrations optimal for tyrosine aminotransferase induction) nor glucose had any effect on the induction caused by AIA and dibutyryl cyclic AMP (Edwards and Elliot, 1974). It is assumed that there was sufficient endogenous hydrocortisone present in the isolated liver cells to produce a "permissive" effect, but the absence of a "glucose effect" in this system is particularly interesting. This finding in isolated rat liver cells and the previous observation by Granick (1966) that glucose did not alter the induction of ALA-synthetase in chick embryo liver cells in vitro suggest that the "glucose effect" does not operate in liver cells in vitro, at least under the conditions examined thus far. Korinek and Moses (1973a) showed that it does operate in chick embryo liver in vivo.

All other studies in rat liver produced no evidence that cyclic AMP is a stimulator of hepatic ALA-synthetase production. AIA markedly lowered hepatic cyclic AMP levels while inducing ALA-synthetase (Pinelli and Capuano, 1973). Injection of dibutyryl cyclic AMP (Pinelli and Capuano, 1973; Bonkowsky et al., 1973) or cyclic AMP (Bonkowsky et al., 1973) depressed the AIA-mediated induction and lowered the activity in control rats (Bonkowsky et al., 1973). These findings contrast with those of the slight enhancement of induction in chick embryo liver (Korinek and Moses, 1973a). Likewise the failure of dibutyrylcyclic AMP to materially alter the "glucose effect" in rat liver (Bonkowsky et al., 1973) contrasts with the finding in chick liver where it blocked the mild "glucose effect" (Korinek and Moses, 1973a). Among a group of nucleotides studied (ATP, ADP, AMP, and cyclic AMP) only cyclic AMP lowered ALA-synthetase activity (Bonkowsky et al., 1973). It was found that dibutyryl cyclic AMP and cyclic AMP both inhibited ALA-synthetase in vitro (57% at 5×10^{-3} M and 14% at 10^{-4} M for dibutyryl cyclic AMP and for cyclic AMP 29% and 22% at the same concentrations and 21% at 10^{-5} M (Bonkowsky et al., 1973). This finding may account for the observation of the lowering of induced ALA-synthetase activity produced by these compounds in some systems.

Other studies have made the picture even more complex. Kim and Kikuchi (1972) found that cyclic AMP acted on the induction of rat hepatic ALA-synthetase in a manner similar to that previously described for hemin (Kurashima et al., 1970). During induction ALA-synthetase is thought to be produced outside the mitochondrion and then taken up into the mitochondria. Cyclic AMP, like heme, when given with an inducer may interfere with enzyme production, but when given 2 h after the inducer appeared to inhibit conversion of the cytosol enzyme to its mitochondrial form.

The xanthine inhibitors of phosphodiesterase have also been studied in attempts to elucidate the relationship between cyclic AMP and induction — repression of hepatic ALA-synthetase further. By increasing cyclic AMP levels, theophylline can induce certain enzymes, such as the 10-fold increase of ornithine decarboxylase which it can produce (Beck et al., 1972). In the case of hepatic ALA-synthetase in both rat liver (Bonkowsky et al., 1973; Pinelli and Capuano, 1973; Korinek and Moses, 1973b) and chick embryo liver (Korinek and Moses 1973a and b) induced activity of the enzyme was lowered considerably by administration of theophylline with or after various inducers such as AIA (Bonkowsky

et al., 1973; PINELLI and CAPUANO, 1973; KORINEK and MOSES, 1973b), phenobarbital or certain steroids (KORINEK and MOSES, 1973b). Thus, although cyclic
AMP acts somewhat differently in its effect on induced hepatic ALA-synthetase
activity in chick embryo and rat liver, slightly stimulating the former and inhibiting the latter, the effect of theophylline appears to be universal in lowering this
activity. This fact, along with the observation that the combination of theophylline
and dibutyrylcyclic AMP impaired ALA-synthetase induction in rat liver in approximately an additive fashion (BONKOWSKY et al., 1973) suggest that the effect
of theophylline on this enzyme may not be mediated through its inhibition of
phosphodiesterase and subsequent change in intracellular cyclic AMP levels. This
contention is further supported by the fact that 1-methyl-3-isobutylxanthine, which
is 15 times more potent as an inhibitor of phosphodiesterase than theophylline,
did not suppress induced ALA-synthetase in chick embryo liver (KORINEK and
MOSES, 1973b). The inhibitory effect of theophylline was not altered by administration of dibutyryl cyclic AMP (KORINEK and MOSES, 1973a).

In summary, at the present time most of the evidence does not suggest cyclic
AMP to be a primary stimulator of rat hepatic ALA-synthetase production as it
is for certain other enzymes. The evidence is even more convincing that the
"glucose effect" in rat liver for all enzymes thus far studied in that regard, is not
mediated by lowering of cyclic AMP levels. It is possible, however, that cyclic
AMP may play a "permissive" role in the induction of ALA-synthetase. In chick
embryo liver there may be differences from rat liver in that some data suggest
that cyclic AMP may block the "glucose effect" on ALA-synthetase.

It is thus necessary that other explanations of the "glucose effect" on ALA-
synthetase must be sought. In the past a number of possibilities have been suggested. These include: (1) that glucose augments glucuronic acid formation, which
in turn removes inducing steroids by glucuronidation (KAPPAS et al., 1968a; KAPPAS
and GRANICK, 1968b), (2) that glucose increases levels of NADPH in liver which
augments drug detoxification (MARVER, 1969), (3) that glucose mediates its effect
via increasing ATP levels (GAJDOS and GAJDOS-TÖRÖK, 1970), and (4) that the
"glucose effect" in liver is mediated by glycogen, deposited on endoplasmic reticulum, which impairs the enzyme-producing activity of these sites (PERAINO et al.,
1966). (This fourth mechanism was not postulated specifically for hepatic ALA-
synthetase.)

A number of aspects of the "glucose effect" in rat liver were studied by
BONKOWSKY et al. (1973) in relation to both ALA-synthetase and tyrosine aminotransferase. Among a number of sugars, glycolytic intermediates, tricarboxylic
acid cycle intermediates, and fatty acids, fructose and glycerol were the most active
in producing a "glucose effect" thus reducing the induction of both hepatic ALA-
synthetase and tyrosine aminotransferase, being approximately equiactive on a
weight basis to glucose. α-Ketoglutarate and succinate also lowered the induction
of hepatic ALA-synthetase, but both of these compounds are known to inhibit this
enzyme significantly at concentrations above 10 mM (MARVER et al., 1966d).

In general metabolites of glucose were much less effective than glucose itself
and tended to decrease in effectiveness the further they were removed from glucose
in the metabolic scheme. The findings of PIPER and TEPHLY (1974) that acetate
administration lowers and also inhibits induced ALA-synthetase activity appears

to be an exception to this finding, but it is not clear how much of this effect relates to competition with succinate for CoA. This fact raises the question of whether glucose must be metabolized to inhibit hepatic ALA-synthetase induction or whether glucose itself can produce the effect. A number of findings in the study of Bonkowsky et al. (1973) are relevant to this question. Glycerol, fructose, and glucose are about equally active in exerting the effect, whereas galactose was less active and ribose and sorbitol inactive. It is possible that the differing efficacy of these carbohydrates in repressing ALA-synthetase induction could relate to the rate and degree to which they are converted to hepatic glucose after oral administration. Ribose and sorbitol are absorbed slowly from the gastrointestinal tract. Rats given these sugars developed diarrhea, whereas those given glucose, fructose, or glycerol did not. On a weight basis fructose and glycerol are as efficient precursors of intracellular hepatic glucose as glucose itself (Webb, 1966). Fructose and glycerol, very active in repressing hepatic ALA-synthetase induction, are much more efficient precursors of hepatic glucose than is pyruvate (Webb, 1966), which was inactive in producing a "glucose effect."

Various procedures which impaired glucose utilization were studied and the results suggest again that glucose is more effective than its metabolites in repressing hepatic ALA-synthetase induction (Bonkowsky et al., 1973). Thus 2-deoxyglucose, a potent inhibitor of glucose-6-phosphate isomerase, markedly impaired AIA-mediated induction of hepatic ALA-synthetase. This compound was shown not to be an inhibitor of the enzyme. Induction of hepatic ALA-synthetase by AIA was markedly impaired in experimental diabetes, whether produced by alloxan, alloxan and hydrocortisone, or large doses of hydrocortisone alone. Glucose administration to diabetic rats impaired the induction further. It is known that under conditions of insulin lack that hepatic cyclic AMP levels are increased, and that these are partly dependent on the ratio of glucagon to insulin (Sutherland and Robison, 1969). Impairment of induction occurs, therefore, in the presence of increased hepatic levels of cyclic AMP, further casting doubt on its decline as the mechanism of the "glucose effect" on hepatic ALA-synthetase. The role of insulin in the control of hepatic ALA-synthetase may extend beyond carbohydrate metabolism, since decreased hepatic protein synthesis due to insulin lack may further impair ALA-synthetase induction. Diazoxide is a compound which has multiple complex effects on carbohydrate metabolism (Tabachnick and Schwartz, 1968) including enhanced glycogenolysis (Tabachnick et al., 1964). This compound was found to be a direct moderate inducer of hepatic ALA-synthetase in the fasted animal, but also markedly diminished AIA-mediated induction and did not impair the "glucose effect" on hepatic ALA-synthetase, but actually augmented it. Pronounced hyperglycemia was demonstrated in the instances where diazoxide impaired induction (Bonkowsky et al., 1973).

In the most recent study of the "glucose effect" it was found that glucose, ATP, cyclic AMP, dibutyryl cyclic AMP, theophylline, insulin, or glucagon, when administered simultaneously with AIA to rats reduced the AIA-mediated induction of hepatic ALA-synthetase and also lowered its activity in normal rats not given an inducer (Kim and Kikuchi, 1974). When these were given after induction was progressing, the level of ALA-synthetase in the cytosol increased greatly while that in mitochondria decreased markedly. The total activity was not reduced under these conditions, except when glucose was given. The half-life of the cytosol enzyme was prolonged by dibutyryl cyclic AMP. These effects are similar to those previously found after administration of hemin to rats untreated or given AIA. It appears that a variety of compounds, as well as hemin, can inhibit the induction of hepatic ALA-synthetase and the conversion of the cytosol form of this enzyme to the mitochondrial enzyme. Dibutyryl cyclic AMP and glucagon also manifested these effects in alloxan-diabetic rats. As the authors of this study point out, it is difficult to explain why both insulin and glucagon exhibited similar effects on the induction of hepatic ALA-synthetase, since these hormones act antagonistically in many respects, including cyclic AMP production in the liver cell (ROBISON et al., 1971). Since catecholamines are known to increase hepatic cyclic AMP levels and induce certain enzymes, their effect on ALA-synthetase induction was also examined (KIM and KIKUCHI, 1974). Epinephrine or isoproterenol (10 – 80 µg/100 g body weight) markedly reduced the AIA-mediated increase of ALA-synthetase and did not cause the accumulation of cytosol ALA-synthetase, whether they were given with the inducer or afterwards. The effects, therefore, differ from those of cyclic AMP and suggest that the effects of catecholamines are not mediated through their stimulation of cyclic AMP formation.

The conclusions about the mechanism by which glucose blocks the induction of hepatic ALA-synthetase must be that it remains unexplained. It is likely that none of the previously proposed mechanisms adequately explains all the data which have been accumulated in the study of this subject. Furthermore the question arises as to what purpose, if any, is served by the "glucose effect" on hepatic ALA-synthetase. What is the physiologic utility of the effect (aside from the treatment of acute attacks of hepatic porphyria in some responsive patients)? It is obviously a means of modulating hepatic heme synthesis downward, but the reason for this effect of diet is not clear.

II. Other Dietary Factors

Two other aspects related to nutrition and diet will be discussed briefly. Pyridoxal phosphate is the cofactor for ALA-synthetase and is the only vitamin derivative known to serve as a cofactor for any of the enzymes of the heme biosynthetic pathway. It might be expected that a profound pyridoxine deficiency could impair hepatic ALA-synthetase induction, but this was not the case in rats (CHABNER et al., 1970). The binding of pyridoxal phosphate to hepatic ALA-synthetase appears to vary in different species, being very strong in the rat liver enzyme.

One of the striking effects of a component of diet is the pronounced synergistic effect on the induction of hepatic ALA-synthetase produced by a large oral dose of iron in the form of ferric citrate (STEIN et al., 1969; STEIN et al., 1970). Ferric citrate is more effective than other forms of iron undoubtedly because of its greater capacity to enter cells. The augmentation of hepatic ALA-synthetase induction by iron might result from effects of iron on decreasing the hepatic heme pool size. This could result from augmenting heme turnover or partially blocking heme synthesis. There is some evidence to suggest that iron may operate in liver by both mechanisms. Thus DE MATTEIS and SPARKS (1973) showed in vivo and in vitro that iron increased heme degradation. KUSHNER et al. (1975) postulated that iron inhibits uroporphyrinogen decarboxylase. If it synergizes hepatic ALA-synthetase induction by diminishing the amount of heme available for repression of this enzyme, it is not clear why it therefore does not act as a direct inducer of the enzyme. These effects on the heme pathway may be related to the etiologic role of iron overload in cutanea tarda porphyria (TSCHUDY, 1974).

C. The Influence of Hormonal Factors

Some aspects of endocrine effects and lack of effects have already been considered in the discussion of the "glucose effect" on hepatic ALA-synthetase. These include glucagon, insulin, and hydrocortisone. Bovine growth hormone slightly enhanced the AIA-mediated induction of hepatic ALA-synthetase (MARVER et al., 1966a), but this has not been investigated further.

Detailed studies of the relationship of triiodothyronine (T_3) and hydrocortisone to AIA-mediated induction of rat hepatic ALA-synthetase were performed by MATSUOKA et al. (1968). It had previously been shown that the induction of this enzyme in rat liver involved two distinct phases with different sensitivities to inhibitors of DNA synthesis. The first phase was not inhibited by mitomycin C or 5-fluorouridine deoxyribose, but the second phase, which occurred only after administration of larger doses of AIA was inhibited by inhibitors of DNA synthesis (NARISAWA and KIKUCHI, 1966). When the lower doses of AIA (150 mg/kg), producing the mitomycin-insensitive first phase of the induction, were administered to intact rats, it was shown that concomitant administration of T_3 or hydrocortisone synergized the induction. The hormones alone produced no induction. The "permissive effect" of hydrocortisone in adrenalectomized rats was confirmed. The significance and mechanism of these synergistic effects of T_3 and hydrocortisone which are exhibited under special conditions are not clear at the present time. They do emphasize the complex series of control mechanisms which operate on hepatic heme synthesis.

Although various effects have been demonstrated, the experimental studies of growth hormone, triiodothyronine (T_3), insulin, glucagon, and epinephrine thus far have not provided a clear answer as to exactly what role these hormones play in hepatic heme synthesis in vivo, if any. The role of hydrocortisone in producing a "permissive effect" in vivo on the induction of hepatic ALA-synthetase is a little clearer. A role of certain steroids in hepatic heme synthesis in vivo is more strongly indicated by consideration of a number of clinical and experimental findings.

Acute intermittent porphyria is transmitted as a Mendelian dominant disorder, but the manifest disease is more frequent in females. The biochemical (increased urinary excretion of porphyrin precursors) and clinical manifestations of this disease almost always occur after puberty. In some women attacks of the disease occur regularly premenstrually and in these women ovulatory suppressants have had therapeutic value (PERLROTH et al., 1965), but in others it is clear that estrogens can be harmful (ZIMMERMAN et al., 1966) and ovulatory suppressants have been implicated in activating the disease in some patients. These clinical facts indicate that there may be some link between sex hormones and porphyrin metabolism.

The first specific link at the enzyme level between sex hormones and the heme biosynthetic pathway was the finding by GRANICK (1966) that progesterone, testosterone, ethinyl estradiol, estradiol, and estrone had weak activity in stimulating excess porphyrin production in primary cultures of chick embryo liver cells. This was related to ALA-synthetase induction. The closed negative feedback loop involved in the control of hepatic ALA-synthetase is a system which can undergo an oscillatory response to certain perturbing factors such as heme (WAXMAN et al., 1966) and estradiol administered i.v. was also shown to be such a perturbing factor (TSCHUDY et al., 1967). Further studies in the in vitro chick embryo liver cell system revealed that many C19 and C21 steroids of the 5β-H configuration can augment porphyrin synthesis (GRANICK and KAPPAS, 1967a; GRANICK and KAPPAS, 1967b; KAPPAS and GRANICK, 1968a; KAPPAS and GRANICK, 1968b). This was shown to result from the induction of ALA-synthetase (KAPPAS et al., 1968b). In contrast to most other inducers of hepatic ALA-synthetase which are active only in liver, these steroids were also shown to augment activity of the heme biosynthetic pathway in erythroid cells. This was shown in the blood islands of chick blastoderm (LEVERE and GRANICK, 1967; LEVERE et al., 1967). Although the 5β-H steroids appear to be direct inducers of ALA-synthetase in both erythroid and hepatic cells of embryonic origin, there are some differences in response to these steroids when adult forms of these two organ systems are examined in vivo. In polycythemic mice steroids with a 5β-H configuration enhanced ^{59}Fe incorporation into circulating erythrocytes (GORSHEIN and GARDNER, 1970; GORDON et al., 1970). Testosterone appeared to stimulate erythropoiesis through production of erythropoietin, whereas the 5β-H steroids were thought to act more directly on blood-forming tissues, presumably by induction of ALA-synthetase, followed by increased heme and hemoglobin synthesis.

Mammalian liver appears to be refractory to these steroids in contrast to avian embryonic liver (WEISSMAN et al., 1973), although slight induction in rats by dehydroepiandrosterone, 17-hydroxypregnenolone, androstenedione, androstenediol, and etiocholanolone has been demonstrated (MOORE et al., 1973; PAXTON et al., 1974). However, pregnanolone, while producing no induction of hepatic ALA-synthetase in mice, did synergize the induction produced by AIA and DDC (WEISSMAN et al., 1973).

The most active ALA-synthetase-inducing steroids are C19 and C21 metabolites of parent hormones such as testosterone and progesterone or of intermediates in the steroid hormone biosynthetic pathway. The specific structural prerequisite for steroids which are inducers of ALA-synthetase is that they be of the 5β-H configuration in which the H on carbon 5 is cis to the methyl on carbon 10, whereas it is in the trans position in 5α-H steroids. Thus 5α-H steroids approach planarity and 5β-H steroids are markedly non-planar. The parent C19 and C21 compounds upon which the nomenclature of the most active derivatives is based are etiocholane and pregnane. Highly active compounds include etiocholanolone, etiocholandiol, etiocholandione, pregnandiol, pregnanolone, pregnandione, and pregnantriol. The most active steroid inducers of ALA-synthetase, therefore, are metabolites of parent steroid hormones such as testosterone and progesterone or are related intermediates in the steroid biosynthetic pathway. Some of these compounds achieve maximal induction in vitro at concentrations as low as 10^{-5} M. Bile acids and C21 hydroxylated hormones such as cortisol and aldosterone are inactive as direct inducers (Kappas and Granick, 1968a).

These findings are significant in two respects. First they demonstrate a biochemical effect (or function) of compounds which were formerly thought to be metabolites with no primary function. Second, they provide a specific link between compounds produced in the adrenals and gonads and alterations in hepatic porphyrin metabolism. They would appear to relate to the clinical observations cited above which implicate endocrine factors in activity of certain hepatic porphyrias and have provided the impetus for further investigation of this relationship. Goldberg et al. (1969) found increased urinary excretion of certain porphyrinogenic steroids in some patients with acute intermittent porphyria. These workers have shown that during attacks and often during remission in acute intermittent porphyria that there is increased excretion of the sulfate and/or glucuronide of dehydroepiandrosterone and etiocholanolone (Moore et al., 1973; Paxton et al., 1974). There was an increased ratio of etiocholanolone to androsterone in the urine of these patients. Since their initial demonstration of the significance of the 5β-H steroid configuration in the induction of ALA-synthetase, Kappas and co-workers have studied its significance in patients with acute intermittent porphyria (Kappas et al., 1971, 1972a and b; Bradlow et al., 1973). Steroids with a double bond in the 4,5 position can undergo reduction in the liver to compounds where the 5H is cis to the 10 methyl (the 5β-H derivatives) or trans to the 10 methyl (the 5α-H derivatives). Two separate enzymes catalyze these reductions—a soluble 5β reductase and an endoplasmic reticular 5α reductase. By administering ^{14}C-testosterone (Kappas et al., 1971, 1972a and b) or ^{14}C-11β-hydroxy Δ^4-androstenedione (Bradlow et al., 1973) and measuring the ratio of 5β to 5α derivatives in the urine, it was shown that patients with acute intermittent porphyria have a significant 5α reductase deficiency. The resultant tendency to preponderant production of 5β-H steroid metabolites may augment the induction of hepatic ALA-synthetase in this disease.

Certain intermediates in bile-acid biosynthesis which have a 5β-H configuration have also been shown to induce ALA-synthetase in cultured liver cells (Javitt et al., 1973). These include dihydroxycoprostane and trihydroxycoprostane, but other 5β-cholestane and cholest-5-ene derivatives were inactive.

The total mechanism for the control of hepatic heme synthesis is quite complex, apparently operating through a closed negative feedback loop on ALA-synthetase in addition to possible other mechanisms, such as feedback inhibition of this enzyme and perhaps alterations in other enzymes of the pathway. Among the many factors which impinge on the control loop are diet and certain hormones. The present discussion shows that the study of these factors is in an incipient phase and that the molecular mechanisms involved represent a vast area for future exploration. The data available thus far are a beautiful example of how clinical and basic biochemical studies have provided a mutual stimulus for progress in each area and how information obtained in each of these areas has complemented the other.

References

Anderson, W.B., Schneider, A.B., Emmer, M., Perlman, R.L., Pastan, I.: Purification of and properties of the cyclic adenosine 3',5'-monophosphate receptor protein which mediates cyclic adenosine 3',5'-monophosphate-dependent gene transcription in *Escherichia coli.* J. biol. Chem. **246**, 5929 – 5937 (1971)

Arditti, R.R., Eron, L., Zubay, G., Tocchini-Valentini, G., Connaway, S., Beckwith, J.: In vitro transcritpion of the lac operon genes. Cold Spr. Harb. Symp. quant. Biol. **35**, 437 – 442 (1970)

Beale, S.I., Gaugh, S.P., Granick, S.: Biosynthesis of δ-aminolevulinic acid from the intact carbon skeleton of glutamic acid in greening barley. Proc. nat. Acad. Sci. (Wash.) **72**, 2719 – 2723 (1975)

Beck, W.T., Bellantone, R.A., Canellakis, E.S.: The in vivo stimulation of rat liver ornithine decarboxylase activity by dibutyryl cyclic adenosine 3',5'-monophosphate, theophylline and dexamethasone. Biochem. biophys. Res. Commun. **48**, 1649 – 1655 (1972)

Bonkowsky, H.L., Collins, A., Doherty, J.M., Tschudy, D.P.: The glucose effect in rat liver: Studies of δ-aminolevulinic synthase and tyrosine aminotransferase. Biochem. biophys. Acta (Amst.) **320**, 561 – 576 (1973)

Bradlow, H.L., Gillette, P.N., Gallagher, T.F., Kappas, A.: Studies in porphyria. II. Evidence for a deficiency of delta 4 – 5 alpha reductase activity in acute intermittent porphyria. J. exp. Med. **138**, 754 – 763 (1973)

Chabner, B.A., Stein, J.A., Tschudy, D.P.: Effect of dietary pyridoxine deficiency on experimental porphyria. Metabolism **19**, 189 – 191 (1970)

Clarke, P.H., Brammar, W.J.: Regulation of bacterial enzyme synthesis by induction and repression. Nature (Lond.) **203**, 1153 – 1155 (1964)

De Crombrugghe, B., Perlman, R.L., Varmus, H.E., Pastan, I.: Regulation of inducible enzyme sinthesis in *Escherichia coli* by cyclic adenosine 3',5'-monophosphate. J. biol. Chem. **244**, 5828 – 5835 (1969)

De Matteis, F.: Increased synthesis of l-ascorbic acid caused by drugs which induce porphyria. Biochem. biophys. Acta (Amst.) **82**, 641 – 644 (1964)

De Matteis, F., Sparks, R.G.: Iron-dependent loss of liver cytochrome P-450 heme in vivo and in vitro. Febs Lett. **29**, 141 – 144 (1973)

Dowdle, E.B., Mustard, P., Eales, L.: δ-aminolevulinic acid synthetase activity in normal and porphyric human livers. S. Afr. med. J. **41**, 1093 – 1096 (1967)

Edwards, M., Elliot, W.H.: Induction of δ-aminolevulinic acid synthetase in isolated rat liver cell suspensions. Adenosine-3',5'-monophosphate dependence of induction by drugs. J. biol. Chem. **249**, 851 – 855 (1974)

Epps, H.M.R., Gale, E.F.: The influence of the presence of glucose during growth on the enzymic activities of *Escherichia coli:* comparison of the effect with that produced by fermentation acids. Biochem. J. **36**, 619 – 623 (1942)

Felsher, B.F., Redeker, A.G.: Acute intermittent porphyria: Effect of diet and griseofulvin. Medicine **46**, 217 – 223 (1967)

Gajdos, A., Gajdos-Török, M.: The role of ATP in the effect of glucose on the excess porphyrin biosynthesis. Biochem. biophys. Acta **215**, 200 – 203 (1970)

Gibson, K.D., Matthew, M., Newberger, A., Thait, G.H.: Biosynthesis of porphyrins and chlorophylls. Nature (Lond.) **192**, 204 – 208 (1961)

Goldberg, A., Moore, M.R., Beattie, A.D., Hall, P.E., McCallum, J., Grant, J.K.: Excessive urinary excretion of certain porphyrinogenic steroids in human acute intermittent porphyria. Lancet **1969 I**, 115 – 118

Gordon, A.S., Zanjani, E.D., Levere, R.D., Kappas, A.: Stimulation of mammalian erythropoiesis by 5β-H steroid metabolites. Proc. nat. Acad. Sci. (Wash.) **65**, 919 – 924 (1970)

Gorshein, D., Gardner, F.H.: Erythropoietic activity of steroid metabolites in mice. Proc. nat. Acad. Sci. (Wash.) **65**, 564 – 568 (1970)

Granick, S.: The induction in vitro of the synthesis of δ-aminolevulinic acid synthetase in chemical porphyria: a response to certain drugs, sex hormones and foreign chemicals. J. biol. Chem. **241**, 1359 – 1375 (1966)

Granick, S., Kappas, A.: Steroid control of porphyrin and heme biosynthesis: a new biological function of steroid hormone metabolites. Proc. nat. Acad. Sci. (Wash.) **57**, 1463 – 1467 (1967a)

Granick, S., Kappas, A.: Steroid induction of porphyrin synthesis in liver cell culture. I. Structural basis and possible physiological role in the control of heme formation. J. biol. Chem. **242**, 4587 – 4593 (1967b)

Granick, S., Urata, G.: Increase in activity of δ-aminolevulinic acid synthetase in liver mitochondria induced by feeding of 3,5-dicarbethoxy-1,4-dihydrocollidine. J. biol. Chem. **238**, 821 – 827 (1963)

Hickman, R., Saunders, S.J., Dowdle, E., Eales, L.: The effect of carbohydrate on δ-aminolevulinic acid synthetase: The role of RNA. Biochem. biophys. Acta (Amst.) **161**, 197 – 204 (1968)

Javitt, N.B., Rifkind, A., Kappas, A.: Porphyrin-heme pathway: regulation by intermediates in bile acid synthesis. Science **182**, 841 – 842 (1973)

Jervell, K.F., Christoffersen, T., Mörland, J.: Studies on the 3-methylcholanthrene induction and carbohydrate repression of rat liver dimethylaminoazobenzene reductase. Arch. Biochem. Biophys. **111**, 15 – 22 (1965)

Kappas, A., Bradlow, H.L., Gillette, P.N., Gallagher, T.F.: Abnormal steroid hormone metabolism in the genetic liver disease acute intermittent porphyria. Ann. N.Y. Acad. Sci. **179**, 611 – 624 (1971)

Kappas, A., Bradlow, H.L., Gillette, P.N., Gallagher, T.F.: Studies in porphyria. I. A defect in the reductive transformation of natural steroid hormones in the hereditary liver disease, acute intermittent porphyria. J. exp. Med. **136**, 1043 – 1053 (1972a)

Kappas, A., Bradlow, H.L., Gillette, P.N., Levere, R.D., Gallagher, T.F.: A defect in steroid hormone metabolism in acute intermittent porphyria. Fed. Proc. **31**, 1293 – 1297 (1972b)

Kappas, A., Granick, S.: Experimental hepatic porphyria: Studies with steroids of physiological origin in man. Ann. N.Y. Acad. Sci. **151**, 842 – 849 (1968a)

Kappas, A., Granick, S.: Steroid induction of porphyrin synthesis in liver cell culture. II. The effects of heme, uridine diphosphate glucuronic acid and inhibitors of nucleic acid and protein synthesis on the induction process. J. biol. Chem. **243**, 346 – 351 (1968b)

Kappas, A., Levere, R.D., Granick, S.: The regulation of porphyrin and heme synthesis. Sem. Hematol. **5**, 323 – 334 (1968a)

Kappas, A., Song, C.S., Levere, R.D., Sachson, R.D., Granick, S.: The induction of δ-aminolevulinic acid synthetase in vivo in chick embryo liver by natural steroids. Proc. nat. Acad. Sci. (Wash.) **61**, 509 – 513 (1968b)

Kim, H.J., Kikuchi, G.: Possible participation of cyclic AMP in the regulation of δ-aminolevulinic acid synthesis in rat liver. J. Biochem. **71**, 923 – 926 (1972)

Kim, H.J., Kikuchi, G.: Mechanism of allylisopropylacetamide-induced increase of δ-aminolevulinate synthetase in liver mitochondria. Effects of administration of glucose, cyclic AMP, and some hormones related to glucose metabolism. Arch. Biochem. Biophys. **164**, 293 – 300 (1974)

Korinek, J., Moses, H.L.: Theophylline suppression of δ-aminolevulinic acid synthetase induction of hepatic δ-aminolevulinic acid synthetase in chick embryo. Fed. Proc. **32**, 865 abs. (1973a)

Korinek, J., Moses, H.L.: Theophylline suppression of Δ-aminolevulinic acid synthetase induction in chick embryo and rat livers. Biochem. biophys. Res. Commun. **53**, 1246 – 1252 (1973b)

Kurashima, Y., Hayashi, N., Kikuchi, G.: Mechanism of inhibition by hemin of increase of δ-aminolevulinate synthetase in liver mitochondria. J. Biochem. **67**, 863 – 865 (1970)

Kushner, J.P., Steinmuller, D.P., Lee, G.P.: The role of iron in the pathogenesis of porphyria cutanea tarda. II. Inhibition of uroporphyrinogen decarboxylase. J. clin. Invest. **56**, 661 – 667 (1975)

Levere, R.D., Granick, S.: Control of hemoglobin synthesis in the cultured chick blastoderm. J. biol. Chem. **242**, 1903 – 1911 (1967)

Levere, R.D., Kappas, A., Granick, S.: Stimulation of hemoglobin synthesis in chick blastoderms by certain 5β androstane and 5β pregnane steroids. Proc. nat. Acad. Sci. (Wash.) **58**, 985 – 990 (1967)

Magasanik, B.: Catabolite repression. Symp. quant. Biol. **26**, 249 – 256 (1961)

Marver, H.S.: In: Microsomes and Drug Oxidations. Gillette, J.R., Conney, A.H., Cosmides, G.J., Estabrook, R.W., Routs, J.R., Mannering, G.J. (eds.), pp. 495. New York: Academic Press 1969

Marver, H.S., Collins, A., Tschudy, D.P.: The "permissive effect" of hydrocortisone on the induction of δ-aminolaevulate synthetase. Biochem. J. **99**, 31 c – 33 c (1966 c)

Marver, H.S., Collins, A., Tschudy, D.P., Rechcigl, M. Jr.: δ-aminolevulinic acid synthetase. II. Induction in rat liver. J. biol. Chem. **241**, 4323 – 4329 (1966 a)

Marver, H.S., Tschudy, D.P., Perlroth, M.G., Collins, A.: Coordinate synthesis of heme and apoenzyme in the formation of tryptophane pyrrolase. Science **154**, 501 – 503 (1966 b)

Marver, H.S., Tschudy, D.P., Perlroth, M.G., Collins, A.: δ-Aminolevulinic acid synthetase. I. Studies in liver homogenates. J. biol. Chem. **241**, 2803 – 2809 (1966 d)

Matsuoka, T., Yoda, B., Kikuchi, G.: Mechanism of allylisopropylacetamide-induced increase of δ-aminolevulinate synthetase in liver mitochondria. III. Effects of triidothyronine and hydrocortisone on the induction process. Arch. Biochem. Biophys. **126**, 530 – 538 (1968)

McLean, A.E.M., McLean, E.K.: The effect of diet and 1,1,1-trichloro-2,2-bis-(-P-chlorophenyl) ethane (DDT) on microsomal hydroxylating enzymes and on sensitivity of rats to carbon tetrachloride poisoning. Biochem. J. **100**, 564 – 571 (1966)

Monod, J.: The phenomenon of enzymatic adaptation. Growth **11**, 223 – 289 (1947)

Moore, M.R., Paxton, J.W., Beattie, A.D., Goldberg, A.: 17-Oxosteroid control of porphyrin biosynthesis. Enzyme **16**, 314 – 325 (1973)

Nakada, D., Magasanik, B.: The roles of inducer and catabolite repressor in the synthesis of β-galactosidase by *Escherichia coli*. J. molec. Biol. **8**, 105 – 127 (1964)

Nakao, K. Wada, O., Kitamura, T., Uono, K., Urata, G.: Activity of aminolevulinic acid synthetase in normal and porphyric livers. Nature (Lond.) **210**, 838 – 839 (1966).

Narisawa, K., Kikuchi, G.: Mechanism of allylisopropylacetamide-induced increase of δ-aminolevulinate synthetase in rat liver mitochondria. Biochim. biophys. Acta (Amst.) **123**, 596 – 605 (1966)

Neidhardt, F.C., Magasanik, B.: Inhibitory effect of glucose on enzyme formation. Nature (Lond.) **178**, 801 – 802 (1956)

Neuberger, A., Turner, J.M.: γ-δ-Dioxovalerate aminotransferase activity in *Rhodopseudomonas spheroides*. Biochim. biophys. Acta (Amst.) **67**, 342 – 345 (1963)

Nissley, S.P., Anderson, W.B., Gottesman, M.E., Perlman, R.L., Pastan, I.: In vitro transcription of the gal operon requires cyclic adenosine monophosphate receptor protein. J. biol. Chem. **246**, 4671 – 4678 (1971)

Paxton, J.W., Moore, M.R., Beattie, A.D., Goldberg, A.: 17-Oxosteroid conjugates in plasma and urine of patients with acute intermittent porphyria. Clin. Sci. molec. Med. **46**, 207 – 222 (1974)

Peraino, C., Lamar, C. Jr., Pitot, H.C.: Studies on the mechanism of carbohydrate repression in rat liver. Advanc. Enzyme Regul. **4**, 199 – 217 (1966)

Peraino, C., Pitot, H.C.: Studies on the induction and repression of enzymes in rat liver. II. Carbohydrate repression of dietary and hormonal induction of threonine dehydrase and ornithine δ-transaminase. J. biol. Chem. **239**, 4308 – 4313 (1964)

Perlroth, M.G., Marver, H.S., Tschudy, D.P.: Oral contraceptive agents and the management of acute intermittent porphyria. J. Amer. med. Ass. **194**, 1037 – 1042 (1965)

Perlroth, M.G., Tschudy, D.P., Ratner, A., Spaur, W., Redeker, A.: The effect of diet in variegate (South African genetic) porphyria. Metabolism **17**, 571 – 581 (1968)

Perlroth, M.G., Tschudy, D.P., Waxman, A., Odell, W.D.: Abnormalities of growth hormone regulation in acute intermittent porphyria. Metabolism **16**, 87 – 90 (1967)

Pestaña, A.: Dietary and hormonal control of enzymes of amino acid catabolism in liver. Europ. J. Biochem. **11**, 400 – 410 (1969)

Pinelli, A., Capuano, A.: ALA-synthetase induction. Inhibitory effect exerted by administration of dibutyryl adenosine-3′,5′-cyclic monophosphate, theophylline and caffeine. Enzyme **16**, 203 – 210 (1973)

Piper, W.N., Tephly, T.R.: The reversal of experimental porphyria and the prevention of induction of hepatic mixed function oxidase by acetate. Arch. Biochem. Biophys. **164**, 351 – 356 (1974)

Pitot, H.C., Peraino, C.: Carbohydrate repression of enzyme induction in rat liver. J. biol. Chem. **238**, P.C. 1910 – 1912 (1963)

Remmer, H.: Drug-induced formation of smooth endoplasmic reticulum and of drug-metabolizing enzymes. Proc. Europ. Soc. Study Drug Toxicity **4**, 57 – 76 (1964)

Robison, G.A., Butcher, R.W., Sutherland, E.W.: Cyclic AMP. New York: Academic Press, 1971, p. 232

Rose, J.A., Hellman, E.S., Tschudy, D.P.: Effect of diet on the induction of experimental porphyria. Metabolism **10**, 514 – 521 (1961)

Shemin, D., Russel, C.S., Abramsky, T.: The succinate-glycine cycle. I. The mechanism of pyrrole synthesis. J. biol. Chem. **215**, 613 – 626 (1955)

Simons, J.: δ-Aminolevulinic acid synthetase: Induction in embryonic chick liver by glucagon. Science **167**, 1378 – 1379 (1970)

Stein, J.A., Berk, P., Tschudy, D.P.: A model for calculating enzyme synthetic rates during induction: application to the synergistic effect of ferric citrate on induction of hepatic δ-aminolevulinic acid synthetase. Life Sci. **8**, 1023 – 1031 (1969)

Stein J.A., Tschudy, D.P.: Acute intermittent porphyria: A clinical and biochemical study of 46 patients. Medicine **49**, 1 – 6 (1970)

Stein, J.A., Tschudy, D.P., Corcoran, L.P., Collins, A.: δ-Aminolevulinic acid synthetase III. Synergistic effect of chelated iron on induction. J. biol. Chem. **245**, 2213 – 2218 (1970)

Sudilovsky, O., Pestaña, A., Hinderakter, P.H., Pitot, H.C.: Cyclic adenosine 3′,5′-monophosphate during glucose repression in the rat liver. Science **174**, 142 – 144 (1971)

Sutherland, E.W., Robison, G.A.: The role of cyclic AMP in the control of carbohydrate metabolism. Diabetes **18**, 797 – 819 (1969)

Tabachnick, I.T.A., Gulbenkian, A., Seidman, F.: The effect of a benzothiadiazine, diazoxide, on carbohydrate metabolism. Diabetes **13**, 408 – 418 (1964)

Tabachnick, I.T.A., Schwartz, H. (conference cochairmen): Diazoxide and the treatment of hypoglycemia. Ann. N.Y. Acad. Sci. **150**, 191 – 467 (1968)

Tschudy, D.P.: Clinical aspects of drug reactions in hereditary hepatic porphyria. Ann. N.Y. Acad. Sci. **151**, 850 – 860 (1968)

Tschudy, D.P.: Porphyrin metabolism and the porphyrias. In: Duncan's Diseases of Metabolism. 7th ed. Philadelphia – London – Toronto: W.B. Saunders 1974

Tschudy, D.P., Perlroth, M.G., Marver, H.S., Collins, A., Hunter, G. Jr., Rechcigl, M. Jr.: Acute intermittent porphyria: the first "overproduction disease" localized to a specific enzyme. Proc. nat. Acad. Sci. (Wash.) **53**, 841 – 847 (1965)

Tschudy, D.P., Waxman, A.D., Collins, A.: Oscillations of hepatic δ-aminolevulinic acid synthetase produced by estrogen: a possible role of "rebound induction" in biological clock mechanisms. Proc. nat. Acad. Sci. (Wash.) **58**, 1944 – 1948 (1967)

Tschudy, D.P., Welland, F.H., Collins, A., Hunter, G.W. Jr.: The effect of carbohydrate feeding on the induction of δ-aminolevulinic acid synthetase. Metabolism **13**, 396 – 406 (1964)

Varmus, H.E., Perlman, R.I., Pastan, I.: Regulation of lac transcription in *Escherichia coli* by cyclic adenosine-3′,5′-monophosphate. J. biol. Chem. **245**, 6366 – 6372 (1970)

Waxman, A.D., Collins, A., Tschudy, D.P.: Oscillations of hepatic δ-aminolevulinic acid synthetase produced in vivo by heme. Biochem. biophys. Res. Commun. **24**, 675 – 683 (1966)

Waxman, A., Schalch, D.S., Odell, W.D., Tschudy, D.P.: Abnormalities of carbohydrate metabolism in acute intermittent porphyria. J. clin. Invest. **46**, 1129 (1967)

Webb, J.L.: Enzyme and Metabolic Inhibitors, Vol. II, pp. 386 – 403. New York: Academic Press 1966

Weissman, E.B., Cheng, L.C., Orten, J.M.: The role of certain 5β-H steroids in the regulation of porphyrin-heme formation. Enzyme **16**, 286 – 294 (1973)

Welland, F.H., Hellman, E.S., Gaddis, E.M., Collins, A., Hunter, G.W. Jr., Tschudy, D.P.: Factors affecting the excretion of porphyrin precursors by patients with acute intermittent porphyria. I. The effect of diet. Metabolism **13**, 232 – 250 (1964)

Wicks, W.D.: Tyrosine-α-ketoglutarate transaminase: Induction by epinephrine and adenosine-3′,5′-cyclic phosphate. Science **160**, 997 – 998 (1968)

Wicks, W.D., Kenney, F.T., Lee, K.L.: Induction of hepatic enzyme synthesis in vivo by adenosine 3′,5′-monophosphate. J. biol. Chem. **244**, 6008 – 6013 (1969)

Young, J.W., Shrago, E., Lardy, H.A.: Metabolic control of enzymes involved in lipogenesis and gluconeogenesis. Biochemistry **3**, 1687 – 1692 (1964)

Yuwiler, A., Wetterberg, L., Geller, E.: Alterations in induction of tyrosine aminotransferase and tryptophan oxygenase by glucose pretreatment. Biochem. biophys. Acta (Amst.) **208**, 428 – 433 (1970)

Zimmerman, T.S., McMillin, J.M., Watson, C.J.: Onset of manifestations of hepatic porphyria in relation to the influence of female sex hormones. Arch. intern. Med. **118**, 229 – 240 (1966)

Zubay, G., Schwartz, D., Beckwith, J.: The mechanism of activation of catabolite sensitive genes. Cold Spr. Harb. Symp. quant. Biol. **35**, 433 – 435 (1970)

CHAPTER 10

Effects of Drugs on Bilirubin Metabolism

H.L. Rayner, B.A. Schacter and L.G. Israels

Definition of Certain Abnormalities of Bilirubin Metabolism

Crigler-Najjar Syndrome

Type I: A hereditary disorder of bilirubin metabolism in which bilirubin glucuronyl transferase activity is lacking and the bile is free of bilirubin glucuronide. Severe unconjugated hyperbilirubinemia usually leads to kernicterus in infancy.

Type II: In these patients glucuronyl transferase deficiency is incomplete, and the bile contains bilirubin glucuronide. Plasma bilirubin levels are lower than in the type I disorder, and kernicterus is unusual.

Gilbert's Syndrome

A common, benign hyperbilirubinemia with plasma unconjugated bilirubin only slightly above normal. Bilirubin glucuronyl transferase activity is diminished and hepatic uptake of bilirubin is impaired.

Dubin-Johnson Syndrome

A hereditary defect in hepatic excretion of certain organic anions, including bilirubin glucuronide.

Gunn rat

A mutant strain of Wistar rat. The homozygote is hyperbilirubinemic due to complete deficiency of bilirubin glucuronyl transferase. Heterozygotes have about half the normal glucuronyl transferase activity and are not hyperbilirubinemic.

A. Introduction

Bilirubin is a tetrapyrrolic degradation product of heme. Hemoproteins play important roles in electron and oxygen transport, and a considerable amount of heme is synthesized daily to support these functions. Upon catabolism of these proteins, the heme moiety is not reutilized but is degraded and excreted. The principal mechanism of heme degradation involves opening of the tetrapyrrole ring and loss of the iron atom, with the eventual formation of bilirubin. This lipid soluble molecule is usually of no pathologic significance as its intracellular concentration is low. A complex and adaptable series of mechanisms protects tissues from high concentrations of bilirubin and leads to its excretion as a water soluble glucuronide conjugate.

Normally the rate of hemoprotein turnover and hence of bilirubin production is relatively constant, and about 3.75 mg/kg/day of bilirubin are produced. In man, the concentration of unconjugated bilirubin in plasma is maintained below 1 mg/dl, with a smaller amount of conjugated bilirubin also present.

A variety of foreign substances including many therapeutic agents interact with the systems which produce bilirubin or with those which effect its conjugation and disposal. These are the subject of the present review. Many environmental and therapeutic agents may produce hyperbilirubinemia by causing dysfunction of hepatocytes either directly or by hypersensitivity reactions. These drug-induced hyperbilirubinemias are due to hepatocellular injury rather than to known specific alterations of bilirubin metabolism (PEREZ et al., 1972; KLATSKIN, 1974) and will not be considered here.

A number of chemicals influence bilirubin metabolism by specific mechanisms. Certain drugs inhibit bilirubin disposal, lead to elevated tissue bilirubin concentrations, and may contribute to bilirubin toxicity. Others facilitate the conjugation and excretion of bilirubin, and are of benefit in the treatment of certain hyperbilirubinemic states. Still other interactions between drugs and bilirubin are of no pathological or therapeutic significance but provide experimental approaches to the study of normal bilirubin metabolism. The present discussion will be limited to those chemicals which interact in a relatively specific manner with the mechanisms for bilirubin production, transport, or excretion.

The data reviewed are subject to several limitations. The drugs which have been examined for effects upon bilirubin metabolism are mostly those which cause jaundice in man, and few systematic surveys of drug effects upon the various stages of bilirubin metabolism have been done. Much of the available information was obtained some time ago with rather imperfect techniques, and there is a need for re-examination of many of the observed drug effects with the more specific methods now available. The quantitative relationships between the in vitro methods used in the study of bilirubin metabolism and the functional capacity of this system in the intact animal are poorly defined even in the absence of drug effects. Many in vitro techniques have utilized high drug concentrations, and are of unknown relevance to clinical drug use. Several of the drugs to be discussed influence bilirubin metabolism at several stages and it is unknown which effect is of most significance in the intact animal.

Various aspects of the interactions between drugs and bilirubin metabolism have been surveyed by DONE (1964), DUTTON (1966, 1971), BILLING and BLACK (1971), OSTROW (1972b) BERTHELOT (1974), and KLATSKIN (1974).

B. Normal Bilirubin Metabolism

I. Sources of Bilirubin

Bilirubin is derived primarily from the catabolism of hemoglobin of senescent erythrocytes (VIRCHOW, 1847; RICH, 1925; ASCHOFF, 1922; WHIPPLE and HOOPER, 1917; TARCHANOFF, 1874; McNEE, 1923; MANN et al., 1926; FISCHER and ORTH, 1937). It is known on the basis of studies of glycine-^{15}N incorporation into heme that approximately 20% of the labeled bile pigment produced is excreted soon after labelling, at a time before it could be derived from the labeled hemoglobin of senescent red cells (LONDON et al., 1950; GRAY et al., 1950). Subsequent studies utilizing glycine-2-^{14}C and delta-aminolevulinic acid-4-^{14}C (ALA) have demonstrated that this early labeled bilirubin has two major components (ISRAELS et al., 1963a; YAMAMOTO et al., 1965; IBRAHIM et al., 1966; ROBINSON et al., 1966). The first component appears within minutes of administration of labeled precursor, quickly reaches maximal specific activity and is largely excreted within 24 h; the later component reaches peak specific activity two to five days after administration of glycine-^{14}C. Since factors which stimulate erythropoiesis (ISRAELS et al., 1963b; IBRAHIM et al., 1966; ROBINSON et al., 1966; PERUGINI et al., 1971) produce increases in the second component while hypertransfusion, marrow irradiation (ISRAELS et al., 1963b; IBRAHIM et al., 1966) and marrow aplasia (PATRIGNANI et al., 1971) decrease ^{14}C-glycine incorporation into this component, it is likely that the second component is largely of erythropoietic origin. It may be derived from heme or hemoglobin synthesized in excess of requirements of individual erythroid cells, or from erythrocyte precursors or red cells destroyed in the bone marrow prior to entering the circulation (ineffective erythropoiesis) (GRAY et al., 1950; LONDON et al., 1950), from catabolism of hemoglobin attached to nuclei extruded from mature normoblasts (BESSIS et al., 1961), or (in rats) from hemolysis of circulating reticulocytes (ROBINSON and KOEPPEL, 1971; ROBINSON and TSONG, 1970). The initial component of early bilirubin production appears to be primarily of hepatic origin on the basis of studies which demonstrate that the size of this component can be influenced by changes in hepatic heme turnover (SCHMID et al., 1966; LEVITT et al., 1968; ROBINSON, 1969) and not by nephrectomy (LEVITT et al., 1968); that liver homogenates (WHITE et al., 1966), isolated perfused rat liver (ROBINSON et al., 1965), and cultured hepatoma cells (ROBINSON et al., 1971a) will produce labeled bilirubin from labeled precursors, and that labeled ALA, which is poorly incorporated into hemoglobin heme but is very effectively incorporated into liver heme (NEUBERGER and SCOTT, 1953), appears only in the first component. However, GLASS et al. (1975) have detected labeled heme in both hepatic and erythroid cells one hour after ^{14}C-glycine administration, suggesting that both tissues may contribute to the earlier component.

II. Enzymatic Degradation of Heme

A mechanism for enzymatic catabolism of heme is provided by the heme oxygenase system (TENHUNEN et al., 1968, 1969). This microsomal enzyme system promotes the oxidative fission of the α-methene bridge of heme to form equimolar amounts of biliverdin-IXα and carbon monoxide. Because of its microsomal localization, absolute requirement for NADPH and molecular oxygen, inhibition by carbon monoxide (TENHUNEN et al., 1972), immunochemically-demonstrated requirement for NADPH-cytochrome c reductase (SCHACTER et al., 1972), and stoichiometric considerations, it was thought that this enzyme was dependent on the microsomal electron transport system comprised of cytochrome P-450 and the flavoprotein enzyme NADPH-cytochrome c reductase. The recent isolation by detergent solubilization and column chromatography of a factor from pig spleen microsomes which is devoid of cytochrome P-450 (but not entirely free of other hemoprotein) and which will in the presence of NADPH-cytochrome c reductase and NADPH catalyze the conversion of heme to biliverdin (YOSHIDA et al., 1974) now suggests that this enzymatic process may not require cytochrome P-450 as the terminal oxidase. Additional evidence for this view is provided by the recent observations that cytochrome c reductase alone will catalyze biliverdin formation from heme (MASTERS and SCHACTER, 1976) and that cobalt and other heavy metal ions potently induce hepatic heme oxygenase while concomitantly decreasing hepatic cytochrome P-450 content (MAINES and KAPPAS, 1974). Further work is required to clarify the essential components and mechanism of this reaction.

Heme oxygenase activity is found primarily but not exclusively in organs which contain reticuloendothelial cells, (TENHUNEN et al., 1970a) with the highest specific activity found in spleen, followed in order by bone marrow, liver, brain, kidney, and lung (TENHUNEN et al., 1970a). Chick embryo heart contains heme oxygenase activity comparable in amount to that found in rat liver (ISRAELS et al., 1974) and duodenal mucosa has also been found to possess heme oxygenase activity (RAFFIN et al., 1974). With isolated preparations of hepatic parenchymal and sinusoidal cells, it has been possible to demonstrate that hepatic parenchymal cells contain heme oxygenase activity and may take up and catabolize circulating hemoglobin. Hepatic sinusoidal cells phagocytose and catabolize the hemoglobin of damaged or effete red cells (BISSELL et al., 1972). Heme oxygenase activity in liver (TENHUNEN et al., 1970a; SCHACTER et al., 1972), macrophages (PIMSTONE et al., 1971a), and kidney (PIMSTONE et al., 1971b) is inducible by its substrate, heme. Induction is dependent on protein synthesis, since it is inhibited in kidney and macrophages by cycloheximide and actinomycin D (PIMSTONE et al., 1971b) and in rat liver by cycloheximide (SCHACTER, 1975). Heme oxygenase has an absolute requirement for iron in the tetrapyrrole ring for activity (SCHACTER and WATERMAN, 1974). Heme bound as methemalbumin and those hemoproteins in which heme is loosely bound (i.e. methemoglobin, isolated α and β chains of hemoglobin) are good substrates for heme oxygenase. However, where heme is more tightly bound to protein as in oxyhemoglobin, carboxyhemoglobin, myoglobin, and haptoglobin-heme complexes, heme oxygenase activity for these substrates is extremely low (TENHUNEN et al., 1968). These data regarding the tissue distribution, relative activities, induction properties, and substrate specificity of microsomal heme oxygenase suggest that it is of primary importance in the catabolism of hemoglobin to biliverdin in reticuloendothelial cells and at other sites, and mediates the production of bile pigment due to hemoprotein turnover in liver and other tissues. Biliverdin-IXα produced as the result of heme oxygenase activity is rapidly and quantitatively converted to bilirubin-IXα by a cytosol enzyme, NADPH-dependent biliverdin reductase (TENHUNEN et al., 1970b) which is present in excess in relation to microsomal heme oxygenase (TENHUNEN, 1972).

III. Albumin Binding of Bilirubin

There is no information regarding the mechanism by which unconjugated bilirubin formed as the result of heme catabolism in various tissues reaches the circulation.

Once there, up to two (BEAVEN et al., 1973; KAMISAKA et al., 1974) or three (JACOBSEN, 1969a) molecules of bilirubin bind with each molecule of plasma albumin. The dissociation constant of the reaction between the first bilirubin molecule and albumin is 7×10^{-9} M, and that for subsequent molecules is 2×10^{-6} M (JACOBSEN, 1969a). Albumin interacts in a comparable fashion with fatty acids (GOODMAN, 1958; ASHBROOK et al., 1975), heme (BEAVEN et al., 1974), certain hormones (SOLOMON, 1971), and other low molecular weight molecules. Because of the high affinity of albumin for bilirubin and the low solubility of bilirubin in aqueous media at physiologic pH, virtually all the bilirubin in plasma is protein bound.

IV. Hepatocellular Uptake

The mechanism by which bilirubin is transported from plasma across the cell membrane into the hepatocyte is not clearly understood. Examination of the hepatic uptake of radio-labeled unconjugated bilirubin and albumin suggests that bilirubin dissociates from albumin prior to transport across the membrane, since significant amounts of labeled bilirubin appear within the liver as compared with minimal albumin entry (BROWN et al., 1964; BERNSTEIN et al., 1966), and the rate of entry of albumin into liver cells is insufficient to account for the rate of bilirubin uptake (GORESKY, 1964). It has been shown that there is a rapid bidirectional flux of bilirubin between liver and plasma (BILLING et al., 1964; GORESKY, 1965). While bilirubin does not bind to hepatocyte plasma membranes (CORNELIUS et al., 1967), recent work has demonstrated a saturable mechanism for uptake to liver cells (GORESKY, 1975; SCHARSCHMIDT et al., 1975) which is probably distinct from the intracellular storage mechanisms. In rat (BROWN et al., 1964) and man (BERK et al., 1969), the unconjugated bilirubin concentration is higher inside the hepatocyte than in plasma, despite lower affinity of intrahepatic binding proteins for bilirubin than that demonstrated for albumin (SCHMID, 1967; BLOOMER et al., 1972). It has been suggested that these findings can be explained by the relationship of the amount and the binding affinities of plasma albumin and Y and Z proteins in hepatocyte cytoplasm (ARIAS, 1972). In this model, influx of bilirubin to the hepatocyte is determined by the amount dissociated from albumin in plasma and occurs by nonionic diffusion across the hepatocyte plasma membrane. Efflux of bilirubin is determined by the relative availability and binding affinities of Y and Z protein. Since bilirubin is constantly being conjugated and excreted by the hepatocyte, continual availability of vacant intracellular binding sites for bilirubin would influence bilirubin movement towards a net influx.

V. Intracellular Binding

Y and Z proteins have been characterized as hepatic cytoplasmic proteins which may be responsible for binding and transport of bilirubin and other organic anions (LEVI et al., 1969). Y protein is thought to be the principal binding protein because it is present in higher concentration and has higher organic anion binding affinity than Z both in vitro and in vivo (LEVI et al., 1969). Y is a basic protein with a molecular weight of 44,000 comprised of two identical subunits (LEVI et al., 1968;

LITWACK et al., 1971). It constitutes 5% of the cytoplasmic protein of hepatic parenchymal cells (LITWACK et al., 1971; FLEISCHNER et al., 1971).

The proposed role of these binding proteins (particularly Y) in hepatic bilirubin uptake and transport is based on the following observations: (1) the high concentration of Y and Z proteins in hepatic cytosol (LEVI et al., 1969); (2) observation of in vitro binding and in vivo hepatic uptake of bilirubin and other organic anions by these proteins (LEVI et al., 1969; REYES et al., 1971); (3) a correlation between the appearance of Y protein in neonatal liver and an increase in selective hepatic uptake of organic anions during that period (LEVI et al., 1970); (4) phylogenetic studies showing a correlation between hepatic uptake of sulfobromophthalein (BSP) and the presence of Y and Z proteins (LEVINE et al., 1971). However, the circumstantial nature of the evidence for the functional importance of these proteins in hepatic uptake and transport of bilirubin leaves their place in the physiology of bilirubin transport unsettled (ARIAS, 1972). There is good evidence for a hepatic storage compartment for bilirubin in rats (BILLING et al., 1963) and man (BILLING et al., 1964; BERK et al., 1969; RAYMOND and GALAMBOS, 1971), and Y and Z proteins may be involved in this process.

By analysis of subcellular radiobilirubin distribution (BROWN et al., 1964; BERNSTEIN et al., 1966), a small proportion of the intracellular unconjugated bilirubin pool has been found to be associated with the microsomal fraction. Presumably it is this pool that is bound on the microsomal membrane either to conjugating enzymes or to another binding site which facilitates access of bilirubin to the conjugation site. The method of transfer of bilirubin from cytosol to the smooth endoplasmic reticulum remains unknown.

VI. Conjugation of Bilirubin

Bilirubin is converted to an ester glucuronide by a hepatic microsomal enzyme, UDP-glucuronyl transferase (GT) which catalyzes the transfer of glucuronic acid from UDP-glucuronic acid to the propionic acid side chains of bilirubin (DUTTON, 1966), to form bilirubin glucuronide. The enzymatic activity has been demonstrated in liver slices (LATHE and WALKER, 1958), homogenates (LATHE and WALKER, 1958; GRODSKY and CARBONE, 1957; ARIAS, 1959), and microsomal preparations (SCHMID et al., 1957; VANROY and HEIRWEGH, 1968; LAGE and SPRATT, 1968). While most of the ester glucuronide formed with bilirubin in many species studied is the diglucuronide (BILLING et al., 1957; TALAFANT, 1956; SCHMID, 1956; ISSELBACHER and MCCARTHY, 1959; SCHMID et al., 1958; BROWN and ZUELZER, 1958), there has been controversy regarding the formation and excretion of small amounts of bilirubin monoglucuronide (BILLING et al., 1957; COLE et al., 1954; SCHMID, 1957). Some evidence has suggested that this entity is a mixture of bilirubin and bilirubin diglucuronide (NOSSLIN, 1960; WEBER et al., 1963). Studies of bilirubin conjugation in vitro have demonstrated the formation of bilirubin β-D-monoglucuronide (VANROY and HEIRWEGH, 1968; BLACK et al., 1970; STREBEL and ODELL, 1969), and more recent work has shown the presence of bilirubin monoglucuronide in bile (JACOBSEN, 1969b; OSTROW and MURPHY, 1970; JANSEN and BILLING, 1971), which may comprise as much as 22% of total bile pigments in man (FEVERY et al., 1972).

Uncertainty exists as to whether there is a specific bilirubin GT since many drugs, steroids, cholecystographic agents, and thyroxin are conjugated in a similar manner. It is likely that there are a variety of conjugating enzymes including one specific for bilirubin (DUTTON, 1966, 1971). Evidence for this includes: (1) the fact that N-linked glucuronides are formed by an enzyme separate from bilirubin GT (ARIAS, 1961; ISSELBACHER et al., 1962; HOWLAND et al., 1971); (2) studies suggesting the existence of several GT enzymes in homogenates (VANLEUSDEN et al., 1962); (3) evidence for a specific bilirubin GT on the basis of differing responses in conjugation rates to various manipulations (VESSEY et al., 1973a); (4) the development of a specific assay for bilirubin GT (VANROY and HEIRWEGH, 1968). Resolution of this problem must await purification of the purported specific enzyme.

The activity of GT increases along with that of other components of the smooth endoplasmic reticulum following treatment in vivo with phenobarbital and other xenobiotics known to cause proliferation of the smooth endoplasmic reticulum (ARIAS et al., 1969; DELEON et al., 1967; GLAUMANN, 1970; GRAM et al., 1967, 1968; ZEIDENBERG et al., 1967).

Many other bilirubin conjugates, including complexes with sulfate (ISSELBACHER and McCARTHY, 1959; NOIR et al., 1970; SCHOENFIELD et al., 1962), glycine (JIRSA and VECEREK, 1958; TENHUNEN, 1965; ISSELBACHER and McCARTHY, 1959), phosphate, taurine (TENHUNEN, 1965), other sugars (i.e. glucoside and xyloside conjugates) (HEIRWEGH et al., 1970, 1971; WONG, 1971) and acyl glycosides of acidic disaccharides (KUENZLE, 1970a, b, c) have been described. However, these conjugates appear to be present in small amounts and their functional importance appears uncertain since in disorders characterized by GT deficiency, no compensatory formation of these products has been observed (FEVERY et al., 1972).

VII. Excretion to Bile

Little conjugated bilirubin is found within the hepatocyte (BERNSTEIN et al., 1966), suggesting that conjugated bilirubin is rapidly transported across the cell membrane into the bile canaliculi. The excretory mechanism is poorly understood, but since it may occur against a concentration gradient and is a saturable process subject to competitive inhibition, it is thought to be an energy-dependent carrier-mediated process (GORESKY, 1965). While it has not been possible to positively associate any intracellular organelles with this process (BERNSTEIN et al., 1966), the presence of endoplasmic reticulum active in bilirubin conjugation close to the canalicular membrane may be of importance in facilitating excretion of conjugated bilirubin (GREGORY and STRICKLAND, 1972). Studies with continuous intravenous administration of increasing amounts of unconjugated bilirubin have shown an initial rise in biliary excretion of bilirubin to a maximal rate (ARIAS et al., 1961; WEINBREN and BILLING, 1956) followed by a rise in conjugated bilirubin levels in plasma with no further increase in the rate of biliary bilirubin excretion (ARIAS et al., 1961; SNYDER et al., 1967). These data suggest that excretion is the rate-limiting step in the movement of bilirubin from plasma to bile. However, conjugation of bilirubin is essential for its biliary excretion (ARIAS et al., 1961; SCHMID et al., 1958), and there is evidence linking bilirubin GT activity and the maximal rate of bilirubin excretion in rats (ROBINSON et al., 1971b).

The higher bilirubin concentration in the canaliculus as compared with the hepatocyte suggests an energy-dependent process. Although there is a lower bilirubin concentration in the cell than in the bile canaliculus, it is probably necessary to examine the state of the bilirubin outside the cell before inferring that this secretion is against a gradient (Goresky et al., 1974). Bile contains mixed micelles made up of cholesterol, bile acids, and lecithin (Carey and Small, 1970), which bind all the bilirubin present in gall bladder bile in a macromolecular complex (Verschure and Mijnlieff, 1956). Thus the bilirubin in the canaliculus probably exists in a bound form and the amount of free conjugated bilirubin on either side of the hepatocyte membrane may be equivalent, or may be higher within the cell, allowing a non-energy-dependent excretory process.

Bilirubin glucuronide excretion is dependent on bile flow, the physiology of which has been reviewed by Erlinger (1972) and Wheeler (1975). Bile flow into the canaliculi is driven by a metabolic process rather than by hydrostatic pressure, as the bile secretion pressure exceeds that of the vascular perfusion pressure (Brauer et al., 1954). Hepatocytes excrete four classes of substances probably by different pathways: (1) the bile acids; (2) organic anions including conjugated bilirubin, rose bengal, BSP, and indocyanine green (ICG); (3) organic cations; (4) neutral substances such as cardiac glycosides (Erlinger, 1972). Competition for biliary excretion occurs within (Hunton et al., 1961; Sperber, 1959; Wheeler et al., 1958), but not between (Alpert et al., 1969; Gutstein et al., 1968) these groups.

VIII. Intestinal Fate of Bilirubin

Bilirubin reaches the gastrointestinal tract in the conjugated glucuronide form which cannot be reabsorbed (Lester and Schmid, 1963a, b). Although unconjugated bilirubin may be formed and absorbed in appreciable amounts from the gastrointestinal tract of newborn infants due to the high activity of intestinal β-glucuronidase (Brodersen and Herman, 1963) and absence of bacteria (Elder et al., 1972), there is no deconjugation of bilirubin and thus no enterohepatic circulation of bilirubin in adults (Lester and Schmid, 1963b). In the terminal ileum and colon, bilirubin is converted by bacterial flora to a group of reduced products collectively known as urobilinogens (Gray, 1961; Watson, 1963; Troxler et al., 1968; Watson et al., 1958). These compounds are no longer glucuronides, but the site and mechanism of deconjugation have not been characterized. While most of the urobilinogens are excreted in the feces, some are reabsorbed and then either excreted by the kidney (in amounts of $1-3$ mg/day) (Bourke et al., 1965; Levy et al., 1968) or re-excreted by the liver into the intestine (Lester and Klein, 1966; Lester and Schmid, 1965; Lester et al., 1965; Stumpf and Lester, 1966).

C. Drug-Mediated Alterations in Bilirubin Metabolism

I. Increased Bilirubin Production Due to Erythrocyte Destruction

Hyperbilirubinemia due to circulating unconjugated bilirubin may be due to increased red cell destruction. This may be related to congenital abnormalities of

red cell shape or structure, or to abnormal hemoglobins or abnormalities of hemoglobin synthesis. Alternately the cause may be external to the cell which may be
destroyed by immune, mechanical, or metabolic mechanisms. In this section we
are concerned only with examples of how drugs may induce a hemolytic process.

Increased bilirubin production from hemoglobin occurs with shortening of the
red cell life span. Although decreased red cell survival may result from a direct
drug effect on the normal red cell, such as the hemolytic effects of phenylhydrazine,
dapsone, or arsine, the commonest forms of drug-induced hemolysis are associated with congenital abnormalities of red cell metabolism, abnormal unstable
hemoglobins, or drug-induced immunohemolytic responses (BEUTLER, 1969a).

1. Hemolysis Related to Impaired Erythrocyte Metabolism

The erythrocyte is a metabolically active cell dependent on glucose as its energy
source. Glycolysis provides energy for the enzyme systems required for cell function including those which maintain the sodium-potassium cell-plasma gradient
and those which maintain hemoglobin in its reduced and functional state. About
90% of the glucose is metabolized through the Embden-Meyerhof pathway which
produces energy in the form of ATP, the remaining glucose going through the
hexose monophosphate shunt which provides NADPH to maintain reduced glutathione (GSH). GSH is a requisite for the protection of hemoglobin and other proteins from oxidation by peroxides which may be generated by a number of oxidant
drugs. The four linked enzyme systems which are required to reduce the peroxides
are glucose-6-phosphate dehydrogenase (G-6-PD) and 6-phosphogluconate, phos-
phogluconic dehydrogenase (PGD) to reduce NADP to NADPH, glutathione reductase which utilizes NADPH to reduce oxidized glutathione to GSH, and glutathione peroxidase which reduces peroxide with the oxidation of GSH. Reduced
function at any step makes the red cell susceptible to hemolysis by oxidant drugs.
The commonest defect is reduction of G-6-PD activity due to genetic variants with
reduced enzyme activity. Much rarer are patients with deficient activity of glutathione synthetase (MOHLER et al., 1970) or glutathione reductase (WALLER, 1968).
Glutathione reductase deficiency may result from the absence of its co-factor flavin
adenine dinucleotide (BEUTLER, 1969b). Of less established clinical significance are
congenital deficiences of glutathione peroxidase (BEUTLER, 1971) or PGD (BREWER
and DERN, 1964). The lower levels of glutathione peroxidase in the newborn may
be one factor in the increased sensitivity of these erythrocytes to oxidant drugs
(GROSS et al., 1967). Clinically significant red cell destruction in patients with
G-6-PD deficiency may be caused by the drugs listed in Table 1. Large doses of
phenacetin have been observed to cause the formation of Heinz bodies, sulfhemoglobinemia and hemolysis in patients with no evidence of G-6-PD, glutathione
reductase or GSH deficiency (MILLAR et al., 1972).

Enzyme defects in the Embden-Meyerhof pathway are often associated with
shortening of red cell survival. GLADER (1976) demonstrated that salicylates caused
a sharp depletion of ATP in pyruvate-kinase deficient erythrocytes. This was associated with a loss in red cell potassium and water and an inhibiton of the ascor-
bate-induced stimulation of glucose-1-^{14}C oxidation. These changes might aggravate the in vivo hemolysis associated with pyruvate kinase deficiency although this
as yet has not been documented.

2. Hemolysis and Unstable Hemoglobins

The normal hemoglobin of adults consists of two alpha chains and two beta chains each of which is bound to the heme iron through two histidine sites. Mutations involving amino acid substitution at or near these histidine sites may result in abnormal hemoglobins which are susceptible to oxidant drugs with the production of oxidized heme products which compromise red cell survival (Nagel and Ranney, 1973). Drug-induced hemolytic anemia has been observed in patients with hemoglobins Zurich (Frick et al., 1962), Torino (Prato et al., 1970), Peterborough (King et al., 1972), and Shepherd's Bush (White et al., 1970). Some of the drugs documented as responsible are sulfonamides, primaquine, and sulfonic acid (Beutler, 1969a), but other oxidant drugs might also be expected to produce hemolysis.

3. Drug-Induced Immune Hemolysis

Drugs may induce hemolytic anemia by acting as foreign antigens which induce an immunologic response which causes red cell destruction. The recognized mechanisms are three in number (Beutler, 1969a; Worledge, 1973).
a) The immune complex type. Here the induced antibody complexes with the antigenic drug and forms antigen-antibody complexes. These complexes may interact with a number of cell membranes including that of the red cell, fix complement, and produce lysis. The erythrocyte is not specifically immunologically involved, serving only as a receptor for the immune complex, and is affected as an

Table 1. Some agents which have been implicated in the production of hemolysis in patients with G-6-PD deficiency

Analgesics	Acetanilid (Dern et al., 1955)
	Acetophenetidin (phenacetin) (Dern et al., 1955)
	Acetylsalicylic acid (Kellermeyer et al., 1962)
Antimalarials	Primaquine (Dern et al., 1955)
	Pamaquine (Beutler, 1959)
	Pentaquine (Beutler, 1959)
	Quinacrine (Kellermeyer et al., 1962)
	Quinocide (Kellermeyer et al., 1962)
Sulfonamides	Sulfanilamide (Dern et al., 1955)
	Sulfapyridine (Zail et al., 1962)
	Sulfisoxazole (Kellermeyer et al., 1962)
Nitrofurans	Nitrofurazone (Robertson, 1961)
	Nitrofurantoin (Kellermeyer et al., 1962)
Sulfones	Diaphenylsulfone (Degowin et al., 1966)
	Thiazosulfone (Dern et al., 1955)
Vitamin K	Vitamin K (Zinkham, 1963)
	Menadione sodium diphosphate (Zinkham, 1963)
Others	Phenylhydrazine (Dern et al., 1955)
	Naphthalene (Zinkham and Childs, 1958)
	Fava beans (Dacie, 1967)

"innocent bystander." Besides stibophen (HARRIS, 1956), other drugs which produce an immunohemolytic anemia by a similar mechanism are acetophenetidin, quinine, (MUIRHEAD et al., 1958) quinidine (FREEDMAN et al., 1956), p-amino-salicylic acid (MACGIBBON et al., 1960), isoniazid (ROBINSON and FOADI, 1969), sulfonamides (DACIE, 1967), insecticides (MUIRHEAD et al., 1959), chlorpromazine (LINDBERG and NORDEN, 1961) rifampicin (LAKSHMINARAYAN et al., 1973), and others (WORLLEDGE, 1973).

b) The hapten, or penicillin type. This may follow the use of large doses of penicillin, cephalothin, or cephaloridine, with fixation of the drug to the red cell membrane. The antibodies are usually IgG and are directed against a number of antigenic groups on the molecule of which the major determinant for penicillin is the benzylpenicilloyl group (SWANSON et al., 1966; GRALNICK et al., 1971; LEVINE, 1966; WORLLEDGE, 1973).

c) The autoimmune, or alpha-methyl dopa type. Here the drug directly induces the formation of an antibody which reacts with the Rh locus on the cell membrane (WORLLEDGE, 1973). A similar phenomenon has been described in patients given L dopa (TERRITO et al., 1973) or mefenamic acid (SCOTT et al., 1968).

II. Effect of Drugs on Hepatic Hemoprotein Turnover

Studies summarized in section BI indicated that the first component of early-labeled bilirubin is largely derived from the rapid turnover of hepatic heme. This source has been estimated to account for $13-21\%$ of daily bilirubin production in three patients with acute intermittent porphyria (JONES et al., 1971). This may be a valid index of nonerythropoietic heme degradation in normal man as well, since similar values are found for total and early-labeled bilirubin production in acute intermittent porphyria and normal individuals (BLOOMER et al., 1971).

The liver contains many hemoproteins, including mitochondrial cytochromes, catalase, tryptophan pyrrolase, and the microsomal cytochromes P-450 and b_5 which could potentially contribute to the heme catabolic pool. The fractional catabolic rate of mitochondrial cytochromes is too low (DRABKIN, 1951; FLETCHER and SANADI, 1961) and the hepatic concentrations of tryptophan pyrrolase and cytochrome b_5 are too small (SCHMID et al., 1966) for these hemoproteins to serve as a significant source of the hepatic component of early-labeled bilirubin. The contribution from catalase turnover must also be small in view of its low turnover rate (SCHMID et al., 1966; LEVITT et al., 1968). Studies of hepatic cytochrome P-450 by pulse radio-labeling of the heme moiety of this hemoprotein with ALA have demonstrated a bi-phasic decay in radioactivity in cytochrome P-450 heme, the first phase having a halflife of $8-10$ h and the second phase having a halflife of $24-48$ h (BOCK and SIEKEVITZ, 1970; MEYER and MARVER, 1971; GARNER and McLEAN, 1969; LEVIN and KUNTZMAN, 1969; GREIM et al., 1970). However, labeled bilirubin can be detected within minutes of i.v. injection of glycine-^{14}C or ALA-^{14}C and the peak excretion of early-labeled bilirubin occurs within 2 h of injection of ALA-^{14}C (ISRAELS et al., 1963a; YAMAMOTO et al., 1965; SCHMID et al., 1966). Therefore the rate of turnover of cytochrome P-450 would appear to be too slow to account for this rapid labeling of bilirubin. Moreover, significant inhibition of synthesis of hepatic protein and hepatic cytochrome P-450 by cycloheximide is associated with a slight increase in early bilirubin formation (Levitt et al., 1968). This observation led to the suggestion that a significant proportion of the hepatic early bilirubin production might originate from the rapid turnover of a hepatic heme pool either not associated with or present in excess of requirements for hemoprotein synthesis (Levitt et al., 1968).

1. Drugs and Bilirubin Production

Most studies of drug effects on bilirubin metabolism and hepatic heme turnover have used phenobarbital. Phenobarbital and other xenobiotics are known to stimulate proliferation of hepatic smooth endoplasmic reticulum in association with enhancement of various microsomal enzymes and cytochromes and induction of drug-metabolizing activity (Conney, 1967; Remmer and Merker, 1963, 1965). Phenobarbital induces ALA-synthetase, the initial and rate limiting step in heme biosynthesis (Granick, 1966; Baron and Tephly, 1969; Marver et al., 1968), and produces increased hepatic heme and hemoprotein synthesis as judged by incorporation of radioactive precursors (Tephly et al., 1971; Marver, 1969). These changes are accompanied by increased levels of the microsomal cytochromes P-450 and b_5 (Remmer and Merker, 1965; Schmid et al., 1966; Levitt et al., 1968) and enhanced hepatic microsomal drug oxidation (Conney, 1967). A two- to threefold increase in early-labeled bilirubin production (Levitt et al., 1968; Landaw et al., 1970; Robinson, 1969; Gisselbrecht and Berk, 1974) and labeled carbon monoxide production (Landaw et al., 1970) from glycine-2-^{14}C following phenobarbital treatment of rats has been amply demonstrated. In contrast, the incorporation into early-labeled bilirubin of ALA-4-^{14}C was only minimally enhanced by phenobarbital (Levitt et al., 1968). This observation led to the suggestion that the major effect of phenobarbital in increasing early-labeled bilirubin production is the induction of hepatic ALA-synthetase with increased heme synthesis and turnover (Levitt et al., 1968), rather than enhanced microsomal hemoprotein turnover (Schmid et al., 1966). The failure of cycloheximide (added to suppress protein and cytochrome P-450 synthesis) to reduce early bilirubin formation (Levitt et al., 1968), together with the lack of correlation between the catabolic rates of the microsomal cytochromes and the rapid initial appearance of early-labeled bilirubin suggest that hemoprotein turnover is a minor source of this component.

Early-labeled bilirubin formation from glycine-2-^{14}C in Gunn rats was only slightly increased by phenobarbital (Robinson, 1971). A small increase in the labeling of the hepatic component of early-labeled bilirubin in rats was also described after hydrocortisone or chronic carbon tetrachloride administration (Robinson, 1969).

Studies of phenobarbital effects on bilirubin and carbon monoxide production in man have yielded conflicting results. Coburn (1970) reported an up to twofold increase in carbon monoxide production in nine normal human subjects given a 7-day course of phenobarbital or diphenylhydantoin, and small increases in carbon monoxide dilution indicating an increase in the total body heme pool. It was concluded that phenobarbital and diphenylhydantoin enlarge hepatic heme pools with subsequent increased catabolism sufficient to account for at least 50% of the total carbon monoxide production. In contrast, Blaschke et al. (1974a) reported that administration of phenobarbital or glutethimide to a group of 19 patients with Gilbert's syndrome and 11 normal subjects resulted in enhanced hepatic bilirubin clearance associated with a modest decrease in both plasma bilirubin turnover and endogenous carbon monoxide production with no change in CO space. The reason for the discrepancy between these two studies is not clear. The observation of an isolated fall in bilirubin turnover following phenobarbital or glutethimide therapy, sufficient to account for a 30 per cent reduction in bilirubin concentration in normals (BLASCHKE et al., 1974a), may be an important new factor to consider in determining the causes of decreases in plasma bilirubin concentration following drug therapy.

While an initial limited study had suggested that phenobarbital administration in rats produced a twofold increase in bile bilirubin excretion (SCHMID et al., 1966), other studies of bile bilirubin excretion (LEVITT et al., 1968; GISSELBRECHT and BERK, 1974) and isotopic bilirubin turnover in Gunn rats (ROBINSON, 1969) and bilirubin turnover in man (BLASCHKE et al., 1974a) have failed to show any consistent increase in total bilirubin excretion following phenobarbital treatment. These discrepancies may simply reflect the wide range of variation in bile bilirubin excretion in rats (GISSELBRECHT and BERK, 1974; LEVITT et al., 1968), but leave unresolved the paradox of enhancement of early-labeled bilirubin production by phenobarbital without significant increase in total bilirubin or carbon monoxide production. Since hepatic bilirubin production may account for approximately 10–20% of total daily bilirubin production in man (JONES et al., 1971), a doubling of this fraction by phenobarbital treatment may only result in a 10–20% increase in total bilirubin excretion, which is a difference that might be difficult to verify experimentally. In fact, the published studies do demonstrate a statistically non-significant 15–20% increase in bile bilirubin excretion in phenobarbital-treated rats (LEVITT et al., 1968; GISSELBRECHT and BERK, 1974) and this difference may explain the paradox mentioned above.

α-naphthylisothiocyanate (ANIT) has been shown to increase bile bilirubin content and to increase incorporation of ALA-^{14}C into bile bilirubin in experimental animals. This drug has complex effects upon the liver, including BSP retention and prolongation of pentobarbital sleeping time which occur 1–4 h after ANIT administration (BECKER and PLAA, 1965a, b) and hyperbilirubinemia and cholestasis, which have a late onset 12–16 h after ANIT (ELIAKIM et al., 1959; BECKER and PLAA, 1965a; INDACOCHEA-REDMOND and PLAA, 1971). The microsomal enzyme inducers phenobarbital and chlorpromazine potentiate (ROBERTS and PLAA, 1965) while inhibitors of RNA and protein synthesis reduce the hyperbilirubinemia and cholestasis produced by ANIT (INDACOCHEA-REDMOND et al., 1973). It has been suggested on the basis of such studies that hepatic protein synthesis may be necessary for the production of enzymes which convert ANIT to metabolites responsible for these effects (ROBERTS and PLAA, 1965; CAPIZZO and ROBERTS, 1971; INDACOCHEA-REDMOND et al., 1973), although ANIT-induced cholestasis and hyperbilirubinemia can be inhibited by much lower doses of inhibitors than those commonly used to inhibit protein or RNA synthesis (INDACOCHEA-REDMOND et al., 1974). The effect of ANIT upon ALA-^{14}C incorporation to bilirubin occurs prior to the onset of cholestasis (ROBERTS and PLAA, 1968) suggesting stimulation of hepatic heme turnover as one cause for the hyperbilirubinemia observed. This effect is also inhibited by pretreatment with inhibitors of RNA and protein synthesis (TRAIGER et al., 1974). The mechanism of this phenomenon is uncertain.

Nicotinic acid, which leads to increased blood carbon monoxide levels (GYDELL, 1960), also causes an increase in serum-unconjugated bilirubin levels. Heme oxygenase activity has not been studied after administration of this drug. The mechanism of this effect is unknown but it has been suggested that increased bilirubin production is involved (FROMKE and MILLER, 1972; LUNDH et al., 1975).

2. Drugs and Heme Oxygenase

Administration of phenobarbital to rats has no significant effect on hepatic or splenic heme oxygenase activity (SCHACTER and MASON, 1974; ROTHWELL et al., 1973) nor on the activity of heme oxygenase of hepatic parenchymal or sinusoidal cells isolated from treated rats (HUPKA and KARLER, 1973). 3-Methylcholanthrene administration was associated with a significant decrease in rat hepatic and splenic heme oxygenase activity (SCHACTER and MASON, 1974). No change in activity in isolated rat hepatic parenchymal and sinusoidal cells was observed by HUPKA and KARLER (1973). 3,4-Benzpyrene and pregnenolone-16α-carbonitrile (PCN) administration produced no significant change in hepatic and splenic heme oxygenase activity (SCHACTER and MASON, 1974). Dicarbethoxydihydrocollidine, an agent known to inhibit heme synthesis at the ferrochelatase step (TEPHLY et al., 1971) also had no effect on rat hepatic or splenic heme oxygenase activity (ROTHWELL et al., 1973). Although phenobarbital is known to increase hepatic early-labeled bilirubin production (SCHMID et al., 1966; LEVITT et al., 1968; LANDAW et al., 1970), this increase is not accompanied by an increase in the specific activity of hepatic heme oxygenase (SCHACTER and MASON, 1974; ROTHWELL et al., 1973). These contradictory observations may be reconciled if basal hepatic heme oxygenase activity is not rate limiting for hepatic heme and hemoprotein catabolism. In addition, it is known that phenobarbital induces an increase in hepatic parenchymal cell mass with a proliferation of smooth endoplasmic reticulum and an increase in microsomal protein per gram of liver (CONNEY, 1967), so that although the specific activity of hepatic heme oxygenase is not increased, the total amount of enzyme may be greater following phenobarbital.

Although phenobarbital, polycyclic hydrocarbons, and PCN are known inducers of various functions of the microsomal electron transport system with which heme oxygenase is thought to be associated, no inductive effect on heme oxygenase activity by these agents has been observed. On the other hand, heme, while promoting induction of hepatic heme oxygenase (TENHUNEN et al., 1970a; SCHACTER et al., 1972) produces a concomitant decrease in hepatic cytochrome P-450 (MARVER et al., 1968; MARVER, 1969; SCHACTER et al., 1972) and hepatic drug metabolism (MARVER, 1969) with no change in hepatic microsomal NADPH-cytochrome c reductase activity (SCHACTER et al., 1972). This dichotomy suggests that factors other than those associated with the microsomal electron transport system might regulate heme oxygenase activity. The existence of a specific microsomal binding protein for heme which facilitates its oxidative catabolism or of a unique enzyme associated with the components of the microsomal electron transport system but responsible specifically for heme catabolism have been proposed (SCHACTER and MASON, 1974). These suggestions were supported by the recent isolation from pig spleen microsomes of a detergent-solubilized protein which facilitates oxidative heme catabolism in the presence of NADPH-cytochrome c reductase (YOSHIDA et al., 1974). This factor might explain the effects of drugs and heme on heme oxygenase activity if it were inducible by heme administration but were not affected by drugs known to stimulate hepatic drug metabolism.

Fasting is known to be associated with induction of hepatic heme oxygenase in rats (BAKKEN et al., 1972; ROTHWELL et al., 1973). This effect can be simulated by hypoglycemia induced by insulin or mannose. Glucagon and epinephrine also cause an increase in rat liver heme oxygenase activity when given parenterally (BAKKEN et al., 1972). Cyclic AMP reproduced this effect, but thyroxin and hydrocortisone did not. None of these manipulations had any effect on splenic heme oxygenase activity. It was suggested on the basis of these data that stimulation of hepatic heme oxygenase activity in response to fasting hypoglycemia may be mediated by release of glucagon and epinephrine acting through cyclic AMP. The suggestion was also made that the induction of hepatic heme oxygenase activity during fasting may thereby increase hepatic heme turnover and bilirubin production and thus contribute to the unconjugated hyperbilirubinemia described in the fasting state (BAKKEN et al., 1972).

3. Heme Catabolism in Drug-Induced Porphyria

Allylisopropylacetamide (AIA), an agent known to produce experimental porphyria in animals (GRANICK, 1966; MARVER et al., 1966) has been shown to cause a rapid decrease in microsomal heme and cytochrome P-450 after in vivo administration (DE MATTEIS, 1970, 1971; LEVIN et al., 1972; MEYER and MARVER, 1971) with formation and accumulation of ill-defined green pigment breakdown products in the liver (SCHWARTZ and IKEDA, 1955). Other barbiturates containing allyl groups (e.g. secobarbital, allobarbital, aprobarbital) have also been shown to produce similar effects (LEVIN et al., 1973) leading to the suggestion that active metabolites, perhaps epoxides, of these allyl-containing compounds may be involved in the formation of green pigments from microsomal heme (LEVIN et al., 1973; DE MATTEIS, 1973). AIA has been found to reduce the fractional conversion of hematin-^{14}C to early-labeled bilirubin and CO, but at the same time the molar ratio of CO/bilirubin recovery was always much greater than unity. Administration of glycine-2-^{14}C to AIA treated animals caused no change or a decrease in early-labeling with a concomitant increase in labeled CO production (LANDAW et al., 1970). The total recovery of radioactivity in bile was not noticeably different. These results were thought to suggest that AIA treatment favors heme degradation to nonbilirubin metabolites (LANDAW et al., 1970) through alternate catabolic pathways. The observation that AIA pre-treatment produces a significant fall in hepatic and splenic heme oxygenase activity (ROTHWELL et al., 1973) supports the suggestion that accelerated heme catabolism following AIA proceeds through pathways different from heme oxygenase. Data are not presently available as to the effects of allyl-containing barbiturates on heme catabolism and bilirubin production in man.

III. Drugs and Protein Binding of Bilirubin

Many drugs are capable of binding with albumin (MEYER and GUTTMAN, 1968; RUDMAN et al., 1971) and certain of these interfere with binding of bilirubin by albumin. Our understanding of such interactions is incomplete. RUDMAN et al. (1971) have suggested several possible mechanisms including direct competition for shared binding sites, electrostatic repulsion between molecules of like charge, and conformational changes in protein structure with alteration of distant binding sites (SPECTOR et al., 1973). Acetylation of albumin, which occurs on exposure to acetylsalicylic acid, alters its affinity for certain drugs (CHIGNELL and STARKWEATHER, 1971; PINCKARD et al., 1973) but not for bilirubin (JACOBSEN, 1972).

Most albumin-bound bilirubin is associated with a single high affinity binding site from which bilirubin is not readily displaced (WOSILAIT, 1974). At very high plasma bilirubin concentrations, which may occur in neonates with hemolytic diseases, high affinity sites become fully saturated and binding sites of lower affinity become significantly loaded with bilirubin. It is the bilirubin bound to low affinity sites which is in significant equilibrium with unbound bilirubin and it is at these sites that most drug-mediated alterations in bilirubin binding probably occur (WOSILAIT, 1974; LEE and COWGER, 1974).

Because vascular and cellular membranes are impermeable to protein-bound bilirubin, it is the plasma concentration of free bilirubin (normally minute) which determines the amount of bilirubin that enters the tissues. Even minor alterations in albumin's ability to bind bilirubin are of significance because small changes in plasma free bilirubin concentration may lead to a relatively large change in tissue bilirubin content. Nonprotein-bound unconjugated bilirubin is toxic and excessive tissue bilirubin in the newborn leads to irreversible central nervous system damage and the syndrome of kernicterus (DIAMOND, 1969).

The danger of drug-induced displacement of unconjugated bilirubin from albumin to the tissues is significant only in patients with severe unconjugated hyperbilirubinemia, particularly if there is also hypoalbuminemia or acidosis. In clinical practice, the sulfonamides are the best known example of drugs which cause *kernicterus* by this mechanism (SILVERMAN et al., 1956; HARRIS et al., 1958) but a number of other drugs have this potential. Studies utilizing newer techniques will be discussed briefly; data obtained with older techniques have been summarized by DONE (1964).

Decreases in serum unconjugated bilirubin in hyperbilirubinemic animals immediately after drug administration generally reflect displacement of albumin-bound bilirubin into the tissues. This can be verified by increased tissue bilirubin concentration in the experimental animal. This method should detect bilirubin displacement by drug metabolites which would not be apparent with in vitro tests and would also be sensitive to agents which might cause bilirubin redistribution by altering cell membrane permeability rather than by displacement from albumin. JOHNSON et al. (1959, 1961) treated young Gunn rats with salicylates and various sulfonamides and demonstrated decreased serum bilirubin and increased tissue bilirubin concentration. A wide variety of drugs have been shown to have this effect, including sodium benzoate, tolbutamide, acetazolamide, penicillin, tetracycline, chloramphenicol, lipid emulsions (JOHNSON et al., 1959, 1961; NATHENSON et al., 1975) probenecid (KENWRIGHT and LEVI, 1973), mefenamic acid, nicotinic acid, oxyphenbutazone, piperazine, and quinidine (YEARY and DAVIS, 1974). Tissue bilirubin assays were not performed in most of these studies and drug dose was often higher than that used in patients. Nevertheless, this in vivo screening method is probably more relevant to the clinical situation than many of the physicochemical methods available.

Several in vitro techniques involve direct measurement of displaced bilirubin. Salicylate, oleate (ODELL, 1966; ODELL et al., 1969), indomethacin, mefenamic acid, phenylbutazone, oxyphenbutazone, and novobiocin (YEARY and DAVIS, 1974) displace unconjugated bilirubin from albumin to rat mitochondria. Others have used similar methods involving displacement of bilirubin from albumin to such acceptors as erythrocytes (BRATLID, 1972a, 1972b) or cholestyramine (ODELL, 1973). Bilirubin bound to albumin can be separated from unbound bilirubin by Sephadex G25 chromatography and using this methodology sulfonamides (JOSEPHSON and FURST, 1966), salicylates, benzoate (COUTINHO et al., 1973; YEARY and DAVIS, 1974), and fatty acids (STARINSKY and SHAFRIR, 1970) have been shown to reduce protein-bound bilirubin. STERN (1972) lists data of CHAN which also demonstrate bilirubin displacement by tolbutamide, furosemide, oxacillin, hydrocortisone, digoxin, and sodium meralluride. SCHIFF et al. (1971) demonstrated that it is the benzoate in parenteral preparations of both diazepam and caffeine sodium benzoate rather than the pharmacologially active agent that displaces bilirubin from albumin.

BRODERSEN (1974) analyzed bilirubin-albumin interaction by determining free bilirubin concentration by oxidation with hydrogen peroxide and peroxidase. Kanamycin, gentamicin, and polymyxin B did not interfere with bilirubin binding to human serum albumin. Fifteen other compounds, including various sulfonamides, sodium salicylate, acetylsalicylic acid, sodium benzoate, diphenylhydantoin, phenobarbital, carbamazepine, benzylpenicillin, and phenylbutazone, displaced bilirubin from albumin. A similar technique was used by THIESSEN et al. (1972) to study displacement of protein-bound bilirubin by fatty acids.

Other methods of estimating bilirubin drug interaction are probably less satisfactory. The amount of certain dyes, such as 2-(4'-hydroxybenzeneazo) benzoic acid (HBABA) (PORTER and WATERS, 1966) or bromphenol blue (HERTZ, 1975) which bind to albumin has been considered an index of the ability of the albumin to bind bilirubin. However, CHAN et al. (1971) demonstrated that HBABA binding sites differ from bilirubin sites. YEARY and DAVIS (1974) found that displacement of HBABA by drugs was not an indicator of the drugs' ability to displace bilirubin. Drug-induced shifts in the optical absorbance maximum of protein bound bilirubin have been extensively studied (ODELL, 1959; ODELL et al., 1969; KHANNA et al., 1969; COUTINHO et al., 1973; ODELL, 1973). The validity of this assay system has been questioned (DONE, 1964) as changes in optical absorbance may occur without a change in free bilirubin concentration as measured by the sensitive peroxidase technique (BRODERSEN, 1974). Drug-induced changes in optical density may therefore be related to simultaneous binding of both ligands by the protein, without alteration in bilirubin binding. WOOLLEY and HUNTER (1970) and KAMISAKA et al. (1974) have utilized changes in circular dichroism to detect interactions between oleate, salicylate, and various dyes with albumin bound bilirubin.

Binding Capacity of Neonatal Albumin

Because of the susceptibility of neonates to bilirubin encephalopathy, there are several studies on the binding of bilirubin and drugs to cord and neonatal plasma albumin. The albumin in cord blood binds with several drugs and with bilirubin in a different manner than the albumin of adult blood (CHIGNELL et al., 1971; KRASNER et al., 1973a; KAPITULNIK et al., 1975). The possibility of intrinsically different binding capacities between fetal and adult serum albumin has not been excluded. It is possible however that the presence in neonatal blood of relatively high concentrations of various small molecules such as bilirubin (RANE et al., 1971), fatty acids (POLACEK et al., 1965; TUILIÉ and LARDINOIS, 1972), and in some circumstances hematin (ODELL et al., 1969) alters the binding characteristics of albumin for other ligands (CHIGNELL et al., 1971; ODELL, 1973).

Table 2. Drugs displacing protein-bound bilirubin

	Analytic technique				
	Change in optical density	Displacement to mitochondria	Peroxidase assay	Sephadex G-25	Gunn rat serum bilirubin
Fatty acids	+	+	+	+	+
Various sulfonamides	+		+	+	+
Sodium salicylate	+	+	+	+	+
Benzoate	+		+	+	+ high dose
Oxacillin	+			+	
Dicloxacillin	+				
Benzylpenicillin			+		
Various other penicillins	−				+ high dose
Tetracycline					+ high dose
Chloramphenicol		−			+ high dose
Gentamicin	+, −		−	+, −	+, −
Novobiocin		+			−
Phenylbutazone		+	+		−
Oxyphenbutazone		+			+
Indomethacin		+			−
Mefenamic acid		+			+
Acetylsalicylic acid			+		
Diphenylhydantoin			+		−
Carbamazepine			+		
Phenobarbital	−		+		−
Diethylnicotinamide	−				
Tolbutamide				+	+
Furosemide				+	
Hydrocortisone				+	
Digoxin				+	
Na meralluride				+	
Acetazolamide					+
Nicotinic acid		−			+
Quinidine					+

+ = displacement demonstrated
− = no displacement demonstrated
+, − = results vary
No symbol = not adequately tested

There is ample evidence that besides sulfonamides, fatty acids, salicylate, benzoate, phenylbutazone, and many other drugs displace bilirubin from albumin. Earlier conflicting data concerning gentamicin was probably due to impurities; this drug does not displace bilirubin (ODELL et al., 1975; WENNBERG and RASMUSSEN, 1975). There is continued need for assessment of the bilirubin-displacing properties of drugs used in neonates by combined use of sensitive in vitro methods such as the peroxidase assay as well as the in vitro Gunn rat assay.

Table 2 lists drugs which have been found by various techniques to displace bilirubin from albumin. The relevant references have been cited.

IV. Drugs and the Hepatocellular Uptake and Storage of Bilirubin

The mechanisms by which bilirubin enters the hepatocyte are incompletely understood (ARIAS, 1972; BERK et al., 1974) but the process can be altered by various drugs. Low albumin concentration and drugs which elevate free bilirubin concentration facilitate entry of bilirubin into cultured hepatoma cells (RUGSTAD and BRATLID, 1974) and perfused rat liver (BARNHART and CLARENBURG, 1973). Low plasma pH may increase bilirubin toxicity by increasing membrane permeability (NELSON et al., 1974) rather than by lowering affinity of albumin for bilirubin (ODELL et al., 1969). Upon entering the cytoplasm, bilirubin is bound to specific proteins which serve as a reservoir and may also transport the bilirubin to the membranes of the endoplasmic reticulum (ARIAS and JANSEN, 1975).

A number of drugs are known to interfere with bilirubin handling at one or more of these steps. These include flavaspidic acid (NOSSLIN, 1963; NOSSLIN and MORGAN, 1965; HAMMAKER and SCHMID, 1967), bunamiodyl and other cholecystographic agents (BOLT et al., 1961; SHOTTON et al., 1961; BILLING et al., 1963; BERTHELOT and BILLING, 1966), and the rifamycin antibiotics (ACOCELLA et al., 1965; ACOCELLA and BILLING, 1965; CAPELLE et al., 1972). Most such interactions are of no pathological significance but they do provide important insight into the mechanisms of bilirubin metabolism.

1. Interference with Transport of Bilirubin Across Membranes

Many experiments have suggested the existence of a common mechanism for hepatic clearance of dyes such as ICG, BSP, rose bengal (HUNTON et al., 1961), rifamycin, and bilirubin (PAUMGARTNER et al., 1970; PAUMGARTNER, 1975). Bilirubin does not bind to the liver cell membrane in vitro or compete with ICG, BSP, flavaspidic acid, or iodipamide for membrane binding (CORNELIUS et al., 1967) but there is recent evidence for the existence of a role for the membrane in bilirubin uptake. Bilirubin uptake by rat intestinal mucosal cells in vitro has been studied by CORCHS et al. (1973) and SERRANI et al. (1973). An uptake pattern consistent with facilitated diffusion was described; low extracellular sodium concentration, ethacrynic acid, and biliverdin inhibited bilirubin uptake. The mechanism of uptake by intestinal cells may well be different from that of hepatocytes. Rifamycin SV and probenecid compete poorly with bilirubin for binding with Y and Z in vitro but decrease Gunn rat cytoplasm bilirubin content in vivo at relatively low doses (KENWRIGHT and LEVI, 1973). Their major effect in vivo is presumably interference with bilirubin uptake at the cell membrane. Evidence for carrier-mediated transport of bilirubin and dyes into the hepatocyte was recently presented by Scharschmidt et al. (1975), who studied the kinetics of plasma clearance of radiolabeled bilirubin in intact rats. The uptake of BSP, ICG and bilirubin is saturable and competitively inhibited by the other compounds. Administration of any of these agents after partial clearance of a load of labeled bilirubin is followed by release of label from the liver. Phenobarbital increased the rate of uptake of each compound by the liver in both normal and Gunn rats verifying the independence from glucuronyl transferase of the uptake mechanism as studied by this technique. The mechanism of this phenobarbital effect is unknown. This direct experimental approach could be applied to other drugs to differentiate drug alterations in membrane transport from other changes in intracellular handling of bilirubin.

2. Interference with Cytoplasmic Binding of Bilirubin

The hepatic cytoplasmic organic anion binding protein Y, or ligandin is capable of binding bilirubin, steroids, and certain carcinogens (Litwack et al., 1971) in addition to a wide variety of other molecules including BSP, ICG, cholecysto-graphic agents, salicylates, hematin, glutathione, probenecid, and various antibiotics (Kunin et al., 1973; Kirsch et al., 1975; Arias and Jansen, 1975). Recently it has been demonstrated that ligandin has glutathione transferase activity (Kaplo-witz et al., 1973; Habig et al., 1974; Kawasaki et al., 1975; Fleischner et al., 1975a). The Z protein binds ICG, BSP, and bilirubin, as well as flavaspidic acid, iodipamide, bunamiodyl (Levi et al., 1969) thyroxine, long chain fatty acids, lactic acid (Arias and Jansen, 1975) and hexachlorophene (Warner and Neims, 1975). While no enzymatic activity has been described for this protein it may play a role in regulating fatty acid metabolism (Ockner and Isselbacher, 1974; O'Doherty and Kuksis, 1975; Mishkin et al., 1975).

As has been discussed previously, it has been suggested that binding by these proteins prevents efflux from the liver of organic anions which enter the cell (Arias, 1972; Arias and Jansen, 1965). If this hypothesis is correct, competition between drugs and bilirubin for sites on Y and Z may be responsible for the impaired bilirubin clearance observed during their administration. Such competition occurs in vitro. Flavaspidic acid, bunamiodyl (Levi et al., 1969), rifamycin SV, and probenecid (Kenwright and Levi, 1973) displace Z-bound BSP or bilirubin, and recent techniques utilizing circular dichroism demonstrate displacement of Y-bound bilirubin by ICG, BSP, iodipamide, flavaspidic acid (Kamisaka et al., 1973), oleic acid, hematoporphyrin, and Evans blue (Kamisaka et al., 1975). In vivo competition of this nature is probably important in some drug effects. Flavaspidic acid readily displaces Z-bound BSP in vitro and the decreases in Y- and Z-bound bilirubin observed in rats given this drug are likely due to competition between flavaspidic acid and bilirubin for intracellular binding sites (Kenwright and Levi, 1974). Other drugs which bind with Y or Z in vitro may also interfere with bilirubin metabolism by competing at these sites. However, there is at present no clear evidence that competition for Y causes hyperbilirubinemia. Both BSP and ICG which compete primarily for Y binding appear to exert at least part of their inhibitory effect at the point of uptake rather than after entry into the cell (Schar-schmidt et al., 1975).

3. Drug-Mediated Increases in Bilirubin Uptake and Storage

Administration of phenobarbital to animals causes increased uptake of bilirubin and BSP and increased liver bilirubin content (ROBERTS and PLAA, 1967; SCHAR-SCHMIDT et al., 1975). Phenobarbital may cause these effects by increasing liver size and blood flow (BRANCH et al., 1974; OHNHAUS and LOCHER, 1975) by as yet undefined effects at the membrane level (SCHARSCHMIDT et al., 1975), and by changes in cytoplasmic proteins. In rats and humans, phenobarbital increases hepatic content of Y protein, but not of Z (REYES et al., 1969; REYES et al., 1971; FLEISCHNER et al., 1972; FLEISCHNER et al., 1975 b). AIA, dieldrin, 3-methylcholanthrene, dichlorodiphenyltrichloroethane (DDT), benzpyrene (REYES et al., 1971), spironolactone, and PCN (KLAASSEN, 1975) also increase hepatic Y concentration in animals. In kidney, phenobarbital and PCN do not increase ligandin concentration, but tetrachloro-dibenzo-p-dioxin does (KIRSCH et al., 1975). Most of these agents have no effect on the Z protein concentration, but DDT and dieldrin diminish Z although they increase BSP clearance (REYES et al., 1971). Only certain hypolipidemic agents (MACHINIST et al., 1975), including clofibrate and nafenopin (FLEISCHNER et al., 1975 b), have been found to elevate liver Z content. The possible contribution of Z induction to bilirubin metabolism has not been studied.

Phenobarbital dependent increases in liver Y content may well contribute to the effects of this drug upon bilirubin metabolism, but certain findings suggest that anion clearance is not related simply to Y or Z content (ARIAS, 1972). For example, hypophysectomy and thyroidectomy in rats increase Y protein but decrease BSP clearance. While phenobarbital further increases Y concentration in these animals, it does not normalize BSP clearance (REYES et al., 1971). Further study of the role of the hepatocyte membrane in bilirubin uptake and development of techniques for the experimental separation of drug effects on membrane and intracellular storage proteins will clarify some of these problems.

Certain hereditary abnormalities of bilirubin handling serve as models for normal and drug-inhibited bilirubin uptake and storage. Mutant Southdown sheep are hyperbilirubinemic because of diminished uptake of bilirubin by the liver (MIA et al., 1970). Hepatic Y and Z concentrations are normal (LEVI et al., 1969) and the defect is presumably at the membrane level. A possibly similar defect was recently described in man (DHUMEAUX and BERTHELOT, 1975). This patient showed no improvement with phenobarbital treatment. In Gilbert's syndrome, uptake of bilirubin by the liver is diminished (BILLING et al., 1964; BERK et al., 1970). Hepatic storage capacity for bilirubin (BLASCHKE et al., 1974 b) and post-uptake handling of BSP (MARTIN et al., 1976) are abnormal in some of these patients and abnormal intracellular binding proteins might be in part responsible for these findings. Hepatic binding proteins have recently been assayed in four patients with Gilbert's syndrome and were found to be normal (FLEISCHNER et al., 1975 a). It is possible that a congenital hyperbilirubinemia syndrome due to deficiency or dysfunction of Y or Z will be identified, but has not as yet been described.

V. Drugs and the Glucuronyl Transferases

Many chemicals influence hepatic GT activity, both in vivo and in vitro and some may alter the rate of bilirubin excretion as mediated by this mechanism. Interpretation of in vitro assays of GT activity is subject to a number of limitations (HEIRWEGH et al., 1973).

1. Glucuronyl Transferase Assay Techniques

Liver contains enzymes capable of transferring glucuronyl residues from UDP-glucuronic acid to many molecules besides bilirubin (DUTTON, 1966). Although the properties and specificities of the various GTs have not been clearly defined, there appears to be a specific transferase for bilirubin which is distinct from those enzymes which glucuronidate other substrates. Because of technical difficulty with the assay of the GT specific for bilirubin, many workers have assayed GT activity with other acceptors, such as *o*-aminophenol, *p*-nitrophenol, and phenolphthalein (ZAKIM and VESSEY, 1973). Similarly, the ability to excrete various chemicals as glucuronides is sometimes used as an index of bilirubin GT activity. Because of the nonidentity of these GTs with the bilirubin GT, the significance of such studies in relation to bilirubin metabolism is unclear. Only recently has it been possible to purify the bilirubin GT in soluble form (GREGORY and STRICKLAND, 1973). In the future, kinetic analysis of purified enzyme should clarify the problems of enzyme multiplicity and specificity (VESSEY et al., 1973a).

Studies of glucuronidation involving intact cells or tissue slices may be misleading because of competition between different metabolic pathways for the disposal of the substrate and because of drug mediated changes in substrate uptake or secretion. Currently most assays utilize microsomal fractions of cell homogenates, with addition of excess UDP-glucuronic acid. Drug-mediated alterations in GT activity in vivo may be partly mediated by alterations in intracellular content of UDP-glucuronic acid (to be discussed later) or perhaps of other regulatory molecules such as UDP-N-acetyl glucosamine (WINSNES, 1971a; STREBEL and ODELL, 1971; VESSEY et al., 1973a, 1973b). Such changes in in vivo enzyme activity would not be detected in vitro.

Because of the low basal activity of bilirubin GT, many assays include microsomal "activation" by detergent, enzyme, or other treatments (HALAC and REFF, 1967; VESSEY and ZAKIM, 1971; WINSNES, 1969, 1971a, 1971b; HEIRWEGH et al., 1972; MARNIEMI, 1974). Such processing increases two- to tenfold the measurable GT activity and makes possible the detection of some drug-mediated changes in enzyme activity which are not demonstrable in native microsomes (WINSNES, 1971b). On activation of the GTs, there is evidence of specificity for both substrate and activating agent (BOCK et al., 1973). Changes in GT kinetics on activation have been described by KRASNER et al. (1973b) and WINSNES and DUTTON (1973). The mechanism of the activation is uncertain but is thought to involve modification of the structure of the microsomal membrane in which the enzyme is situated (WINSNES, 1969; MULDER, 1970; VESSEY and ZAKIM, 1971). The biological significance of the existence of GT activity in this latent form is unclear. Comparisons of enzyme activity for substrates other than bilirubin in perfused liver or in liver slices with that present in microsomal preparations has suggested that the enzyme functions in vivo at an unactivated or only partially activated level (WINSNES and DUTTON, 1973; BOCK, 1974; BOCK and WHITE, 1974). HALAC and REFF (1967) suggested that the bilirubin GT activity of activated microsomes reflects the level of enzyme activity in vivo more closely than the activity of native microsomes, but further study of this relationship is needed.

2. Glucuronyl Transferase Induction

a) *Phenobarbital*

Bilirubin GT is one of many hepatic microsomal enzymes inducible in animals by phenobarbital (CONNEY, 1967; CONNEY et al., 1973). Induction of GT activity involves synthesis of new protein (BOCK et al., 1973) rather than alteration of the activity of pre-existing enzyme or physical changes in microsomal membranes. Latent enzyme activity, as well as activity of nonactivated microsomes is increased by phenobarbital (BOCK and WHITE, 1974). The effect of phenobarbital upon the kinetic properties of the enzyme has been studied and the K_m of the induced enzyme appears to be unaltered (BOCK et al., 1973; KRASNER et al., 1973b).

Phenobarbital and other barbiturates have been shown to increase GT activity for bilirubin in mice (CATZ and YAFFE, 1968; WINSNES, 1971b, BURCHELL, 1973; KRASNER et al., 1973b) and rats (HALAC and SICIGNANO, 1969; DELEON et al., 1967; OKOLICSANYI et al., 1970; ROBINSON et al., 1971b; JANSEN and HENDERSON, 1972; BOCK et al., 1973; VAINIO and HIETANEN, 1974; VAISMAN et al., 1976). Technical differences including activation techniques may in part explain other studies in which phenobarbital did not significantly increase hepatic bilirubin GT specific activity in guinea pigs (POTREPKA and SPRATT, 1971) or rats (WONG, 1972; MAXWELL et al., 1973; ORME et al., 1974).

Phenobarbital also induces GT activity for other substrates including morphine (ROERIG et al., 1974), chloramphenicol (BOCK et al., 1973), o-aminophenol (HANNINEN and AITIO, 1968, CATZ and YAFFE, 1968; WINSNES and DUTTON, 1973), p-nitrophenol (ZEIDENBERG et al., 1967; HALAC and SICIGNANO, 1969; OKOLICSANYI et al., 1970; JANSEN and HENDERSON, 1972, VAINIO and HIETANEN, 1974; ADACHI and YAMAMOTO, 1976), 1-naphthol (BOCK and WHITE, 1974), phenolphthalein and 4-methylumbelliferone (WINSNES, 1971b).

Phenobarbital administered to normal adult humans increases bilirubin clearance and lowers plasma unconjugated bilirubin (BLASCHKE et al., 1974a; BLACK et al., 1974). BLACK et al. (1973) studied bilirubin GT activity in liver biopsies of patients with normal bilirubin metabolism who were undergoing nonbiliary surgery. Subjects who received phenobarbital daily for 1 week prior to surgery had significant elevations of bilirubin GT activity, and plasma bilirubin concentrations were slightly decreased as compared with patients not receiving drugs. FELSHER et al. (1973) found hepatic bilirubin GT levels in viral hepatitis patients receiving phenobarbital to be twice as high as in untreated patients. In normal animals, secretion rather than conjugation of bilirubin is rate limiting (ARIAS et al., 1961). Induction of bilirubin GT by phenobarbital in normal rats is not accompanied by changes in plasma bilirubin or in the rate of bilirubin excretion to bile (ROBINSON et al., 1971b). Drug effects other than GT induction may therefore be responsible for the acceleration of bilirubin clearance observed in phenobarbital treated subjects.

More extensive studies of the effect of phenobarbital upon bilirubin GT have been performed in animals and patients with partial or complete deficiency of this enzyme, in which glucuronidation of bilirubin is likely to be the rate-limiting step in bilirubin excretion. The mutant strain of Gunn rats have unconjugated hyperbilirubinemia due to complete deficiency of bilirubin GT. While GT activity for many other substrates is also low, transferases forming N-linked glucuronides are of normal activity (ARIAS, 1961). Administration of phenobarbital to homozygous Gunn rats does not lower serum bilirubin or induce measurable bilirubin GT activity (DELEON et al., 1967; ROBINSON, 1971; JANSEN and HENDERSON, 1972; VAINIO and HIETANEN, 1974). Although GT activity for other substrates in inducible by phenobarbital, the response of the enzyme to microsomal activation is diminished, perhaps due to a generalized defect of the microsomal membrane (ZAKIM et al., 1973). Heterozygous Gunn rats, with low but detectable GT, respond to phenobarbital with an increase in bilirubin GT activity (ROBINSON et al., 1971 b).

Similar drug effects are observed in humans with GT deficiency. In patients with severe unconjugated hyperbilirubinemia due to the type I Crigler-Najjar syndrome in whom bilirubin GT is absent and the bile is free of conjugated bilirubin phenobarbital administration does not lower serum bilirubin or alter clearance of bilirubin (BLASCHKE et al., 1974 b) or increase hepatic bilirubin GT activity (ARIAS et al., 1969). Patients with the less severe type II Crigler-Najjar syndrome also exhibit impaired glucuronidation but the bile contains some conjugated bilirubin mainly as the monoglucuronide (ARIAS et al., 1969). In these patients phenobarbital produces a drop in plasma bilirubin (though not to normal levels), an increase in bilirubin clearance, and increased fecal excretion of labeled bilirubin (YAFFE et al., 1966; WHELTON et al., 1968; KREEK and SLEISENGER, 1968; CRIGLER and GOLD, 1969; ARIAS et al., 1969; ERTEL and NEWTON, 1969; BLACK et al., 1974; GOLLAN et al., 1975). Nevertheless, hepatic bilirubin GT activity was absent or marginally detectable in the few patients in whom this assay was performed (OKOLICSANYI et al., 1971; BLACK et al., 1974; GOLLAN et al., 1975). These patients' ability to excrete menthol (KREEK and SLEISENGER, 1968; ARIAS et al., 1969) and salicylamide (YAFFE et al., 1966) as glucuronides was improved by phenobarbital therapy. In other patients, hepatic GT activity for 4-methylumbelliferone (ARIAS et al., 1969) and p-nitrophenol (CRIGLER and GOLD, 1969) were increased by phenobarbital.

In patients with the mild unconjugated hyperbilirubinemia of Gilbert's syndrome, in which there is a partial deficiency of bilirubin GT (METGE et al., 1964; BLACK and BILLING, 1969; OKOLICSANYI et al., 1971; FELSHER et al., 1973; BELLET and RAYNAUD, 1974; KUTZ et al., 1975), barbiturate therapy decreases plasma bilirubin concentration (BLACK and SHERLOCK, 1970; HUNTER et al., 1971; MAXWELL et al., 1973) and increases the rate of ^{14}C bilirubin clearance from the plasma (BLACK et al., 1974; BLASCHKE et al., 1974 a). Whether these changes are due to GT induction is uncertain. Hepatic GT activity after phenobarbital therapy was found by BLACK et al. (1974) to be significantly increased in only one of the three patients in whom assays were done before and after therapy. Two others assayed after phenobarbital had GT activity in the normal range, suggesting that induction had occured. FELSHER et al. (1973), however, found no significant increase in GT activity in liver biopsies from seven patients with Gilbert's syndrome treated with phenobarbital. MAXWELL et al. (1973) detected increased glucaric acid excretion, an indirect indicator of microsomal enzyme induction, in patients with Gilbert's syndrome treated with phenobarbital.

BERK (1975) has described a linear relationship between hepatic bilirubin clearance and bilirubin GT activity in untreated patients with Gilbert's syndrome and in normals with and without phenobarbital. The phenobarbital-induced improvement in bilirubin clearance without convincing changes in measurable GT in Gilbert's and in type II Crigler-Najjar syndromes remain unexplained. In vitro GT assays may not reflect in vivo enzyme activity and undetectable GT activity in the latter may be related to the assay's insensitivity to the very low enzyme activity which is present, or to the possibility that the digitonin used in the assay is not a suitable activator for the enzyme in these patients (BLACK et al., 1974). The lack of measurable increases in hepatic GT activity after phenobarbital therapy does not exclude that the improvement in bilirubin clearance may be due to increased enzyme activity, but the possibility that the major effect of phenobarbital on bilirubin clearance is mediated by other mechanisms must be considered.

Phenobarbital is of some therapeutic significance in the treatment of hyperbilirubinemia in the human neonate, particularly in prematures. Impaired neonatal bilirubin clearance may be caused by many factors including deficiency of cytoplasmic binding proteins, low microsomal content of bilirubin GT, impaired production of UDP-glucuronic acid, and impaired bilirubin diglucuronide excretion (MAISELS, 1972; THALER, 1972), some or all of which may be improved by phenobarbital. CATZ and YAFFE (1962, 1968) demonstrated elevation of hepatic bilirubin GT activity in neonatal mice whose mothers had been treated with phenobarbital during gestation, and similar data have been presented by HALAC and SICIGNANO (1969) and KRASNER et al. (1973b). In humans, administration of phenobarbital either to the mother in late pregnancy or to the newborn has been shown to lower neonatal plasma bilirubin, to improve bilirubin clearance, and to decrease the need for exchange transfusion for severe hyperbilirubinemia. The reader is referred to other sources in which an extensive clinical experience with phenobarbital is reviewed (YAFFE et al., 1970; WILSON, 1972; OSTROW, 1972b; MAISELS, 1972; BERK et al., 1974).

b) *Glutethimide*

Glutethimide lowers plasma bilirubin and increases its clearance in Gunn rat heterozygotes with partial bilirubin GT deficiency (BLASCHKE and BERK, 1972), in most normal humans (BLASCHKE et al., 1974a) and in Gilbert's syndrome (BLACK and SHERLOCK, 1970; BERK and BLASCHKE, 1971; BLACK et al., 1974; BLASCHKE et al., 1974a). In normal rats and Gunn heterozygotes, but not Gunn homozygotes, BLASCHKE and BERK (1972) observed significant induction of hepatic bilirubin GT activity. In man, glutethimide-mediated induction of hepatic GT has been demonstrated only by BLACK et al. (1973), who gave the drug to 13 normal persons undergoing nonbiliary surgery. Again, demonstrable enzyme induction is not proof that this change is responsible for the altered bilirubin clearance either in animals or in patients. Aside from the observation that bilirubin turnover was decreased with glutethimide therapy (BLASCHKE et al., 1974a), possible effects of glutethimide at other steps in bilirubin metabolism have not been studied.

c) *Antipyrine*

ORME et al. (1974) have reported that antipyrine (phenazone), another microsomal enzyme inducer, elevates bilirubin GT activity in rats. Treatment of six patients with Gilbert's syndrome significantly decreased plasma unconjugated bilirubin. Hepatic GT assays and bilirubin clearance studies were not performed in these patients and the suggestion that lowered plasma bilirubin is due to increased GT activity in vivo is tentative.

d) Dicophane (DDT)

DDT has been used to lower plasma bilirubin in a patient with type II Crigler-Najjar syndrome (Thompson et al., 1969). This effect was prolonged with lowered plasma bilirubin persisting almost 2 years after DDT was stopped (Williams et al., 1972), presumably due to storage of DDT in body lipids with persistent release to the blood and liver. The ability of this patient to excrete menthol as a glucuronide was depressed before treatment but was normal after DDT administration; GT activity was not directly measured. Thompson et al. (1969) gave DDT to rats and demonstrated increased total hepatic bilirubin GT activity, although the activity of the enzyme per milligram microsomal protein was not changed.

e) Clofibrate

Clofibrate was shown to lower serum bilirubin in patients with Gilbert's syndrome by Kutz et al. (1975). The drug also increased liver bilirubin GT activity in normal rats (Kutz et al., 1975). Its effect on hepatic Z protein concentration has been mentioned previously.

f) Other Agents

Arias et al. (1963) found that chloroquine induced microsomal o-aminophenol and bilirubin GT activity in neonatal rats, and that treatment of pregnant rats led to elevation of neonatal o-aminophenol GT. However, a trial of chloroquine in 16 pregnant women for 1−8 weeks antepartum did not change neonatal serum bilirubin levels.

Sereni et al. (1967) gave neonates diethylnicotinamide for seven days and observed a significant decrease in serum bilirubin compared with their twin controls who received saline. Ertel and Newton (1969) found this drug to reduce serum bilirubin only slightly in two patients with type II Crigler-Najjar syndrome. This drug is said to increase bilirubin GT in rabbits (Careddu et al., 1964; cited by Ertel and Newton, 1969). It does not displace albumin bound bilirubin according to Khanna et al. (1969).

Rifampicin, which is said to improve hepatic bilirubin uptake in Gilbert's syndrome (Okolicsanyi et al., 1972b), induces the GT for p-nitrophenol but not bilirubin in man (Hakim et al., 1973).

Phenylbutazone (Reinicke et al., 1970) and Valium (Heubel and Muhlberger, 1971; Heubel, 1974) have been used in neonates to lower serum bilirubin but the mechanism has not been delineated. Since both are known to displace bilirubin from binding sites on albumin, their use in neonatal hyperbilirubinemia would seem to be contraindicated regardless of whether or not they have an effect upon bilirubin GT activity.

Maternal exposure to certain nontherapeutic agents may influence neonatal bilirubin metabolism. Chronic ethanol intake stimulates microsomal drug metabolising activity (Rubin and Lieber, 1974). Ideo et al. (1971) administered ethanol to rats and found significant induction of hepatic bilirubin GT activity. Human neonates whose mothers had received ethanol ante-partum had lower serum bilirubin levels (WALTMAN et al., 1969). Alcohol given to a single patient with Gilbert's syndrome led to decreased plasma bilirubin (IDEO et al., 1971), but OKOLICSANYI et al. (1972a) observed no consistent change in plasma bilirubin kinetics in 14 patients with Gilbert's syndrome treated with intravenous ethanol. Cigarette smoking during pregnancy has also been shown to be associated with diminished neonatal plasma bilirubin levels (HARDY and MELLITS, 1972) and it has been suggested that induction of GT by unknown substances in the smoke is responsible for this effect (NYMAND, 1974). Neonates born to heroin addicts have been reported to have significantly lower serum bilirubin than normal neonates (ZELSON et al., 1971; NATHENSON et al., 1972). The patients of NATHENSON received Valium (containing sodium benzoate) for withdrawal symptoms; the authors felt it unlikely that the slight changes in albumin binding observed were responsible for the decrease in serum bilirubin. NATHENSON et al. (1972) administered morphine to mice and observed induction of bilirubin GT in liver after 4 – 12 weeks of treatment.

g) GT Induction in Animals

In addition to drugs which have been used in humans, various other agents have been shown to modify GT activity in experimental animals. In rats, spironolactone and PCN induce hepatic bilirubin GT and lower plasma bilirubin levels (SOLYMOSS and ZSIGMOND, 1973; RADZIALOWSKI, 1973). Bilirubin GT activity is increased by chloroquine and various polycyclic hydrocarbons including 3,4-benzpyrene, 3-methylcholanthrene (ARIAS et al., 1963; POTREPKA and SPRATT, 1971) and chrysene (MARNIEMI, 1974). The same agents (INSCOE and AXELROD, 1960; ARIAS et al., 1963; GOLDSTEIN and TAUROG, 1968; HANNINEN and AITIO, 1968; BOCK et al., 1973; BOCK and WHITE, 1974; LAITINEN et al., 1974), as well as diethylnitrosoamine (GREENWOOD and STEVENSON, 1965), chlordane and dieldrin (LUCIER and McDANIEL, 1972), and polychlorinated biphenyls (VAINIO, 1964a) induce the activity of glucuronyl transferases as assayed with other glucuronide acceptors. These agents have not been studied widely in GT deficient animals.

3. Glucuronyl Transferase Inhibition

An obvious mechanism for drug-induced interference with bilirubin metabolism is inhibition of the enzyme responsible for its conjugation, as has been demonstrated for other substrates (MULDER, 1973; HEATH and DINGELL, 1974; LINHART, 1974; BATT et al., 1975; MULDER and PILON, 1975). Despite the multiplicity of the GTs it is possible that other substrates may compete with bilirubin for the enzyme.

Many chemicals and drugs of therapeutic significance have been shown to inhibit bilirubin GT in vitro, although their primary effects in vivo may be at other steps in the metabolism of bilirubin (HAMMAKER and SCHMID, 1967; MULDER, 1973). Many of the in vitro drug effects to be described were observed at relatively high drug concentrations, probably higher than the drug concentration at the microsomal membrane in vivo, and some of these inhibitory effects may be due to nonspecific membrane changes (MULDER, 1974), such as those seen with detergents and organic solvents (POTREPKA and SPRATT, 1972; VAINIO, 1974b). Most of the studies to be discussed were performed before techniques with radiolabeled bilirubin or purified bilirubin GT became available.

Bilirubin GT activity is inhibited in vitro by borneol (GRODSKY and CARBONE, 1957), o-aminophenol (LATHE and WALKER, 1958), anthranilic acid, p-nitrophenol, 4-methylumbelliferone, and phenolphthalein (TOMLINSON and YAFFE, 1966; HARGREAVES and LATHE, 1963; MULDER, 1972; RUGSTAD and DYBING, 1974). 2-diethylaminoethyl 2,2-diphenylvalerate (SKF 525-A), which inhibits many microsomal enzymes, (MANNERING, 1971) inhibits GT activity for bilirubin and other substrates (HARGREAVES, 1967; DYBING and RUGSTAD, 1973). Bilirubin itself has only occasionally been shown to inhibit GT activity towards other glucuronide acceptors (MULDER, 1972); this effect may be nonspecific and related to a detergent effect (SANCHEZ and TEPHLY, 1973). In humans hyperbilirubinemia does not interfere with glucuronidation of drugs in vivo (LEVY and ERTEL, 1971).

a) *Novobiocin*

There is reasonable evidence that direct GT inhibition may contribute to the hyperbilirubinemia caused by novobiocin in humans and animals (SUTHERLAND and KELLER, 1961; LOKIETZ et al., 1963; HSIA et al., 1963; EDMOND et al., 1966; HARBISON and SPRATT, 1967). Novobiocin inhibits in vitro GT activity for bilirubin (HARGREAVES and HOLTON, 1962; HARGREAVES and LATHE, 1963; TOMLINSON and YAFFE, 1966; BERTHELOT et al., 1971) and for other glucuronyl acceptors (LOKIETZ et al., 1963; HSIA et al., 1963). In vivo, novobiocin also inhibits GT activity for o-aminophenol (HSIA et al., 1963) and bilirubin (BERTHELOT et al., 1971).

b) *Vitamin K*

Vitamin K, at the high doses used a number of years ago, caused unconjugated hyperbilirubinemia in human neonates (SILVERBERG et al., 1963). In vitro, menadiol inhibits GT activity for bilirubin (WATERS et al., 1958) and other substrates (HSIA et al., 1963). GT inhibition, however, was probably a minor mechanism for vitamin K-induced hyperbilirubinemia, the major factor being hemolysis due to oxidative erythrocyte damage (ZINKHAM, 1963). Current low-dose vitamin K_1 therapy is not known to interfere with bilirubin metabolism.

c) *Other Agents*

A wide variety of other chemicals have been demonstrated to interfere with glucuronidation of bilirubin and other substrates in vitro. These include chloramphenicol, streptomycin (WATERS et al., 1958), flavaspidic acid (HARGREAVES, 1966), bunamiodyl, BSP, ICG, rose bengal, norethandrolone, methicillin (HARGREAVES and LATHE, 1963), chlorpromazine, promazine (HARGREAVES, 1965), isoniazid, phenelzine, nialamide, isocarboxazid (HARGREAVES, 1968), imipramine (HARGREAVES et al., 1969), iproniazid, benzylhydrazine and harmol (MULDER, 1974). The significance of such inhibition is unclear. Most of these agents, if associated with hyperbilirubinemia, do this by causing hepatitis or cholestasis (KLATSKIN, 1974).

Various hormones affect bilirubin metabolism, primarily by interfering with bilirubin glucuronide secretion, but these may also inhibit bilirubin glucuronidation. Maternal steroids in either plasma or breast milk have been implicated in certain varieties of neonatal jaundice, and breast milk of mothers with icteric infants has been shown to inhibit GT for *o*-aminophenol and for bilirubin. This effect was thought to be due to pregnane-3α 20β-diol (ARIAS et al., 1964; ARIAS and GARTNER, 1964), but subsequent studies have questioned the ability of this steroid to significantly inhibit bilirubin GT in humans (RAMOS et al., 1966; ADLARD and LATHE, 1970; HARGREAVES and PIPER, 1971). Various other steroids, including pregnanediol and estriol and their glucuronides, inhibit rat liver *o*-aminophenol and 4-methylumbelliferone GT in vitro (HSIA et al., 1963; JONES, 1964). HARGREAVES et al. (1971) described inhibition of rat liver bilirubin GT by ethinylestradiol. Low concentrations of unsaturated fatty acids inhibit bilirubin GT in rat liver microsomal suspensions (HARGREAVES, 1973) and slices (BEVAN and HOLTON, 1972).

d) *GT Inhibition in Intact Cells*

HARGREAVES and associates (HARGREAVES and LATHE, 1963; HARGREAVES, 1965, 1967, 1968; HARGREAVES et al., 1969, 1971) have studied many therapeutic agents for their ability to interfere with glucuronidation of bilirubin and *o*-aminophenol in rat liver slices. DYBING has studied the effect of many drugs on glucuronidation of various substrates by MH_1C_1 rat hepatoma cell cultures (DYBING, 1972, 1973; DYBING and RUGSTAD, 1973). As DUTTON (1966) has pointed out, techniques involving intact cells may demonstrate specific or non-specific drug interference with a number of different processes, including uptake, intracellular binding, conjugation, generation of UDP-glucuronic acid, and secretion of the conjugate. Such experiments cannot therefore be interpreted as demonstrating specific inhibition of GT.

4. Alterations in UDP-Glucuronic Acid Availability

The activity of GT is dependent upon an adequate supply of UDP-glucuronic acid, which is synthesized by the enzyme UDP-glucose dehydrogenase with UDP-glucose as substrate. Little is known about the control mechanisms which regulate the concentration of UDP-glucuronic acid, but the K_m of bilirubin GT for this substrate is such that alterations in its intracellular concentration are likely to change in vivo GT activity (VESSEY et al., 1973b; BOCK and WHITE, 1974). A number of drugs are known to increase the concentration of UDP-glucuronic acid or the activity of UDP-glucose dehydrogenase in experimental animals, including barbiturates (ZEIDENBERG et al., 1967), chloretone (HOLLMAN and TOUSTER, 1962; AARTS, 1966), morphine (TAKEMORI, 1960), cinchophen (HANNINEN, 1968) and novobiocin (BROWN and HENNING, 1963). It is not known whether these effects significantly influence the glucuronidation of bilirubin or drugs in vivo.

Because of the possibility that UDP-glucuronic acid availability may limit bilirubin GT activity in neonates, several attempts have been made to treat hyperbilirubinemia by providing this substrate or its precursors. CAREDDU and MARINI (1968) administered UDP-glucose to neonates and found significant lowering of plasma bilirubin levels. Aspartic and orotic acids, intermediates in UDP-glucuronic acid synthesis, lowered serum bilirubin in some but not all studies of full term and premature infants (MATSUDA and SHIRAHATA, 1966; KINTZEL et al., 1971; SCHWARZE et al., 1971; GRAY and MOWAT, 1971). ARROWSMITH et al., (1975) were able to lower serum bilirubin in a child with type I Crigler-Najjar syndrome with aspartic acid, but the probable absence of GT activity in this condition suggests that this effect was not mediated by bilirubin glucuronidation. UDP-glucose was ineffective in this patient, as well as in a number of patients with Gilbert's syndrome (OKOLICSANYI et al., 1972b). Even in the cases in which these agents were successful, there is no direct evidence that their effects were mediated by increasing the conjugation of bilirubin.

VI. Drugs and the Biliary Excretion of Bilirubin

Bile secretion involves at least two partly defined mechanisms; (1) that which is bile acid—dependent and (2) that which is bile acid—independent. Bile acids are potent choleretics and the excretion of bile acids is directly related to bile flow and electrolyte output in the dog (PREISIG et al., 1962), rabbit (ERLINGER et al., 1970), rat (BOYER and KLATSKIN, 1970) and man (SCHERSTEN et al., 1971). Bile flow usually increases with bile acid infusion. If the effects on bile flow mediated by bile acids are osmotic in nature they are probably related to associated ions as the bile acids are normally present as micelles with low osmotic activity.

Bile acid independent secretion may represent in excess of 50% of the total flow in some species including man (ERLINGER et al., 1970; SCHERSTEN et al., 1971; PREISIG et al., 1969), and is associated at least in some species with the active transport of sodium as mediated through the sodium-potassium ATPase membrane transport system. An increase in the bile acid independent flow may be brought about by phenobarbital (ROBERTS and PLAA, 1967), hydrocortisone (MACAROL et al., 1970), cortisol, spironolactone, PCN (SOLYMOSS and ZSIGMOND, 1973), theophylline (ERLINGER and DUMONT, 1973), and cyclic AMP (MORRIS, 1972). The last observation suggests that agents which increase cyclic AMP in the hepatocyte may also increase the bile acid independent flow.

The bile ductules and ducts also contribute to biliary flow. Flow from these sites may be stimulated by secretin, gastrin, histamine (PREISIG et al., 1962; WAITMAN et al., 1969; JONES and GROSSMAN, 1969; ZATEPKA and GROSSMAN, 1966), and insulin hypoglycemia (FRITZ and BROOKS, 1963).

Reduction in bile flow is produced by certain dyes which are excreted in the bile such as BSP and ICG (GROSZMANN et al., 1969), and rose bengal (DHUMEAUX et al., 1970). The latter reduces the bile acid independent flow. Inhibitors of the ATPase mediated sodium-potassium transport system, such as ouabain and etha-crynic acid, reduce bile salt independent bile flow as measured by erythritol clearance in rabbits (ERLINGER et al., 1970).

Although bilirubin excretion depends on bile flow there is no simple relationship between the two. An increase in bile flow is not always associated with an increase in the maximal rate of bilirubin excretion (T_m), and conversely bile flow may drop in response to steroids more than bilirubin excretion (HEIKEL and LATHE, 1970a). GORESKY et al. (1974) using anesthetized dogs with bile flow stabilized by cholinergic blockade found that on infusion of taurocholate and unconjugated bilirubin the T_m of bilirubin increased linearly with flow and taurocholate excretion. They concluded that the capacity for bilirubin transport is linked to the secretion of the bile acids. They postulated that at low rates of supply of exogenous bile acids, little bile acid reaches the centrilobular areas and thus contributes little to bile flow. At higher rates of supply of bile acids to the centrilobular area there is an increased contribution by these areas to bile formation and bilirubin excretion.

1. Drugs Increasing Bilirubin Excretion

ROBERTS and PLAA (1967) found that treatment of mice with phenobarbital significantly enhanced disappearance of exogenously administered bilirubin from the plasma. This was accompanied by an increase in bile flow. The concentration of bilirubin in the bile remained constant and the increased bilirubin excretion was related to the increase in bile volume. Similar studies in dogs (GORESKY and KLUGER, 1969) and sheep (UPSON et al., 1970) demonstrated that the increase in bilirubin T_m was associated with an increase in bile flow. KLAASSEN (1970) found that phenobarbital pre-treatment enhanced plasma disappearance and biliary excretion of a number of agents which are not conjugated prior to their excretion, such as ouabain, amaranth, disulfonate, and phenol 3-6-dibromphthalein. Again, the increased biliary excretion correlated with the increase in bile flow produced by phenobarbital. In rats spironolactone and PCN increased bile flow and T_m for bilirubin, as well as enhancing hepatic microsomal bilirubin GT activity. In contrast cortisol enhances bile flow and the bilirubin T_m without significantly augmenting transferase activity (SOLYMOSS and ZSIGMOND, 1973).

2. Drugs Decreasing Bilirubin Excretion

Sodium dehydrocholate (Decholin) inhibits bilirubin excretion in man despite its choleretic effect (BLOOMER et al., 1973). Novobiocin, which produces variable effects on bile flow, reduces the biliary excretion of organic anions including bilirubin, BSP, morphine glucuronide, organic cations, and neutral compounds such as ouabain and digitoxin (SMITH and FUJIMOTO, 1974). Molecules sharing excretory mechanisms with bilirubin, such as BSP, may interfere with the excretion of bilirubin (CLARENBERG and KAO, 1973).

3. Cholestasis Due to Drugs

Hyperbilirubinemia may result from specific interference with excretory transport of bilirubin from the cell, or from cholestasis with failure of bile formation or bile flow. Cholestasis may be of hepatocytic origin or may result from intrahepatic or extrahepatic obstruction of the bile ducts. Drug induced cholestasis may occur as a pure centrilobular form with little or no portal inflammation or it may be combined with cellular injury of varying degree. It is not known if these cellular changes are directly due to the drug or are secondary to the cholestasis. Pure cholestasis is characterized by visible bile stasis in the form of bile thrombi in dilated bile canaliculi with bile staining of the cytoplasm of some of the hepatocytes. On electron microscopy the dilatation of the bile canaliculi is seen to be associated with shortening or loss of microvilli and deep intracytoplasmic diverticula. Histochemical demonstration of decreased canalicular ATPase activity and increased and spread pericanalicular acid phosphatase activity is also observed (GOLDFISCHER et al., 1962).

Cholestasis may be produced by certain bile acids such as taurolithocholate and taurocholenate which interfere with the bile acid dependent fraction of bile flow (JAVITT and EMERMAN, 1968). Ethinylestradiol reduces bile flow by reducing the bile acid independent fraction of bile water (GUMUSIO and VALDIVIESO, 1971). 17-α-ethinyl substituted estrogens and progestogens reduce basal bile flow in the rat while the parent compounds estradiol-17β and 19-nortestosterone have little effect. The substituted estrogens were eightfold more effective in reducing bile flow than the progestogens (HEIKEL and LATHE, 1970a), and a number of these compounds were shown to inhibit the ATPase activity of rat liver plasma membranes in vitro (HEIKEL and LATHE, 1970b).

Centrilobular cholestasis results from administration of the triterpene acid icterogenin or the 17-alkylated anabolic steroids (ARIAS, 1963). Examples are those compounds with a methyl or ethyl group in the 17α position, such as methyltesterone, norethandrolone, methyltestrenolone, methandrostenolone and 2α,17-α-dimethyl-dihydrotestosterone (ADLERCREUTZ and TENHUNEN, 1970). Although the proportion of patients receiving these agents who develop jaundice is of the order of $1-2\%$, many more patients develop BSP retention. As with bilirubin the capcity for hepatic BSP uptake and conjugation remains intact but the excretory mechanism fails (ARIAS, 1963).

Intrahepatic cholestasis has been noted with synthetic progestogens of the 19- nor type, that is, those lacking the C-19 methyl group. The 17-α-synthetic progestogens lynestrenol and norethindrone both reduced basal bile flow in the rat but did not decrease the bilirubin T_m or produce a rise in serum bilirubin (HEIKEL and LATHE, 1970a), while norethynodrel depressed the maximum hepatic excretion of bilirubin and ICG (HARGREAVES, 1965). HEIKEL and LATHE (1970a) also demonstrated in rats that the 17α-ethinyl substituted estrogens reduced bile flow and bilirubin T_m (mestranol) and produced a rise in serum conjugated bilirubin. BARTOK et al. (1970) suggested that the effects of lynesterol are due to a functional disturbance in the Golgi apparatus.

Oral contraceptives containing both estrogen and a progestogen may produce cholestatic jaundice in a small number of women. A typical histological picture of cholestasis is seen with variable signs of hepatocellular damage. The production of jaundice by these oral contraceptives is more common in women with a history of recurrent benign cholestasis of pregnancy. Challenge of these women with ethinylestradiol or mestranol produces hyperbilirubinemia but challenge with the progestogen component usually does not. This suggests that it is the estrogenic component which is primarily responsible for the cholestasis (ADLERCREUTZ and TENHUNEN, 1970).

A number of drugs produce cholestasis and hyperbilirubinemia associated with parenchymal cellular changes (KLATSKIN, 1974; PEREZ et al., 1972). These include antibiotics, hypoglycemic agents, monoamine oxidase inhibitors, thiazide diuretics and phenothiazines. Clinically, the phenothiazines are the most common cause. It is of interest that various phenothiazines and derived products inhibit Na:K ATPase activity (BRODY et al., 1974).

4. Phenobarbital Therapy for Cholestasis

Stimulation of the bile secretory process probably contributes to the effects of phenobarbital in various cholestatic disorders. Phenobarbital lowers serum bilirubin and facilitates bile salt and dye excretion in some cases of intrahepatic cholestasis (STIEHL et al., 1972, 1973; BLOOMER and BOYER, 1975; ESPINOZA et al., 1974). In some patients with the Dubin-Johnson syndrome in which conjugated hyperbilirubinemia is due to impaired secretion of organic anions into bile, phenobarbital decreases serum bilirubin levels and increases the T_m for BSP (SHANI et al., 1974).

VII. Drugs and Bilirubin in the Intestine

Possible chemical induced alterations of the intestinal stage of bilirubin excretion have not been widely explored. Phenobarbital (OKOLICSANYI et al., 1970), chlordane, dieldrin, benzpyrene, and piperonyl butoxide (LUCIER and MCDANIEL, 1972) have been shown to diminish the activity of hepatic microsomal β-glucuronidase in experimental animals, but the significance of this to bilirubin metabolism is unknown. Neonatal intestinal β-glucuronidase activity has not been specifically studied after phenobarbital or other drugs.

Therapeutic attempts to block enterohepatic circulation of bilirubin have been made with various agents which complex with bilirubin in the intestinal lumen. Agar, which binds bilirubin (POLAND and ODELL, 1974), has been shown to inhibit bacterial degradation of bound bilirubin (POLAND and ODELL, 1971; ARROWSMITH et al., 1975). While no data are available on its possible effect on the activity of human intestinal β-glucuronidase, it might be expected that any unconjugated bilirubin formed by this enzyme would be retained in the lumen and would not be reabsorbed.

In 1962 LESTER et al. demonstrated that chronic administration of cholestyramine to Gunn rats lowered their serum bilirubin. Both agar (ODELL et al., 1974) and polyvinylpyrrolidone (PLOUSSARD et al., 1972) lower serum bilirubin and increase fecal bilirubin, and agar and cholestyramine decrease tissue bilirubin content and protect against bilirubin nephropathy in Gunn rats (ODELL et al., 1974; CALL and TISHER, 1975). The same therapeutic approach has been used in human neonates but with less success. Agar (POLAND and ODELL, 1971) and charcoal (ULSTROM and EISENKLAM, 1964) have lowered serum bilirubin in normal neonates and in the one patient with Crigler-Najjar syndrome treated by ARROWSMITH et al. (1975) cholestyramine lowered serum bilirubin. However agar (BLUM and ETIENNE, 1973; MAURER et al., 1973; MOLLER, 1974; ROMAGNOLI et al., 1975; WINDORFER et al., 1975), cholestyramine (SCHMID et al., 1963), and polyvinylpyrrolidone (PLOUSSARD et al., 1972) have been of no value in normal neonates or prematures and agar (BLASCHKE et al., 1974b) and cholestyramine (WRANNE, 1967; BLUMENSCHEIN et al., 1968; GIROTTI et al., 1969) have been ineffective in several patients with the Crigler-Najjar syndrome. In contrast, in various cholestatic liver disorders with conjugated hyperbilirubinemia, cholestyramine has been shown to lower the serum bilirubin (VISINTINE et al., 1961; LOTTSFELDT et al., 1963; SPIEGEL et al., 1965) although this effect has not always been observed (ENGSTROM et al., 1970; STIEHL et al., 1973).

Various possible explanations for the discrepancies between these studies exist. The bilirubin binding capacity of different agar preparations varies (POLAND and ODELL, 1974). Bilirubin binding and distribution differ between rat and man (SCHMID and HAMMAKER, 1963), with a higher proportion of the Gunn rat's unconjugated bilirubin pool being more loosely bound to albumin and therefore free in the extravascular space from where it may diffuse into the intestinal lumen. Variations in patient populations, diet, gastrointestinal flora, and the practise of breast feeding (MOLLER, 1974) may also be of importance.

VIII. Alternate Paths of Bilirubin Excretion

In animals and humans lacking bilirubin GT, alternate mechanisms for bilirubin disposal do exist with conversion of bilirubin to water soluble diazo negative catabolites which are excreted in bile and urine (SCHMID and HAMMAKER, 1963). Nothing is known about factors regulating the activity of these pathways but it is possible that drugs may influence the proportion of bilirubin degraded and excreted in this manner (KREEK and SLEISENGER, 1968). There is no evidence that drugs have such effects in man. Patients completely lacking bilirubin GT do not respond to phenobarbital with changes in serum bilirubin concentration or clearance rate (BLASCHKE et al., 1974b), while patients with detectable but diminished GT (type II Crigler-Najjar and Gilbert's syndromes) do respond suggesting that the glucuronidation pathway is essential for the phenobarbital effect.

Most studies of drug administration in homozygous Gunn rats have demonstrated no decrease in serum bilirubin or increase in hepatic bilirubin GT activity (DELEON et al., 1967; ROBINSON, 1971; ROBINSON et al., 1971b; JANSEN and HENDERSEN, 1972; VAINIO and HIETANEN, 1974). METGE et al. (1964) described a fall in serum bilirubin in Gunn rats treated with benzpyrene. However, bilirubin GT activity was demonstrable in the rats before and after therapy and it is likely that these were heterozygous Gunn rats. LUDERS (1970) (cited by VAINO and HIETANEN, 1974) administered phenobarbital to Gunn rats for 2 weeks and observed a fall in serum bilirubin. TOPHAM and BROAD (1971) described decreases in serum bilirubin in Gunn rats treated with salicylate or ICI 54450 (2-(4-chlorophenyl) thiazo-4-yl acetic acid). The lower serum bilirubin persisted for a number of weeks after the drugs were discontinued, an effect probably unrelated to alterations in plasma protein binding. The authors suggested but did not demonstrate an alternate excretory pathway.

IX. Bilirubin Photodegradation

Following the initial reports by CREMER et al. (1958) and others (BROUGHTON et al., 1965; OBES-POLLERI, 1967) that exposure of newborn infants to fluorescent light reduces serum bilirubin levels, phototherapy of neonatal jaundice has become a popular mode of therapy whose effectiveness has been confirmed by controlled trials (LUCEY et al., 1968; LUCEY, 1970; HODGMAN and SCHWARTZ, 1970). However, only recently has some progress been made in establishing the identity and mode of excretion of some of the products of bilirubin photodegradation, and there is continuing controversy regarding possible undesirable side-effects and long term safety of this procedure in newborns.

In vitro studies have established that exposure of pure unconjugated bilirubin in organic, alkaline aqueous, and protein containing solutions to a strong light source with maximal emission in the range from 420–490 nm (OSTROW and BRANHAM, 1970; DAVIES and KEOHANE, 1970; SAUSVILLE et al., 1972) results in a progressive loss of yellow color (LATHE et al., 1966). OSTROW et al. (1971) have characterized the products of bilirubin degradation in alkali in the dark, which are the same as the photodegradation products of unconjugated bilirubin formed during photoillumination at neutral pH in the presence of albumin (OSTROW and BRANHAM, 1970). Products of this reaction include in sequence: biliverdin, hydroxy-bilirubins, bilichrysins, and 5,5 -diformyl-dipyrrylmethane (OSTROW et al., 1971). LIGHTNER and QUISTAD (1972a) have isolated methylvinylmaleimide from the products formed from photodegradation of unconjugated bilirubin or biliverdin (LIGHTNER and CRANDALL, 1972) in an oxygenated methanolic solution. MCDONAGH (1971) has proposed that bilirubin photo-oxidation proceeds by a singlet oxygen mechanism in which the light-exposed bilirubin acts as a photosensitizer to form singlet oxygen which then reacts with the double bonds in the bilirubin methene bridges to form the di-pyrrole, 5,5′-diformyldipyrrylmethane, as well as other products. This di-pyrrole has since been isolated (BONNETT and STEWART, 1975) and other major reaction products including propentdyopents (LIGHTNER and QUISTAD, 1972b; LIGHTNER, 1974; BONNETT and STEWART, 1972, 1975), allylic rearrangements of these compounds (BONNETT and STEWART, 1975), and hematinic acid imide (LIGHTNER and QUISTAD, 1972b) and imide hydrolysis products (LIGHTNER, 1974) have also been identified and isolated. Since biliverdin IX-α-dimethylester inhibits the photo-oxidation of bilirubin IXα, MCDONAGH (1972) has suggested that biliverdin is probably not an intermediate in the major pathway of bilirubin photo-oxidation in vitro. LIGHTNER et al. (1973) also found that biliverdin was not a principal product or precursor of other bilirubin photoproducts, although biliverdin would slowly photo-oxidize to form many of the same products as bilirubin (methylvinylmaleimide, hematinic acid and propentdyopents). The relevance of these in vitro findings to in vivo pathways has not been established. The in vitro mechanisms have been fully reviewed (OSTROW, 1972a, b; LIGHTNER, 1974).

Apart from the known clinical effectiveness in reducing hyperbilirubinemia in newborn infants and children, little is known about the nature and disposition of the bilirubin photodegradation products formed in vivo. During phototherapy of jaundiced infants, the urine becomes darker and there is evidence of urinary excretion of di-pyrroles (PORTO, 1970). The stools also have been noted to exhibit a characteristic green or brown color (HODGMAN and SCHWARTZ, 1970; LUCEY, 1970; PORTO, 1970) presumably reflecting the excretion of undefined photodegradation products. In children with Crigler-Najjar syndrome, phototherapy during administration of radio-labeled bilirubin results in rapid excretion of undefined water-soluble photodegradation products principally in the bile and also in the urine

(CALLAHAN et al., 1970; THALER et al., 1973) and promotes excretion of bile bilirubin (THALER et al., 1973). Excretion is sufficiently rapid so that the photo-derivatives do not accumulate in the circulation. Similar results have been obtained in studies with congenitally jaundiced Gunn rats (OSTROW, 1971) and it has also been demonstrated that photoderivatives of bilirubin produced in vitro are rapidly excreted in bile following intravenous administration to normal or Gunn rats (OSTROW, 1967). While the nature of the photo-degradation products of bilirubin formed in vivo in man have not been determined, OSTROW and BERRY (1972a) have isolated a major di-pyrrole product from Gunn rat bile which appears only during phototherapy. This di-pyrrole is not the diformyl dipyrrylmethane formed in vitro. Other degradation products have not yet been fully characterized, but appear to differ from the in vitro products in spectral, chromatographic, and solubility characteristics (OSTROW, 1967, 1971).

Phototherapy of Gunn rats also causes a striking enhancement of biliary excretion of unconjugated bilirubin to levels comparable to excretion of conjugated bilirubin in normal rats (OSTROW, 1971); LUND and JACOBSEN, 1972, 1974; MCDONAGH 1973, 1974, 1975). As much as half of the bilirubin loss during phototherapy in Gunn rats may be accounted for by this phenomenon (OSTROW, 1971; OSTROW and BERRY, 1972b). While it has been suggested that this process might reflect alteration of the hepatocyte canalicular membrane to allow unconjugated bilirubin to passively diffuse from blood to bile, such alteration in membrane permeability is not a general phenomenon involving other substances (OSTROW and BERRY, 1972b).

It is known that the water soluble bilirubin photoderivatives produced in vitro lose the cytotoxic characteristics of bilirubin (BROUGHTON et al., 1965). Since the derivatives produced in vivo are qualitatively different (OSTROW, 1967, 1971), the unequivocal endorsement of the safety of phototherapy is not justified until these derivatives are fully characterized and carefully examined for cytotoxic effects. On the other hand, extensive clinical experience with phototherapy in infants has revealed no serious side-effects nor evidence of long-term neurotoxicity (LUCEY, 1970, 1972). While it is possible that coupled photoreactions could alter bilirubin binding by albumin during phototherapy in vivo (ODELL et al., 1970) there is in fact an increase in bilirubin binding capacity during phototherapy (BROWN, 1970; PORTO et al., 1969), so that displacement of bilirubin from albumin with facilitation of the development of kernicterus is unlikely.

When aged red cells are exposed to light in the presence of bilirubin in vitro, a red cell cation leak with increased osmotic fragility develops (KOPELMAN et al., 1971). There have been isolated reports of massive hemolysis during phototherapy in premature infants with reduced red cell glucose-6-phosphate dehydrogenase (JOHNSON and BOGGS, 1972). However, this complication appears to be rare and is only seen with very high doses of radiation (SAUSVILLE et al., 1972). It is thus unlikely that red cell hemolysis with increased bilirubin production occurs often during phototherapy at usual light intensities (BLACKBURN et al., 1972).

The occasional failure of phototherapy in clinical and experimental situations (CREMER et al., 1958; BROUGHTON et al., 1965; OSTROW, 1971) might be related to the enhanced endogenous bilirubin production described in treated Gunn rats (OSTROW, 1971). The source of increased pigment formation is unclear, but could represent hemolysis, increased early bilirubin formation, or mobilization of a sequestered bilirubin pool. The occasional observation of interruption of bile flow during phototherapy to Gunn rats, without mechanical obstruction of the biliary passages (OSTROW, 1972a) suggests that the hepatic secretory apparatus may be damaged in this situation. This complication should be carefully sought in humans.

Abbreviations

AIA	Allylisopropylacetamide
ALA	Δ-aminolevulinic acid
ANIT	α-Naphthylisothiocyanate
BSP	Sulfobromophthalein
DDT	Dichlorodiphenyltrichlorethane
G-6-PD	Glucose-6-phosphate dehydrogenase
GSH	Reduced glutathione
GT	UDP—glucuronyl transferase
HBABA	2-(4-Hydroxybenzeneazo) benzoic acid
ICG	Indocyanine green
PCN	Pregnenolone-16-α-carbonitrile
PGD	Phosphogluconic dehydrogenase
T_m	Maximal rate of excretion into bile

References

Aarts, E.M.: Differentiation of the barbiturate stimulation of the glucuronic acid pathway from de novo enzyme synthesis. Biochem. Pharmacol. **15**, 1469 – 1477 (1966)

Acocella, G., Billing, B.H.: The effect of rifamycin SV on bile pigment excretion in rats. Gastroenterology **49**, 526 – 530 (1965)

Acocella, G., Nicolis, F.B., Tenconi, L.T.: The effect of an intravenous infusion of rifamycin SV on the excretion of bilirubin, bromsulphalein and indocyanine green in man. Gastroenterology **49**, 521 – 525 (1965)

Adachi, Y., Yamamoto, T.: Influence of drugs and chemicals upon hepatic enzymes and proteins. I. Structure-activity relationship between various barbiturates and microsomal enzyme induction in rat liver. Biochem. Pharmacol. **25**, 663 – 668 (1976)

Adlard, B.P.F., Lathe, G.H.: Breast milk jaundice: Effect of 3α20β-pregnanediol on bilirubin conjugation by human liver. Arch. Dis. Childh. **45**, 186 – 189 (1970)

Adlercreutz, H., Tenhunen, R.: Some aspects of the interaction between natural and synthetic female sex hormones and the liver. Amer. J. Med. **49**, 630 – 648 (1970)

Alpert, S., Mosher, M., Shanske, A., Arias, I.M.: Multiplicity of hepatic excretory mechanisms for organic anions. J. gen. Physiol. **53**, 238 – 247 (1969)

Arias, I.M.: A defect in microsomal function in nonhemolytic acholuric jaundice. J. Histochem. Cytochem. **7**, 250 – 252 (1959)

Arias, I.M.: Ethereal and N-linked glucuronide formation by normal and Gunn rats in vitro and in vivo. Biochem. biophys. Res. Commun. **6**, 81 – 84 (1961)

Arias, I.M.: Effects of a plant acid (icterogenin) and certain anabolic steroids on the hepatic metabolism of bilirubin and sulfobromophthalein. Ann. N.Y. Acad. Sci. **104**, 1014 – 1025 (1963)

Arias, I.M.: Transfer of bilirubin from blood to bile. Semin. Hematol. **9**, 55 – 70 (1972)

Arias, I.M., Gartner, L.M.: Production of unconjugated hyperbilirubinemia in full-term new born infants following administration of pregnane-3(alpha), 20(beta)-diol. Nature (Lond.) **203**, 1292 – 1293 (1964)

Arias, I.M., Gartner, L.M., Cohen, M., Ben Ezzer, J., Levi, A.J.: Chronic nonhemolytic unconjugated hyperbilirubinemia with glucuronyl transferase deficiency. Amer. J. Med. **47,** 395 − 409 (1969)

Arias, I.M., Gartner, L., Furman, M., Wolfson, S.: Studies of the effect of several drugs on hepatic glucuronide formation in newborn rats and humans. Ann. N.Y. Acad. Sci. **111,** 274 − 280 (1963)

Arias, I.M., Gartner, L.M., Seifter, S., Furman, M.: Prolonged neonatal unconjugated hyperbilirubinemia associated with breast feeding and a steroid, pregnane-3 (alpha), 20 (beta)-diol, in maternal milk that inhibits glucuronide formation in vitro. J. clin. Invest. **43,** 2037 − 2047 (1964)

Arias, I.M., Jansen, P.: Protein binding and conjugation of bilirubin in the liver cell In: Jaundice. Goresky, C.A., and Fisher, M.M. (eds.), pp. 175 − 193. New York: Plenum Press 1975

Arias, I.M., Johnson, L., Wolfson, S.: Biliary excretion of injected conjugated and un conjugated bilirubin by normal and Gunn rats. Amer. J. Physiol. **200,** 1091 − 1094 (1961)

Arrowsmith, W.A., Payne, R.B., Littlewood, J.M. Comparison of treatments for congenital nonobstructive nonhemolytic hyperbilirubinemia. Arch. Dis. Childh. **50,** 197 − 201 (1975)

Aschoff, L.: Das reticulo-endotheliale System und seine Beziehungen zur Gallenfarbstoffbildung. Münch. med. Wschr. **69,** 1352 (1922)

Ashbrook, J.D., Spector, A.A., Santos, E.C., Fletcher, J.E.: Long chain fatty acid binding to human plasma albumin. J. biol. Chem. **250,** 2333 − 2338 (1975)

Bakken A.F., Thaler M.M., Schmid, R.: Metabolic regulation of heme catabolism and bilirubin production. I. Hormonal control of hepatic heme oxygenase activity. J. clin. Invest. **51,** 530 − 536 (1972)

Barnhart, J.L., Clarenburg, R.: Factors determining clearance of bilirubin in perfused rat liver. Amer. J. Physiol. **225,** 497 − 507 (1973)

Baron, J., Tephly, T.R.: The role of heme synthesis during the induction of hepatic microsomal cytochrome P-450 and drug metabolism produced by benzpyrene. Biochem. biophys. Res. Commun. **36,** 526 − 532 (1969)

Bartok, I., Varga, L., Varga, G.: Elektronenmikroskopische Veränderungen in der Rattenleber nach Verabreichung von dem oralen Antikonzeptionsmittel Lynestrenol. Acta hepato. splenol. (Stuttg.) **17,** 1 (1970)

Batt, A.M., Ziegler, J.M., Siest, G.: Competitive inhibition of glucoronidation by p-hydro-xyphenyl hydantoin. Biochem. Pharmacol. **24,** 152 − 154 (1975)

Beaven, G.H., Chen, S.H., D'Albis, A., Gratzer, W.B.: A spectroscopic study of the haemin-human serum albumin system. Europ. J. Biochem. **41,** 539 − 546 (1974)

Beaven, G.H., D'Albis, A., Gratzer, W.B.: The interaction of bilirubin with human serum albumin. Europ. J. Biochem. **33,** 500 − 510 (1973)

Becker, B.A., Plaa, G.L.: The nature of α-naphthylisothiocyanate-induced cholestasis. Toxicol. appl. Pharmacol. **7,** 680 − 685 (1965a)

Becker, B.A., Plaa, G.L.: Quantitative and temporal delineation of various parameters of liver dysfunction due to α-naphthylisothiocyanate. Toxicol. appl. Pharmacol. **7,** 708 − 718 (1965b)

Bellet, H., Raynaud, A.: An assay of bilirubin UDP-glucuronyl transferase on needle-biopsies applied to Gilbert's syndrome. Clin. chim. Acta **53,** 51 − 55 (1974)

Berk, P.D.: Total body handling of bilirubin. In: Jaundice. Goresky, C.A., and Fisher, M.M. (eds.), pp. 135 − 157. New York: Plenum Press 1975

Berk, P.D., Blaschke, T.: Effect of glutethimide on the plasma concentration of unconjugated bilirubin. Clin. Res. **19,** 347 (1971) (Abstract)

Berk, P.D., Bloomer, J.R., Howe, R.B., Berlin, N.I.: Constitutional hepatic dysfunction (Gilbert's syndrome). A new definition based on kinetic studies with unconjugated radio-bilirubin. Amer. J. Med. **49,** 296 − 305 (1970)

Berk, P.D. Howe, R.B., Berlin, N.I.: Disorders of bilirubin metabolism. pp. 841 − 880, In: Duncan's Diseases of Metabolism. Bondy, P.K. and Rosenberg, L.E. (eds.). Philadelphia − London − Toronto: Saunders 1974

Berk, P.D., Howe, R.B., Bloomer, J.R., Berlin, H.I.: Studies of bilirubin kinetics in normal adults. J. clin. Invest. **48,** 2176 − 2190 (1969)

Bernstein, L.H., Ben-Ezzer, J., Gartner, L., Arias, I.M.: Hepatic intracellular distribution of tritium-labelled unconjugated and conjugated bilirubin in normal and Gunn rats. J. clin. Invest. **45,** 1194 − 1201 (1966)

Berthelot, P.: Influence of drugs on bilirubin disposal. In: International Symposium on Hepatoxicity. M. Eliakim., J. Eshchar and H.J. Zimmermann (eds.), pp. 69–74. New York: Academic Press 1974

Berthelot, P., Billing, B.H.: Effect of bunamiodyl on hepatic uptake of sulfobromphthalein in the rat. Amer. J. Physiol. **211**, 395–399 (1966)

Berthelot, P., Erlinger, S., Dhumeaux, D., Preaux, A.M.: Effect of rifamycin, bunamiodyl, and novobiocin on bilirubin UDP-glucuronyl transferase. Digestion **4**, 134–135 (1971)

Bessis, M., Breton-Gorius, J., Thiery, J.P.: Role possible de l'hemoglobine accompagnant le noyau des erythroblastes dans l'origine de la stercobiline eliminée precocement. C.R. Acad. Sci. (Paris) **252**, 2300–2302 (1961)

Beutler, E.: The hemolytic effect of primaquine and related compounds: A review. Blood **14**, 103–139 (1959)

Beutler, E: Drug induced hemolytic anemia. Pharmacol. Rev. **21**, 73–103 (1969a)

Beutler, E.: Effect of flavin compounds on glutathione reductase activity: in vivo and in vitro studies. J. clin. Invest. **48**, 1957–1966 (1969b)

Beutler, E.: Abnormalities of the hexose monophosphate shunt. Semin. Hemat. **8**, 311–347 (1971)

Bevan, B.R., Holton, J.B.: Inhibition of bilirubin conjugation in rat liver slices by free fatty acids, with relevance to the problem of breast milk jaundice. Clin. chim. Acta **41**, 101–107 (1972)

Billing, H.B., Black, M.: The action of drugs on bilirubin metabolism in man. Ann. N.Y. Acad. Sci. **179**, 403–410 (1971)

Billing, B.H., Cole, P.G., Lathe, G.H.: The excretion of bilirubin as a diglucuronide giving the direct van den Bergh reaction. Biochem. J. **65**, 774–784 (197)

Billing, B.H., Maggiore, Q., Cartter, M.A.: Hepatic transport of bilirubin. Ann. N.Y. Acad. Sci. **111**, 319–324 (1963)

Billing, B.II., Williams, R., Richards, T.G.: Defects in hepatic transport of bilirubin in congenital hyperbilirubinemia. An analysis of plasma bilirubin disappearance curves. Clin. Sci. **27**, 245–257 (1964)

Bissell, D.M., Hammaker, L., Schmid, R.: Hemoglobin and erythrocyte catabolism in rat liver: The separate roles of parenchymal and sinusoidal cells. Blood **40**, 812–822 (1972)

Black, M., Billing, B.H.: Hepatic bilirubin UDP-glucuronyl transferase activity in liver disease and Gilbert's syndrome. New Engl. J. Med. **280**, 1266–1271 (1969)

Black, M., Billing, B.H., Heirwegh, K.P.M.: Determination of bilirubin UDP-glucuronyl transferase activity in needle-biopsy specimens of human liver. Clin. chim. Acta **29**, 27–35 (1970)

Black, M., Fevery, J., Parker, D., Jacobson, J., Billing, B.H., Carson, E.R.: Effect of phenobarbitone on plasma (^{14}C) bilirubin clearance in patients with unconjugated hyperbilirubinaemia. Clin. Sci. molec. Med. **46**, 1–17 (1974)

Black, M., Perret, R.D., Carter, A.E.: Hepatic bilirubin UDP-glucuronyl transferase activity and cytochrome P-450 content in a surgical population and the effects of preoperative drug therapy. J. Lab. clin. Med. **81**, 704–712 (1973)

Black, M., Sherlock, S.: Treatment of Gilbert's syndrome with phenobarbitone. Lancet **1970 I**, 1359–1362

Blackburn, M.G., Orzalesi, M.M., Pigram, P.: Effect of light on fetal red blood cells in vivo. J. Pediat. **80**, 640–643 (1972)

Blaschke, T.F., Berk, P.D.: Augmentation of bilirubin UDP glucuronyl transferase activity in rat liver homogenates by glutethimide. Proc. Soc. exp. Biol. (N.Y.) **140**, 1315–1318 (1972)

Blaschke, T.F., Berk, P.D., Rodkey, F.L., Scharschmidt, B.F., Collison, H.A., Waggoner, J.G.: Drugs and the liver—I. Effects of glutethimide and phenobarbital on hepatic bilirubin clearance, plasma bilirubin turnover and carbon monoxide production in man. Biochem. Pharmacol. **23**, 2795–2806 (1974a)

Blaschke, T.F., Berk, P.D., Scharschmidt, B.F., Guyther, J.R., Vergalla, J.M., Waggoner, J.G.: Crigler-Najjar syndrome: An unusual course with development of neurologic damage at age eighteen. Pediat. Res. **8**, 573–590 (1974b)

Bloomer, J.R., Berk, P.D., Berlin, N.I.: Albumin and hepatic uptake of bilirubin. Clin. Res. **20**, 449 (1972) (Abstract)

Bloomer, J.R., Berk, P.D., Bonkowsky, H.L., Stein, J.A., Berlin, N.I., Tschudy, D.P.: Blood volume and bilirubin production in acute intermittent porphyria. New Engl. J. Med. **284,** 17−20 (1971)

Bloomer, J.R., Boyer, J.L.: Phenobarbital effects in cholestatic liver disease. Ann. intern. Med. **82,** 310−317 (1975)

Bloomer, J.R., Boyer, J.L., Klatskin, G.: Inhibition of bilirubin excretion in man during dehydrocholate choleresis. Gastroenterology **65,** 929−935 (193)

Blum, D., Etienne, J.: Agar in control of hyperbilirubinemia. J. Pediat. **83,** 345 (1973)

Blumenschein, S.D., Kallen, R.J., Storey, B., Natzschka, J., Odell, G.B., Childs, B.: Familial nonhemolytic jaundice with late onset of neurological damage. Pediatrics **42,** 786−792 (1968)

Bock, K.W.: Oxidation of barbiturates and the glucuronidation of 1-naphthol in perfused rat liver and in microsomes. Naunyn-Schmiedeberg's Arch. Pharmacol. **283,** 319−330 (1974)

Bock, K.W., Frohling, W., Remmer, H., Rexer, B.: Effects of phenobarbital and 3-methylcholanthrene on substrate specificity of rat liver microsomal UDP-glucuronyltransferase. Biochim. biophys. Acta (Amst.) **327,** 46−56 (1973)

Bock, K.W., Siekevitz, P.: Turnover of heme and protein moieties of rat liver microsomal cytochrome b_5. Biochem. biophys. Res. Commun. **41,** 374−380 (1970)

Bock, K.W., White, I.N.H.: UDP-glucuronyltransferase in perfused rat liver and in microsomes: Influence of phenobarbital and 3-methylcholanthrene. Europ. J. Biochem. **46,** 451−459 (1974)

Bolt, R.J., Dillon, R.S., Pollard, H.M.: Interference with bilirubin excretion by a gall-bladder dye. (Bunamiodyl). New Engl. J. Med. **265,** 1043−1045 (1961)

Bonnett, R., Stewart, J.C.M.: Photo-oxidation of bilirubin in hydroxylic solvents. Propentdyopent adducts as major products. Chem. Commun. **1972,** 596−597

Bonnett, R., Stewart, J.C.M.: The photo-oxidation of bilirubin in hydroxylic solvents. J. chem. Soc. [Perkin I] **1,** 224−231 (1975)

Bourke, E., Milne, M.D., Stokes, G.S.: Mechanism of renal excretion of urobilinogen. Brit. med. J. **1965 II,** 1510−1514

Boyer, J.L., Klatskin, G.: Canalicular bile flow and bile secretory pressure. Evidence for a non-bile salt dependent fraction in the isolated perfused rat liver. Gastroenterology **59,** 853−859 (1970)

Branch, R.A., Shand, D.G., Wilkinson, G.R., Nies, A.S.: Increased clearance of antipyrine and d-propranolol after phenobarbital treatment in the monkey. J. clin. Invest. **53,** 1101−1107 (1974)

Bratlid, D.: The effect of free fatty acids, bile acids, and hematin on bilirubin binding by human erythrocytes. Scand. J. clin. Lab. Invest. **30,** 107−112 (1972a)

Bratlid, D.: The effect of antimicrobial agents on bilirubin binding by human erythrocytes. Scand. J. clin. Lab. Invest. **30,** 331−337 (1972b)

Brauer, R.W., Leong, G.F., Holloway, R.J.: Mechanics of bile secretion. Effect of perfusion pressure and temperature on bile flow and bile secretion pressure. Amer. J. Physiol. **177,** 103−119 (1954)

Brewer, J.G., Dern, P.J.: A new inherited enzymatic deficiency of human erythrocytes: 6-phosphogluconate dehydrogenase deficiency. Amer. J. hum. Genet. **16,** 472−476 (1964)

Brodersen, R.: Competitive binding of bilirubin and drugs to human serum albumin studied by enzymatic oxidation. J. clin. Invest. **54,** 1353−1364 (1964)

Brodersen, R., Hermann, L.S.: Intestinal reabsorption of unconjugated bilirubin: A possible contributing factor in neonatal jaundice. Lancet **1963 I,** 1242

Brody, T.M., Akera, T., Baskin, S.I., Gubitz, R., Lee, C.Y.: Interaction of Na, K-ATPase with chlorpromazine free radical and related compounds. Ann. N.Y. Acad. Sci. **242,** 527−542 (1974)

Broughton, P.M.G., Rossiter, E. Jr., Warren, C.B.M., Goulis, G., Lord, P.S.: Effect of blue light on hyperbilirubinemia. Arch. Dis. Childh. **40,** 666−671 (1965)

Brown, A.K.: Variations in the management of neonatal hyperbilirubinemia; Impact on our understanding of fetal and neonatal physiology. In: Bilirubin Metabolism in the Newborn. D. Bergsma, D.Y.Y. Hsia, and C. Jackson (eds.), pp. 22−30. New York: National Foundation for Birth Defects (Original Article Series) 1970

Brown, A.K., Henning, G.: The effect of novobiocin on the development of the glucuronide conjugating system in newborn animals. Ann. N.Y. Acad. Sci. **111**, 307 – 318 (1963)

Brown, A.K., Zuelzer, W.W.: Studies on the neonatal development of the glucuronide conjugating system. J. clin. Invest. **37**, 332 – 340 (1958)

Brown, W.R., Grodsky, G.M., Carbone, J.: Intracellular distribution of tritiated bilirubin during hepatic uptake and excretion. Amer. J. Physiol. **207**, 1237 – 1241 (1964)

Burchell, B.: Observations of uridine diphosphate glucuronyltransferase activity towards oestriol and xenobiotics in developing and cultured tissues from mouse and man. Biochem. Soc. Trans. **1**, 1212 – 1214 (1973)

Call, N.B., Tisher, C.C.: The urinary concentrating defect in the Gunn strain of rat. J. clin. Invest. **55**, 319 – 329 (1975)

Callahan, E.W. Jr., Thaler, M.M., Karon, M., Bauer, K., Schmid, R.: Phototherapy of severe unconjugated hyperbilirubinemia: Formation and removal of labelled bilirubin derivatives. Pediatrics **46**, 841 – 848 (1970)

Capelle, P., Dhumeaux, D., Mora, M., Feldmann, G., Berthelot, P.: Effect of rifamycin on liver function in man. Gut **13**, 366 – 371 (1972)

Capizzo, F., Roberts, R.J.: Effect of phenobarbital, chlorpromazine, actinomycin D and chronic α-Napthylisothiocyanate administration on α-Naphthylisothiocyanate-^{14}C disposition and α-Naphthylisothiocyanate-induced hyperbilirubinemia. J. Pharmacol. exp. Ther. **179**, 455 – 464 (1971)

Careddu, P., Marini, A.: Stimulating bilirubin conjugation. Lancet **1968 I**, 982 – 983

Careddu, P., Piceni Sereni, L., Guinta, A., Sereni, F.: Sulle possibilita di attivare i processe di coniugazione e di escrezione epatica della bilirubina mediante alcuni farmaci. Richerche sperimentali con la dietilamide dell'acido nicotinico (Coramina) e con l'acido fenil-etil-barbiturico (Gardenale). Minerva pediat. **55**, 2559 – 2562 (1964)

Carey, M.C., Small, D.M.: The characteristics of mixed micellar solutions with particular reference to bile. Amer. J. Med. **49**, 590 – 608 (1970)

Catz, C., Yaffe, S.J.: Pharmacological modification of bilirubin conjugation in the newborn. Amer. J. Dis. Child. **104**, 516 – 517 (1962) (Abstract)

Catz, C., Yaffe, S.J.: Barbiturate enhancement of bilirubin conjugation and excretion in young and adult animals. Pediat. Res. **2**, 361 – 370 (1968)

Chan, G., Shiff, D., Stern, L.: Competitive binding of free fatty acids and bilirubin to albumin: Differences in HBABA dye versus Sephadex G-25 interpretation of results. Clin. Biochem. **4**, 208 – 214 (1971)

Chignell, C.F., Starkweather, D.K.: Optical studies of drug-protein complexes. V. The interaction of phenylbutazone, flufenamic acid, and dicoumarol with acetylsalicylic acid-treated human serum albumin. Molec. Pharmacol. **7**, 229 – 237 (1971)

Chignell, C.F., Vessell, E.S., Starkweather, D.K., Berlin, C.M.: The binding of sulfaphenazole to fetal, neonatal, and adult human plasma albumin. Clin. Pharmacol. Ther. **12**, 897 – 901 (1971)

Clarenburg, R., Kao, L.: Shared and separate pathways for biliary excretion of bilirubin and BSP in rats. Amer. J. Physiol. **225**, 192 – 199 (1973)

Coburn, R.F.: Enhancement by phenobarbital and diphenylhydantoin of carbon monoxide production in normal man. New Engl. J. Med. **283**, 512 – 515 (1970)

Cole, P.G., Lathe, G.H., Billing, B.H.: Separation of the bile pigments of serum, bile, and urine. Biochem. J. **57**, 514 – 518 (1954)

Conney, A.H.: Pharmacological implications of microsomal enzyme induction. Pharmacol. Rev. **19**, 317 – 366 (1967)

Conney, A.H., Levin, W., Jacobson, M., Kuntzman, R.: Effects of drugs and environmental chemicals on steroid metabolism. Clin. Pharmacol. Ther. **14**, 727 – 741 (1973)

Corchs, J.L., Serrani, R.E., Rodriguez Garay, E.: Bilirubin uptake in vitro by the rat intestinal mucosa. Biochim. biophys. Acta (Amst.) **291**, 308 – 314 (1973)

Cornelius, C.E., Ben-Ezzer, J., Arias, I.M.: Binding of sulfobromphthalein sodium (BSP) and other organic anions by isolated hepatic cell plasma membranes in vitro. Proc. Soc. exp. Biol. (N.Y.) **124**, 665 – 667 (1967)

Coutinho, C.B., Lucek, R.W., Cheripko, J.A., Kuntzman, R.: A new approach to the determination of protein-bound bilirubin displacement and its applications. Ann. N.Y. Acad. Sci. **226**, 238 – 246 (1973)

Cremer, R.J., Perryman, P.W., Richards, D.H.: Influence of light on the hyperbilirubinemia of infants. Lancet **1958 I,** 1094 – 1097

Crigler, J.F. Jr., Gold, N.I.: Effect of sodium phenobarbital on bilirubin metabolism in an infant with congenital nonhemolytic, unconjugated hyperbilirubinemia and kernicterus. J. clin. Invest. **48,** 42 – 55 (1969)

Dacie, J.V.: The Haemolytic Anaemias. Congenital and Acquired. Part IV. Drug-induced haemolytic anaemias, paroxysmal nocturnal haemoglobinuria, hemolytic disease of the newborn. London: J. & A. Churchill Ltd. 1967

Davies, R.E., Keohane, S.J.: Some aspects of the photochemistry of bilirubin. Boll. chim.-farm. **109,** 589 – 598 (1970)

Degowin, R.L., Eppes, R.B., Powell, R.D., Carson, P.E.: The hemolytic effects of diaphenyl-sulfone (DDS) in normal subjects and in those with glucose-6-phosphate dehydrogenase deficiency. Bull. Wld. Hlth. Org. **35,** 165 – 179 (1966)

Deleon, A.L., Gartner, M., Arias, I.M.: The effect of phenobarbital on hyperbilirubinemia in glucuronyl transferase deficient rats. J. Lab. clin. Med. **70,** 273 – 278 (1967)

De Matteis, F.: Rapid loss of cytochrome P-450 and heme caused in the liver microsomes by the porphyrinogenic agent 2-allyl-2-isopropylacetamide. FEBS Lett. **6,** 343 – 345 (1970)

De Matteis, F.: Loss of heme in rat liver caused by the porphyrinogenic agent 2-allyl-2-iso-propylacetamide. Biochem. J. **124,** 767 – 777 (1971)

De Matteis, F.: Drug-induced destruction of cytochrome P-450. Drug Metab. Dispos. **1,** 267 – 274 (1973)

Dern, R.J., Beutler, E., Alving, A.S.: The hemolytic effect of primaquine. V. Primaquine sensitivity as a manifestation of a multiple drug sensitivity. J. Lab. clin. Med. **45,** 30 – 39 (1955)

Dhumeaux, D., Berthelot, P.: Chronic hyperbilirubinemia associated with hepatic uptake and storage impairment. Gastroenterology **69,** 988 – 993 (1975)

Dhumeaux, D., Erlinger, S., Benhamou, J.P., Fauvert, R.: Effects of rose bengal on bile secretion in the rabbit: Inhibition of bile salt independent fraction. Gut **11,** 134 – 140 (1970)

Diamond, I.: Bilirubin binding and kernicterus. Advanc. Pediat. **16,** 99 – 119 (1969)

Done, A.K.: Developmental pharmacology. Clin. Pharmacol. Ther. **5,** 432 – 479 (1964)

Drabkin, D.L.: Independent biosynthesis of different hemin chromoproteins-cytochrome c in various tissues. Proc. Soc. exp. Biol. (N.Y.) **76,** 527 – 530 (1951)

Dutton, G.J.: The biosynthesis of glucuronides. In: Glucuronic Acid Free and Combined. Dutton, G.J. (ed.), pp. 186 – 299. New York: Academic Press 1966

Dutton, G.J.: Glucuronide forming enzymes. In: Handbook of Experimental Pharmacology XXVIII/2 pp. 378 – 400. Berlin – Heidelberg – New York. Springer 1971

Dybing, E.: Chlorpromazine inhibition of p-aminophenol glucuronidation by rat hepatoma cells in culture. Acta pharmacol. (Kbh.) **31,** 287 – 295 (1972)

Dybing, E.: Effects of membrane stabilizers on glucuronidation and amino acid transport in cultures of rat hepatoma cells. Acta pharmacol. (Kbh.) **32,** 481 – 486 (1973)

Dybing, E., Rugstad, H.E.: The inhibiting effect of diethylaminoethyl diphenylvalerate (SKF 525-A) on glucuronidation by cultures of rat hepatoma cells. Acta pharmacol. (Kbh.) **32,** 112 – 118 (1973)

Edmond, M., Erlinger, S., Berthelot, P., Benhamou, J.P., Fauvert, R.: Effets de la novobiocine sur la fonctionnement du foie: I. Etude clinique. Canad. med. Ass. J. **94,** 900 – 904 (1966)

Elder, G., Gray, C.H., Nicholson, D.C.: Bile pigment fate in gastrointestinal tract. Semin. Hematol. **9,** 71 – 89 (1972)

Eliakim, M., Eisner, M., Ungar, H.: Experimental intrahepatic obstructive jaundice following ingestion of alpha-naphthyl-isothiocyanate. Bull. Res. Coun. Israel E, **8,** 7 – 17 (1959)

Engstrom, J., Hellstrom, K., Posse, N., Sjovall, J.: Recurrent cholestasis of pregnancy. Acta obstet. gynec. scand. **49,** 29 – 34 (1970)

Erlinger, S.: Physiology of bile flow. Progr. Liver Dis. **IV,** 63 – 82 (1972)

Erlinger, S., Dhumeaux, D., Berthelot, P., Dumont, M.: Effect of inhibitors of sodium transport on bile formation in the rabbit. Amer. J. Physiol. **219,** 416 – 422 (1970)

Erlinger, S., Dumont, M.: Influence of theophylline on bile formation in the dog. Biomedicine **19,** 27 – 32 (1973)

Ertel, I.J., Newton, W.A.: Therapy in congenital hyperbilirubinemia. Phenobarbital and diethylnicotinamide. Pediatrics **44**, 43−48 (1969)

Espinoza, J., Baranafi, L., Schnaidt, E.: The effect of phenobarbital on intrahepatic cholestasis of pregnancy. Amer. J. Obstet. Gynec. **119**, 234−238 (1974)

Felsher, B.F., Craig, J.R., Carpio, N.: Hepatic bilirubin glucuronidation in Gilbert's syndrome. J. Lab. clin. Med. **81**, 829−837 (1973)

Fevery, J., Van Damme, B., Michiels, R., De Groote, J., Heirwegh, K.P.M.: Bilirubin conjugates in bile of man and rat in the normal state and in liver disease. J. clin. Invest. **51**, 2482−2492 (1972)

Fischer, H., Orth, H.: Die Chemie des Pyrrols. Leipzig: Akademische Verlagsgesellschaft 1973

Fleischner, G., Kamisaka, K., Habig, W., Jakoby, W., Arias, I.M.: Human ligandin: Characterization and quantitation. Gastroenterology **69**, 821 (1975a) (Abstract)

Fleischner, G., Meijer, D.K.F., Levine, W.G., Gatmaitan, Z., Gluck, R., Arias, I.M.: Effect of hypolipidemic drugs, nafenopin and clofibrate, on the concentration of ligandin and Z protein in rat liver. Biochem. biophys. Res. Commun. **67**, 1401−1407 (1975b)

Fleischner, G., Robbins, J., Arias, I.M.: Immunological studies of Y protein. J. clin. Invest. **51**, 677−684 (1972)

Fleischner, G., Robbins, J., Reyes, H., Levi, A.J., Arias, I.M.: Immunologic studies of Y, the major organic anion-binding protein in rat liver cytosol. Gastroenterology **60**, 185 (1971) (Abstract)

Fletcher, M.J., Sanadi, D.R.: Turnover of rat liver mitochondria. Biochim. biophys. Acta (Amst.) **51**, 356−360 (1961)

Freedman, A.L., Barr, P.S., Brody, E.A.: Hemolytic anemia due to quinidine: Observations on its mechanism. Amer. J. Med. **20**, 806−816 (1956)

Frick, P.G., Hitzig, W.H., Betke, L.: Hemoglobin Zurich. Blood. **20**, 261−271 (1962)

Fritz, M.E., Brooks, F.P.: Control of bile flow in the cholecystectomized dog. Amer. J. Physiol. **204**, 825−828 (1963)

Fromke, V.L., Miller, D.: Constitutional hepatic dysfunction (CHD; Gilbert's disease); a review with special reference to a characteristic increase and prolongation of the hyperbilirubinemic response to nicotinic acid. Medicine **51**, 451−464 (1972)

Garner, R.C., McLean, A.E.M.: Separation of heme incorporation from protein synthesis in liver microsomes. Biochem. biophys. Res. Commun. **37**, 883−887 (1969)

Girotti, F., Finocchi, G., Sartori, L., Boscherini, B.: Congenital non-haemolytic jaundice in a four year old girl without disease of the central nervous system. Helv. paediat. Acta **4**, 399−403 (1969)

Gisselbrecht, C., Berk, P.D.: Failure of phenobarbital to increase bilirubin production in the rat. Biochem. Pharmacol. **23**, 2895−2905 (1974)

Glader, B.E.: Salicylate-induced injury of pyruvate-kinase-deficient erythrocytes. New Engl. J. Med. **294**, 916−918 (1976)

Glass, J., Yannoni, C.Z., Robinson, S.H.: Rapidly synthesized heme: Relationship to erythropoiesis and hemoglobin production. Blood Cells **1**, 557−571 (1975)

Glaumann, H.: Chemical and enzymatic composition of microsomal subfractions from rat liver after treatment with phenobarbital and 3-methylcholanthrene. Chem. biol. Interact. **2**, 369−380 (1970)

Goldfischer, S., Arias, I.M., Essner, E., Novikoff, A.B.: Cytochemical and electronmicroscopic studies of rat liver with reduced capacity to transport conjugated bilirubin. J. exp. Med. **115**, 467−474 (1962)

Goldstein, J.A., Taurog, A.: Enhanced biliary excretion of thyroxine glucuronide in rats pretreated with benzpyrene. Biochem. Pharmacol. **17**, 1049−1065 (1968)

Gollan, J.L., Huang, S.N., Billing, B., Sherlock, S.: Prolonged survival in three brothers with severe type 2 Crigler-Najjar syndrome: Ultrastructural and metabolic studies. Gastroenterology **68**, 1543−1555 (1975)

Goodman, D.S.: The interaction of human serum albumin with long-chain fatty acid anions. J. Amer. chem. Soc. **80**, 3892−3898 (1958)

Goresky, C.A.: Initial distribution and rate of uptake of sulfobromophthalein in the liver. Amer. J. Physiol. **207**, 13−26 (1964)

Goresky, C.A.: The hepatic uptake and excretion of sulfobromophthalein and bilirubin. Canad. med. Ass. J. **92,** 851–857 (1965)

Goresky, C.A.: The hepatic uptake process: Its implications for bilirubin transport. In: Jaundice. Goresky, C.A. and Fisher, M.M. (eds.), pp. 159–174. New York: Plenum Press 1975

Goresky, C.A., Haddad, H.H., Kluger, W.S., Nadeau, B.E., Bach, G.G.: The enhancement of maximal bilirubin excretion with taurocholate-induced increments in bile flow. Canad. J. Physiol. Pharmacol. **52,** 389–403 (1974)

Goresky, C.A., Kluger, S.W.: The relation between bile flow and transport maximum for bilirubin in the dog. Gastroenterology **56,** 398 (1969) (Abstract)

Gralnick, H.R., McGinness, M., Elton, W., McCurdy, P.: Hemolytic anemia associated with cephalothin. J. Amer. med. Ass. **217,** 1193–1197 (1971)

Gram, T.E., Hansen, A.R., Fouts, J.R.: The submicrosomal distribution of hepatic uridine diphosphate glucuronyl transferase in the rabbit. Biochem. J. **106,** 587–591 (1968)

Gram, T.E., Rogers, L.A., Fouts, J.R.: Effect of pretreatment of rabbits with phenobarbital or 3-methylcholanthrene on the distribution of drug-metabolizing enzyme activity in subfractions of hepatic microsomes. J. Pharmacol. exp. Ther. **157,** 435–445 (1967)

Granick, S.: The induction in vitro of the synthesis of delta-aminolevulinic acid synthetase in chemical porphyria: A response to certain drugs, sex hormones and foreign chemicals. J. biol. Chem. **241,** 1359–1375 (1966)

Gray, C.H.: Bile Pigments in Health and Disease. Springfield Ill.: Ch. C. Thomas 1961

Gray, C.H., Neuberger, A., Sneath, P.H.A.: Studies in congenital porphyria. 2. Incorporation of ^{15}N in the stercobilin in the normal and in the porphyric. Biochem. J. **47,** 87–92 (1950)

Gray, D.W.G., Mowat, A.P.: Effects of aspartic acid, orotic acid, and glucose on serum bilirubin concentrations in infants born before term. Arch. Dis. Childh. **46,** 123–124 (1971)

Greenwood, D.T., Stevenson, I.H.: The stimulation of glucuronide formation in vitro and in vivo by a carcinogen diethylnitrosamine. Biochem. J. **96,** 37P (1965) (Abstract)

Gregory, D.H., Strickland, R.D.: Preparation characterization and partial purification of soluble bilirubin UDP-glucuronyl transferase. Gastroenterology **62,** 171 (1972) (Abstract)

Gregory, D.H., Strickland, R.D.: Solubilization and characterization of hepatic bilirubin-UDP-Glucuronyltransferase. Biochim. biophys. Acta (Amst.) **327,** 36–45 (1973)

Greim, H., Schenkman, J.B., Klotzbucher, M., Remmer, H.: The influence of phenobarbital on the turnover of hepatic microsomal cytochrome b_5 and cytochrome P-450 hemes in the rat. Biochim. biophys. Acta (Amst.) **201,** 20–25 (1970)

Grodsky, G.M., Carbone, J.V.: The synthesis of bilirubin glucuronide by tissue homogenates. J. biol. Chem. **226,** 449–458 (1957)

Gross, R.T., Bracci, R., Rudolph, N., Schroeder, E., Kochen, J.A.: Hydrogen peroxide toxicity and detoxification in erythrocytes of newborn infants. Blood **29,** 481–493 (1967)

Groszmann, R.J., Kotelanski, B., Kendler, J., Zimmerman, H.J.: Effect of sulfobromophthalein and indocyanine green on bile excretion. Proc. Soc. exp. Biol. (N.Y.) **132,** 712–714 (1969)

Gumusio, J.J., Valdivieso, V.D.: Studies on the mechanism of ethynylestradiol impairment of the bile flow and bile salt excretion in the rat. Gastroenterology **61,** 339–344 (1971)

Gutstein, S., Alpert, S., Arias, I.M.: Studies of hepatic excretory function. IV. Biliary excretion of sulfobromophthalein sodium in a patient with the Dubin–Johnson syndrome and a biliary fistula. Israel J. med. Sci. **4,** 36–40 (1968)

Gydell, K.: Transient effect of nicotinic acid on bilirubin metabolism and formation of carbon monoxide. Acta med. scand. **167,** 431–441 (1960)

Habig, W.H., Pabst, M.J., Fleischner, G., Gatmaitan, Z., Arias, I.M., Jakoby, W.B.: The identity of glutathione S-transferase B with ligandin, a major binding protein of liver. Proc. nat. Acad. Sci. (Wash.) **71,** 3879–3882 (1974)

Hakim, J., Feldmann, G., Boivin, P., Troube, H., Boucherot, J., Penaud, J., Guibot, P., Kreis, B.: Étude comparative des activités bilirubine et paranitrophenolglucuronyl transferases hépatique. III. Effet de la rifampicine seule ou associée à la streptomycine et à l'isoniazide chez l'homme. Path. et Biol. **21,** 255–263 (1973)

Halac, E., Reff, A.: Studies on bilirubin UDP-glucuronyltransferase. Biochim. biophys. Acta (Amst.) **139,** 328–343 (1967)

Halac, E., Sicignano, C.: Re-evaluation of the influence of sex, age, pregnancy and pheno-barbital on the activity of UDP-glucuronyl transferase in rat liver. J. Lab. clin. Med. **73**, 677–685 (1969)

Hammaker, L., Schmid, R.: Interference with bile pigment uptake in the liver by flavaspidic acid. Gastroenterology **53**, 31–37 (1967)

Hanninen, O.: Repression in the glucuronic acid pathway in the different tissues in the rat. Acta med. scand., Suppl. **101**, 8 (1968) (Abstract)

Hanninen, O., Aitio, A.: Enhanced glucuronide formation in the different tissues following drug administration. Biochem. Pharmacol. **17**, 2307–2311 (1968)

Harbison, R.D., Spratt, J.L.: Novobiocin-induced hyperbilirubinemia and its reduction by phenobarbital pretreatment. Toxicol. appl. Pharmacol. **11**, 257–263 (1967)

Hardy, J.B., Mellits, E.D.: Does maternal smoking during pregnancy have a long term effect on the child? Lancet **1972 II**, 1332–1336

Hargreaves, T.: Cholestatic drugs and bilirubin metabolism. Nature (Lond.) **206**, 154–156 (1965)

Hargreaves, T.: The effect of male fern extract on biliary secretion. Brit. J. Pharmacol. **26**, 34–40 (1966)

Hargreaves, T.: The effect of diethylaminoethyl diphenylpropylacetic acid (SKF 525-A) on uridine 5-pyrophosphate glucuronyltransferase. Biochem. Pharmacol. **16**, 1481–1488 (1967)

Hargreaves, T.: The effect of monoamine oxidase inhibitors on conjugation. Experientia (Basel) **24**, 157–158 (1968)

Hargreaves, T.: Effect of fatty acids on bilirubin conjugation. Arch. Dis. Childh. **48**, 446–450 (1973)

Hargreaves, T., Holton, J.B.: Jaundice of the newborn due to novobiocin. Lancet **1962 I**, 839

Hargreaves, T., Lathe, G.H.: Inhibitory aspects of bile secretion. Nature (Lond.) **200**, 1172–1176 (1963)

Hargreaves, T., Piper, R.F.: Breast milk jaundice. Effect of inhibitory breast milk and 3α, 20β-pregnanediol on glucuronyl transferase. Arch. Dis. Childh. **46**, 195–198 (1971).

Hargreaves, T., Piper, R.F., Cam, J.: Effect of oral contraceptives on glucuronyl transferase. Nature (Lond.) New Biol. **234**, 110–111 (1971)

Hargreaves, T., Piper, R.F., Trickey, R.: The effect of imipramine and desipramine on UDP-glucuronyl transferase. Experientia (Basel) **25**, 725–726 (1969)

Harris, J.W.: Studies on the mechanism of a drug induced hemolytic anemia. J. Lab. clin. Med. **47**, 760–775 (1956)

Harris, R.C., Lucey, J.F., MacLean, J.R.: Kernicterus in premature infants associated with low concentration of bilirubin in the plasma. Pediatrics **21**, 875–884 (1958)

Heath, E.C., Dingell, J.V.: The interaction of foreign chemical compounds with the glucuronida-tion of estrogens in vitro. Drug Metab. Dispos. **2**, 556–565 (1974)

Heikel, T.A.J., Lathe, G.H.: The effect of oral contraceptive steroids on bile secretion and bilirubin T_m in rats. Brit. J. Pharmacol. **38**, 593–601 (1970a)

Heikel, T.A.J., Lathe, G.H.: The effect of 17α-ethinyl substituted steroids on adenosine tri-phosphatases of rat liver plasma membrane. Biochem. J. **118**, 187–189 (1970a)

Heirwegh, K.P.M., Meuwissen, J.A.T.P., Fevery, J.: Enzymic formation of β-D-monoglucu-ronide, β-D-monoglucoside and mixtures of β-D-monoxyloside and β-D-dixyloside of bili-rubin by microsomal preparations from rat liver. Biochem. J. **125**, 28p–29p (1971)

Heirwegh, K.P.M., Meuwissen, J.A.T.P., Fevery, J.: Critique of the assay and significance of bilirubin conjugation. In: Advances in Clin. Chem. O. Bodansky and A.L. Latner (eds.). Vol. 16, pp. 239–289. New York: Academic Press 1973

Heirwegh, K.P.M., Van de Vijver, M., Fevery, J.: Assay and properties of digitonin activated bilirubin uridine diphosphate glucuronyl transferase from rat liver. Biochem. J. **129**, 605–618 (1972)

Heirwegh, K.P.M., Vanhees, G.P., Leroy, P., Vanroy, F.P., Jansen, F.H.: Heterogeneity of bile pigment conjugation as revealed by chromatography of their ethyl anthranilate azo-pigments. Biochem. J. **120**, 877–890 (1970)

Hertz, H.: A direct spectrometric method for determination of the concentration of available bilirubin binding sites in serum using bromphenol blue. Scand. J. clin. Lab. Invest. **35**, 545–559 (1975)

Heubel, F.: Diazepam und Phenobarbital bei der Senkung des Neugeborenen-Bilirubinspiegels durch nichtsedierende Dosen. Int. J. clin. Pharmacol. **9**, 210–219 (1974)

Heubel, F., Muhlberger, G.: Senkung des Neugeborenen Bilirubinspiegels durch Diazepam. Int. J. clin. Pharmacol. **6**, 332–341 (1971)

Hodgman, J.E., Schwartz, A.: Phototherapy and hyperbilirubinemia of the premature. Amer. J. Dis. Child. **119**, 473–477 (1970)

Hollman, S., Touster, O.: Alterations in tissue levels of uridine diphosphate glucose dehydrogenase, uridine diphosphate glucuronic acid pyrophosphatase and glucuronyl transferase induced by substances influencing the production of ascorbic acid. Biochim biophys. Acta (Amst.) **62**, 338–352 (1962)

Howland, R.D., Burkhalter, A., Trevor, A.J., Hegman, S., Shirachi, D.Y.: Properties of lubrol-extracted uridine diphosphate glucuronyl transferase. Biochem. J. **125**, 991–997 (1971)

Hsia, D.Y., Dowben, R.M., Riabov, S.: Inhibitors of glucuronyl transferase in the newborn. Ann. N.Y. Acad. Sci. **111**, 326–336 (1963)

Hunter, J., Thompson, R.P.H., Rake, M.O., Williams, R.: Controlled trial of phetharbital, a non-hypnotic barbiturate, in unconjugated hyperbilirubinemia. Brit. med. J. **1971 II**, 497–499

Hunton, D.B., Bollman, J.L., Hoffman, H.N.H.: The plasma removal of indocyanine green and sulfobromophthalein: Effect of dosage and blocking agents. J. clin. Invest. **40**, 1648–1655 (1961)

Hupka, A.L., Karler, R.: Biotransformation of ethylmorphine and heme by isolated parenchymal and reticuloendothelial cells of rat liver. RES: J. reticuloendoth. Soc. **14**, 225–241 (1973)

Ibrahim, G.W., Schwartz, S., Watson. C.J.: Early labeling of bilirubin from glycine and Δ-aminolevulinic acid in bile fistula dogs, with special reference to stimulated versus suppressed erythropoiesis. Metabolism **15**, 1129–1139 (1966)

Ideo, G., Defranchis, R., Del Ninno, E., Dioguardi, N.: Ethanol increases liver uridine diphosphate glucuronyl transferase. Experientia (Basel) **27**, 24–25 (1971)

Indacochea-Redmond, N., Plaa, G.L.: Functional effects of α-naphthylisothiocyanate in various species. Toxicol. appl. Pharmacol. **19**, 71–80 (1971)

Indacochea-Redmond, N., Witschi, H.P., Plaa, G.L.: Effect of inhibitors of protein and ribonucleic acid synthesis on the hyperbilirubinemia and cholestasis produced by α-naphthylisothiocyanate. J. Pharmacol. exp. Ther. **184**, 780–786 (1973)

Indacochea-Redmond, N., Witschi, H., Plaa, G.L.: Effects of inhibitors of protein and ribonucleic acid synthesis on α-naphthylisothiocyanate-induced hyperbilirubinemia, sulfobromophthalein retention and prolongation of pentobarbital hypnosis. J. Pharmacol. exp. Ther. **189**, 278–284 (1974)

Inscoe, J.K., Axelrod, J.: Some factors affecting glucuronide formation in vitro. J. Pharmacol. exp. Ther. **129**, 128–133 (1960)

Israels, L.G., Schacter, B.A., Yoda, B., Goldenberg, G.J.: Delta-aminolevulinic acid transport and synthesis, porphyrin synthesis and heme catabolism in chick embryo liver and heart cells. Biochim. biophys. Acta (Amst.) **372**, 32–38, (1974)

Israels, L.G., Skanderberg, J., Guyda, H., Zingg, W., Zipursky, A.: A study of the early-labeled fraction of bile pigment. The effect of altering erythropoiesis on the incorporation of $(2\text{-}^{14}\text{C})$ glycine into heme and bilirubin. Brit J. Haemat. **9**, 50–62 (1963b)

Israels, L.G., Yamamoto, T., Skanderberg, J., Zipursky, A.: Shunt bilirubin: Evidence for two components. Science **139**, 1054–1055 (1963a)

Isselbacher, K.J., Chrabas, M.F., Quinn, R.C.: The solubilization and partial purification of a glucuronyl transferase from rabbit liver microsomes. J. biol. Chem. **237**, 3033–3036 (1962)

Isselbacher, K.J., McCarthy, E.A.: Studies on bilirubin sulphate and other non-glucuronide conjugates of bilirubin. J. clin. Invest. **38**, 645–651 (1959)

Jacobsen, C.: Chemical modification of the high affinity bilirubin binding site of human serum albumin. Europ. J. Biochem. **27**, 513–519 (1972)

Jacobsen, J.: Binding of bilirubin to human serum albumin-determination of the dissociation constants. FEBS Lett. **5**, 112–114 (1969a)

Jacobsen, J.: A chromatographic separation of bilirubin glucuronides from human bile. Acta chem. scand. **23**, 3023 – 3026 (1969 b)

Jansen, F.H., Billing, B.H.: The identification of mono-conjugates of bilirubin in bile as amide derivatives. Biochem. J. **125**, 917 – 919 (1971)

Jansen, P.L., Henderson, P.T.: Influence of phenobarbital treatment on p-nitrophenol and bilirubin glucuronidation in Wistar rat, Gunn rat, and cat. Biochem. Pharmacol. **21**, 2457 – 2462 (1972)

Javitt, N.B., Emerman, S.: Effect of sodium taurolithocholate on bile flow and bile acid excretion. J. clin. Invest. **47**, 1002 – 1014 (1968)

Jirsa, M., Vecerek, B.: Neue Bilirubinderivate. I. Ihr Vergleich mit Gallen- und Serum-Bilirubin. Hoppe Seylers Z. physiol. Chem. **311**, 87 92 (1958)

Johnson, L., Boggs, T.R.: In Ostrow, J.D.: Photochemical and biochemical basis of the treatment of neonatal jaundice. Progress in Liver Disease. H. Popper and F. Schaffner (eds.). Vol. IV, p. 452. New York: Grune and Stratton 1972

Johnson, L., Garcia, M.L., Figueroa, E., Sarmiento, F.: Kernicterus in rats lacking glucuronyl transferase. II. Factors which alter bilirubin concentration and frequency of kernicterus. Amer. J. Dis. Child. **101**, 322 – 349 (1961)

Johnson, L., Sarmiento, F., Blanc, W.A., Day, R.: Kernicterus in rats with an inherited deficiency of glucuronyl transferase. Amer. J. Dis. Child. **97**, 591 – 608 (1959)

Jones, B.: Glucuronyl transferase inhibition by steroids. J. Pediat. **64**, 815 – 821 (1964)

Jones, E.A., Bloomer, J.R., Berlin, N.I.: The measurement of the synthetic rate of bilirubin from hepatic heme in patients with acute intermittent porphyria. J. clin. Invest. **50**, 2259 – 2265 (1971)

Jones, R.S., Grossman, M.I.: Choleretic effects of secretin and histamine in the dog. Amer. J. Physiol. **217**, 532 – 535 (1969)

Josephson, B., Furst, P.: Sulfonamides competing with bilirubin for conjugation to albumin. Scand. J. clin. Lab. Invest. **18**, 51 – 63 (1966)

Kamisaka, K., Listowsky, I., Arias, I.M.: Circular dichroism studies of Y protein (ligandin), a major organic anion binding protein in liver, kidney, and small intestine. Ann. N.Y. Acad. Sci. **226**, 148 – 153 (1973)

Kamisaka, K., Listowsky, I., Betheil, J.J., Arias, I.M.: Competitive binding of bilirubin, sulfobromophthalein, indocyanine green and other organic anions to human and bovine serum albumin. Biochim. biophys. Acta (Amst.) **365**, 169 – 180 (1974)

Kamisaka, K., Listowsky, I., Gatmaitan, Z., Arias, I.M.: Interactions of bilirubin and other ligands with ligandin. Biochemistry **14**, 2175 – 2180 (1975)

Kapitulnik, J., Horner-Mibashan, R., Blondheim, S.H., Kaufmann, N.A., Russell, A.: Increase in bilirubin binding affinity of serum with age of infant. J. Pediat. **86**, 442 – 445 (1975)

Kaplowitz, N., Percy-Robb, I.W., Javitt, N.B.: Role of hepatic anion-binding protein in bromsulphthalein conjugation. J. exp. Med. **138**, 483 – 487 (1973)

Kawasaki, H., Sakaguchi, S., Arimura, K., Irisa, T., Tominaga, K., Hirayama, C., Ibayashi, H.: Studies on the relationship of hepatic anion-binding proteins and sulfobromophthalein-glutathione conjugation in normal and phenobarbital-treated rats. Biochim. biophys. Acta (Amst.) **385**, 334 – 342 (1975)

Kellermeyer, R.W., Tarlov, A.R., Brewer, G.J., Carson, P.E., Alving, A.S.P.: Hemolytic effect of therapeutic drugs. Clinical consideration of the primaquine-type hemolysis. J. Amer. med. Ass. **180**, 388 – 394 (1962)

Kenwright, S., Levi, A.J.: Impairment of hepatic uptake of rifamycin antibiotics by probenicid and its therapeutic implications. Lancet **1973 II**, 1401 – 1405

Kenwright, S., Levi, A.J.: Sites of competition in the selective hepatic uptake of rifamycin-SV, flavaspidic acid, bilirubin and bromsulphthalein. Gut **15**, 220 – 226 (1974)

Khanna, N.N., Harpur, E.R., Stern, L.: In vitro effect of sodium phenobarbital and diethyl-nicotinamide (Coramine) on the protein binding of bilirubin. Clin. Biochem. **2**, 349 – 356 (1969)

King, M.A.R., Wiltshire, B.G., Lehmann, H., Morimoto, H.: An unstable haemoglobin with reduced oxygen affinity. Haemoglobin Peterborough. Brit. J. Haemat. **22**, 125 – 134 (1972)

Kintzel, H.W., Hinkel, G.K., Schwarze, R.: The decrease in the serum bilirubin level in premature infants by orotic acid. Acta paediat. scand. **61**, 1 – 5 (1971)

Kirsch, R., Fleischner, G., Kamisaka, K., Arias, I.M.: Structural and functional studies of ligandin, a major renal organic anion-binding protein. J. clin. Invest. **55**, 1009–1019 (1975)

Klaassen, C.D.: Effects of phenobarbital on the plasma disappearance and biliary excretion of drugs in rats. J. Pharmacol. exp. Ther. **175**, 289–300 (1970)

Klaassen, C.D.: Biliary excretion of drugs: Role of ligandin in newborn immaturity and in the action of microsomal enzyme inducers. J. Pharmacol. exp. Ther. **195**, 311–319 (1975)

Klatskin, G.: Drug-induced hepatic injury. In: The Liver and its Disease. Schaffner, F., Sherlock, S., and Leevy, C.M. (eds.), pp. 163–178. New York: Intercontinental Med. Book Corp. 1974

Kopelman, A.E., Brown, R.S., Odell, G.B.: The bronze baby; a complication of phototherapy. Trans. Amer. pediat. Soc. **81**, 3 (1971) (Abstract)

Krasner, J., Giacoia, G.P., Yaffe, S.J.: Drug-protein binding in the newborn infant. Ann. N.Y. Acad. Sci. **226**, 101–114 (1973a)

Krasner, J., Juchau, M.R., Yaffe, S.J.: Postnatal developmental changes in hepatic bilirubin UDP-glucuronyl transferase. Studies on the solubilized enzyme. Biol. Neonat. (Basel) **23**, 381–390 (1973b)

Kreek, M.J., Sleisenger, M.H.: Reduction of serum unconjugated bilirubin with phenobarbital in adult congenital non-haemolytic unconjugated hyperbilirubinemia. Lancet **1968 II**, 73–78

Kuenzle, C.C.: Bilirubin conjugates of human bile. Isolation of phenylazo derivatives of bile bilirubin. Biochem. J. **119**, 387–394 (1970a)

Kuenzle, C.C.: Bilirubin conjugates of human bile. Nuclear magnetic-resonance, infrared and optical spectra of model compounds. Biochem. J. **119**, 395–409 (1970b)

Kuenzle, C.C.: Bilirubin conjugates of human bile. The excretion of bilirubin as the acyl glycosides of aldobiouronic acid, pseudoaldobiouronic acid and hexuronosylhexuronic acid, with a branched-chain hexuronic acid as one of the components of the hexuronosylhexuronide. Biochem. J. **119**, 411–435 (1970c)

Kunin, C.M., Craig, W.A., Kornguth, M., Monson, R.: Influence of binding on the pharmacologic activity of antibiotics. Ann. N.Y. Acad. Sci. **226**, 214–224 (1973)

Kutz, K., Loffler, A., Kandler, H., Fevery, J.: Clofibrate: A potent serum bilirubin lowering agent in subjects with Gilbert's syndrome. Digestion **12**, 255 (1975)

Lage, G.L., Spratt, J.L.: Bilirubin conjugation by hepatic microsomes from adult male guinea pigs. Arch. Biochem. Biophys. **126**, 175–180 (1968)

Laitinen, M., Lang, M., Hanninen, O.: Changes in the protein lipid interaction in rat liver microsomes after pretreatment of the rat with barbiturates and polycyclic hydrocarbons. Int. J. Biochem. **5**, 747–751 (1974)

Lakshminarayan, S., Sahn, S.A., Hudson, L.D.: Massive haemolysis caused by rifampicin. Brit. med. J. **1973 II**, 282–283

Landaw, S.W., Callahan, E.W. Jr., Schmid, R.: Catabolism of heme in vivo: Comparison of the simultaneous production of bilirubin and carbon monoxide. J. clin. Invest. **49**, 914–925 (1970)

Lathe, G.H., Lord, P., Toothill, C.: Bilirubin transport by plasma protein. In: Desgrez, P. and De Traverse, P.M. (eds.). Transport Functions of Plasma Protein. Vol. V, p. 129. New York: Elsevier 1966

Lathe, G.H., Walker, M.: The synthesis of bilirubin glucuronide in animal and human liver. Biochem. J. **70**, 705–712 (1958)

Lee, J.J., Cowger, M.L.: Bilirubin albumin binding and a possible mechanism of kernicterus. Res. Commun. chem. Path. Pharmacol. **8**, 327–339 (1974)

Lester, R., Hammaker, L., Schmid, R.: A new therapeutic approach to unconjugated hyperbilirubinemia. Lancet **1962 II**, 1257

Lester, R., Klein, P.D.: Bile pigment excretion: a comparison of the biliary excretion of bilirubin and bilirubin derivatives. J. clin. Invest. **45**, 1839–1846 (1966)

Lester, R., Schmid, R.: Intestinal absorption of bile pigments. I. The enterohepatic circulation of bilirubin in the rat. J. clin. Invest. **42**, 736–746 (1963a)

Lester, R., Schmid, R.: Intestinal absorption of bile pigments. II. Bilirubin absorption in man. New Engl. J. Med. **269**, 178–182 (1963b)

Lester, R., Schmid, R.: Intestinal absorption of bile pigments. III. The enterohepatic circulation of urobilinogen in the rat. J. clin. Invest. **44**, 722 – 730 (1965)

Lester, R., Schumer, W., Schmid, R.: Intestinal absorption of bile pigments. IV. Urobilinogen absorption in man. New Engl. J. Med. **272**, 939 – 943 (1965)

Levi, A.J., Gatmaitan, Z., Arias, I.M.: Two cytoplasmic proteins from rat liver and their role in hepatic uptake of sulfobromophthalein (BSP) and bilirubin. J. clin. Invest. **47**, 61 a (1968)

Levi, A.J., Gatmaitan, Z., Arias, I.M.: Two hepatic cytoplasmic protein fractions, Y and Z and their possible role in the hepatic uptake of bilirubin, sulfobromophthalein, and other anions. J. clin. Invest. **48**, 2156 – 2167 (1969)

Levi, A.J., Gatmaitan, Z., Arias, I.M.: Deficiency of hepatic organic anion-binding protein, impaired organic anion uptake by liver and "physiologic" jaundice in newborn monkeys. New Engl. J. Med. **283**, 1136 – 1139 (1970)

Levin, W., Jacobson, M., Kuntzman, R.: Incorporation of radioactive delta-aminolevulinic acid into microsomal cytochrome P-450: Selective breakdown of the hemoprotein by allylisopropylacetamide and carbon tetrachloride. Arch. Biochem. Biophys. **148**, 262 – 269 (1972)

Levin, W., Jacobson, M., Sernatinger, E., Kuntzman, R.: Breakdown of cytochrome P-450 heme by secobarbital and other allyl-containing barbiturates. Drug Metab. Dispos. **1**, 275 – 285 (1973)

Levin, W., Kuntzman, R.: Biphasic decrease of radioactive hemoprotein from liver microsomal CO-binding particles. Effect of 3-methylcholanthrene. J. biol. Chem. **244**, 3671 – 3676 (1969)

Levine, B.B.: Immunochemical mechanisms of drug allergy. Ann. Rev. Med. **17**, 23 – 38 (1966)

Levine, R.I., Reyes, H., Levi, A.J., Gatmaitan, Z., Arias, I.M.: Phylogenetic study of organic anion transfer from plasma into the liver. Nature (Lond.) New Biol. **231**, 277 – 279 (1971)

Levitt, M., Schacter, B.A., Zipursky, A., Israels, L.G.: The non-erythropoietic component of early bilirubin. J. clin. Invest. **47**, 1281 – 1294 (1968)

Levy, G., Ertel, I.J.: Effect of bilirubin on drug conjugations in children. Pediatrics **47**, 811 – 817 (1971)

Levy, M., Lester, R., Levinsky, N.G.: Renal excretion of urobilinogen in the dog. J. clin. Invest. **47**, 2117 – 2124 (1968)

Lightner, D.A.: In vitro photooxidation products of bilirubin. In: Phototherapy in the Newborn. An Overview. Odell, G.B., R. Shaffer and A.P. Simopoulos (eds.), pp. 34 – 35. Washington, D.C.: U.S. National Academy of Sciences 1974

Lightner, D.A., Crandall, D.C.: Biliverdin photo-oxidation. In vitro formation of methylvinylmaleimide. FEBS Lett. **20**, 53 – 56 (1972)

Lightner, D.A., Crandall, D.C., Gertler, S., Quistad, G.B.: On the formation of biliverdin during photooxygenation of bilirubin in vitro. FEBS Lett. **30**, 309 – 312 (1973)

Lightner, D.A., Quistad, G.B.: Methylvinylmaleimide from bilirubin photo-oxidation. Science **175**, 324 (1972)

Lightner, D.A., Quistad, G.B.: Hematinic acid and propentdyopents from bilirubin photo-oxidation in vitro. FEBS Lett. **25**, 94 – 96 (1972b)

Linberg, L.G., Norden, A.: Severe hemolytic reaction to chlorpromazine. Acta med. scand. **170**, 195 – 199 (1961)

Linhart, P.: Affinity of UDP-glucuronyl-transferase for several substrates and for chloramphenicol. Res. exp. Med. **163**, 241 – 249 (1974)

Litwack, G., Ketterer, B., Arias, I.M.: Ligandin: A hepatic protein which binds steroids, bilirubin, carcinogens and a number of exogenous anions. Nature (Lond.) **234**, 466 – 467 (1971)

Lokietz, H., Dowben, R.M., Hsia, D.Y.: Studies on the effect of novobiocin on glucuronyl transferase. Pediatrics **32**, 47 – 51 (1963)

London, I.M., West, R., Shemin, D., Rittenberg, D.: On the origin of bile pigment in normal man. J. biol. Chem. **184**, 351 – 358 (1950)

Lottsfeldt, F.I., Krivit, W., Aust, J.B., Carey, J.B.: Cholestyramine therapy in intrahepatic biliary atresia. New Engl. J. Med. **269**, 186 – 189 (1963)

Lucey, J.F.: Phototherapy of jaundice. In: Bilirubin Metabolism in the Newborn. D. Bergsma, D.Y.Y. Hsia, and C. Jackson (eds.), pp. 63–70. New York: National Foundation for Birth Defects (Original article series) 1970

Lucey, J.F.: Neonatal phototherapy: Uses, problems and questions. Semin. Hematol. **9**, 127–135 (1972)

Lucey, J.F., Ferreiro, M., Hewitt, J.: Prevention of hyperbilirubinemia of prematurity by phototherapy. Pediatrics **41**, 1047–1054 (1968)

Lucier, G.W., McDaniel, O.S.: Alterations in rat liver microsomal and lysosomal β-glucuronidase by compounds which induce hepatic drug metabolizing enzymes. Biochim. biophys. Acta (Amst.) **261**, 168–176 (1972)

Luders, D.: Einfluss von Phenobarbital auf den Bilirubinstoffwechsel bei Gunnratten. Versuche mit inaktivem und ¹⁴C-markiertem Bilirubin. Z. Kinderheilk. **109**, 149–168 (1970)

Lund, H.T., Jacobsen, J.: Influence of phototherapy on unconjugated bilirubin in duodenal bile of newborn infants with hyperbilirubinemia. Acta paediat. scand. **61**, 693–696 (1972)

Lund, H.T., Jacobsen, J.: Influence of phototherapy on the biliary bilirubin excretion pattern in newborn infants with hyperbilirubinemia. Pediatrics **85**, 262–267 (1974)

Lundh, B., Cavallin-Stahl, E., Mercke, C.: Nicotinic acid and the endogenous production of carbon monoxide. Acta med. scand. **197**, 173–176 (1975)

Macarol, V., Morris, T.Q., Baker, K.J., Bradley, S.E.: Hydrocortisone choleresis in the dog. J. clin. Invest. **49**, 1714–1723 (1970)

MacGibbon, B.H., Loughbridge, L.W., Hourihane, D.O., Boyd, D.W.: Autoimmune haemolytic anemia with acute renal failure due to phenacetin and p-aminosalicylic acid. Lancet **1960 I**, 7

Machinist, J.M., Ahn, K., Becker, B.A.: The induction of hepatic Z cytoplasmic protein by hypolipidemic drugs. Gastroenterology **69**, 843 (1975) (Abstract)

Maines, M.D., Kappas, A.: Cobalt induction of hepatic heme oxygenase; with evidence that cytochrome P-450 is not essential for this enzyme activity. Proc. nat. Acad. Sci. (Wash.) **71**, 4293–4297 (1974)

Maisels, M.J.: Bilirubin. On understanding and influencing its metabolism in the newborn infant. Pediat. Clin. N. Amer. **19**, 447–501 (1972)

Mann, F.C., Sheard, C., Bollman, J.L., Blades, E.J.: The formation of bile pigment from hemoglobin. Amer. J. Physiol. **76**, 306–315 (1926)

Mannering, G.J.: Inhibition of drug metabolism. In: Handbook Exp. Pharmacol., Vol. XXVIII/2, pp. 452–476. Berlin–Heidelberg–New York: Springer 1971

Marniemi, J.: Bilirubin UDP-glucosyl and UDP-glucuronosyltransferase of rat liver. A comparative study of the effects of membrane perturbants in vitro and of chrysene administration in vivo. Chem. biol. Interact. **9**, 135–145 (1974)

Martin, J.F., Vierling, J.M., Wolkoff, A.W., Scharschmidt, B.F., Vergalla, J., Waggoner, J.G., Berk, P.D.: Abnormal hepatic transport of indocyanine green in Gilbert's syndrome. Gastroenterology **70**, 385–391 (1976)

Marver, H.S.: The role of heme in the synthesis and repression of microsomal protein. In: Microsomes and Drug Oxidations (eds. J.R. Gillette, A.H. Conney, G.J. Cosmides, R.W. Estabrook, J.R. Fouts, and G.J. Mannering), pp. 495–511. New York: Academic Press 1969

Marver, H.S., Collins, A., Tschudy, D.P., Rechcigl, J. Jr.: Delta-aminolevulinic acid synthetase. II. Induction in rat liver. J. biol. Chem. **241**, 4323–4329 (1966)

Marver, H.S., Schmid, R., Schutzel, H.: Heme and methemoglobin: Naturally occurring repressors of microsomal cytochrome. Biochem. biophys. Res. Commun. **33**, 969–974 (1968)

Masters, B.S.S., Schacter, B.A.: Catalysis of heme degradation by purified NADPH-cytochrome c reductase in the absence of other microsomal proteins. Ann. clin. Res. 8, Suppl. **17**, 18–27 (1976)

Matsuda, I., Shirahata, T.: Effects of aspartic acid and orotic acid upon serum bilirubin level in newborn infants. Tohuku J. exp. Med. **90**, 133–136 (1966)

Maurer, H.M., Shumway, C.N., Draper, D.A., Hossaini, A.A.: Controlled trial comparing agar, intermittent phototherapy, and continuous phototherapy for reducing neonatal hyperbilirubinemia. J. Pediat. **82**, 73–76 (1973)

Maxwell, J.D., Hunter, J., Stewart, D.A., Carrella, M., Williams, R.: Effect of phenobarbitone on bile flow and bilirubin metabolism in man and the rat. Digestion 9, 138 – 148 (1973)

McDonagh, A.F.: The role of singlet oxygen in bilirubin photo-oxidation. Biochem. biophys. Res. Commun. 44, 1306 – 1311 (1971)

McDonagh, A.F.: Evidence for singlet oxygen quenching by biliverdin IX-α dimethyl ester and its relevance to bilirubin photo-oxidation. Biochem. biophys. Res. Commun. 48, 408 – 415 (1972)

McDonagh, A.F.: Thermal and photochemical reactions of bilirubin IX-α. Conference on the biological role of porphyrins and related structures. Ann. N.Y. Acad. Sci. 244, 553 – 569 (1973)

McDonagh, A.F.: The photochemistry and photometabolism of bilirubin. In: Phototherapy in the Newborn. An Overview. Odell, G.B., Schaffer, R., and Simopoulos, A.P. (eds.), pp. 56 – 73. Washington, D.C.: U.S. National Acad. Sci. 1974

McDonagh, A.F.: Phototherapy and hyperbilirubinaemia. Lancet 1975 I, 339

McNee, N.W.: Jaundice: a review of recent work. Quart. J. Med. 16, 390 – 420 (1923)

Metge, W.R., Owen, C.A., Foulk, W.T., Hoffman, H.N.: Bilirubin glucuronyl transferase activity in liver disease. J. Lab. clin. Med. 64, 89 – 98 (1964)

Meyer, M.C., Guttman, D.E.: The binding of drugs by plasma proteins. J. pharm. Sci. 57, 895 – 918 (1968)

Meyer, U., Marver, H.S.: Chemically induced porphyria. Increased microsomal heme turnover after treatment with allylisopropylacetamide. Science 171, 64 – 66 (1971)

Mia, A.S., Gronwall, R.R., Cornelius, C.E.: Bilirubin-^{14}C turnover. Studies in normal and mutant Southdown sheep with congenital hyperbilirubinemia. Proc. Soc. exp. Biol. (N.Y.) 133, 955 – 959 (1970)

Millar, J., Peloquin, R., De Leeuw, N.K.M.: Phenacetin-induced hemolytic anemia. Canad. med. Ass. J. 106, 770 – 775 (1972)

Mishkin, S., Stein, L., Fleischner, G., Gatmaitan, Z., Arias, I.M.: Z protein in hepatic uptake and esterification of long-chain fatty acids. Amer. J. Physiol. 228, 1634 – 1640 (1975)

Mohler, D.N., Majerus, P.W., Minnich, V., Hess, C.E., Garrick, M.D.: Glutathione synthetase deficiency as a cause of hereditary hemolytic disease. New Engl. J. Med. 283, 1253 – 1257 (1970)

Moller, J.: Agar ingestion and serum bilirubin values in newborn infants. Acta obstet. gynec. scand. 53, 61 – 63 (1974)

Morris, T.Q.: Choleretic responses to cyclic AMP and theophylline in the dog. Gastroenterology. 62, 187 (1971) (Abstract)

Muirhead, E.E., Groves, M., Guy, R., Halden, E.R., Bass, R.K.: Acquired hemolytic anemia, exposures to insecticides and positive Coombs test dependent on insecticide preparations. Vox Sang. (Basel) 4, 277 – 292 (1959)

Muirhead, E.E., Halden, E.R., Groves, M.P.: Drug-dependent Coombs (antiglobulin) test and anemia. Observations on quinine and acetophenetidin. Arch. intern. Med. 101, 87 – 96 (1958)

Mulder, G.J.: The effect of phenobarbital on the submicrosomal distribution of uridine diphosphate glucuronyl transferase from rat liver. Biochem. J. 117, 319 – 324 (1970)

Mulder, G.J.: Bilirubin and the heterogeneity of microsomal uridine diphosphate glucuronyl transferase from rat liver. Biochim. biophys. Acta (Amst.) 289, 284 – 292 (1972)

Mulder, G.J.: The rate-limiting step in the biliary elimination of some substrates of uridine diphosphate glucuronyl transferase in the rat. Biochem. Pharmacol. 22, 1751 – 1763 (1973)

Mulder, G.J.: On nonspecific inhibition of rat liver microsomal UDP-glucuronyl transferase by some drugs. Biochem. Pharmacol. 23, 1283 – 1291 (1974)

Mulder, G.J., Pilon, A.H.E.: UDP glucuronyltransferase and phenolsulfotransferase from rat liver in vivo and in vitro. III. The effect of phenolphthalein and its sulfate and glucuronide conjugate on conjugation and biliary excretion of harmol. Biochem. Pharmacol. 24, 517 – 521 (1975)

Nagel, R.L., Ranney, H.M.: Drug induced oxidative denaturation of hemoglobin. Semin. Hematol 10, 269 – 278 (1973)

Nathenson, G., Cohen, M.I., Litt, I.F., McNamara, H.: The effect of maternal heroin addiction on neonatal jaundice. J. Pediat. 81, 899 – 903 (1972)

Nathenson, G., Cohen, M.I., McNamara, H.: The effect of Na benzoate on serum bilirubin of the Gunn rat. J. Pediat. **86**, 799 – 803 (1975)

Nelson, T., Jacobsen, J., Wennberg, R.P.: Effect of pH on the interaction of bilirubin with albumin and tissue culture cells. Pediat. Res. **8**, 963 – 967 (1974)

Neuberger, J.A., Scott, J.J.: Aminolevulinic acid and porphyrin biosynthesis. Nature (Lond.) **172**, 1093 – 1094 (1953)

Noir, B.A., Dewalz, A.T., Rodriguez-Garay, E.A.: Studies on the bilirubin sulphate conjugate excreted in human bile. Biochim. biophys. Acta (Amst.) **222**, 15 – 27 (1970)

Nosslin, B.: The direct diazo reaction of bile pigments in serum. Experimental and clinical studies. Scand. J. clin. Lab. Invest. **12**, Suppl. 49, pp. 1 – 176 (1960)

Nosslin, B.: Bromsulphalein retention and jaundice due to unconjugated bilirubin following treatment with male fern extract. Scand. J. clin. Lab. Invest. **15**, Suppl. 69, 206 – 212 (1963)

Nosslin, B., Morgan, E.H.: The effect of phloroglucinol derivatives from male fern on dye excretion by the liver in the rabbit and rat. J. Lab. clin. Med. **65**, 891 – 902 (1965)

Nymand, G.: Maternal smoking and neonatal hyperbilirubinemia. Lancet **1974 II**, 173

Obes-Polleri, J.: Phototherapy in neonatal hyperbilirubinemia. Arch. Pediat. Urug. **38**, 77 – 81 (1967)

Ockner, R.K., Isselbacher, K.J.: Recent concepts of intestinal fat absorption. Rev. Physiol. Biochem. Pharmacol. **71**, 107 – 146 (1974)

Odell, G.B.: The dissociation of bilirubin from albumin and its clinical implications. J. Pediat. **55**, 268 – 279 (1959)

Odell, G.B.: The distribution of bilirubin between albumin and mitochondria. J. Pediat. **68**, 165 – 180 (1966)

Odell, G.B.: Influence of binding on the toxicity of bilirubin. Ann. N.Y. Acad. Sci. **226**, 225 – 237 (1973)

Odell, G.B., Bolen, J.L., Poland, R.L., Seungdamrong, S., Cukier, J.O.: Protection from bilirubin nephropathy in jaundiced Gunn rats. Gastroenterology **66**, 1218 – 1224 (1974)

Odell, G.B., Brown, R.S., Holtzmann, N.A.: Dye-sensitized photo-oxidation of albumin associated with a decreased capacity for protein-binding of bilirubin. In: Bilirubin Metabolism in the Newborn. D. Bergsma, D.Y.Y. Hsia, and C. Jackson (eds.), pp. 31 – 36. New York: National Foundation for Birth Defects (Original Article Series) 1970

Odell, G.B., Cohen, S.N., Kelly, P.C.: Studies in kernicterus. II. The determination of the saturation of serum albumin with bilirubin. J. Pediat. **74**, 214 – 230 (1969)

Odell, G.B., Cukier, J.O., Maglalang, A.C.: Commentary: Albumin binding of bilirubin. J. Pediat. **86**, 614 (1975)

O'Doherty, P.J.A., Kuksis, A.: Stimulation of triacylglycerol synthesis by Z protein in rat liver and intestinal mucosa. FEBS Lett. **60**, 256 – 258 (1975)

Ohnhaus, E.E., Locher, J.T.: Liver blood flow and blood volume following chronic phenobarbitone administration. Europ. J. Pharmacol. **31**, 161 – 165 (1975)

Okolicsanyi, L., Cartei, G., Naccarato, R.: Effects of ethanol on Gilbert's hyperbilirubinemia. Lancet **1972 I**, 450

Okolicsanyi, L., Cortelazzo, S., Carluccio, A., Naccarato, R.: Effects of rifampicin, UDPG and phenobarbital on bilirubin metabolism in Gilbert's syndrome. Digestion **6**, 295 (1972) (Abstract)

Okolicsanyi, L., Frei, J., Magnenat, P.: Multiplicity and specificity of UDP glucuronyl transferase. II. Influence of phenobarbital and cholestasis on the activity of glucuronyl transferase and beta glucuronidase in rat liver. Enzym. biol. clin. **11**, 402 – 411 (1970)

Okolicsanyi, L., Frei, J., Magnenat, P., Naccarato, R.: Multiplicity and specificity of UDP glucuronyl transferase. 3. UDP-glucuronyl transferase and β-glucuronidase activities assayed with different substrates in inherited and acquired human liver diseases. Enzyme **12**, 658 – 673 (1971)

Orme, M.L'E., Davies, L., Breckenridge, A.: Increased glucuronidation of bilirubin in man and rat by administration of antipyrine (phenazone). Clin. Sci. molec. Med. **46**, 511 – 518 (1974)

Ostrow, J.D.: Photo-oxidation derivatives of ^{14}C-bilirubin and their excretion by the Gunn rat. In: Bilirubin Metabolism. I.A.D. Bouchier and B.H. Billing (eds.), pp. 117 – 127. Oxford: Blackwell 1967

Ostrow, J.D.: Photocatabolism of labeled bilirubin in the congenitally jaundiced Gunn rat. J. clin. Invest. **50**, 707–718 (1971)

Ostrow, J.D.: Mechanism of bilirubin photodegradation. Semin. Hematol. **9**, 113–125 (1972a)

Ostrow, J.D.: Photochemical and biochemical basis of the treatment of neonatal jaundice. Progr. Liver Dis. **IV**, 447–462 (1972b)

Ostrow, J.D., Berry, C.S.: Characterization of bilirubin photoderivatives in Gunn rat bile. J. clin. Invest. **51**, 71a (1972a) (Abstract)

Ostrow, J.D., Berry, C.S.: Effect of phototherapy on hepatic excretory function in normal and Gunn rats. Gastroenterology **62**, 168 (1972b) (Abstract)

Ostrow, J.D., Branham, R.V.: Photodecomposition of bilirubin and biliverdin in vitro. Gastroenterology **58**, 15–25 (1970)

Ostrow, J.D., Murphy, N.H.: Isolation and properties of conjugated bilirubin from bile. Biochem. J. **120**, 311–327 (1970)

Ostrow, J.D., Nicholson, D.C., Stoll, M.S.: Derivatives of the alkaline degradation of bilirubin. Gastroenterology **60**, 186 (1971) (Abstract)

Patrignani, A., Sternieri, E., Perugini, S.: Ricerche sulla bilirubina precocemente marcata: II. Incorporazione della glicina-2-^{14}C e del $\varDelta$-ALA-3,5-^{3}H nella bilirubina del plasma, nell emina e nella globina degli eritrociti in pazienti affetti de aplasia midollare. Haematologica **56**, 65–72 (1971)

Paumgartner, G.: The handling of indocyanine green by the liver. Schweiz. med. Wschr. **105**, Supplement (1975)

Paumgartner, G., Probst, P., Kraines, R., Leevy, C.M.: Kinetics of indocyanine green removal from the blood. Ann. N.Y. Acad. Sci. **170**, 134–147 (1970)

Perez, V., Schaffner, F., Popper, H.: Hepatic drug reactions. Progr. Liver Dis. **IV**, 597–625 (1972)

Perugini, S., Patrignani, A., Sternieri, E., Mucci, P.: Ricerche sulla bilirubina precocemente marcata: I. Incorporazione della glicina-2-^{14}C e del $\varDelta$-ALA-3,5-^{3}H nella bilirubina del plasma, nell emina e nella globinadegli eritrociti, in condizioni di eritropoiesi normale e stimolata. Haematologica **56**, 21–35 (1971)

Pimstone, N.R., Engel, P., Tenhunen, R., Seitz, P.T., Marver, H.S., Schmid, R.: Inducible heme oxygenase in the kidney: A model for the homeostatic control of hemoglobin catabolism. J. clin. Invest. **50**, 2042–2050 (1971b)

Pimstone, N.R., Tenhunen, R., Seitz, P.T., Marver, H.S., Schmid, R.: The enzymatic degradation of hemoglobin to bile pigments by macrophages. J. exp. Med. **133**, 1264–1281 (1971a)

Pinckard, R.N., Hawkins, D., Farr, R.S.: The influence of acetylsalicylic acid on the binding of acetrizoate to human albumin. Ann. N.Y. Acad. Sci. **226**, 341–354 (1973)

Ploussard, J.P., Foliot, A., Christoforov, B., Petite, J.P., Alison, F., Etienne, J.P., Housset, L.: Interet et limite de l'utilisation d'un capteur intestinal de la bilirubine non conjugée (polyvinylpyrrolidone) dans l'ictere du premature. Arch. franç. Pédiat. **29**, 373–390 (1972)

Polacek, K., Novak, M., Melichar, V.: Influence of free fatty acids on the distribution of bilirubin and its clinical significance in the newborn. Rev. Czech. Med. **11**, 161–169 (1965)

Poland, R.L., Odell, G.B.: Physiologic jaundice: the enterohepatic circulation of bilirubin. New Engl. J. Med. **284**, 1–6 (1971)

Poland, R.L., Odell, G.B.: The binding of bilirubin to agar. Proc. Soc. exp. Biol. (N.Y.) **146**, 1114–1118 (1974)

Porter, E.G., Waters, W.J.: A rapid micromethod for measuring the reserve albumin binding capacity in serum from newborn infants with hyperbilirubinemia. J. Lab. clin. Med. **67**, 660–668 (1966)

Porto, S.O.: In vitro and in vivo studies on the effect of phototherapy upon bilirubin. In: Bilirubin metabolism in the newborn. D. Bergsma, D.Y.Y. Hsia, and C. Jackson (eds.), pp. 83–89. New York: National Foundation for Birth Defects (Original Article Series) 1970

Porto, S.O., Pildes, R.S., Goodman, H.: Studies on the effect of phototherapy on neonatal hyperbilirubinemia among low birthweight infants. II. Protein binding capacity. J. Pediat. **75**, 1048–1050 (1969)

Potrepka, R.F., Spratt, J.L.: Effect of phenobarbital and 3-methylcholanthrene pretreatment on guinea pig hepatic microsomal bilirubin glucuronyl transferase activity. Biochem. Pharmacol. **20**, 861 –867 (1971)

Potrepka, R.F., Spratt, J.L.: A study on the enzymatic mechanism of guinea pig hepatic microsomal bilirubin glucuronyl transferase. Europ. J. Biochem. **29**, 433 –439 (1972)

Prato, V., Gallo, E., Ricco, G., Mazza, H., Bianco, G., Lehmann, H.: Haemolytic anemia due to hemoglobin Torino. Brit. J. Haemat. **19**, 105 –115 (1970)

Preisig, R., Bucher, H., Stirnemann, H., Tauber, J.: Postoperative choleresis following bile duct obstruction in man. Rev. franç. Ét. clin. biol. **14**, 151 –158 (1969)

Preisig, R., Cooper, H.L., Wheeler, H.O.: The relationship between taurocholate secretion rate and bile production in the unanesthetized dog during cholinergic blockade and during secretin administration. J. clin. Invest. **41**, 1152 –1162 (1962)

Radzialowski, F.M.: Effect of spironolactone and pregnenolone—16-α carbonitrile on bilirubin metabolism and plasma levels in male and female rats. Biochem. Pharmacol. **22**, 1607 –1611 (1973)

Raffin, S.B., Woo, C.H., Roost, K.T., Price, D.C., Schmid, R.: Intestinal absorption of hemoglobin iron—heme cleavage by mucosal heme oxygenase. J. clin. Invest. **54**, 1344 –1352 (1974)

Ramos, A., Silverberg, M., Stern, L.: Pregnanediols and neonatal hyperbilirubinemia. Amer. J. Dis. Child. **111**, 353 –356 (1966)

Rane, A., Lunde, P.K.M., Jalling, B., Yaffe, S.J., Sjoqvist, F.: Plasma protein binding of diphenylhydantoin in normal and hyperbilirubinemic infants. J. Pediat. **78**, 877 –882 (1971)

Raymond, G.D., Galambos, J.T.: Hepatic storage and excretion of bilirubin in man. Amer. J. Gastroent. **55**, 135 –144 (1971)

Reinicke, C., Rogner, G., Frenzel, J., Maak, B., Klinger, W.: The effect of phenylbutazone and phenobarbital on the elimination of amidopyrine, the concentration of bilirubin in blood serum and various blood clotting factors in the newborn. Pharmacol. Clin. **2**, 167 –172 (1970)

Remmer, H., Merker, J.: Drug-induced changes in the liver endoplasmic reticulum: Association with drug metabolizing enzymes. Science **142**, 1657 –1658 (1963)

Remmer, H., Merker, H.J.: Effect of drugs on the formation of smooth endoplasmic reticulum and drug metabolizing enzymes. Ann. N.Y. Acad. Sci. **123**, 79 –97 (1965)

Reyes, H., Levi, A.J., Gatmaitan, Z., Arias, I.M.: Organic anion-binding protein in rat liver: drug induction and its physiologic consequence. Proc. nat. Acad. Sci. (Wash.) **64**, 168 –170 (1969)

Reyes, H., Levi, A.J., Gatmaitan, Z., Arias, I.M.: Studies of Y and Z, two hepatic cytoplasmic organic anion-binding proteins: Effect of drugs, chemicals, hormones, and cholestasis. J. clin. Invest. **50**, 2242 –2252 (1971)

Rich, A.R.: The formation of bile pigment. Physiol. Rev. **5**, 182 –224 (1925)

Roberts, R.J., Plaa, G.L.: Potentiation and inhibition of α-naphthylisothiocyanate-induced hyperbilirubinemia and cholestasis. J. Pharmacol. exp. Ther. **150**, 499 –506 (1965)

Roberts, R.J., Plaa, G.L.: Effect of phenobarbital on the excretion of an exogenous bilirubin load. Biochem. Pharmacol. **16**, 827 –835, (1967)

Roberts, R.J., Plaa, G.L.: Alteration in biliary bilirubin content and non-erythropoietically-derived bilirubin synthesis in rats after alpha-naphthylisothiocyanate administration. J. Pharmacol. exp. Ther. **161**, 382 –388 (1968)

Robertson, D.H.H.: Nitrofurazone-induced hemolytic anemia in a refractory case of trypanosoma rhodesiense sleeping sickness: The hemolytic trait and self-limiting hemolytic anemia. Ann. trop. Med. Parasit. **55**, 49 –64 (1961)

Robinson, M.G., Foadi, M.: Hemolytic anemia with positive Coombs test. Association with isoniazid therapy. J. Amer. med. Ass. **208**, 656 –658 (1969)

Robinson, S.H.: Increased bilirubin formation from nonhemoglobin sources in rats with disorders of the liver. J. Lab. clin. Med. **73**, 668 –676 (1969)

Robinson, S.H.: Production and excretion of bilirubin in Gunn rats treated with phenobarbital. Proc. Soc. exp. Biol. (N.Y.) **138**, 281 –284 (1971)

Robinson, S.H., Koeppel, E.: Preferential hemolysis of immature erythrocytes in experimental iron deficiency anemia: source of erythropoietic bilirubin formation. J. clin. Invest. **50**, 1847 –1853 (1971)

Robinson, S.H., Owen, C.A. Jr., Flock, E.V., Schmid, R.: Bilirubin formation in the liver from non-hemoglobin sources. Blood **26**, 825 – 829 (1965)

Robinson, S.H., Rugstad, H.E., Yannoni, C., Tashijian, A.H., Jr.: Labeled bilirubin production by a clonal strain of rat hepatoma cells. Proc. Soc. exp. Biol. (N.Y.) **136**, 684 – 686 (1971a)

Robinson, S.H., Tsong, M.: Hemolysis of stress reticulocytes: A source of erythropoietic bilirubin formation. J. Clin. Invest. **49**, 1025 – 1035 (1970)

Robinson, S.H., Tsong, M., Brown, B.W., Schmid, R.: The sources of bile pigment in the rat: studies of the "early-labeled" fraction. J. clin. Invest. **45**, 1569 – 1586 (1966)

Robinson, S.H., Yannoni, C., Nagasawa, S.: Bilirubin excretion in rats with normal and impaired bilirubin conjugation. Effect of phenobarbital. J. clin. Invest. **50**, 2606 – 2613 (1971b)

Roerig, D.L., Hasegawa, A.T., Peterson, R.E., Wang, R.I.H.: Effect of chloroquine and phenobarbital on morphine glucuronidation and biliary excretion in the rat. Biochem. Pharmacol. **23**, 1331 – 1339 (1974)

Romagnoli, G., Polidori, G., Foschini, M., Cataldi, L., De Turris, P., Tortorolo, G., Mastrangelo, R.: Agar in the management of hyperbilirubinemin in the premature baby. Arch. Dis. Childh. **50**, 202 – 204 (1975)

Rothwell, J.D., Lacroix, S., Sweeney, G.D.: Evidence against a regulatory role for heme oxygenase in hepatic heme synthesis. Biochim. biophys. Acta (Amst.) **304**, 871 – 874 (1973)

Rubin, F., Lieber, C.S.: The effects of alcohol on the human liver. In: The Liver and its Diseases. Schaffner, F., Sherlock, S., and Leevy, C.M. (eds.), pp. 236 – 244. New York: Intercontinental Med. Book Corp. 1974

Rudman, D., Bixler, T.J., Del Rio, A.E.: Effect of free fatty acids on binding of drugs by bovine serum albumin, by human serum albumin and by rabbit serum. J. Pharmacol. exp. Ther. **176**, 261 – 272 (1971)

Rugstad, H.E., Bratlid, D.: The effect of sulfisoxazole (Gantrisin) and albumin on bilirubin conjugation in cultures of a clonal cell line with liver like functions. Biochem. Pharmacol. **23**, 1432 – 1436 (1974)

Rugstad, H.E., Dybing, E.: Competition between p-aminophenol. p-nitrophenol and bilirubin for glucuronidation in cultures of rat hepatoma cells and homogenates of the same cells Acta pharmacol. (Kbh.) **34**, 65 – 75 (1974)

Sanchez, E., Tephly, T.R.: Activation of hepatic microsomal glucuronyl transferase by bilirubin. Life Sci **13**, 1483 – 1490 (1973)

Sausville, J.W., Sisson, T.R.C., Berger, D.: Blue lamps in phototherapy of hyperbilirubinemia. J. Illum Engin. Soc. **1**, 112 – 118 (1972)

Schacter, B.A.: Induction mechanisms for bile pigment formation. In: Jaundice. Goresky, C.A., and Fisher, M.M. (eds.), pp. 85 – 102. New York: Plenum Press 1975

Schacter, B.A., Mason, J.I.: The effect of phenobarbital, 3-methylcholanthrene, 3,4-benzyprene, and pregnenolone-16α carbonitrile on microsomal heme oxygenase and splenic cytochrome P-450. Arch. Biochem. Biophys. **160**, 274 – 278 (1974)

Schacter, B.A., Nelson, E.B., Marver, H.S., Masters, B.S.S.: Immunochemical evidence for an association of heme oxygenase with the microsomal electron transport system. J. biol. Chem. **247**, 3601 – 3607 (1972)

Schacter, B.A., Waterman, M.R.: Activity of various metalloporphyrin protein complexes with microsomal heme oxygenase. Life Sci. **14**, 47 – 53 (1974)

Scharschmidt, B.F., Waggoner, J.G., Berk, P.D.: Hepatic organic anion uptake in the rat. J. clin. Invest. **56**, 1280 – 1292 (1975)

Schersten, T., Nilsson, S., Cahlin, E., Filipson, M., Brodina-Persson, G.: Relationship between the biliary excretion of bile acids and the excretion of water, lecithin and cholesterol in man. Europ. J. clin. Invest. **1**, 242 – 247 (1971)

Schiff, D., Chan, G., Stern, L.: Fixed drug combinations and the displacement of bilirubin from albumin. Pediatrics **48**, 139 – 141 (1971)

Schmid, R.: Direct-reacting bilirubin, bilirubin glucuronide in serum bile and urine. Science **124**, 76 (1956)

Schmid, R.: The identification of "direct-reacting" bilirubin as bilirubin glucuronide. J. biol. Chem. **229**, 881 – 888 (1957)

Schmid, R.: Discussion of Grodsky, G. Studies in the uptake and intrahepatic transport of ³H-bilirubin. In: Bilirubin Metabolism. I.A.D. Bouchier and B.H. Billing (eds.), p. 171. Oxford: Blackwell Scientific Publications 1967

Schmid, R., Axelrod, J., Hammaker, L., Swarm, R.L.: Congenital jaundice in rats due to a defect in glucuronide formation. J. clin. Invest. **37**, 1123 – 1130 (1958)

Schmid, R., Forbes, A., Rosenthal, I.M., Lester, R.: Lack of effect of cholestyramine resin on hyperbilirubinemia of premature infants. Lancet **1963 II**, 938 – 939

Schmid, R., Hammaker, L.: Metabolism and disposition of ¹⁴C-bilirubin in congenital non-hemolytic jaundice. J. clin. Invest. **42**, 1720 – 1734 (1963)

Schmid, R., Hammaker, L., Axelrod, J.: The enzymatic formation of bilirubin glucuronide. Arch. Biochem. Biophys. **70**, 285 – 288 (1957)

Schmid, R., Marver, H.S., Hammaker, L.: Enhanced formation of rapidly labeled bilirubin by phenobarbital: Hepatic microsomal cytochromes as a possible source. Biochem. biophys. Res. Commun. **24**, 319 – 328 (1966)

Schoenfield, L.J., Bollman, J.L., Hoffman, H.N.: Sulphate and glucuronide conjugates of bilirubin in experimental liver injury. J. clin. Invest. **41**, 133 – 140 (1962)

Schwartz, S., Ikeda, K.: Studies of porphyrin synthesis and interconversion with special reference to certain green porphyrins in animals with experimental hepatic porphyria. In: Ciba Foundation Symposium on porphyrin biosynthesis and metabolism. G.E.W. Wolstenholme and E.C.P. Millar (eds.), p. 209. London: J & A Churchill 1955

Schwarze, R., Kintzel, H.W., Hinkel, G.K.: The influence of orotic acid on the serum bilirubin level of mature newborn. Acta pediat. scand. **60**, 705 – 708 (1971)

Scott, C.L., Myles, A.B., Bacon, P.A.: Autoimmune hemolytic anemia and mefenamic acid therapy. Brit. med. J. **3**, 534 – 535 (1968)

Sereni, F., Perletti, L., Marini, A.: Influence of diethylnicotinamide on the concentration of serum bilirubin of newborn infants. Pediatrics **40**, 446 – 449 (1967)

Serrani, R.E., Corchs, J.L., Rodriguez Garay, E.A.: Sodium effect on bilirubin uptake by the rat intestinal mucosa. Biochim. biophys. Acta (Amst.) **330**, 186 – 191 (1973)

Shani, M., Seligsohn, U., Ben-Ezzer, J.: Effect of phenobarbital on liver functions in patients with Dubin-Johnson syndrome. Gastroenterology **67**, 303 – 308 (1974)

Shotton, D., Carpenter, M., Rinehart, W.B.: Bromsulfalein retention due to administration of gall-bladder dye (Bunamiodyl). New Engl. J. Med. **264**, 550 – 552 (1961)

Silverberg, M., Desforges, J., Gellis, S.: Mechanisms underlying vitamin K induced hyperbilirubinemia in premature infants. Ann. N.Y. Acad. Sci. **111**, 472 – 482 (1963)

Silverman, W.A., Anderson, D.H., Blanc, W.A., Crozier, D.N.: A difference in mortality rate and incidence of kernicterus among premature infants alloted to two prophylactic antibacterial regimens. Pediatrics **18**, 614 – 625 (1956)

Smith, D.S., Fujimoto, J.M.: Alterations produced by novobiocin during biliary excretion of morphine, morphine-3-glucuronide and other compounds. J. Pharmacol. exp. Ther. **188**, 504 – 515 (1974)

Snyder, A.L., Satterlee, W., Robinson, S.H., Schmid, R.: Conjugated plasma bilirubin in jaundice caused by pigment overload. Nature (Lond.) **213**, 93 (1967)

Solomon, H.M.: Competition between drugs and normal substrates for plasma and tissue binding sites. In: Handbook of Experimental Pharmacology, Vol. 28, part 1, pp. 234 – 239. Berlin – Heidelberg – New York: Springer 1971

Solymoss, B., Zsigmond, G.: Effect of various steroids on the hepatic glucuronidation and biliary excretion of bilirubin. Canad. J. Physiol. Pharmacol. **51**, 319 – 323 (1973)

Spector, A.A., Santos, E.C., Ashbrook, J.D., Fletcher, J.E.: Influence of free fatty acid concentration on drug binding to plasma albumin. Ann. N.Y. Acad. Sci. **226**, 247 – 258 (1973)

Sperber, I.: Secretion of organic anions in the formation of urine and bile. Pharmacol. Rev. **11**, 109 – 134 (1959)

Spiegel, E.L., Schubert, W., Perrin, E., Schiff, L.: Benign recurrent intrahepatic cholestasis with response to cholestyramine. Amer. J. Med. **39**, 682 – 688 (1965)

Starinsky, R., Shafrir, E.: Displacement of albumin-bound bilirubin by free fatty acids. Implications for neonatal hyperbilirubinemia. Clin. chim. Acta **29**, 311 – 318 (1970)

Stern, L.: Drugs, the newborn infant, and the binding of bilirubin to albumin. Pediatrics **49**, 916–918 (1972)

Stiehl, A., Thaler, M.M., Admirand, W.H.: The effects of phenobarbital on bile salts and bilirubin in patients with intrahepatic and extrahepatic cholestasis. New Engl. J. Med. **286**, 858–866 (1972)

Stiehl, A., Thaler, M.M., Admirand, W.H.: Effects of phenobarbital on bile salt metabolism in cholestasis due to intrahepatic bile duct hypoplasia. Pediatrics **51**, 992–997 (1973)

Strebel, L., Odell, G.B.: UDP glucuronyl transferase in rat liver. Genetic variation and maturation. Pediat. Res. **3**, 351–352 (1969)

Strebel, L., Odell, G.B.: Bilirubin uridine diphosphoglucuronyl transferase in rat liver microsomes: genetic variation and maturation. Pediat. Res. **5**, 548–559 (1971)

Stumpf, W.E., Lester, R.: Secretion and absorption of mesobilirubinogen-^{3}H studied by autoradiography. Lab. Invest. **15**, 1156–1162 (1966)

Sutherland, J.M., Keller, H.H.: Novobiocin and neonatal hyperbilirubinemia. Amer. J. Dis. Child. **101**, 447–453 (1961)

Swanson, M.A., Chanmougan, D., Schwartz, R.S.: Immunohemolytic anemia due to antipenicillin antibodies: report of a case. New Engl. J. Med. **274**, 178–181 (1966)

Takemori, A.E.: Enzymic studies on morphine glucuronide synthesis in acutely and chronically morphinized rats. J. Pharmacol. exp. Ther. **130**, 370–374 (1960)

Talafant, E.: Properties and composition of the bile pigment giving a direct diazo reaction. Nature (Lond.) **178**, 312 (1956)

Tarchanoff, J.F.: Über die Bildung von Gallenpigment aus Bluifarbstoff im Thierkoerper. Arch. ges. Physiol. **9**, 53 (1874)

Tenhunen, R.: Studies on bilirubin and its metabolism. Ann. Med. exp. Fenn. **43**, Suppl. 6, 1–45 (1965)

Tenhunen, R.: The enzymatic degradation of heme. Semin. Hematol. **9**, 19–29 (1972)

Tenhunen, R., Marver, H., Pimstone, N.R., Trager, W.F., Cooper, D.Y., Schmid, R.: Enzymatic degradation of heme. Oxygenative cleavage requiring cytochrome P-450. Biochemistry **11**, 1716–1720 (1972)

Tenhunen, R., Marver, H.S., Schmid, R.: The enzymatic conversion of heme to bilirubin by microsomal heme oxygenase. Proc. nat. Acad. Sci. (Wash.) **61**, 748–755 (1968)

Tenhunen, R., Marver, H.S., Schmid, R.: Microsomal heme oxygenase: Characterization of the enzyme. J. biol. Chem. **244**, 6388–6394 (1969)

Tenhunen, R., Marver, H.S., Schmid, R.: The enzymatic catabolism of hemoglobin: stimulation of microsomal heme oxygenase by hemin. J. Lab. clin. Med. **75**, 410–421 (1970a)

Tenhunen, R., Ross, M., Marver, H.S., Schmid, R.: Reduced nicotinamide-adenine dinucleotide phosphate dependent biliverdin reductase: Partial purification and characterization. Biochemistry **9**, 298–303 (1970b)

Tephly, T.R., Hasegawa, E., Baron, J.: Effect of drugs on heme synthesis in the liver. Metabolism **20**, 200–214 (1971)

Territo, M.C., Peters, R.W., Tanaka, K.P.: Autoimmune hemolytic anemia due to levodopa therapy. J. Amer. med. Ass. **226**, 1347–1348 (1973)

Thaler, M.M.: Perinatal bilirubin metabolism. Advanc. Pediat. **19**, 215–235 (1972)

Thaler, M.M., Dawber, N.H., Krasner, J., Mosovich, L., Yaffe, S.: Effects of phototherapy on bilirubin (B) metabolism and sulfobromphthalein (BSP) excretion in unconjugated hyperbilirubinemia. Pediat. Res. **7**, 34 (1973) (Abstract)

Thiessen, H., Jacobsen, J., Brodersen, R.: Displacement of albumin bound-bilirubin by fatty acids. Acta paediat. scand. **61**, 285–288 (1972)

Thompson, R.P.H., Stathers, G.M., Pilcher, C.W.T., McLean, A.E.M., Robinson, J., Williams, R.: Treatment of unconjugated jaundice with dicophane. Lancet **1969 II**, 4–6

Tomlinson, G.A., Yaffe, S.J.: The formation of bilirubin and p-nitrophenyl glucuronides by rabbit liver. Biochem. J. **99**, 507–512 (1966)

Topham, J.C., Broad, R.D.: Persistent reduction of serum bilirubin levels after treatment of Gunn rats with some acidic compounds. Biochem. Pharmacol. **20**, 718–720 (1971)

Traiger, G.J., Derepentigny, L., Plaa, G.L.: Effect of inhibitors of protein and ribonucleic acid synthesis on the alteration in biliary bilirubin excretion and non-erythropoietically derived bilirubin synthesis in rats after α-naphthylisothiocyanate administration. Biochem. Pharmacol. **23**, 2845–2856 (1974)

Troxler, R.F., Dawber, N.H., Lester, R.: Synthesis of urobilinogen by broken cell preparation of intestinal bacteria. Gastroenterology **54**, 568–574 (1968)

Tuilié, M., Lardinois, R.: The binding of unconjugated bilirubin by human sera and purified albumins. Biol. Neonate **21**, 447–462 (1972)

Ulstrom, R.A., Eisenklam, E.: The enterohepatic shunting of bilirubin in the newborn infant. J. Pediat. **65**, 27–37 (1964)

Upson, D.W., Gronwall, R.R., Cornelius, C.E.: Maximal hepatic excretion of bilirubin in sheep. Proc. Soc. exp. Biol. (N.Y.) **134**, 9–12 (1970)

Vainio, H.: Enhancement of microsomal drug oxidation and glucuronidation in rat liver by an environmental chemical, polychlorinated biphenyl. Chem. Biol. Interact. **9**, 379–387 (1974a)

Vainio, H.: Activation and inactivation of membrane-bound UDP-glucuronosyltransferase by organic solvents in vitro. Acta pharmacol. (Kbh.) **34**, 152–156 (1974b)

Vainio, H., Hietanen, E.: Drug metabolism in Gunn rats: Inability to increase bilirubin glucuronidation by phenobarbital treatment. Biochem. Pharmacol. **23**, 3405–3512 (1974)

Vaisman, S.L., Lee, K.S., Gartner, L.M.: Various bilirubin conjugates in pregnant and non-pregnant rats with and without phenobarbital treatment. Pediat. Res. **10**, 111–113 (1976)

Vanleusden, H.A.I.M., Bakkeren, J.A.J.M., Zilliken, F., Stolte, L.A.M.: p-Nitrophenyl-glucuronide formation by homozygous adult Gunn rats. Biochem. biophys. Res. Commun. **7**, 67–69 (1962)

Vanroy, F.P., Heirwegh, K.P.M.: Determination of bilirubin glucuronide and assay of glucuronyltransferase with bilirubin as acceptor. Biochem. J. **107**, 507–518 (1968)

Verschure, J.C.M., Mijnlieff, P.F.: The dominating macromolecular complex of human gallbladder bile. Clin. chim. Acta. **1**, 154–166 (1956)

Vessey, D.A., Goldenberg, J., Zakim, D.: Differentiation of homologous forms of hepatic microsomal UDP-glucuronyl transferase. II. Characterization of the bilirubin conjugating form. Biochim. biophys. Acta (Amst.) **309**, 75–82 (1973a)

Vessey, D.A., Goldenberg, J., Zakim, D.: Kinetic properties of microsomal UDP-glucuronyltransferase. Evidence for cooperative kinetics and activation by UDP-N-acetylglucosamine. Biochim. biophys. Acta (Amst.) **309**, 58–66 (1973b)

Vessey, D.A., Zakim, D.: Regulation of microsomal enzymes by phospholipids II. Activation of hepatic uridine diphosphate-glucuronyltransferase. J. biol. Chem. **246**, 4649–4656 (1971)

Virchow, R.: Die pathologischen Pigmente. Arch. path. Anat. Physiol. klin. Med. **1**, 379 (1847)

Visintine, R.E., Michaels, G.D., Fukanama, G., Conklin, J., Kinsell, L.W.: Xanthomatous biliary cirrhosis treated with cholestyramine, a bile acid absorbing resin. Lancet **1961 II**, 341–343

Waitman, A.M., Dyck, W.P., Janowitz, H.D.: Effect of secretion and acetazolamide on the volume and electrolyte composition of hepatic bile in man. Gastroenterology **56**, 286–294 (1969)

Waller, H.D.: Glutathione reductase deficiency. In: Hereditary Disorders of Erythrocyte Metabolism. Beutler, E. (ed.), pp. 185–208. New York: Grune & Stratton 1968

Waltman, R., Bonura, F., Nigrin, G., Pipat, C.: Ethanol in prevention of hyperbilirubinemia in the newborn. Lancet **1969 II**, 1265–1267

Warner, M., Neims, A.H.: Studies on Z-Fraction. I. Isolation and partial characterization of low molecular weight ligand—binding protein from rat hepatic cytosol. Canad. J. Physiol. Pharmacol. **53**, 493–500 (1975)

Waters, W.J., Dunham, R., Bowen, W.R.: Inhibition of bilirubin conjugation in vitro. Proc. Soc. exp. Biol. (N.Y.) **99**, 175–177 (1958)

Watson, C.J.: Recent studies of the urobilin problem. J. clin. Path. **16**, 1–11 (1963)

Watson, C.J., Campbell, M., Lowry, P.T.: Preferential reduction of conjugated bilirubin to urobilinogen by normal fecal flora. Proc. Soc. exp. Biol. (N.Y.) **98**, 707–711 (1958)

Weber, A.P., Schalm, L., Witmans, J.: Bilirubin monoglucuronide (pigment I): A complex. Acta med. scand. **173**, 19–24 (1963)

Weinbren, K., Billing, B.H.: Hepatic clearance of bilirubin as an index of cellular function in the regenerating rat liver. Brit. J. exp. Path. **37**, 199–204 (1956)

Wennberg, R.P., Rasmussen, L.F.: Effects of gentamicin on albumin binding of bilirubin. J. Pediat. **86,** 611 – 613 (1975)

Wheeler, H.O.: Principles of biliary secretion. In: Jaundice. Goresky, C.A. and Fisher, M.M. (eds.), pp. 195 – 215. New York: Plenum Press 1975

Wheeler, H.O., Cranston, W.I., Meltzer, J.I.: Hepatic uptake and biliary excretion of indocyanine green in the dog. Proc. Soc. exp. Biol. (N.Y.) **99,** 11 – 14 (1958)

Whelton, M.J., Krustev, L.P., Billing, B.H.: Reduction in serum bilirubin by phenobarbital in adult unconjugated hyperbilirubinemia. Amer. J. Med. **45,** 160 – 164 (1968)

Whipple, G.H., Hooper, C.W.: Bile pigment output influenced by hemoglobin injections, anemia and blood regeneration. Amer. J. Physiol. **43.** 258 – 274 (1917)

White, J.M., Brain, M.C., Lorkin, P.A., Lehmann, H., Smith, M.: Mild "unstable haemoglobin haemolytic anaemia" caused by haemoglobin Shepherds' Bush. Nature (Lond.) **225,** 939 – 941 (1970)

White, P., Silvers, A.A., Rosher, M.L., Shafer, B.C., Williams, W.J.: Hepatic production of bilirubin and carbon monoxide in vitro. J. clin. Invest. **45,** 1085 – 1086 (1966) (Abstract)

Williams, R., Maxwell, J.D., Hunter, J.: Some clinical implications of hepatic enzyme induction, pp. 44 – 51. Proc. Europ. Soc. for the Study of Drug Toxicity, Vol. XIII. Amsterdam: Excerpta Medica 1972

Wilson, J.T.: Developmental pharmacology: A review of its application to clinical and basic science. Ann. Rev. Pharmacol. **12,** 423 – 450 (1972)

Windorfer, A., Kunzer, W., Bolze, H., Ascher, K., Wilcken, F., Hoehne, K.: Studies on the effect of orally administered agar on the serum bilirubin level of premature infants and mature newborns. Acta paediat. scand. **64,** 699 – 702 (1975)

Winsnes, A.: Studies on the activation in vitro of glucuronyltransferase. Biochim. biophys. Acta (Amst.) **191,** 279 – 291 (1969)

Winsnes, A.: Age and sex dependent variability of the activation characteristics of UDP-glucuronyltransferase in vitro. Biochem. Pharmacol. **20,** 1249 – 1258 (1971 a)

Winsnes, A.: Variable effect of phenobarbital treatment of mice on hepatic UDP-glucuronyltransferase activity when judged by slightly different enzyme-assay techniques. Biochem. Pharmacol. **20,** 1853 – 1857 (1971 b)

Winsnes, A., Dutton, G.J.: Comparison between o-aminophenol glucuronidation in liver slices and homogenates from control and phenobarbital treated Wistar and Gunn rats. Biochem. Pharmacol. **22,** 1765 – 1771 (1973)

Wong, K.P.: Formation of bilirubin glucoside. Biochem. J. **125,** 929 – 934, (1971)

Wong, K.P.: Bilirubin glucosyl and glucuronyltransferase. A comparative study and the effect of drugs. Biochem. Pharmacol. **21,** 1485 – 1491 (1972)

Woolley, P.V., Hunter, M.J.: Binding and circular dichroism data on bilirubin-albumin in the presence of oleate and salicylate. Arch. Biochem. Biophys. **140,** 197 – 209 (1970)

Worlledge, S.: Immune drug-induced hemolytic anemias. Semin. Hematol. **10,** 327 – 344, (1973)

Wosilait, W.D.: A theoretical analysis of the binding of bilirubin by human serum albumin: The contribution of the two binding sites. Life Sci. **14,** 2189 – 2198 (1974)

Wranne, L.: Congenital nonhaemolytic jaundice. Acta paediat. scand. **56,** 552 – 556 (1967)

Yaffe, S.J., Catz, C.S., Stern, L., Levy, G.: The use of phenobarbital in neonatal jaundice. In: Bilirubin Metabolism in the Newborn. D. Bergsma, D.Y.Y. Hsia, and C. Jackson (eds.), pp. 37 – 45. New York: National Foundation for Birth Defects, Original Article Series **VI** 1970

Yaffe, S.J., Levy, G., Matsuzawa, T., Baliah, T.: Enhancement of glucuronide-conjugating capacity in a hyperbilirubinemic infant due to apparent enzyme induction by phenobarbital. New Engl. J. Med. **275,** 1461 – 1466 (1966)

Yamamoto, T., Skanderbeg, J., Zipursky, A., Israels, L.G.: The early appearing bilirubin: Evidence for two components. J. clin. Invest. **44,** 31 – 41 (1965)

Yeary, R.A., Davies, D.R.: Protein binding of bilirubin: Comparison of in vitro and in vivo measurements of bilirubin displacement by drugs. Toxicol. appl. Pharmacol. **28,** 269 – 283 (1974)

Yoshida, T., Takahashi, S., Kikuchi, G.: Partial purification and reconstitution of the heme oxygenase system from pig spleen microsomes. J. Biochem. (Tokyo) **75,** 1187 – 1191 (1974)

Zail, S.S., Charlton, R.W., Bothwell, T.H.: The hemolytic effect of certain drugs in Bantu subjects with a deficiency of glucose-6-phosphate dehydrogenase. S. Afr. J. med. Sci. **27,** 95 – 99 (1962)

Zakim, D., Goldenberg, J., Vessey, D.A.: Regulation of microsomal enzymes by phospholipids. VI. Abnormal enzyme lipid interactions in liver microsomes from Gunn Rats. Biochim. biophys. Acta (Amst.) **297,** 497 – 502 (1973)

Zakim, D., Vessey, D.A.: Techniques for the characterization of UDP-glucuronyltransferase, glucose-6-phosphatase and other tightly bound microsomal enzymes. In: Methods of Biochemical Analysis, Vol. 21. Glick, D. (ed.). New York: Interscience 1973, pp. 1 – 37

Zatepka, S., Grossman, M.I.: The effect of gastrin and histamine on secretion of bile. Gastroenterology **50,** 500 – 505 (1966)

Zeidenberg, P., Orrenius, S., Ernster, L.: Increase in levels of glucuronylating enzymes and associated rise in activities of mitochondrial oxidative enzymes upon phenobarbital administration in the rat. J. Cell Biol. **32,** 528 – 531 (1967)

Zelson, C., Rubio, E., Wasserman, E.: Neonatal narcotic addiction: 10 year observation. Pediatrics **48,** 178 – 189 (1971)

Zinkam, W.H.: Peripheral blood and bilirubin values in normal full-term primaquine-sensitive Negro infants: Effect of Vitamin K. Pediatrics **31,** 983 – 995 (1963)

Zinkham. W.H., Childs, B.: A defect of glutathione metabolism in erythrocytes from patients with a naphthalene-induced hemolytic anemia. Pediatrics **22,** 461 – 471 (1958)

CHAPTER 11

Toxic Effects of Lead, with Particular Reference to Porphyrin and Heme Metabolism[1]

Shigeru Sassa[2]

Lead has been shown to interfere with the biosynthesis of heme in a number of in vitro systems and in experimental animals as well as in human beings. Several steps of the heme biosynthetic chain are subject to the toxic effects of lead. ALA-dehydratase and ferrochelatase, in particular, are two enzymes which are strongly inhibited by lead, leading to decreased heme synthesis.

A. Biosynthesis of Heme

The major steps of heme biosynthesis have been clarified by a number of studies in photosynthetic bacteria, avian, and mammalian erythrocytes and liver. Enzymes which catalyze the initial and the two terminal reactions are present in the mitochondria, but other enzymes are present in the cytoplasm (MAUZERALL, 1964). Studies on heme biosynthesis in bacteria (BURNHAM and LASCELLES, 1963), avian erythrocytes (SHEMIN et al., 1948; DRESEL and FALK, 1956a, b; GIBSON et al., 1958), rabbit reticulocytes (KARIBIAN and LONDON, 1965), or avian (GRANICK, 1966) and mammalian liver cells (MARVER et al., 1966a, b; NARISAWA and KIKUCHI, 1965), all show a striking resemblance in the metabolic reactions of heme biosynthesis, i.e., the enzymes that convert ALA to porphyrins are usually present at non-limiting activities and the enzyme that limits the rate of the porphyrin-heme pathway appears to be the first one in the biosynthetic chain, ALA-synthetase, which forms ALA from glycine and succinyl CoA (GRANICK, 1966).

Since a more detailed discussion of heme biosynthesis is given in the chapter by TAIT, we shall consider here only the enzymes which are most affected by lead. Two major steps in the heme biosynthetic pathway that are affected by lead are the conversion of ALA to PBG and the insertion of iron into protoporphyrin IX.

I. Conversion of ALA to Porphobilinogen (PBG)

ALA formed in the mitochondria is subsequently transferred into the cytoplasm where 2 mol of ALA are condensed to form a monopyrrole, porphobilinogen (PBG). This reaction is catalyzed by ALA-dehydratase. ALA-dehydratase has been purified from a number of sources including photosynthetic bacteria (NANDI et al., 1968), mammalian erythrocytes (WEISSBERG and VOYTEK, 1974), liver (GIBSON et al., 1955; WILSON

---

[1] Supported by a USPHS grant ES01055 and an ACS grant BC 180.
[2] Recipient of a Career Scientist Award (I-768) of the Health Research Council of the City of New York.

et al., 1972) and human erythrocytes (CALISSANO et al., 1966). All the enzyme preparations require sulfhydryl groups such as reduced glutathione, cysteine, β-mercaptoethanol or dithiothreitol for maximal activity. ALA-D from beef liver has been reported to contain 56 sulfhydryl groups per mole of enzyme (WILSON et al., 1972). The enzyme activity is markedly inhibited by lead, inorganic mercury salts, pCMB, and N-ethylmaleimide (SHEMIN, 1975) with the exception of the mouse enzyme which is stimulated with mercury or pCMB (COLEMAN, 1966). The enzyme is also inhibited by a number of metal chelating agents including EDTA (GIBSON et al., 1955; GRANICK and MAUZERALL, 1958; SHETTY and MILLER, 1969; KOMAI and NEILANDS, 1969; GURBA et al., 1972) suggesting that some divalent heavy metals may be involved in its active site. In fact recent studies have shown that bovine liver ALA-dehydratase contains approximately one mole of Zn per 1 unit of enzyme of mol wt. 275,000 (GURBA et al., 1972). It has also been reported that the activity of ALA-dehydratase in the erythrocytes and the liver is decreased in animals fed with a low Zn diet (FINELLI et al., 1974). ALA-dehydratase purified from *Rhodopseudomonas spheroides*, on the other hand, requires K^+, Li^+, Rb^+, NH_4^+, or Mg^{++} for activation of the enzyme. These ions, however, have little effect on the mammalian enzyme.

The molecular weight is in the range of 240,000 to 280,000 for the enzyme preparation from all sources. It appears that the bovine liver enzyme consists of six subunits of identical size (mol. wt. of each subunit = 42,250). More recent evidence on the bacterial enzyme, however, favors eight subunits of identical size which are arranged in dihedral (D_4) symmetry (SHEMIN, 1975).

Human erythrocyte ALA-dehydratase has a rather low K_m of 8×10^{-5} M, (CALISSANO et al., 1966); however, the enzyme preparations from other sources have K_m's in the range of $1.4 \sim 7 \times 10^{-4}$ M (GIBSON et al., 1955; CALISSANO et al., 1966; TOMIO et al., 1968; DOYLE and SCHIMKE, 1969; WILSON et al., 1972; SHEMIN, 1975).

The determination of PBG can be made by the reaction of the pyrrole with Ehrlich reagent. It should be pointed out that there are two kinds of Ehrlich reagents which yield different extinction coefficients. The regular Ehrlich reagent is the usual 2% (wt/vol) p-dimethylaminobenzaldehyde (DMBA) in 6 N HCl. The reaction of PBG with equal volumes of the regular Ehrlich reagent gives a molar extinction coefficient of 3.6×10^4 at 555 nm (MAUZERALL and GRANICK, 1956).

The modified Ehrlich reagent contains 4 N perchloric acid. The color salt developed from PBG with this reagent has a molar extinction coefficient of 6.1×10^4 at 555 nm (MAUZERALL and GRANICK, 1956). The advantage of the modified Ehrlich reagent is that the color salt with PBG is more stable and more intense.

II. Conversion of PBG to Uroporphyrinogen III

This reaction involves two cytosol enzymes, uroporphyrinogen-I synthetase (URO-I S) and uroporphyrinogen-III cosynthetase (URO-III CoS). URO-III CoS which can be inactivated completely at 60°C for 15 min appears to be present in excess, and the rate of uroporphyrinogen-III formation is determined by URO-I S activity which is heat-stable (STRAND et al., 1972 b; SASSA et al., 1974). This enzyme has an optimum pH at around 7.8 (JORDAN and SHEMIN 1971, 1973). Sulfhydryl reagents have been reported to inhibit the activity of the enzyme. (LLAMBIAS and DEL C. BATTLE, 1971; JORDAN and SHEMIN, 1973). Lead has been shown to inhibit the activity of URO-I S but rather at high concentrations (PIPER and TEPHLY, 1974).

III. Formation of Protoporhyrin IX

Protoporphyrinogen-IX is formed from coproporphyrinogen-III by the action of coproporphyrinogen (COPRO) decarboxylase. COPRO-decarboxylase is not only specific for the type III isomer, but oxidatively decarboxylates two specific propionic acid side chains of the four to form vinyl groups; thus yielding only one type of protoporphyrin isomer, i.e., protoporphyrin-IX. Unlike URO-decarboxylase, COPRO-decarboxylase is present in the mitochondria (SANO and GRANICK, 1961).

The reaction that is catalyzed by COPRO-decarboxylase involves the decarboxylation and oxidation of the propionate groups at positions 2 and 4 to yield two vinyl groups; by the subsequent removal of six hydrogen atoms, protoporphyrin-IX is formed. The reaction requires molecular oxygen. No cofactor for this enzyme has been described.

The only reagents found to inhibit COPRO-decarboxylase are o-phenanthroline and α, α'-dipyridyl (SANO and GRANICK, 1961). Since other metal chelators, e.g., 8-hydroxyquinoline-5-sulfonic acid, sodium diethyldithiocarbamate, EDTA, do not inhibit the enzyme activity, ferrous iron may be involved in the reaction. Sulfhydryl reagents, e.g., iodoacetamide, p-chloromercuribenzoate (p-CMB), Na_2AsO_3 are without appreciable effect.

Small amounts of protoporphyrin are found in many tissues, e.g., in erythrocytes, liver, and feces. Protoporphyrin is also found in bacteria, yeasts, and plant cells. Rat Harderian gland is known to contain large amounts of protoporphyrin IX (GRAFFLIN, 1942). In humans, it is known that erythrocyte protoporphyrin is decreased in folic acid and vitamin B_{12} deficiency anemia (SCHWARTZ, 1953; WINTROBE, 1949–1950); red cell protoporphyrin is increased in iron deficiency anemia, hemolytic anemia and particularly increased in chronic lead poisoning and erythropoietic protoporphyria (CHISOLM et al., 1975a; GRANICK et al., 1972). Protoporphyrin as well as other porphyrins emit an intense reddish fluorescence, when excited by the light in the long wavelength range and thus small amounts can be readily recognized by fluorescence determination.

IV. Formation of Heme

The final reaction to form heme from protoporphyrin-IX and ferrous iron is catalyzed by the mitochondrial enzyme, ferrochelatase (GOUDY et al., 1967; JONES, 1968; OYAMA et al., 1961; LABBE and HUBBARD, 1960; PORRA and JONES, 1963a, b).

The determination of this enzyme activity has presented a number of problems. The major problem is that iron can be inserted into protoporphyrin-IX in the absence of the enzyme to a certain extent under appropriate conditions—usually including anaerobic incubations in the presence of strong acid (FALK, 1964) or in hot pyridine (BAUM, 1965) or in the presence of sodium lauryl sulfate (TOKUNAGA and SANO, 1972). However, under physiological pH and temperature, particularly in the presence of air, the nonenzymatic insertion of iron into protoporphyrin IX is far less than that produced by the enzymic reaction. The enzyme has rather low specificity for the metal substrate, since cobalt or other metal ions (PORRA and JONES, 1963a, b; TEPHLY et al., 1971) can be incorporated instead of iron, and mesoporphyrin (PORRA and JONES, 1963a, b) is usually a better substrate than protoporphyrin presumably because of its greater water solubility.

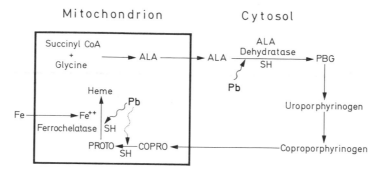

Fig. 1 Effect of lead on the biosynthesis of heme

Usually the enzyme activity is determined by one of the three different methods. One is based on the rate of disappearance of the substrate, protoporphyrin-IX; this method is least sensitive and probably has the greatest error when the enzyme activity is low. The second is based on the determination of the product, heme, by the pyridine hemochromogen method; though this method is more accurate than the first, it still lacks sensitivity. The third method is the determination of radioiron incorporation into heme; this method is probably the most sensitive among the three, but is time consuming. In all assays, iron has to be present in ferrous form, therefore almost all the assays are made under anaerobic conditions and include reducing agents, such as reduced glutathione, cysteine or ascorbate. The enzyme assay is often carried out by using cobaltous ion and mesoporphyrin as the substrates in order to increase its sensitivity, however, the relevance of such activities obtained in vitro to in vivo levels of the enzyme is not clear.

B. Effect of Lead on the Heme Biosynthetic Pathway

It is well known that in human and experimental lead poisoning, there is a highly increased excretion of ALA and coproporphyrin in urine and a marked accumulation of protoporphyrin-IX in erythrocytes (HARRIS and KELLERMEYER, 1970). PBG and uroporphyrin may also appear in the urine and in the bone marrow in severe lead intoxication. The accumulations of porphyrins and their precursors are largely due to the inhibition by lead of the two enzymes, ALA-dehydratase and ferrochelatase (SASSA et al., 1975). Compartmentalization of the enzymes in heme biosynthesis within the cell and the effect of lead on them are shown in Figure 1.

I. Inhibition of ALA-Dehydratase (ALA-D) Activity

Lead inhibits most of the enzymes which carry a single functional SH. Usually mercury or cadmium have a higher affinity than lead toward monovalent sulfhydryl groups in proteins; however, the inhibition of ALA-dehydratase in erythrocytes by

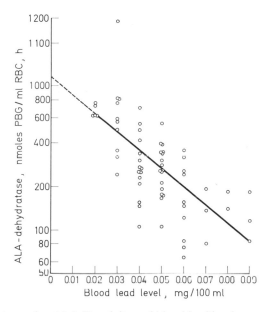

Fig. 2 Correlation between log ALA-D activity and blood lead level

low concentrations of lead is highly remarkable (DeBruin et al., 1967; Hernberg and Nikkanen, 1970; Haeger-Aronsen et al., 1971; Granick et al., 1973), whereas cadmium (Roels et al., 1975a) or mercury (Wada et al., 1969) has considerably less effect. This is probably related to the preferential binding of lead to the red blood cells. The inhibition of ALA-D in the red blood cells by lead is generally recognized as the most sensitive index of the individual's exposure to this environmental chemical. A significant decrease in the enzyme's activity in erythrocytes occurs even at blood lead levels in the so-called upper "normal" ranges (20–40 µg/100 ml blood) (Millar et al., 1970; Granick et al., 1973) (Fig. 2). Hernberg and Nikkanen (1970) described the significant reduction of ALA-D activity in the red cells in 26 healthy medical students who had never been exposed to lead occupationally. Although the effect of lead on the overall health of the human population is not clear, this finding raises a question as to the degree to which the normal population is affected by environmental lead. Inhibition of ALA-D activity occurs not only in the erythrocytes, but also in the brain, liver, kidney, and bone marrow of experimentally lead-poisoned rats (Gibson and Goldberg, 1970).

The enzyme activity is markedly inhibited in vitro by lead, inorganic mercury salts, p-CMB, and N-ethylmaleimide (Gibson et al., 1955). Inhibition of the enzyme activity caused by lead or sulfhydryl reagents can be overcome by the addition in vitro of sulfhydryl containing compounds such as reduced glutathione, cysteine or dithiothreitol. In vivo administration of GSH to occupationally lead poisoned workers also increased lead-inhibited erythrocyte ALA-D activity toward normal levels (Nakao et al., 1968). Lead inhibition of erythrocyte Na^+/K^+ ATPase is also reversed by cysteine, while lead-inhibition of membrane acetylcholine esterase is not altered (Galzigna et al., 1969; Tice, 1969; Rosenthal et al., 1969).

Zinc appears to play an important role in ALA-D activity. The purified enzyme preparation from bovine liver has been shown to contain Zn in a stoichiometric relation of 1 mole of Zn per mole of the enzyme (Gurba et al., 1972). Meredith et al. (1974) have reported that in vitro addition of zinc (1.8×10^{-4} M) to rat erythrocytes activated the ALA-D activity by 240%. ALA-D activity in the red cells from rats fed with low Zn diet was found to be decreased by 60% (Finelli et al., 1974). Moreover, in vitro addition of Zn to isolated erythrocytes from rats previously exposed to lead reactivated the enzyme activity to control levels (Finelli et al., 1975). It has been also reported that erythrocyte ALA-D activity was increased in a lead poisoned man receiving orally $30 - 40$ mg zinc per day for a 4-week period (Abdulla and Haeger-Aronsen, 1971). It is therefore tempting to assume that Zn is involved at the active site, probably in close relation to the SH group and that lead and zinc may compete for the same binding site.

The stability constant of the lead-enzyme complex may be relatively low, since the inhibition of ALA-D activity by lead in human erythrocytes can be overcome completely by the addition of agents containing SH groups, or partially, by the addition of EDTA, or by dilution with phosphate buffer (Sassa et al., 1975). Incubation of lead-poisoned hemolysates at higher temperatures (e.g. 55° C) in the presence of the substrate reactivates the enzyme activity to the normal level suggesting that lead-enzyme complex may be thermally dissociable (Tomokuni and Kawanishi, 1975). The affinity constant of Zn for the enzyme may be low, since a high concentration of Zn is required to reactivate lead-poisoned ALA-D activity (Finelli et al., 1975).

1. Assay of ALA-D Activity

ALA-D activity is determined by the quantitation of PBG by its reaction with Ehrlich reagent after incubation of the enzyme with ALA. The activity of ALA-D in red cells depends on the availability of the sulfhydryl groups of the enzyme (Sassa et al., 1975). Therefore, in order to screen for lead poisoning, the ALA-D assay must be performed in the absence of added SH, without affecting the endogenous level of sulfhydryl groups. For example, fresh blood or blood stored at 4° C for two days, or in liquid nitrogen for an indefinite period is usually satisfactory for analysis, but frozen blood samples stored under air lose enzyme activity within hours apparently because of the oxidation of SH groups of the enzyme. Any substance which might chelate lead, such as EDTA or citrate should be avoided. The use of a low volume of phosphate buffer (50 mM, pH 6.3) (e.g. hemolysate : buffer = 1 : 1, vol/vol) is satisfactory but a greater dilution with the same buffer leads to a loss of the good inverse correlation between blood lead and ALA-D activity (Sassa et al., 1975), presumably due to the formation of insoluble lead phosphate. The solubility of lead phosphate at room temperature is approximately 1/20th of that of lead sulfide. When $NaHCO_3$—CO_2 buffer is used, an inverse correlation between the enzyme activity and blood lead is observed (Bonsignore et al., 1965; Sassa et al., 1975; Weissberg et al., 1971). However, it is difficult to maintain an optimum pH of $6.3 - 6.8$ for the enzyme reaction at the recommended concentration of the bicarbonate (Bonsignore et al., 1965) and without gassing. SH groups of the enzyme appear to be protected from oxidation in the presence of substrate, since the enzyme activity is stable for at least 2 h at 37° C in the presence of ALA. The pH optimum

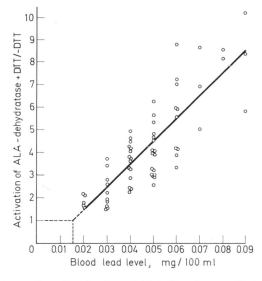

Fig. 3 Correlation between the ratio of activated ALA-D and non-activated ALA-D activity and blood lead level.
+ DTT: Activated ALA-D activity by the addition of dithiothreitol
− DTT: Non-activated ALA-D activity

for human erythrocyte ALA-D is 6.3 (GRANICK et al., 1973; TOMOKUMI, 1974) in phosphate buffer, 6.4 in 2-(N-morpholino)ethane sulfonic acid buffer (COLLIER, 1971), and 6.7 in citrate phosphate buffer (BURCH and SEGEL, 1971). Heme has been claimed to inhibit ALA-D activity (CALISSANO, et al., 1966; COLEMAN, 1966), but only at high concentrations. V_{max} for the human erythrocyte ALA-D has a wide distribution with a mean value of 2.5 μmol PBG formed (ml RBC), h, 37°C (SASSA et al., 1973a).

2. Inhibition Kinetics

Kinetic studies show that lead does not change the K_m of ALA-D appreciably, indicating that affinity of the enzyme for the substrate ALA is not affected (GRANICK et al., 1973). On the other hand, the V_{max} is greatly reduced by lead. Therefore lead inhibition of ALA-D activity is primarily of the non-competitive type (SASSA et al., 1975; WILSON et al., 1972).

Assuming simple Michaelis-Menten kinetics of the non-competitive inhibition type, the inhibitor constant K_i for ALA-D is derived from the following equation:

$$V_0/V_i = 1 + \frac{1}{K_i} \, [I]$$

V_0 = Maximum activity of the enzyme
V_i = Velocity in the presence of lead
$[I]$ = Lead concentration

A plot of the ratio of activated/non-activated ALA-D on the ordinate vs. blood lead concentration in the abscissa is shown in Figure 3. The apparent K_i for lead can be determined from the figure, since 1/slope of the regression line equals to $K_i = 0.5\,\mu M$ or 0.01 mg Pb/100 ml blood.

3. Genetic Factors Which Affect ALA-D Levels

Levels of ALA-D are controlled not only by chemicals such as lead but also by genetic factors. The activity of ALA-D in mouse tissue has been shown to be under the genetic control of two alleles at the levulinate locus (Russell and Coleman, 1963). The levulinate locus appears to control the amount rather than the structure of ALA-D (Coleman, 1966). In humans the levels of erythrocyte ALA-D activity are also regulated by genetic factors (Sassa et al., 1973a; Sassa et al., 1975). The range of ALA-D activity in normal human red cells is approximately fourfold, but erythrocytes from identical twins show a very small variation. The rather wide distribution of ALA-D activity in the normal human population may partially explain a large scatter of ALA-D activity vs. blood lead around the regression line (Fig. 2). A genetically high level of ALA-D may result in a relatively high activity for a given lead concentration. In support of this idea, a better correlation has been obtained when the ratio of activated/non-activated ALA-D activity is plotted vs. blood lead concentration (Fig. 3). The ratio of activated/non-activated ALA-D activity obviously depends less on genetic variation than on the fraction of the enzyme activity inhibited primarily by lead.

The regression line in Fig. 3 theoretically should end at one on the ordinate, at zero lead concentration; however, it intercepts the ordinate level of 1 at a lead concentration of 0.015 mg/100 ml of blood. This fact would imply that blood lead below this concentration may be bound to some other lead binding site without an inhibitory effect on the activity of ALA-D.

4. Erythrocyte GSH Concentration in Lead Poisoning

GSH concentration in the normal erythrocytes is approximately $2-2.5$ mmol/l of packed erythrocytes, or 0.4 to 0.5 mol/mol of hemoglobin (Beutler et al., 1955; Roels et al., 1975a). This high concentration of GSH is maintained by the action of glucose-6-phosphate dehydrogenase and glutathione synthetase. The rate of turnover $(T/2)$ of red cell GSH is approximately 4 days (Dimant et al., 1955). Decreased G-6-PD activity is reported to increase susceptibility to the toxic effects of lead (Granzoni and Rhomberg, 1965; McIntire and Angle, 1972; Saita and Lussana, 1971; Steiger, 1968).

It might be expected that ALA-D activity in lead-poisoned erythrocytes may inversely correlate with the intracellular levels of GSH. In fact, the endogenous GSH concentration in erythrocytes was reported to be decreased slightly in lead workers (Batolska and Marinova, 1970; Bonsignore et al., 1967; Rubino et al., 1963; Shiraishi, 1952; Vasiliu et al., 1962). Its reduction is also known to occur in rabbits experimentally poisoned with lead (Nagai et al., 1956; Vergnano et al., 1967). However, from a careful study in 110 individuals of the concentration of erythrocyte GSH with various blood lead levels, Roels et al. (1975a) have concluded that inhibition of ALA-D in vivo by lead is not due to decreased levels of endogenous erythrocyte GSH. They have also shown that the overall activity of the glutathione oxidation-reduction pathway is not impaired in lead exposed workers. These data are consistent with the findings by ANGLE and McINTYRE (1974), and PAGLIA et al. (1975a).

Mercury is another heavy metal which occurs as an environmental pollutant and is known to inhibit sulfhydryl enzymes in vitro. However, mercury has little effect on erythrocyte ALA-D in vivo (LAUWERYS & BUCHET, 1973). WADA et al. (1969) reported that only slight inhibition of erythrocyte ALA-D was observed among severely mercury exposed workers who were excreting more than 200 μg Hg/g urinary creatinine/day. Another heavy metal which is known to inhibit SH enzymes in vitro is cadmium. In vitro, cadmium inhibits glutathione reductase, an enzyme which possesses SH groups at its active site (ICEN, 1967) at concentrations of 10^{-6} M and ALA-D at concentrations around 10^{-4} M (WILSON et al., 1972). However, erythrocyte ALA-D activity is scarcely affected in subjects with cadmium poisoning (ROELS et al., 1975a). Thus the decrease of erythrocyte ALA-D is rather specifically related to increased absorption of lead. It is worth noting that erythrocyte ALA-D activity was not affected among patients with a variety of neurological and hematological disorders (BATTISTINI et al.; 1971; NAKAO et al., 1968).

II. Inhibition of Ferrochelatase

Another important site of lead inhibition of the heme biosynthetic pathway is ferrochelatase. This enzyme, like ALA-D, is activated by cysteine and 2-mercaptoethanol (KAGAWA et al., 1959). However, the action of sulfhydryl compounds on ferrochelatase is not only to protect SH groups of the protein, but also to maintain the substrate, iron, in the reduced form (PORRA and JONES, 1963a, b). The enzyme also requires lipid factors for maximal activity (LABBE et al., 1968; SAWADA et al., 1969; YONEYAMA et al., 1969). Sulfhydryl compounds may also protect against phospholipid peroxidation of the enzyme (LABBE et al., 1968). Unlike ALA-D, this enzyme has never been purified to homogeneity. The enzyme catalyzes the formation of the iron-protoporphyrin-IX complex from ferrous iron and protoporphyrin-IX, but can also insert other metal ions, e.g., cobalt, or act on other porphyrins, e.g., mesoporphyrin.

Ferrochelatase has been demonstrated to be directly inhibited by lead in fowl erythrocytes (DRESEL and FALK, 1956a, b; GOLDBERG et al., 1956; GRINSTEIN et al., 1959) and in bone marrow erythrocytes obtained from human subjects with lead poisoning (WADA et al., 1972). However, lead inhibition of ferrochelatase in vitro was observed only when rather high concentrations of lead ($10^{-4} - 10^{-3}$ M) were added to homogenates (GIBSON and GOLDBERG, 1970). It appears that this terminal enzyme of the heme pathway is not as sensitive to lead as is ALA-D. In agreement with this idea, STRAND et al. (1972a) found that the addition of lead to chick embryo liver cells in culture decreased porphyrin formation from ALA. If the inhibition by lead of ferrochelatase was greater than the inhibition of ALA-D, then the addition of lead to cell culture should have resulted in an increase in protoporphyrin accumulation rather than the observed decrease in concentration.

Although in the liver the inhibition of ferrochelatase by lead is relatively smaller than the inhibition of ALA-D, the increased erythrocyte protoporphyrin caused by lead must be due to the inhibition of ferrochelatase in erythroblasts in the bone marrow. In addition to chronic lead poisoning, increased erythrocyte protoporphyrin

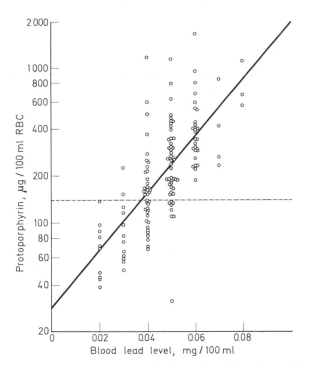

Fig. 4 Scatter diagram for erythrocyte protoporhyrin vs. blood lead level. The solid line is the least squares best fit regression line. The correlation coefficient for log protoporphyrin vs. lead concentration is 0.72. The broken line at a protoporhyrin level of 140 μg/100 ml RBC is a useful level for lead screening

is also found in iron deficiency anemia (Chisolm et al., 1975a; McLaren et al., 1975) and erythropoietic protoporphyria, but for different reasons. In erythropoietic protoporphyria, protoporphyrin accumulates because of a genetic defect of ferro-chelatase activity (Bonkowsky et al., 1975; Bottomley et al., 1975; De Goeiji et al., 1975) and because of increased activity of prior steps in the heme biosynthetic activity (Porter, 1963). In iron deficiency anemia, however, protoporphyrin accumulates because of the shortage of iron, another substrate for the ferrochelatase reaction. Increased protoporphyrin production in response to lead is higher in children and in adult females than in adult males. This point will be discussed in more detail under section E. IV.

1. Assay of Erythrocyte Protoporphyrin

Erythrocyte protoporphyrin concentration can be readily determined by various microfluorometric techniques (Granick et al., 1972; Kammholz et al., 1972; Piomelli, 1973; Sassa et al., 1973b; Chisolm and Brown, 1975). It is possible now to determine erythrocyte protoporphyrin by using only 2 μl of whole blood (Sassa et al., 1973b). The correlation between blood lead and erythrocyte proto-porphyrin is shown in Figure 4. The correlation coefficient of the regression line is

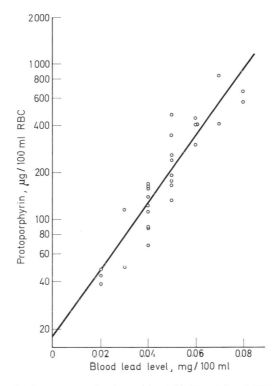

Fig. 5 Scatter diagram for log protoporhyrin vs. blood lead level for children with constant lead level for 3 months or longer. The regression line shown has a correlation coefficient of 0.91

0.72. Since circulating erythrocytes are devoid of mitochondria, increased erythrocyte protoporphyrin must be a reflection of the lead effect on bone marrow erythroblasts which still contain mitochondria and which actively synthesize heme. Thus the level of erythrocyte protoporphyrin in blood is an index of the chronic effect of lead on erythroid cells while they are still in the bone marrow.

The relation of erythrocyte protoporphyrin formation in bone marrow to that of blood lead can be more clearly depicted in Figure 5. This scatter diagram was obtained from a group of children whose blood lead levels remained constant for 3 months or longer on several repeated determinations. In other words, their lead levels in the blood have achieved equilibrium with lead in the bone marrow. The resulting decrease in scatter around the regression line is obvious and the correlation coefficient is increased to 0.91. This suggests that erythrocyte protoporphyrin may correlate better with bone marrow lead, rather than with the lead of the circulating blood. In experimentally lead-poisoned rats, the increase in erythrocyte protoporphyrin is found only in chronic intoxication but not in acute poisoning (Sassa et al., 1973b). Thus low levels of erythrocyte protoporphyrin are often found in acute lead encephalopathy among children at the time of detection, and the blood protoporphyrin may continue to rise even after lead chelation therapy, due to mobilization of red cells from the bone marrow to the circulation. All these data are compatible with the idea that an increase in erythrocyte protoporphyrin is caused primarily by lead affecting the ferrochelatase of erythroid cells in the bone marrow. As will be discussed later, globin synthesis may also be impaired by lead but probably only at very high blood levels of the metal (WHITE and HARVEY, 1972). At concentrations of 0.06 mg lead per 100 ml blood or less, there is little or no associated anemia, suggesting that the overall rate of heme or hemoglobin synthesis is not appreciably affected (SASSA et al., 1975). Although erythrocyte protoporphyrin is extremely high in chronic lead poisoning, the actual molar ratio of protoporphyrin to the heme present in hemoglobin is still only 1/3000 (SASSA et al., 1973b). Because the mean corpuscular hemoglobin concentration is hardly affected, it is probable that the over-all rate of insertion of iron into protoporphyrin is scarcely interfered with at this blood lead level. However, at such a lead concentration, the inhibition of ALA-D and the increase in erythrocyte protoporphyrin can both be readily observed. Thus these parameters are very useful for the early detection of excessive lead exposure before serious pathological effects take place.

The reason for the correlation of the logarithm of erythrocyte protoporphyrin rather than of the concentration itself to blood lead (Figs. 4, 5, 6) is not clear. One possible explanation is that there may be several kinds of binding sites of increasing affinity for lead. As the lead concentration increases, the tighter binding sites are saturated first and the extra ,,free" lead will then increase logarithmically to cause an inhibition of protoporphyrin conversion to heme. Another explanation may be that the correlation curve between erythrocyte protoporphyrin and lead follows the law of biological random variation, which expression is quasi-logarithmic up to a certain lead concentration (CHISOLM et al., 1975b; KJELLSTRÖM and ENG, 1975).

2. Increased Protoporphyrin is Chelated with Zinc

Among the recent developments in microfluorometric assays for erythrocyte protoporphyrin, a useful method is the assay of Zn-protoporphyrin by a portable hematofluorometer (LAMOLA et al., 1975a). In this device, fluorescence is determined in a drop of blood deposited on a glass slide. The concentration of protoporphyrin is displayed as micrograms per 100 ml blood. No extraction or volume correction is required. From the fluorescence emission spectrum, porphyrin thus determined in the red cells was identified as Zn-protoporphyrin. A comparison was made between the regular microfluorometric method for protoporphyrin and the Zn-protoporphyrin method (BLUMBERG et al., 1975; FISCHBEIN et al., 1975). It was found that there is complete agreement between the two methods, suggesting that protoporphyrin in the erythrocytes exists in the form of Zn-protoporphyrin and that Zn is readily removed by the acid extraction used in the regular microfluorometric methods.

Zn-protoporphyrin is also found in erythrocytes from patients with iron deficiency anemia (LAMOLA and YAMANE, 1974), but not in erythrocytes from patients with erythropoietic protoporphyria. In erythropoietic protoporphyria, erythrocyte protoporphyrin is predominantly free protoporphyrin (PIOMELLI et al., 1975). Zn-protoporhyrin is bound to globin peptide tightly at the heme pocket, and does not elute from the red cell (LAMOLA et al., 1975b). On the other hand, free erythrocyte protoporphyrin is readily eluted from the red cell. This explains the increase of protoporphyrin in plasma of patients with erythropoietic protoporphyria, with a significant amount of protoporphyrin reaching the skin where it induces photosensitivity. In lead-poisoned erythrocytes, on the other hand, the increased Zn-protoporphyrin sits in the heme pocket of hemoglobin and is hardly depleted during the life span of the red cell (LAMOLA et al., 1975b). Hence it does not appear in plasma, nor in the skin, nor in feces. Thus in lead poisoning, plasma and fecal protoporphyrin remain normal, and no skin photosensitivity develops.

III. Effects of Lead on ALA-Synthetase

Effects of lead on ALA-synthetase activity, the rate limiting enzyme of the heme biosynthetic pathway, have not been clearly established. A single administration of a toxic dose of lead acetate (100 mg/kg) to a rabbit did not cause an increase in the activity of ALA-synthetase (GAJDOS, 1971) in the liver and in the bone marrow. However, one single dose of lead acetate (60 mg/kg) administered i.p. induced the activity of rat liver ALA-synthetase by twofold (MAINES and KAPPAS, 1976a). The same dose also increased rat kidney ALA-synthetase activity by the same magnitude (MAINES and KAPPAS, 1976b). Studies in chick embryo liver cells in culture (STRAND, 1972a) also indicates that lead induces ALA-synthetase approximately two-fold at 10 µM, and threefold at 50 µM lead concentration. The increase of ALA-synthetase in the liver appears to be the result of de novo synthesis of the enzyme, since it is completely blocked by the addition of cycloheximide. Actinomycin D prevents effectively the induction of ALA-synthetase by 2-allyl-2-isopropylacetamide, but it does not interfere with the induction of ALA-synthetase by lead. Lead strongly inhibits ALA-D and ferrochelatase activity in chick embryo liver cells in culture (STRAND, 1972a). It has been proposed that induction of ALA-synthetase may be due to a derepression of the enzyme synthesis by the impaired heme formation due to lead. However, the increased ALA-synthetase activity caused by lead could also be due to the decrease in the breakdown of the enzyme or to the enhancement of the catalytic activity of the enzyme. These possibilities may be distinguished by the use of the specific antibody generated against chick embryo liver ALA-synthetase (WHITING and GRANICK, 1976).

Other in vivo studies demonstrate that ALA-synthetase activity is not enhanced in lead poisoning — rather it is progressively inhibited with increasing lead concentration (MORROW et al., 1969). Therefore, increased urinary excretion of ALA in lead-poisoned subjects must be largely due to the inhibition of ALA-D activity by lead in bone marrow red cells, liver and prob bly kidney, rather than due to the induction of ALA-synthetase activity.

IV. Effects on Other Enzymes of the Heme Biosynthetic Pathway

Partially purified preparations of uroporphyrinogen-I synthetase (URO-S) from ox liver, avian erythrocytes (LLAMBIAS and DEL C. BATTLE, 1971; STEVENS et al., 1968) and from *Rhodopseudomonas spheroides* (JORDAN and SHEMIN, 1973) were reported to be sensitive to sulfhydryl reagents. Therefore, it might be expected that URO-S activity would be inhibited by lead in human subjects with lead poisoning. However, the levels of erythrocyte URO-S are not appreciably altered in lead-poisoned patients up to blood lead concentration of 90 µg/100 ml blood (Sassa, unpublished). Since erythrocyte ALA-D activity is markedly reduced and erythrocyte protoporphyrin is increased in a logarithmic fashion at these lead concentrations, one must assume preferential binding of lead to the SH group of ALA-D or ferrochelatase.

Only when human hemolysates were incubated with as high as 10^{-5} M lead, was URO-S activity inhibited by 40% (Piper and Tephly, 1974). In a few very severely affected human subjects it has been reported that urinary PBG as well as URO excretion was increased (Gibson et al., 1968; Haeger-Aronsen, 1960). Since both PBG and URO were increased in severe lead poisoning, if URO-S is inhibited by lead, then its activity cannot be decreased to the rate limiting level. In fact, Kreimer-Birnbaum and Grinstein (1965) showed by using rabbit reticulocytes and a radiochemical technique that lead may inhibit a step after URO-S, probably between 7-COOH porphyrinogen and coproporphyrinogen-III.

Coproporphyrinogen decarboxylase is an enzyme in the heme biosynthetic pathway which is frequently referred as a sulfhydryl enzyme and which is inhibited by lead (Committee on Biol. Effects of Atm. Poll., 1972; Waldron, 1974). It is localized in the mitochondria and has been purified approximately 20-fold (Sano and Granick, 1961). The enzyme is not inhibited by sulfhydryl reagents (Sano and Granick, 1961). Therefore it is not clear whether or not increased urinary coproporphyrin in lead poisoned subjects is due to the inhibition of COPRO-decarboxylase. The increased coproporphyrin excretion in lead-poisoned subjects might also represent a back-up accumulation of coproporphyrin as a result of protoporphyrin accumulation.

V. Effect of Lead on Heme Degradation

Lead acetate (60 mg/kg) when administered intraperitoneally to rats causes an increase of about 300% in the heme oxygenase activity of liver (Maines and Kappas, 1976a) and 200% increase in kidney heme oxygenase activity with no appreciable effect on heme oxygenase activity in the heart (Maines and Kappas, 1976b). The same dose of lead when given subcutaneously is only half as effective in altering hepatic or renal heme oxidation activity.

C. Toxic Effects of Exposure to Lead

The toxic effects of this environmental chemical on various organs and tissues will now be considered. Several of them are probably not directly related to effects of lead on heme biosynthesis.

I. Effects on the Red Blood Cells

1. Distribution of Lead Between Red Cells and Plasma

When human blood was incubated in vitro with increasing concentrations of inorganic lead, the lead was essentially all taken up by red cells, whereas plasma lead content remained relatively constant (Clarkson and Kench, 1958). Plasma lead levels among subjects with variable degree of lead poisoning were found to be remarkably constant (ROSEN et al., 1974). A recent study showed that the lead was mostly localized within the red cell matrix rather than in the stromal fraction (BARLTROP and SMITH, 1971).

Once lead binds to the red blood cells, it is no longer dialyzable (CLARKSON and KENCH, 1958), suggesting the formation of an insoluble complex of lead. This is most likely a lead-phosphate complex which is highly insoluble at neutral pH. Tri-phosphates are abundantly present in red cells but not in the plasma. It has been suggested that plasma lead exists as a peptized lead phosphate sol which readily precipitates out if its concentration exceeds over 3 μg lead/100 ml plasma (CLARKSON and KENCH, 1958).

BARLTROP and SMITH (1971) found that there is a macromolecule within the red cells which tightly binds lead. The molecular weight of this lead binding protein is approximately 240,000, whereas none of the stromal proteins have such a high molecular weight (ROSENBERG and GUIDOTTI, 1969). The nature of this macromolecule is not clear; however, it is interesting to note that this protein has a molecular weight similar to ALA-D.

2. Effect of Lead on Globin Synthesis

In addition to its inhibitory effect on heme biosynthesis in erythroid precursor cells, lead may also have a direct inhibitory effect on globin synthesis (KASSENAAR et al., 1957). Lead interferes with amino acid incorporation into nascent polypeptides on the polyribosomes (TRAKETELLER et al., 1965); when reticulocytes are incubated with lead, polyribosomes are disaggregated leading to a marked depression of globin formation. The inhibitory effect of lead is prevented by the addition of hemin in vitro (WAXMANN and RABINOVITZ, 1966). Since the hemin effect has been shown to prevent a binding of a translational repressor to the met-tRNA$_f^{MET}$-40S ribosomal subunit complex, it would be tempting to assume that lead may have a similar effect as the translational repressor for globin synthesis or that lead displaces hemin so as to facilitate the binding of the repressor to the initiation complex (CLEMENS et. al., 1974).

The basophilic stippling frequently found in red cells from patients with lead poisoning has been shown to be due at least in part to altered ribosomes (JENSEN et al., 1965) (see later). Therefore, it is possible that the lead effect on polyribosomes found in vitro may well be taking place in erythroid precursor cells or reticulocytes, and that disaggregation of polyribosomes may lead to irreversible denaturation of ribosomes. Lead inhibits not only the synthesis of globin peptides, but it has been shown to interfere with the assembly of globin chains (WHITE and HARVEY, 1972). However it should be noted that all these effects of lead on globin synthesis are observed only at high concentrations of the metal.

3. Fast Hemoglobin

A unique hemoglobin with fast migration during electrophoresis at pH 8.6 has been described in some children with chronic lead poisoning (TUTTLE and FITCH, 1958). Its incidence was approximately 40% in preschool children with chronic lead poisoning (Charache and Weatherall, 1966). The component disappears after recovery (Tuttle and Fitch, 1958). The nature of this hemoglobin Pb has not been established. Charache and Weatherall (1966) have suggested that some small ligands which carry a negative charge may be attached to hemoglobin Pb. It is tempting to speculate that the negatively charged molecule may be Zn-proto-porphyrin, since it has been shown that Zn-protoporphyrin is increased in the red cells from patients with lead poisoning, and since Zn-protoporphyrin may bind to the heme pocket of globin peptides. Hemoglobin Pb is found more often in lead-poisoned subjects if they are simultaneously affected by iron deficiency anemia. This finding is also consistent with the idea that hemoglobin Pb may be the hemoglobin-Zn-protoporphyrin complex since both lead poisoning and iron deficiency anemia lead to an increase in erythrocyte Zn-protoporphyrin.

4. Basophilic Stippling of Erythrocytes in Lead Poisoning

Electron micrographic studies have demonstrated extensive accumulation of iron in the mitochondria in the form of "ferruginous micelles" (Bessis and Breton-Gorius, 1959). Erythrocytes which are loaded with ferruginous micelles are called "ringed side-roblasts" which are characteristic of sideroblastic anemias. Dense aggregations of ferritin are also found in damaged mitochondria in sideroblasts (Bessis and Jensen, 1965; Sano, 1958). These depositions of altered cytoplasmic elements, including ribosomal RNA and mitochondrial fragments, are responsible for the basophilic stippling of erythrocytes which is also often found in human and experimental lead poisoning (Bessis and Jensen, 1965; Cartwright and Deiss, 1975; Sano, 1958). Recently, Valentine et al. (1974) reported that basophilic stippling of erythrocytes is frequently found in patients with deficient pyrimidine 5'-nucleotidase activity. This enzyme is sensitive to lead and its activity is inhibited at lead concentrations of 10^{-6} M which have little effects on many other erythrocyte enzymes (Paglia et al., 1975). The basophilic granules in this disorder is caused from the retarded degradation of RNA secondary to the inability to dephosphorylate and render diffusible the pyrimidine degradation products of RNA (Paglia and Valentine, 1975). These data suggest that inhibition of pyrimidine 5'-nucleotidase activity by lead may result in the formation of basophilic stippling.

5. Effects of Lead on Mitochondria

Obviously lead interferes with the utilization of iron for heme formation within the mitochondria leading to the excessive accumulation of iron and the destruction of the mitochondria. It has been suggested that the deposition of iron in the mitochondria is not only due to the decrease in its utilization, but also due to the increased uptake of iron from the cytoplasm (Borová et al., 1973; Poňka and Neuwirt, 1975).

Also the associated Zn-protoporphyrin accumulation in lead poisoning contributes to a loss of mitochondrial enzyme activities. Metalloporphyrins in concentrations of 10^{-5} M and 10^{-6} M were reported to inhibit the activities of intramitochondrial enzymes, such as succinate dehydrogenase, isocitrate dehydrogenase, L-glutamate dehydrogenase and DPNH cytochrome c reductase (Silverstein, 1962). Stippled erythrocytes found in lead-poisoning are known to actively synthesize porphyrins (SANO, 1958). It was also shown that lead itself may enter the mitochondria, thus directly inhibiting some mitochondrial function. When isotopically labeled lead was administered to dogs, the label was found to accumulate in the mitochondria of various organs (MIANI and VITERBO, 1958).

6. Anemia in Lead Poisoning

The nature of anemia in lead poisoning is rather complex. Anemia is usually mild in the adult (GRIGGS, 1964; RUBINO et al., 1959; WALDRON, 1966), but frequently severe in the child (WATSON et al., 1958). It is most often normocytic and normochromic, but in some severely affected children, it may be microcytic and hypochromic (FULLERTON, 1952). The hypochromicity of the lead-induced anemia in children is sometimes due to a concurrent state of iron deficiency anemia. The reticulocytes are usually elevated to 2 to 7 per cent (HARRIS and KELLERMEYER, 1970). The mean corpuscular hemoglobin concentration is usually normal in the adult (BERK et al., 1970), or only slightly decreased in children (MOOSA and HARRIS, 1969). Although lead inhibits ALA-D, ferrochelatase and some other steps in the heme pathway, lead inhibition of hemoglobin formation is so small that it cannot be the major cause of the anemia.

Lead effects on the development of anemia can be considered to occur at two different sites, namely at the formation of red cells in the bone marrow and at the destruction of red cells in the peripheral circulation. It is known that lead is preferentially deposited in the bone marrow and its concentration in fresh marrow may reach 50 times that which is present in the blood (ALBAHARY, 1972). By comparison liver contains only three times, and kidney 2 times as much lead as blood (ALBAHARY, 1972). Therefore bone marrow cells, particularly premature erythroid precursor cells, are most liable to the toxic effects of lead. Such toxic effects are expressed in some patients as erythroid hypoplasia. LEIKEN and ENG (1963) suggested that there is a defect in erythroid differentiation and maturation in patients with lead anemia. Studies in hypoxic plethoric mice also suggest that lead administration produces a transient erythroid hypoplasia and disturbances in intracellular iron transport. Part of the depressed erythropoiesis may be a result of impairment of erythropoietin production in lead-poisoned animals (LANDOW et al., 1973). However, in a single case study of an anemic adult patient with lead poisoning, BERK et al. (1970) have reported completely effective erythropoiesis as determined by ferrokinetic studies, thus excluding the possibility of erythroid hypoplasia. They have further commented that an increased early labeled bilirubin peak found in this patient in addition to the effective erythropoiesis even indicates an increase in heme biosynthesis in the lead-poisoned subject. However, the origin of the early labeled bilirubin peak has not been established, hence it is not possible to make a firm conclusion on this patient. This case is probably the only reported case of lead poisoning with effective erythropoiesis, since most lead-poisoned subjects have a variable degree of erythroid hypoplasia. A severe erythroid hypoplasia (Hb 4.8 g/100 ml, PCV 16%, MCHC 30%, reticulocyte 1%) has been reported in a 3-year-old boy with lead poisoning and the anemia was completely alleviated after treatment with CaEDTA (MOOSA and HARRIS, 1969). Erythroid hypoplasia was apparently the predominant cause of the anemia in this subject and was treatable with chelation therapy. Since patients with erythroid hypoplasia of other origin usually have a poor prognosis, it is important to establish whether a condition of lead-induced hypoplasia exists in a patient because of the controllable nature of this intoxication.

Another mechanism of lead anemia can be attributed to the metal's effect on the red cell membrane, leading to an early destruction of red cells. When red cells are removed from a patient with lead poisoning, labeled with ^{51}Cr, and reinfused into the donor, the life span of the labeled red cells is significantly reduced ($T_{\frac{1}{2}} = 18 \sim 26$ days; compared with normal $T_{\frac{1}{2}} = 30$ days) (GRIGGS and HARRIS, 1958; WALDRON, 1966). When red cells from a normal subject were treated with lead in vitro for a short period, labeled with ^{51}Cr, and reinfused back to the same subject, it was also found that the survival of lead-treated cells was diminished ($T_{\frac{1}{2}} = 18 - 30$ days) (FRATIANNE et al., 1958). These data indicate that there is a shortening of the survival of lead-poisoned red blood cells is most likely due to the direct effect of lead on the cell membrane. For example, it has been shown in vitro that lead binds tightly to phosphatidylcholine in the membranes (HOOGEVEEN, 1970).

It is known that red cells incubated with high concentrations of lead in vitro leak out a large amount of potassium (ØRSKOV, 1935). This loss of erythrocyte potassium is irreversible and is caused by lead interference with an energy-requiring pump (JOYCE et al., 1954; PASSOW and TILLMAN, 1955; PASSOW et al., 1961; VINCENT and BLACKBURN, 1958a, b). Concomitant with a loss of potassium, a reduction of the erythrocyte Na^+/K^+ ATPase activity was also found in blood samples of patients with lead poisoning (HASAN et al., 1967). Not only lead, but also other heavy metals like Hg and Au have been shown to evoke a large efflux of potassium from the red cells (GRIGARZIK and PASSOW, 1958; JOYCE et al., 1954). However, Ni, Co, and Cd have no effect on red cell potassium efflux (PASSOW, 1964). Although the potassium efflux is increased several hundred-fold by lead, lead scarcely affects sodium influx. Since the loss of potassium is associated with the shrinkage of the cells, consequently the sodium concentration rises in lead-poisoned erythrocytes. In contrast, Hg, or N-ethylmaleimide also produce similar rapid losses of potassium from the red cells, but these are associated with a nearly equivalent sodium entry (PASSOW, 1964). Also the action of mercury can be completely prevented by equimolar amounts of SH (WEED et al., 1962), but the lead effect on potassium loss is not reversible even in the presence of 200-fold excess of cysteine (PASSOW and TILLMAN, 1955).

Whether the potassium loss occurs more extensively in reticulocytes or in stippled cells than in older red cells is not known. However, this disturbance in membrane permeability caused by lead certainly leads to an increased mechanical fragility of the red blood cells (HARRIS and GREENBERG, 1954).

Another interesting feature of lead is its pseudoimmunological effect on the red cell membrane. When lead was infused into a dog, a positive direct Coombs' test was observed within 24 h (MUIRHEAD et al., 1954). Coombs' test is based on the principle that antibody molecules in the serum bind strongly to antigenic sites on the red cells. When such "antibody-coated" red cells are incubated with the Coombs' serum (antihuman globulin antibody generated in a rabbit), the sensitized red cells aggregate, giving a positive Coombs' test. A positive direct Coombs' test was also found in the reticulocyte-rich fraction of blood obtained from lead poisoned subjects (SUTHERLAND and EISENTRAUT, 1956). These effects of lead are similar to those found in the case of phenylhydrazine-induced hemolytic anemia (MUIRHEAD et al., 1954). The nature of the induced agglutinability of red cells is not clear. However, it has been postulated that transferrin adhering to the cell surface or a hapten formation by lead-protein complex may be responsible for these changes (JANDL, 1960).

II. Lead Effect on the Immune System

Except the induction of the positive direct Coombs test by lead which may be considered to be pseudoimmunological phenomenon, lead has generally an inhibitory effect on body defences against infection, including the immunological system. For example, treatment of mice with lead nitrate enhanced the mortality to *Salmonella typhimurium* (HEMPHILL et al., 1971). The lifespan of the leukocytes from lead-poisoned animals has been reported to be shorter than controls (SAWINSKY et al., 1971). By using a plaque-forming assay (CUNNINGHAM and SZENBERG, 1968), KOLLER and KOVACIC (1974) examined the number of antibody producing cells in mice which had been orally treated with lead in drinking water. They found that even at the lowest test dose in drinking water (13.8 ppm, which is 10 times more than the lead present in the regular diet), lead reduced the number of 7S-plaque-forming cells, or γ-globulin producing cells, i.e., suppressed the secondary response mediated by IgG. A reduction in the number of 19S-plaque-forming cells which synthesize macroglobulin was also produced but at much higher lead concentrations. These data suggest that chronic lead exposure produces a significant decrease in antibody synthesis, particularly IgG, indicating that the "memory cells" are impaired. The results of this study offer some clue to the increased mortality from bacterial and viral diseases in animals which are chronically exposed to lead. Whether the decrease in antibody formation by lead is due to decreased heme biosynthesis in the immuno-competent cells is not known.

III. Drug Metabolizing System

Metabolism of a wide variety of chemicals, drugs, and steroids is carried out by the mixed function oxidase system which is present in the liver, adrenal cortex, placenta, lung, and in other tissues (KAPPAS and ALVARES, 1975). The key enzyme of the mixed function oxidase system is cytochrome P-450. Cyt. P-450 as well as other enzymes in the mixed function oxidase system are known to be inducible upon exposure to a variety of environmental agents and drugs that act as substrates for the system.

Many, if not all, chemical inducers which bring about enhanced synthesis of cyt. P-450 in the liver appear to cause increased synthesis of ALA-synthetase. In many instances, the increase in ALA-S level is earlier and greater than the increase in cyt. P-450. Since cyt. P-450 is the major hemoprotein in the liver (ESTABROOK et al., 1968) and has the shortest half-life among hepatic cytochromes, it is expected that lead may significantly interfere with the formation of cyt. P-450 via the inhibition of heme biosynthesis. Such studies were carried out in experimental animals and in men, and the results indicate that lead may have entirely different effects depending on whether it is administered acutely or chronically.

When lead chloride (5 mg/kg) was administered to weanling rats intravenously, it was found that cyt. P-450, ethylmorphine N-demethylase, aniline hydroxylase activities were all decreased by approximately 50% in 24 h after the chemical treatment. Methyl mercury, which is also known to interfere with the heme biosynthetic pathway had a very similar effect (ALVARES et al., 1972). Inhibition by lead of the mixed function oxidase system including cyt. P-450 was greatest at 24th hour and restored to normal levels between the 5th and 7th day after the treatment (SCOPPA et al. 1973). In acute lead poisoning, the impairment of the hepatic drug metabolizing system appears to be the result of the inhibition of heme biosynthesis, rather than the result of lead inhibition of drug hydroxylases, since the lead concentrations found in tissues in experimental animals were much too low to inhibit hydroxylase activities in vitro (SCOPPA et al., 1973). On the other hand, ALA-D activity in the livers of lead-poisoned rats was practically absent in the first 2 days and only recovered to 54% of the control level on the 5th day (SCOPPA et al., 1973).

Although these experiments provided evidence for the inhibition of drug metabolism by acute lead intoxication, the effects of chronic lead poisoning on the drug metabolizing system in humans are entirely different. ALVARES et al. (1975) examined drug metabolism among children with chronic lead poisoning of environmental origin by following the rate of disappearance of antipyrine and phenylbutazone from the circulation. They found that the mean antipyrine or phenylbutazone half life in chronically lead poisoned children was not appreciably different from that of normal children. However, in two cases of acutely lead-poisoned children, the antipyrine half-lives were significantly prolonged above normal and were restored toward normal 1 week after lead chelation therapy with CaEDTA. Thus it appears that lead inhibits the metabolism of antipyrine only in the case of acute intoxication but not under conditions of chronic intoxication.

It can be concluded that in chronic lead intoxication some adaptive mechanism develop which abolishes the effects of lead on cyt. P-450 and associated enzymes. Such adaptation has also been reported in mice (YOSHIKAWA, 1968) and rats (SANAI et al., 1972).

IV. Lead Neuropathy

1. Encephalopathy

Acute encephalopathy is the most serious toxic effect of lead, often seen among children. Lead encephalopathy is rather rare among adults, but occasionally described in drinkers of illicitly distilled whiskey (WHITFIELD et al., 1972). Papilloedema, retinal hemorrhages, optic atrophy, and other lesions of the cranial nerves have been described in lead encephalopathy.

In lead encephalopathy lead content increases more than 10-fold in the cerebrospinal fluid. Knowledge of concentrations of porphyrins or their precursors in the cerebrospinal fluid would be of considerable interest, but no data on this have so far been reported. Lead encephalopathy can be induced in neonatal rats from lead in mother's milk (PENTSCHEW and GARRO, 1966). Suckling rats were apparently more susceptible to lead effects than adult animals since the fostering mothers did not show any clinical signs of lead poisoning. It has been also reported that the lead retention can be many times greater in young animals than in older animals (FORBES and REINO, 1972; KOSTIAL and McMCILOVIC, 1975). A similar situation is also observed among human subjects. The lowest toxic blood concentration of lead has been suggested to be 80 µg/100 ml blood for adults, but blood lead levels as low a 50 µg/100 ml sometimes are associated with clinical symptoms in children (LIN-FU, 1972). This fact suggests that children may have also increased sensitivity to lead.

Surprisingly, very few studies have been made on the effects of lead on heme biosynthetic capacity in nerve cells, though this is obviously an important problem in relation to the pathogenesis of lead encephalopathy. In the case of acutely lead-poisoned rabbits, the activity of ALA-D has been found somewhat diminished in the brain, as well as in the liver, kidney and bone marrow (GIBSON and GOLDBERG, 1970). A possible inference of this finding may be that children with slightly elevated blood lead levels have some decrease in the formation of cytochromes in the brain which might lead to an irreversible impairment of brain function.

2. Neuropathy in Lead Poisoning and in Acute Intermittent Porphyria

There is a remarkable clinical similarity between lead poisoning and acute intermittent porphyria (DAGG et al., 1965). Abdominal pain, constipation, vomiting, paralysis, or paresis are very common symptoms observed in both clinical disorders. Neuropsychiatric symptoms are sometimes observed in lead intoxication, but less frequently than in acute intermittent porphyria. In lead poisoning, the paresis is entirely that of the lower motor neuron type, but 10% of acute intermittent porphyrics show signs of upper motor neuron involvement and organic brain disorders (GOLDBERG, 1968). Lead encephalopathy is predominantly found in children, but porphyric symptoms are only found at or after puberty. The disorder of heme biosynthesis in lead poisoning is entirely acquired, whereas in acute intermittent porphyria there is a genetic defect of uroporphyrinogen-1 synthetase leading to impairment of heme biosynthesis (STRAND et al., 1912b; MEYER and SCHMID, 1973; SASSA et al., 1974; SASSA et al., 1975). The abnormalities of porphyrin metabolism in lead poisoning originate largely in the bone marrow and in acute intermittent porphyria in the liver. On the other hand, the clinical manifestations of both disorders can mostly be explained by their effects on the nervous system. Although the biochemical effects of lead on the hematopoietic system and the disturbances of hepatic heme synthesis in acute intermittent porphyria have been elucidated, the agent responsible for the pathologic lesion in the nervous system for both disorders has not been identified.

The effects of porphyrin precursors on the nervous system have been examined, however, no firm conclusion was reached. It is true that ALA has been reported to interfere with certain aspects of nerve functions in experimental systems (BECKER et al., 1971), but the neurological disturbances of lead poisoning or porphyria cannot be ascribed to the elevated ALA concentration in the tissue (JARRETT et al., 1956; GOLDBERG et al., 1954). For example, the serum levels of ALA or PBG do not correlate with the neurologic manifestation in patients with acute intermittent porphyria (MIYAGI et al., 1971). It has also been debated whether ALA can penetrate the blood brain barrier (GOLDBERG and McGILLION 1973; SHANLEY et al., 1975). Porphobilin, the oxidized product of porphobilinogen, has been shown to inhibit nerve end-plate potential in a rat diaphragm preparation (FELDMAN et al., 1971);

however, its biological significance is not yet established. Capsular degeneration and segmental demyelination have been described in lead encephalopathy, but their pathognomonic significance is not clear, since these lesions can be observed in other diseases such as diabetic neuropathy (Greenbaum et al., 1964; Thomas and Lascelles, 1966) or hypertrophic neuritis (Thomas and Lascelles, 1967).

V. Lead Effects on the Kidney

Acute renal effects of lead poisoning are different from those encountered in patients with chronic lead nephropathy. Acute lead nephropathy is usually associated with non-specific degeneration of renal tubular cells, particularly of the proximal convoluted tubular cells. One of the most notable changes in the renal tubular cells is the formation of intranuclear inclusion bodies. These inclusion bodies vary considerably in size and in ratio of core to fibrils (Beaver, 1961; Bracken et al., 1958; Richter et al., 1968), but are always distinct from nucleoli. The most common type of intranuclear inclusion is a compact core and a circumferential fringe (Richter et al., 1968). The latter consists largely of a loose mesh of fibrils that varies considerably in thickness (100 – 130 Å).

The formation of inclusion bodies has been reported not only in humans but also in swine (Watrach, 1964), rabbits (Hass et al., 1964), fowls (Simpson et al., 1970), and rats (Goyer, 1968). The inclusion bodies are composed of protein stainable with fast green, suggesting that they do not contain histones (Richter et al., 1968). Studies using isolated inclusion bodies show that they are composed of a lead-protein complex containing approximately 50 µg of lead per mg protein. Lead within the inclusion bodies amounts to 60 to 100 times more than lead in the whole kidney (Goyer et al., 1970). Intranuclear inclusion bodies are observed at very low kidney concentrations of lead, in fact at lower concentrations of lead than those which are associated with any biochemical signs of lead exposure. For example, inclusion bodies in the rat kidney were observed when the kidney lead concentration was 10 µg/g wet weight, whereas increased urinary ALA excretion was observed only after the lead concentration was higher than 20 µg/g wet weight (Goyer et al., 1970). It has been suggested that inclusion bodies function as a depot of non-diffusible lead (Goyer, 1971), thus reducing the cytoplasmic concentration of lead and toxic effects on the cells. Inclusion bodies have also been found in the leaves of moss plants exposed to lead (Skaar et al., 1973).

It has been shown by Bessis and Jensen (1965) that mitochondria of reticulocytes of bone marrow of lead-poisoned rats are swollen and contain excess iron as ferruginous micelles. These ultrastructural changes of mitochondria also occur in cells of liver and kidney. Amino-aciduria is well known to occur as a consequence of acute renal effects of lead. Since renal tubular reabsorption of small organic molecules including amino acids is an energy-requiring process, it is possible that amino-aciduria in lead poisoning is a result of disturbances in energy-metabolism caused by the toxic effects of lead. In support of this idea, isolated mitochondria from lead poisoned rats show impairment of respiration and phosphorylation despite the presence of phosphate (Goyer, 1971), notably in the presence of ATP (Parr and Harris, 1975), which acts as a chelating agent.

Amino-aciduria observed in lead poisoning is of a non-specific type. Namely there is no specific pattern for the excretion of amino acids. Plasma amino acid levels are not elevated. This suggests that lead-induced amino-aciduria is of renal origin (WILSON et al., 1953). Amino-aciduria is most marked in children with severe lead poisoning, but rather rare in adult subjects with lead intoxication. Since urinary ALA is increased in both cases, the excretion of ALA is a far more sensitive index of lead exposure than is amino-aciduria.

It has been shown that a mercurial diuretic, mercaptomerin inhibits heme synthesis in the rat kidney as determined by ^{14}C-ALA incorporation into heme (ISRAELS, 1972). The inhibitory effect of mercaptomerin is most likely on the SH containing enzymes, ALA-D and ferrochelatase. Since lead can be expected to inhibit ALA-D, like mercury, increased urinary excretion of ALA in plumbism may well be due to lead-inhibition of ALA-D in the proximal tubule cells. Inhibition of heme synthesis in the kidney may be an important aspect of the pharmacological and toxicological effects of lead on the excretion of ALA or coproporphyrin in urine.

Chronic lead effects on the kidney are usually those of a slowly contracting organ with arteriosclerotic features. Most of these cases have been found among occupational workers. An increased incidence of hypertension is described among lead workers; however a renal basis for the hypertension has not been established (GOYER, 1971).

VI. Tumorigenic and Teratogenic Effects of Lead

Another important aspect of lead intoxication is the appearance of tumors in lead-exposed animals. Repeated injection of lead phosphate into rats is known to cause kidney tumors (VAN ESCH et al., 1962, ZOLLINGER, 1953). Lead-induced tumors have been also described in mice (EPSTEIN and MANTEL, 1968). Tumor cells do not contain intranuclear inclusion bodies and lead content of the tumors is less than that of adjacent renal cortex. In contrast to inorganic lead, tetraethyl lead administration causes lymphoma in mice, but not renal tumors nor nephropathy (EPSTEIN and MANTEL, 1968). It is interesting to note that newborn mice are notably more resistant to the toxic effects of tetraethyl lead. This fact may be related to immaturity of their hepatic microsomal mixed function oxidases with consequent failure to dealkylate tetraethyl lead to triethyl lead which is known to be more toxic (CREMER, 1965).

Lead treatment in pregnant female hamsters causes tail bud malformation in the offspring (FERM and CARPENTER, 1967a). Cadmium, on the other hand, causes anterior malformation (FERM and CARPENTER, 1968). It appears that lead and cadmium interact with each other at the cellular level in a different fashion depending on the tissue. For example cadmium potentiates the tail bud malformation caused by lead, and lead blocks the effect of cadmium on the differentiation of the visceral arch system preventing facial abnormalities (FERM, 1969).

The direct relevance of these tumorigenic and teratogenic effects of lead observed in rodents to humans is not clear, since an increased incidence of renal tumors has not been reported in industrial workers with chronic lead poisoning, nor is an increased incidence of congenital malformation known among this population.

D. Biological Defense Mechanisms Against Lead

YOSHIKAWA (1968) showed that pretreatment of mice with a small dose of lead protected them from the subsequent lethal effects of lead. A similar finding was also reported in rats by SANAI et al. (1972). These experiments indicate that biological adaptation develops against the toxic effects of lead. The development of biological defense mechanisms against lead may explain the difference in the inhibitory effects of lead on the drug metabolism between acute and chronic lead poisoning.

The mechanism of adaptation to lead is not understood; also whether the adaption to other metals also occurs by lead is not clear. However, chronic administration of lead brings about a number of changes which are not encountered in acute lead intoxication. Some of these changes may confer protection against the toxic effects of lead. For example, lead stimulates nuclear DNA synthesis and cell proliferation in the tubular epithelium of rat kidneys within 2 days (CHOIE and RICHTER, 1973). It has been also shown that, after many intraperitoneal injections of lead, given over a period of 6 months, ^{3}H-thymidine incorporation was enhanced in the renal tubular cells of the rat (CHOIE and RICHTER, 1972a, b). Together with the increase in nuclear DNA-synthesis, intranuclear inclusion bodies develop in the renal tubules and in liver parenchymal cells in lead poisoned animals (BLACKMAN, 1936; CHOIE and RICHTER, 1972c; WACHSTEIN, 1949). GOYER has suggested that renal intranuclear inclusion bodies may serve as a scavenger for lead by binding to it, thus removing lead from toxic sites of action (GOYER et al., 1970).

Another mechanism of adaptation to lead is probably due to the induction of synthesis of metallothionein, a protein induced in response to heavy metals. Metallothionein is a polypeptide containing a large number of SH groups and is assumed to play an important role in a biological defense mechanism against heavy metals (ULMER and VALLEE, 1969). For example, the protein fraction extracted from kidneys of cadmium-treated mice contains $21-25$-fold more SH groups (moles per unit weight) than the control kidney and as much as 85% of the SH groups in the protein fraction were shown to be due to metallothionein (ONO et al., 1973a). It has been shown that the intraperitoneal administration of lead acetate into mice caused a marked increase in SH concentration in the kidney (ONO et al., 1973b).

E. Factors Affecting the Toxic Effects of Lead

I. Alcohol

Lead is a common contaminant in illicitly distilled whiskey which is produced in certain regions of the United States. Lead is leached into the distilling alcohol from automobile radiators which are frequently used as condensors, with other parts connected by lead-containing solder. The concentration of lead in such whiskey preparations may exceed 1 mg/l in one-third of the samples tested (Comm. on Biologic Effects of Atmospheric Pollutants, 1972).

Frequent occurrence of lead toxicity among drinkers of moonshine whiskey may in part be due to the synergism between lead and alcohol at the cellular level. Both lead and alcohol lead to mitochondrial dysfunction. Mitochondria isolated from ethanol-treated rats show decreased oxidative properties and increased membrane permeability (FRENCH and TODOROFF, 1970). Lead also induces mitochrondrial injury in reticulocytes of the bone marrow (BESSIS and JENSEN, 1965), liver (WATRACH, 1964), and kidney (GOYER, 1968), yielding impairment of mitochondrial function (GOYER, 1968; LESSLER et al., 1968; TERAS and KAKHN, 1967). The most important synergism between lead and ethanol may take place at the level of ALA-D, since this enzyme activity is inhibited by both compounds (MOORE, 1972). Lead workers who consume alcohol (legally distilled whiskey) regularly (7.5 l or more of strong liquor per month) were found to have a definitely higher incidence of lead poisoning than those with lower liquor consumption (CRAMER, 1966). On the other hand, MOORE (1972) has made a curious observation in rats. A significant depression of ALA-D in the red cells was observed in rats which were treated with either lead or ethanol; however, the enzyme activity was elevated over the two separate depressed activities when they were administered together. The mechanism for this paradoxical effect of lead and ethanol on ALA-D activity in rats is not understood.

II. Sickle Cell Anemia

Children with hemoglobin S-S or S-C disease were found to have a significantly increased incidence of lead encephalopathy (ERENBERG et al., 1974). The S-S or S-C hemoglobinopathy alone does not cause neuropathy (GREER and SCHOTLAND, 1962). Therefore, the toxic effects of lead appear to be potentiated by the accompanying hemoglobinopathy. Increased turnover of red cells may mobilize lead from bones to the central nervous system. In this regard the association of lead poisoning with other forms of hemolytic anemias should also be expected to be clinically severe; however, no such cases have been reported.

Patients with sickle cell disease have been shown to be zinc deficient (SCHOOMAKER et al., 1973). The zinc deficiency appears to be the result of increased excretion of zinc into urine secondary to hemolysis. Zinc is an important metal for the activity of ALA-D, particularly in lead-poisoned animals, since the lead-inhibited enzyme activity can be restored to normal by the addition of zinc in vitro (FINELLI et al., 1975) and by zinc administration in vivo (FINELLI et al., 1974). Therefore, the toxic effect of lead may be potentiated by zinc deficiency in patients with sickle cell anemia. It is interesting to note that zinc inhibits cadmium-induced teratogenic, embryocidal and neoplastic effects (FERM and CARPENTER 1967b; GUNN et al., 1967). Whether zinc protects against lead-induced tumorigenicity has not been studied.

In patients with lead poisoning, it has been recently reported that erythrocyte Zn-protoporphyrin is increased. The occurrence of zinc protoporphyrin would not be expected in S-S hemoglobinopathy or in other zinc deficiency syndromes. Therefore it would be interesting to examine Zn-protoporhyrin concentration in the red cells from subjects with Hb S-S who also show other signs and symptoms of lead poisoning.

III. Diet

Lead poisoning among children in the United States is known to be more frequent in the economically poor populations including Blacks and Puerto Ricans (GRIGGS,

1964). It has been suggested that poor diets and low nutritional state may be responsible for pica which then lead to lead poisoning (CARLANDER, 1959; LANZKOW-SKY, 1959). However, in a recent study where matched groups of children were examined for their dietary intake, it appears that there is no direct correlation between the dietary intake and the occurrence of lead poisoning (MOOTY et al., 1975). Therefore, dietary effects on the occurrence of lead poisoning among humans have not been firmly established.

However, it is well decomented in rats, that low dietary clalcium (0.1%) enhances the toxicity of lead significantly (SIX and GOYER, 1970, 1972) whereas high dietary calcium reduces the retention of lead in the body (QUARTERMAN et al., 1975). The amount of lead found in femur and kidney is consistently greater in rats on a low calcium diet than in animals on a normal calcium diet at any concentrations of lead (SIX and GOYER, 1972). Although the exact mechanisms of the low calcium diet in facilitating enhanced lead absorption is not known, the enhanced lead toxicity by low calcium diet is most likely due to the increased concentration of lead in soft tissues, including brain, kidney, liver, or bone marrow.

IV. Iron Deficiency

It is known that female subjects have higher erythrocyte protoporhyrin concentration than males at a given blood level of lead (ROELS et al., 1975b). The increase of erythrocyte protoporphyrin in females (STUIK, 1974) and children (LAMOLA et al., 1975a) occurs at lower blood lead levels and the slope of increase in protoporphyrin concentrations is steeper than in males. Since children and women have less iron stores in the body (FAIRBANKS and BEUTLER, 1972), it appears that iron deficiency may potentiate the toxic effects of lead.

Pica is a well-known problem which occurs both in iron deficiency anemia and in lead poisoning. However, there are some disputes about the nature of pica observed in lead poisoning. Some investigators feel that lead pica is the result of malnutrition and of the accompanying iron deficiency and that it can be relieved by treatment of iron deficiency (BER and VALERO, 1961; CARLANDER, 1959; LANZ-KOWSKY, 1959; STETSON, 1947; WEIPPL, 1959), while others do not agree (BARLTROP, 1966; FERGUSON and KEATON, 1950; GUTELIUS et al., 1962, 1963). Thus disturbance of heme biosynthesis as a predisposing factor in developing pica has not yet been established. However, inasmuch as both lead and iron deficiency strongly impair heme biosynthesis, this problem merits further investigation.

F. Diagnosis of Lead Poisoning

The diagnosis of lead poisoning has been based on the blood lead determination. However, this assay is an exacting one and is subject to significant errors introduced at any step in the procedure such as sampling, shipping, and analysis of the sample. For example, even in the most competent laboratories, there is a $\pm 15\%$ error in the determination on multiple runs of the same blood sample (BALOH, 1974).

Comparison between different laboratories reveal even greater discrepancies. Nevertheless, the blood lead level has been preferred to levels of lead in urine, in hair, and in teeth, on practical as well as theoretical grounds.

The levels of blood lead which are generally accepted as the safe upper limit are approximately 80 µg/100 ml blood for adults and 60 µg/100 ml for children (HSMHA, 1971; KEHOE, 1964; NIOSH, 1972). Although clinical symptoms may not appear below these lead concentrations, biochemical abnormalities are very often present. For example, VITALE et al. (1975) demonstrated that 23 out of 26 occupationally lead-exposed workers had lead excretion in excess of 650 µg/day when challenged with EDTA, indicating excessive body burden of lead. However, only 2 of them had blood lead levels which would be considered above the safe level. Thus blood lead determination alone is not an adequate test for the diagnosis of lead poisoning, since it does not measure any of the toxic effect of lead.

In contrast to blood lead determination, microfluorometric assay of protoporphyrin (KAMMHOLZ et al., 1972; LAMOLA and YAMANE, 1974; PIOMELLI, 1973; SASSA et al., 1973b) and spectrophotometric assay of ALA-D (GRANICK et al., 1973; WEISSBERG et al., 1971) in capillary blood samples are simple and rapid. Moreover, these methods reflect the biological effects of lead rather than the lead concentration in the tissue. As a screening test for chronic lead toxicity, the flurometric assay of protoporhyrin is most suitable, since erythrocyte protoporhyrin increases in a curvilinear fashion with the increase in blood lead concentration and its determination is simple. Microassay procedures can be adapted to simple fluoromcters by using proper filters and detectors. It is possible to analyze approximately 30 samples in duplicates in a hour by using a simple flurometer and probably more, by using a hematofluorometer. Therefore, it is possible to perform this test on-site. A recently developed hematofluorometer (BLUMBERG et al., 1975) is extremely useful for this purpose. In contrast to protoporphyrin which is increased both in lead poisoning and iron deficiency anemia, the determination of ALA-D activity establishes the diagnosis of lead poisoning, since the enzyme is rather specifically inhibited by lead. In acute lead poisoning, ALA-D is inhibited but little increase in protoporphyrin takes place, while in chronic lead poisoning, both inhibition of ALA-D and elevation of protoporphyrin are observed. A widely cited statement (Comm. Biol. Effects of Atmospheric Pollutants, 1972) with regard to ALA-D for the range of blood lead up to 40 µg/100 ml blood that "its biological significance is dubious, because it is unaccompanied by any detectable effects on the biological function of intact man", should be challenged since ALA-D activity is the most sensitive indicator of a metabolic response to increased lead absorption.

Determination of urinary ALA or coproporphyrin is considered less accurate in identifying children with mild-to-moderate increases in lead absorption (SPECTOR et al., 1971).

There are a few other parameters which are obviously the expression of toxic effects of lead, but their correlation with increased lead absorption has not been established. For example, changes of nerve conduction velocities due to lead do not correlate with blood lead levels (SEPPELAINEN, 1974); nor is the potassium efflux from erythrocytes caused by lead proportional to blood lead concentration (PASSOW, 1970).

G. Summary

A large body of evidence in a variety of systems in vivo or in vitro indicates that lead inhibits the biosynthesis of heme at various steps. Major sites which are inhibited by lead are ALA-D and ferrochelatase. Both enzymes require sulfhydryl groups for the maximal activity and lead interferes with the catalytic activity of the enzyme by binding to SH groups. Lead-inhibited activity of ALA-D can be restored to normal by SH donors or by zinc or by chelation therapy with EDTA in vitro or in vivo. There is no evidence which indicates that lead inhibits the synthesis or accelerates the degradation of these enzymes.

Erythrocyte ALA-D activity is significantly correlated with the blood lead level. The logarithm of ALA-D activity decreases linearly with the increase in blood lead concentration. The reduction of ALA-D activity occurs both in acute and chronic lead poisoning and it is a very sensitive index of lead exposure. Unlike the inhibition of ALA-D activity, increased erythrocyte protoporhyrin is found only in chronic lead exposure. It is a reflection of lead effects on bone marrow erythroblasts, and is an extremely useful index for the biological effects of lead.

Clinically, children with blood lead levels at or higher than 60 μg/100 ml blood or adults at or higher than 80 μg/100 ml are considered as lead-poisoned subjects and should be treated. However, increased erythrocyte protoporhyrin and inhibition of erythrocyte ALA-D activity or increased urinary ALA excretion can be observed in subjects with blood lead levels lower than these concentrations. These subjects may be termed a "subclinically lead-poisoned" subjects. No adverse effects of lead have been described in any red cell enzyme systems at lead concentrations lower than 15 μg/100 ml blood. It appears that this figure represents the body's reserve capacity for binding lead to remove it from functionally important sites. However, a linear increase of blood lead levels above 40 μg/100 ml blood results in an exponential increase of erythrocyte protoporphyrin, an exponential decrease in ALA-D activity, and exponential increase in urinary ALA concentration.

These data suggest that lead has some toxic effects on the heme biosynthetic pathway even in the subclinical range or "normal" range. At or above 60 μg/100 ml in children or 80 μg/100 ml in adults, lead effects on hematopoietic tissues can no longer be compensated, yielding usually mild, but sometimes severe anemia. Lead inhibition of heme biosynthesis is most evident in hematopoietic tissues; however, acute administration of massive doses of lead in the rat is known to cause reduction of hepatic cyt. P-450 and related drug hydroxylase activities. ALA-D activity in the brain of lead-poisoned rat is also known to decrease. Whether the lead-inhibited ALA-D activity may lead to decreased formation of cytochromes in brain cells is yet to be determined.

Lead has also a number of other toxic effects in addition to its adverse effects on heme biosynthesis. Lead affects the red cell membrane to cause rapid loss of potassium, leading to an early destruction of the cells. It reduces the number of immunocompetent cells as well as antibody formation. It causes encephalopathy as well as peripheral neuropathy. It forms intranuclear inclusion bodies in the convoluted proximal tubule cells in the kidney and sometimes yields amino-aciduria due to nephropathy.

It should be pointed out that toxic effects of lead can be modified by a number of factors. For example, coexisting iron deficiency anemia potentiates the toxic effects of lead. Thus even low lead exposure may become toxic in iron-deficient subjects. The toxic effects of lead also appear to be potentiated in subjects with abnormal hemoglobinopathy. On the other hand, pretreatment with a small dose of lead apparently confers a tolerance to an animal against a larger dose of lead through a mechanism which is not clear. Thus it is important to understand these interplays between lead and other factors in order to characterize fully the biological effects of lead.

Toxic effects of lead on heme biosynthesis have been well elucidated. On the other hand, lead-poisoned subjects suffer from neurological disturbances rather than from derangement of heme biosynthesis. There is much to be learned as to the toxic effects of lead, in the nervous system in particular, whether they are the direct results of lead toxicity or secondary effects due to derangements of heme synthesis in these tissues.

Acknowledgment : The author is indebted to Doctors S. GRANICK, A KAPPAS and P. SINCLAIR of the Rockfeller University, New York. N. Y., for their critical reading of the manuscript. Secretarial assistance of Mrs. HEIDI ROBINSON and Miss SUSAN VANDERPOOL is also acknowledged with gratitude.

Abbreviations

ALA	δ-Aminolevulinic Acid
ALA-D	δ-Aminolevulinic Acid Dehydratase
PBG	Porphobilinogen
URO	Uroporphyrinogen
COPRO	Coproporphyrinogen
PROTO	Protoporhyrin
Hb	Hemoglobin
PCV	Packed cell volume
MCHC	Mean corpuscular hemoglobin concentration
IgG	Immunoglobulin G
p-CMB	*p*-Chloromercuribenzoate

References

Abdulla, M., Haeger-Aronsen, B.: ALA-dehydratase activation by zinc. Enzyme **12**, 708 – 710 (1971)

Albahary, C.: Lead and hemopoiesis. The mechanism and consequences of the erythropathy of occupational lead poisoning. Amer. J. Med. **52**, 367 – 378 (1972)

Alvares, A.P., Kapelner, S., Sassa, S., Kappas, A.: Drug metabolism in normal children, lead-poisoned children, and normal adults. Clin Pharmacol. Ther. **17**, 179 – 183 (1975)

Alvares, A.P., Leigh, S., Cohn, J., Kappas, A.: Lead and methyl mercury; Effects of acute exposure on cytochrome P-450 and the mixed function oxidase system in the liver. J. exp. Med. **135**, 1406 – 1409 (1972)

Angle, C.R., McIntyre, M.S.: Red cell lead, whole blood lead, and red cell enzymes. Environ. Hlth Persp. **7**, 133 – 137 (1974)

Baloh, R.W.: Laboratory diagnosis of increased lead absorption. Arch. environ. Hlth **28**, 198 – 208 (1974)

Barltrop, D.: The prevalence of pica. Am. J. Dis. Child. **112**, 116 – 123 (1966)

Barltrop, D., Smith, A.: Interaction of lead with erythrocytes. Experientia (Basel) **27**, 92 – 93 (1971)

Batolska, A., Marinova, H.: Modifications du glutathion chez les travailleurs d'une entreprise metallurgique minière. Arch. Mal. prof. **31**, 117 – 122 (1970)

Battistini, V., Morrow, J.J., Ginsburg, D., Thompson, G., Moore, M.R., Goldberg, A.: Erythrocyte delta-aminolaevulinic acid dehydratase activity in anaemia. Brit. J. Haemat. **20**, 177 – 184 (1971)

Baum, S.: Incorporation of magnesium ion into porphyrins. Ph. D. Dissertation, Cornell University, Ithaca, N.Y. 1965

Beaver, D.L.: The ultrastructure of the kidney in lead intoxication with particular reference to intranuclear inclusions. Amer. J. Path. **39**, 195 – 208 (1961)

Becker, D., Viljoen, D., Kramer, S.: The inhibition of red cell and brain ATPase by δ-aminolevulinic acid. Biochim. Biophys. Acta **25**, 26 – 34 (1971)

Ber, R., Valero, A.: Pica and hypochromic anemia: A survey of 14 cases seen in Israel. Hebrew med. J. **61**, 35 – 39 (1961)

Berk, P.D., Tschudy, D.P., Shepley, L.A., Waggoner, J.G., Berlin, N.I.: Hematologic and biochemical studies in a case of lead poisoning. Amer. J. Med. **48**, 137 – 144 (1970)

Bessis, M.C., Breton-Gorius, J.: Ferritin and ferruginous miscelles in normal erythroblasts and hypochromic hypersideremic anemias. Blood **14**, 423 – 432 (1959)

Bessis, M.C., Jensen, W.N.: Sideroblastic anemia, mitochondria and erythroblastic iron. Brit. J. Haemat. **11**, 49 – 51 (1965)

Beutler, E., Dern, R.J., Flanagan, C.L., Alving, A.S.: The hemolytic effect of primaquine VII. Biochemical studies of drug-sensitive erythrocytes. J. Lab. clin. Med. **45**, 286 – 295 (1955)

Blackman, S.S., Jr.: Intranuclear inclusion bodies in the kidney and liver caused by lead poisoning. Bull. Johns Hopk. Hosp. **58**, 384 – 404 (1936)

Blumberg, W.E., Eisinger, J., Lamola, A.A., Zuckerman, D.M.: A new quick test for lead poisoning: A dedicated portable hematofluorometer. J. Lab. clin. Med. **89**, 712 – 723 (1977)

Bogorad, L.: The enzymatic synthesis of porphyrins from porphyrinogen III. Uroporphyrinogens as intermediates. J. biol. Chem. **233**, 516 – 519 (1958)

Bonkowsky, H.L., Bloomer, J.R., Ebert, P.S., Mahoney, M.J.: Heme synthetase deficiency in human protoporphyria. Demonstration of the defect in liver and cultured skin fibroblasts. J. clin. Invest. **56**, 1139 – 1148 (1975)

Bonsignore, D., Calissano, P., Cartasegna, C.: Un semplice metodo per la determinazione della δ-amino-levulinicodeidratasi nel sangue: comportamento dell'enzima nell'intossicazione saturnina. Med. d. Lavoro **56**, 199 – 205 (1965)

Bonsignore, B., Cartasegna, C., Ardoino, V., Vergnano, C.: Glutatione ridotto eritrocitario nel saturnismo. Lav. um. **19**, 97 – 102 (1967)

Borová J., Ponka, P., Neuwirt, J.: Study of intracellular iron distribution in rabbit reticulocytes with normal and inhibited heme synthesis. Biochim. biophys. Acta **320**, 143 – 156 (1973)

Bottomley, S.S., Tanaka, M., Everett, M.A.: Diminished erythroid ferrochelatase activity in protoporphyria. J. Lab. clin. Med. **86**, 126 – 131 (1975)

Bracken, E.C., Beaver, D.L., Randall, C.C.: Histochemical studies of viral and lead-induced intranuclear bodies. J. Path. Bact. **75**, 253 – 256 (1958)

Burch, H.B., Siegel, A.L.: Improved method for measurement of delta-aminolevulinic acid dehydratase activity of human erythrocytes. Clin. Chem. **17**, 1038 – 1041 (1971)

Burnham, B., Lascelles, J.: Control of porphyrin biosynthesis through a negative-feedback mechadism. Studies with preparations of δ-aminolevulinate synthetase and δ-aminolaevulate dehydratase from *Rhodopseudomonas spheroides*. Biochem. J. **87**, 462 – 472 (1963)

Calissano, P., Bonsignore, D., Cartasegna, C.: Control of heme synthesis by feedback inhibition on human-erythrocyte δ-aminolaevulinate dehydratase. Biochem. J. **101**, 550 – 552 (1966)

Carlander, O.: Aetiology of pica. Lancet **1959 II**, 569

Cartwright, G.E., Deiss, A.: Sideroblasts, siderocytes and sideroblastic anemia. New Engl. J. Med. **292**, 185 – 193 (1975)

Charache, S., Weatherall, D.J.: Fast hemoglobin in lead poisoning. Blood **28**, 377 – 386 (1966)

Chisolm, J.J., Jr., Barrett, M.B., Mettits, E.D.: Dose-effect and dose-response relationships for lead in children. J. Pediat. in press (1975b)

Chisolm, J.J., Jr., Brown, D.H.: Micro-scale photofluorometric determination of "free erythro-cyte porphyrin" (Protoporphyrin IX). Clin. Chem. in press (1975a)

Choie, D.D., Richter, G.W.: Cell proliferation in rat kidneys after prolonged treatment with lead. Amer. J. Path. **68**, 359–367 (1972a)

Choie, D.D., Richter, G.W.: Cell proliferation in rat kidney by lead acetate and effects of uninephrectomy on the proliferation. Amer. J. Path. **66**, 265–276 (1972b)

Choie, D., Richter, G.: Lead poisoning: Rapid formation of intranuclear inclusions. Science **177**, 1194–1195 (1972c)

Choie, D.D., Richter, G.W.: Stimulation of DNA synthesis in rat kidney by repeated administra-tion of lead. Proc. Soc. exp. Biol. (N.Y.) **142**, 446–449 (1973)

Clarkson, T.W., Kench, J.E.: Uptake of lead by human erythrocytes in vitro. Biochem. J. **69**, 432–439 (1958)

Clemens, M.J., Henshaw, E.C., Rahamimoff, H., London, I.M.: Met-tRNA$_{met}$ binding to 40S ribosomal subunits: A site for the regulation of initiation of protein synthesis by hemin. Proc. nat. Acad. Sci. (Wash.) **71**, 2946–2950 (1974)

Coleman, D.L.: Purification and properties of δ-aminolevulinate dehydratase from tissues of two strains of mice. J. biol. Chem. **241**, 5511–5517 (1966)

Collier, H.B.: A study of the determination of δ-aminolevulinate hydrolyase (δ-aminolaevulinate dehydratase) activity in hemolysates of human erythrocytes. Clin. Biochem. **4**, 222–232 (1971)

Committee on Biologic Effects of Atmospheric Pollutants. Lead; airborne lead in perspective. Nat. Acad. Sci. 1972, p. 81–84, Washington, D.C.

Cramér, K.: Predisposing factors for lead poisoning. Acta med. scand. **179** (Suppl. 445), 56–59 (1966)

Cremer, J.E.: Toxicology and biochemistry of alkyl lead compounds. Occup. Hlth Rev. **17**, 14–19 (1965)

Cunningham, A.G., Szenberg, A.: Further improvements in the plaque technique for detecting single antibody-forming cells. Immunology **14**, 599–601 (1968)

Dagg, J.H., Goldberg, A., Lockhead, A., Smith J.A.: The relationship of lead poisoning to acute intermittent porphyria. Quart. J. Med. **34**, 163–175 (1965)

De Bruin, A., Hoolboom, H.: Early signs of lead exposure. A comparative study of laboratory tests. Brit. J. industr. Med. **24**, 203–212 (1967)

De Goeiji, A.F.P.M., Christianse, K., Van Steveninck, J.: Decreased haem synthetase activity in blood cells of patients with erythropoietic protoporphyria. Europ. J. clin. Invest. **5**, 397–400 (1975)

Dimant, E., Landerg, E., London, I.M.: The metabolic behavior of reduced glutathione in human and avian erythrocytes. J. biol. Chem. **213**, 769–776 (1955)

Doyle, D., Schimke, R.T.: The genetic and developmental regulation of hepatic δ-aminolevulinate dehydratase in mice. J. Biol. Chem. **244**, 5449–5459 (1969)

Dresel, E.I.B., Falk, J.D.: Studies on the biosynthesis of blood pigments. 2. Haem and porphyrin formation in intact chicken erythrocytes. Biochem. J. **63**, 72–79 (1956a)

Dresel, E.I.B., Falk, J.D.: Studies on the biosynthesis of blood pigments. 3. Haem and porphyrin formation from δ-aminolaevulinic acid and from porphobilinogen in haemolysed chicken erythrocytes. Biochem. J. **63**, 80–87 (1956b)

Epstein, S.S., Mantel, N.: Carcinogenicity of tetraethyl lead. Experientia (Basel) **24**, 580–581 (1968)

Erenberg, G., Rinsler, S.S., Fish, B.G.: Lead neuropathy and sickle cell disease. Pediatrics **54**, 438–441 (1974)

Estabrook, R.W., Hildebrandt, A., Remmer, H., Schenkman, J.B., Rosenthal, O., Cooper, D.Y.: The role of cytochrome P-450 in microsomal mixed function oxidation reactions. In: Hess and Staudinger 19th Colloquium der Gesellschaft für Biologische Chemie. Berlin: Springer 1968

Fairbanks, V.F., Beutler, E.: Iron deficiency. In: Hematology. New York: McGraw-Hill 1972

Falk, J.E.: Porphyrins and Metalloporphyrins, Vol. 2. New York: Elsevier 1964

Feldman, D.S., Levere, R.D., Lieberman, J.S., Cardinal, R.A., Watson, C.J.: Presynaptic neuromuscular inhibition by porphobilinogen and porphobilin. Proc. nat. Acad. Sci (Wash.) **68**, 383–386 (1971)

Ferguson, J.H., Keaton, A.G.: Studies of the diets of pregnant women in Mississipi: Ingestion of clay and laundry starch. New Orleans med. surg. J. **102**, 460 – 463 (1950)

Ferm, V.H.: The synteratogenic effect of lead and cadmium. Experientia (Basel) **25**, 56 – 57 (1969)

Ferm, V.H., Carpenter, S.J.: Developmental malformations resulting from the administration of lead salts. J. cxp. molec. Path. **7**, 208 – 213 (1967a)

Ferm, V.H., Carpenter, S.J.: Teratogenic effect of cadmium and its inhibition by zinc. Nature (Lond.) **216**, 1123 (1967b)

Ferm, V.H., Carpenter, S.J.: The relationship of cadmium and zinc in experimental mammalian teratogenesis. Lab. Invest. **18**, 429 – 432 (1968)

Finelli, V.N., Klauder, D.S., Karaffa, M.A., Petering, H.G.: Interaction of zinc and lead on δ-aminolevulinate dehydratase. Biochem. biophys. Res. Commun. **65**, 303 – 311 (1975)

Finelli, V.N., Murthy, L., Peirano, W.B., Petering, H.G.: δ-aminolevulinate dehydratase, a zinc dependent enzyme. Biochem. biophys. Res. Commun. **60**, 1418 – 1424 (1974)

Fischbein, A., Sassa, S., Eisinger, J., Blumberg, W.: Blood lead and protoporphyrin levels in lead exposed workers. The application of a new method for the detection of lead poisoning. Proc. Int. Conf. on Heavy Metals in the Environment. Toronto, Ontario, Canada, Oct., 1975

Forbes, G.B., Reino, J.C.: Effect of age on gastrointestinal absorption (Fe, Sr, Pb) in the rat. J. Nutr. **102**, 647 – 652 (1972)

Fratianne, R.B., Griggs, R.C., Harris, J.W.: Autosurvival of erythrocytes treated in vitro with lead chlorides. Clin. Res. **7**, 384 (1958)

French, S.W., Todoroff, T.: Hepatic mitochondrial fragility and permeability. Arch. Path. (Chicago) **89**, 329 – 336 (1970)

Fullerton, J.M.: Value of hematology in diagnosis of chronic plumbism. Brit. med. J. **1952 II**, 117 – 119

Gajdos, A., Gajdos-Török, M.: Delta-aminolevulinic acid synthetase and adenosine triphosphate activity in acute saturnine intoxication in rabbits. Arch. environ. Hlth. **23**, 270 – 274 (1971)

Galzigna, L., Corsi, G.C., Saia, B., Rizzoli, A.A.: Inhibitory effect of triethyl lead on serum choline esterase in vitro. Clin. chim. Acta **26**, 391 – 393 (1969)

Gibson, S.M., Goldberg, A.: Defects in heme synthesis in mammalian tissues in experimental lead poisoning and experimental porphyria. Clin. Sci. **38**, 63 – 72 (1970)

Gibson, K.D. Laver, W.G., Neuberger, A.: Initial stages in the biosynthesis of porphyrins. 2. The formation of δ-aminolaevulinic acid from glycine and succinyl coenzyme A by particles from chicken erythrocytes. Biochem. J. **70**, 71 – 81 (1958)

Gibson, S.L.M., MacKenzie, G.C., Goldberg, A.: The diagnosis of industrial lead poisoning. Brit. J. industr. Med. **26**, 40 – 51 (1968)

Gibson, K.D., Neuberger, A., Scott, J.J.: The purification and properties of δ-aminolaevulinic acid dehydratase. Biochem. J. **61**, 618 – 629 (1955)

Goldberg, A.: Lead poisoning as a disorder of heme synthesis. Semin. Hemat. **5**, 424 – 433 (1968)

Goldberg, A., Ashenbrucker, G.E., Cartwright, G.E., Wintrobe, M.M.: Studies on the biosynthesis of heme in vitro by avian erythrocytes. Blood **11**, 821 – 833 (1956)

Goldberg, A., McGillion, F.B.: Central uptake and cardiovascular effects of δ-aminolaevulinic acid. Brit. J. Pharmacol. **49**, 178 (1973)

Goldberg, A., Paton, W.D.M., Thompson, J.W.: Pharmacology of porphyrins and porphobilinogen. Brit. J. Pharmacol. **9**, 91 – 94 (1954)

Goudy, B., Dawes, E., Wilkinson, A.E., Wills, E.D.: Ferrochelatase activity in normal and irradiated animal tissues. Europ. J. Biochem. **3**, 208 – 212 (1967)

Goyer, R.A.: The renal tubule in lead poisoning. I. Mitochondrial swelling and aminoaciduria. Lab. Invest. **19**, 71 – 77 (1968)

Goyer, R.A.: Lead and the kidney. Curr. Top. Path. **55**, 147 – 176 (1971)

Goyer, R.A., Leonard, D., Moore, J.F., Rhyne, B., Krigman, M.R.: Lead dosage and the role of the intranuclear inclusion body. Arch environ. Hlth **20**, 705 – 711 (1970)

Grafflin, A.L.: Histological observations upon the porphyrin excreting Harderian gland of the albino rat. Amer. J. Anat. **71**, 43 – 64 (1942)

Granick, S.: The induction in vitro of the synthesis of δ-aminolevulinic acid synthetase in chemical porphyria. A response to certain drugs, sex hormones, and foreign chemicals. J. biol. Chem. **241**, 1359 – 1375 (1966)

Granick, S., Mauzerall, D.: Porphyrin biosynthesis in erythrocytes. II. Enzymes converting δ-aminolevulinic acid to coproporphyrinogen. J. biol. Chem. **232**, 1119 – 1140 (1958)

Granick, S., Sassa, S., Granick, J.L., Levere, R.D., Kappas, A.: Assays for porphyrins, δ-aminolevulinic acid dehydratase, and porphyrinogen synthetase in microliter samples of whole blood: Applications to metabolic defects involving the heme pathway. Proc. nat. Acd. Sci. (Wash.) **69**, 2381 – 2385 (1972)

Granick, J.L., Sassa, S., Granick, S., Levere, R.D., Kappas, A.: Studies in lead poisoning. II. Correlation between the ratio of activated to inactivated δ-aminolevulinic acid dehydratase of whole blood and the blood lead level. Biochem. Med. **8**, 149 – 159 (1973)

Granzoni, A., Rhomberg, F.: Hämolytische Krise bei Mangel an Glukose-6-phosphatdehydrogenase und Bleiintoxikation. Acta hemat. (Basel) **34**, 338 – 346 (1965)

Greenbaum, D., Richardson, P.C., Salmon, M.V., Urich, H.: Pathological observation on six cases of diabetic neuropathy. Brain **87**, 201 – 214 (1964)

Greer, M., Schotland, D.: Abnormal hemoglobin as a cause of neurologic disease. Neurology (Minneap.) **12**, 114 – 123 (1962)

Grigarzik, H., Passow, H.: Versuche zum Mechanismus der Bleiwirkung auf die Kaliumpermeabilität roter Blutkörperchen. Pflügers Arch. ges. Physiol. **267**, 73 – 92 (1958)

Griggs, R.C.: Lead poisoning. Hematologic aspects. Progr. Hemat. **4**, 117 – 137 (1964)

Griggs, R.C., Harris, J.W.: Erythrocyte survival and heme synthesis in lead poisoning. Clin. Res. **6**, 188 (1958)

Grinstein, M., Bannerman, R.M., Moore, C.V.: The utilization of protoporphyrin IX in heme synthesis. Blood **14**, 476 – 489 (1959)

Gunn, S.A., Gould, T.C., Anderson, W.A.D.: Specific response of mesenchymal tissue to carcinogenesis by cadmium. Arch. Path. (Chicago) **83**, 493 – 499 (1967)

Gurba, P.E., Sennet, R.E., Kobes, R.D.: Studies on the mechanism of action of δ-aminolevulinate dehydratase from bovine and rat liver. Arch. Biochem. **150**, 130 – 136 (1972)

Gutelius, M.F., Millican, F.K., Layman, E.M., Cohen, G.J., Dublin, C.C.: Nutritional studies of children with pica: I. Controlled study evaluating nutritional status. Pediatrics **29**, 1012 – 1023 (1962)

Gutelius, M.F., Millican, Y.K., Layman, E.M., Cohen, G.J., Dublin, C.C.: Treatment of pica with a vitamin and mineral supplement. Amer. J. clin. Nutr. **12**, 388 – 393 (1963)

Haeger-Aronsen, B.: Studies on urinary excretion of δ-aminolevulinic acid and other heme precursors in lead workers and lead-intoxicated rabbits. Scand. J. clin. Lab. Invest. **12** (Suppl. 47) 1 – 28 (1960)

Haeger-Aronsen, B., Abdulla, M., Fristedt, B.I.: Effect of lead on δ-aminolevulinic acid dehydratase in red blood cells. Arch. environ. Hlth **23**, 440 – 445 (1971)

Harris, J.W., Greenberg, M.S.: Erythrocyte fragilities in plumbism. Clin. Res. Proc. **2**, 55 (1954)

Harris, J.W., Kellermeyer, R.W.: The Red Cell. Production, Metabolism, Destruction: Normal and Abnormal. Cambridge, Mass.: Harvard University Press 1970

Hasan, J., Vihko, V., Hernberg, S.: Deficient red cell membrane $(Na^+ + K^+)$-ATPase in lead poisoning. Arch. environ. Hlth. **14**, 313 – 318 (1967)

Hass, G.M., Brown, D.V.L., Eisenstein, R., Hemmens, A.: Relations between lead poisoning in rabbit and man. Amer. J. Path. **45**, 691 – 727 (1964)

Hemphill, F.E., Kaeberle, M.L., Buck, W.B.: Lead suppression of mouse resistance to *Salmonella typhimurium*. Science **172**, 1031 – 1032 (1971).

Hernberg, S., Nikkanen, G.: Enzyme inhibition by lead under normal urban conditions. Lancet **1970 I**, 63 – 64

Hoogeveen, J.T.: Thermoconductometric investigation of phosphatidylcholine in aqueous tertiary butanol solutions in the absence and presence of metal ions. In: Effect of Metals on Cells, Subcellular Elements and Macromolecules. Springfield, Ill.: Thomas 1970

HSMHA: Medical aspects of childhood poisoning. HSMHA Hlth Rep. **86**, 140 – 143 (1971)

Icen, A.: Glutathione reductase of human erythrocytes. Purification and properties. Scand. J. clin. Lab. Invest. Suppl. **96**, 1 – 67 (1967)

Israels, L.G.: Inhibition of heme synthesis in the kidney by organic mercurials. Biochem. Pharmacol. **21**, 434 – 435 (1972)

Jandl, J.H.: The agglutination and sequestration of immature red cells. J. Lab. clin. Med. **55**, 663 – 681 (1960)

Jarrett, A., Rimington, C., Willoughby, D.A.: δ-aminolaevulinic acid and porphyria. Lancet **1956 I,** 125 – 127

Jensen, W.N., Moreno, G.D., Bessis, M.C.: An electron microscopic description of basophilic stippling in red cells. Blood **25,** 933 – 943 (1965)

Jones, O.T.G.: Ferrochelatase of spinach chloroplasts. Biochem. J. **107,** 113 – 119 (1968)

Jordan, P.M., Shemin, D.: Uroporphyrinogen I synthetase from *R. spheroides.* Purification and properties. Fed. Proc. **30,** 1260 (1971)

Jordan, P.M., Shemin, D.: Purification and properties of uroporphyrinogen I synthetase from *Rhodopseudomonas spheroides.* J. biol. Chem. **248,** 1019 – 1024 (1973)

Joyce, C.R.B., Moore, H.L., Weatherall, M.: Effects of lead, mercury and gold on the potassium turnover of rabbit blood cells. Brit. J. Pharmacol. **9,** 463 – 470 (1954)

Kagawa, Y., Minakami, S., Yoneyama, Y.: Heme synthesis in the soluble preparation from avian erythrocytes. J. Biochem. **46,** 771 – 780 (1959)

Kammholz, L.P., Thatcher, L.G., Blodgett, F.M., Good, T.A.: Rapid protoporphyrin quantitation for detection of lead poisoning. Pediatrics **50,** 625 – 631 (1972)

Kappas, A., Alvares, A.P.: How the liver metabolizes foreign substances. Sci. Amer. **232,** 22 – 31 (1975)

Karibian, D., London, I.M.: Control of heme synthesis by feedback inhibition. Biochem. biophys. Res. Commun. **18,** 243 – 249 (1965)

Kassenaar, A., Morell, H., London, I.M.: The incorporation of glycine into globin and the synthesis of heme in vitro in duck erythrocytes. J. biol. Chem. **229,** 423 – 435 (1957)

Kehoe, R.A.: Normal metabolism of lead. Arch. environ. Hlth **8,** 232 – 235 (1964)

Kjellström, T., Eng, M.: Mathematical and statistical approaches in evaluating dose-response relationships for metals. In: Effects and Dose-Response Relationships of Toxic Metals. Amsterdam: Elevier 1975

Koller, L.D., Kovacic, S.: Decreased antibody formation in mice exposed to lead. Nature (Lond.) **250,** 148 – 150 (1974)

Komai, H., Neilands, J.B.: The metalloprotein nature of Ustilago δ-aminolevulinate dehydratase. Biochim. biophys. Acta **171,** 311 – 320 (1969)

Kostial, K., McMcilovic, B.: Transport of lead[203] and calcium[47] from mother to offspring. Arch. environ. Hlth **29,** 28 – 30 (1975)

Kreimer-Birnbaum, M., Grinstein, M.: Porphyrin biosynthesis III. Porphyrin metabolism in experimental lead poisoning. Biochim. biophys. Acta **111,** 110 – 123 (1965)

Labbe, P., Volland, C., Chaix, P.: Etude de l'activité ferrochélatase des mitochondries de levure. Biochim. biophys. Acta **159,** 527 – 539 (1968)

Labbe, R.F., Hubbard, N.: Preparation and properties of iron-proto chelating enzyme. Biochim. biophys. Acta **41,** 185 – 191 (1960)

Lamola, A.A., Joselow, M., Yamane, T.: Zinc protoporphyrin (ZPP): A simple sensitive, fluorometric screening test for lead poisoning. Clin. Chem. **21,** 93 – 97 (1975a)

Lamola, A.A., Piomelli, S., Poh-Fitzpatrick, M., Yamane, T., Harber, L.: Erythropoietic protoporphyria and Pb intoxication: The molecular basis for difference in cutaneous photosensitivity. II. Different binding of erythrocyte protoporphyrin to hemoglobin. J. clin. Invest. **56,** 1528 – 1535 (1975b)

Lamola, A.A., Yamane, T.: Zinc protoporhyrin in the erythrocytes of patients with lead intoxication and iron deficiency anemia. Science **186,** 936 – 938 (1974)

Landow, S.A., Schooley, J.C., Arroyo, F.L.: Decreased erythropoietin synthesis and impaired erythropoiesis in acutely lead-poisoned rats. Clin. Res. **21,** 559 (1973)

Lanzkowsky, P.: Investigation into the aetiology and treatment of pica. Arch. Dis. Childh. **34,** 140 – 148 (1959)

Lauwerys, R., Buchet, J.P.: Relationship between occupational exposure to mercury vapors and biological action. Arch. environ. Hlth **27,** 65 – 68 (1973)

Leiken, S., Eng, G.: Erythrokinetic studies of the anemia of lead poisoning. Pediatrics **31,** 996 – 1002 (1963)

Lessler, M.A., Cardona, E., Padilla, F., Jensen, W.N.: Effect of lead on reticulocyte respiratory activity. J. Cell Biol. **39,** 171 a (1968)

Lin-Fu, J.S.: Undue absorption of lead among children – A new look at an old problem. New Engl. J. Med. **286,** 702 – 710 (1972)

Llambias, E.B.C., Del C. Battle, A.M.: Porphyrin biosynthesis VIII. Avian erythrocyte porphobilinogen deaminase. Uroporphyrinogen III cosynthetase, its purification, properties and the separation of its components. Biochim. biophys. Acta **227**, 180 – 191 (1971)

Maines, M.D., Kappas, A.: Studies on the mechanism of induction of heme oxygenase by cobalt and other metal ions. Biochem. J. **154**, 125 – 131 (1976a)

Maines, M.D., Kappas, A.: The induction of heme oxidation in various tissues by trace metals: Evidence for the catabolism of endogenous heme by hepatic heme oxygenase. Procedings of the International Conference on Porphyrin Metabolism, Sannas, Finland (1976b)

Marver, H.S., Collins, A., Tschudy, D.P., Rechcigl, M.Jr.: δ-Aminolevulinic acid synthetase. II. Induction in rat liver. J. biol. Chem. **241**, 4323 – 4329 (1966b)

Marver, H.S., Tschudy, D.P., Perlroth, M.G., Collins, A.: δ-Aminolevulinic acid synthetase. I. Studies in liver homogenates. J. biol. Chem. **241**, 2803 – 2809 (1966a)

Mauzerall, D.: Normal porphyrin metabolism. J. Pediatr. **64**, 5 – 16 (1964)

Mauzerall, D., Granick, S.: The occurrence and determination of δ-aminolevulinic acid and porphobilinogen in urine. J. biol. Chem. **219**, 435 – 446 (1956)

McIntire, M.S., Angle, C.R.: Air lead; relation to lead in blood of black school children deficient in glucose-6-phosphate dehydrogenase. Science **177**, 520 – 522 (1972)

McLaren, G.D., Carpenter, J.T.Jr., Nino, H.V.: Erythrocyte protoporhyrin in the detection of iron deficiency. Clin. Chem. **21**, 1121 – 1127 (1975)

Meredith, P.A., Moore, M.R., Goldberg, A.: Effects of aluminum, lead, and zinc on delta-aminolaevulinic acid dehydratase. Biochem. Soc. Trans. **2**, 1243 – 1245 (1974)

Meyer, U.A., Schmid, R.: Hereditary hepatic porphyrias. Fed. Proc. **32**, 1649 – 1655 (1973)

Miani, N., Viterbo, B.: Studio isoautoradiografico sulla localizzazione del piombo (RaD) in vari organi di cane. Z. Zellforsch. **49**, 188 – 208 (1958)

Millar, J.A., Battistini, V., Cumming, R.L.C., Carswell, F., Goldberg, A.: Lead and δ-aminolevulinic acid dehydratase levels in mentally retarded children and in lead-poisoned suckling rats. Lancet **1970 II**, 695 – 698

Miyagi, K., Cardinal, R., Bossenmaier, I., Watson, C.J.: The serum porphobilinogen and hepatic porphobilinogen deaminase in normal and porphyric individuals. J. Lab. clin. Med. **78**, 683 – 695 (1971)

Moore, M.R.: Lead, ethanol and δ-aminolaevulinate dehydratase. Biochem. J. **129**, 43P – 44P (1972)

Moore, A., Harris, F.: Erythrocyte hypoplasia due to lead poisoning. A devastating, yet curable disease. Clin. Pediat. **8**, 400 – 402 (1969)

Mooty, J., Ferrand, C.F.Jr., Harris, P.: Relationship of diet to lead poisoning in children. Pediatrics **55**, 636 – 639 (1975)

Morrow, J.J., Urata, G., Goldberg, A.: The effect of lead and ferrous and ferric iron on δ-aminolevulinic acid synthetase. Clin. Sci. **37**, 533 – 538 (1969)

Muirhead, E.E., Groves, M., Bryan, S.: Positive direct Coombs test induced by phenylhydrazine. J. clin. Invest. **33**, 1700 – 1711 (1954)

Nagai, T., Huse, T., Saikawa, S.: On the change of blood glutathione level in experimentally lead-poisoned rabbits. Sci. Labour (Japan) **32**, 390 – 403 (1956)

Nakao, K., Wada, O., Yano, Y.: δ-aminolevulinic acid dehydratase activity in erythrocytes for the evaluation of lead poisoning. Clin. chim. Acta **19**, 319 – 325 (1968)

Nandi, D.L., Baker-Cohen, K.F., Shemin, D.: δ-aminolevulinic acid dehydratase of *Rhodopseudomonas spheroides*. I. Isolation and properties. J. biol. Chem. **243**, 1224 – 1230 (1968)

Narisawa, K., Kikuchi, G.: Effect of inhibitors of DNA synthesis on allylisopropylacetamide induced increases of δ-aminolevulinc acid synthetase and other enzymes in rat liver. Biochim. biophys. Acta **99**, 580 – 583 (1965)

NIOSH: Criteria for a recommended standard, occupational exposure to inorganic lead. U.S. Department of Health, Education, and Welfare, Public Health Service. National Institute for Occupational Safety and Health, 1972.

Ono, T., Wada, O., Nagahashi, M., Yamaguchi, N., Toyokawa, K.: Maximum levels of the increased sulfhydryl group in a special protein fraction extracted from kidney of mice administered with cadmium. Industr. Hlth **11**, 243 – 244 (1973a)

Ono, T., Wada, O., Nagahashi, M., Yamaguchi, N., Toyokawa, K.: Increase of sulfhydryl group in proteins from kidney of mice administered with various heavy metals. Industr. Health **11**, 73 – 74 (1973b)

Ørskov, S.L.: Untersuchungen über den Einfluss von Kohlensäure und Blei auf die Permeabilität der Blutkörperchen für Kalium and Rubidium. Biochem. Z. **279**, 250—261 (1935)

Oyama, H., Sugita, Y., Yoneyama, Y., Yoshikawa, H.: Stoichiometry of heme synthesis by partially purified enzyme prepared from duck erythrocytes. Biochim. biophys. Acta **47**, 413—414 (1961)

Paglia, D.E., Valentine, W.N.: Characteristics of a pyrimidine-specific 5'-nucleotidase in human erythrocytes. J. biol. Chem. **250**, 7973—7979 (1975)

Paglia, D.E., Valentine, W.N., Dahlgren, J.G.: Effects of low-level lead exposure on pyrimidine 5'-nucleotidase and other erythrocyte enzymes. Possible role of pyrimidine 5'-nucleotidase in the pathogenesis of lead-induced anemia. J. clin. Invest. **56**, 1164—1169 (1975)

Parr, D.R., Harris, E.J.: Enhancement by chelating agents of lead toxicity to mitochondria in the presence of inorganic phosphate. FEBS Lett. **59**, 92—95 (1975)

Passow, H.: Ion and water permeability of the red blood cell. In: The Red Blood Cell: A Comprehensive Treatise. New York: Academic Press 1964

Passow, H.: The red blood cell: Penetration, distribution, and toxic actions of heavy metals. In: Effects of Metals on Cells, Subcellular Elements, and Macromolecules. Springfield, Ill.: Thomas 1970

Passow, H., Rothstein, A., Clarkson, T.W.: The general pharmacology of the heavy metals. Pharmacol. Rev. **13**, 185—224 (1961)

Passow, H., Tillman, K.: Untersuchungen über den Kaliumverlust bleivergifteter Menschenerythrocyten. Pflügers Arch. ges. Physiol. **262**, 23—26 (1955)

Pentschew, A., Garro F.: Lead encephalomyelopathy of suckling rat and implications on the porphyrinopathic nervous diseases. Acta neuropath. (Berl.) **6**, 266—278 (1966)

Piomelli, S.: A micromethod for free erythrocyte porphyrins: The FEP test. J. Lab. clin. Med. **81**, 932—940 (1973)

Piomelli, S., Lamola, A.A., Poh-Fitzpatrick, M.B., Seaman, C., Harber, L.C.: Erythropoietic protoporphyria and Pb intoxication: The molecular basis for difference in cutaneous photosensitivity. I. Different rates of diffusion of protoporhyrin from the erythrocytes, both in vivo and in vitro. J. clin. Invest. **56**, 1519—1527 (1975)

Piper, W.N., Tephly, T.R.: Differential inhibition of erythrocyte and hepatic uroporphyrinogen I synthetase activity by lead. Life Sci. **14**, 873—876 (1974)

Poňka, P., Neuwirt, G.: Mitochondrial iron overload. New Engl. J. Med. **293**, 406 (1975)

Porra, R.J., Jones, O.T.G.: Studies on ferrochelatase. I. Assay and properties of ferrochelatase from a pig-liver mitochondrial extract. Biochem. J. **87**, 181—185 (1963 a)

Porra, R.J., Jones, O.T.G.: Studies on ferrochelatase II. An investigation of the role of ferrochelatase in the biosynthesis of various heme prosthetic groups. Biochem. J. **87**, 186—192 (1963 b)

Porter, S.: Congenital erythropoietic protoporhyria. II. An experimental study. Blood **22**, 532—544 (1963)

Quaterman, J., Morrison, J.N., Humphries, W.R.: The influence of high dietary intakes of calcium on lead retention and release in rats. Proc. Nutr. Soc. **34**, 89—90 A (1975)

Richter, G.W., Kress, Y., Cornwall, C.C.: Another look at lead inclusion bodies. Amer. J. Path. **53**, 189—217 (1968)

Roels, H.A., Buchet, J.P., Lauwerys, R.R., Sonnett, J.: Comparison of in vivo effect of inorganic lead and cadmium on glutathione reductase system and δ-aminolevulinate dehydratase in human erythrocytes. Brit. J. industr. Med. **32**, 181—192 (1975a)

Roels, H.A., Lauwerys, R.R., Buchet, J.P., Vrelust, M.TH.: Response of free erythrocyte porphyrin and urinary δ-aminolevulinic acid in men and women moderately exposed to lead. Int. Arch. Arbeitsmed. **34**, 97—108 (1975b)

Rosen, J.F., Zarate-Salvador, C., Trinidad, E.E.: Plasma lead levels in normal and lead-intoxicated children. J. Pediatr. **84**, 45—48 (1974)

Rosenberg, S.A., Guidotti, G.: Fractionation of the protein components of human erythrocyte membranes. J. biol. Chem. **244**, 5118—5124 (1969)

Rosenthal, A.S., Moses, H.L., Tice, L., Ganote, C.E.: Lead ion and phosphatase histochemistry. III. The effects of lead and adenosine triphosphate concentration on the incorporation of phosphate into fixed tissue. J. Histochem. Cytochem. **17**, 608—616 (1969)

Rubino, G.F., Coscia, G.C., Perrelli, G., Parigi, A.: Comportamento del glutatione del test di stabilita del glutatione e dell'attivita glucosio-6-fosfato-deidrogenasica nel saturnismo. Minerva med. (Torino) **54**, 930 – 932 (1963)

Rubino, G.F., Prato, V., Fiorina, L.: Anemia of lead poisoning: Its nature and pathogenesis. Folia med. (Napoli) **42**, 1 – 20 (1959)

Russell, R.L., Coleman, D.L.: Genetic control of hepatic δ-aminolevulinate dehydratase in mice. Genetics **48**, 1033 – 1039 (1963)

Saita, G., Lussana, S.: Intossicazione da piombo in portatrice de emazie fabiche. Med. d. Lavoro **62**, 22 – 27 (1971)

Sanai, G.H., Hasegawa, T., Yoshikawa, H.: Pretreatment of rats with lead in experimental acute lead poisoning. J. occup. Med. **14**, 301 – 305 (1972)

Sano, S.: The effect of mitochondria on porphyrin and heme biosynthesis in red blood cells. Acta hemat. jap. **21** (Suppl. 2), 337 – 351 (1958)

Sano, S., Granick, S.: Mitochondrial coproporphyrinogen oxidase and protoporphyrin formation. J. biol. Chem. **236**, 1173 – 1180 (1961)

Sassa, S., Granick, J. L., Granick, S., Kappas, A., Levere, R.D.: Studies in lead poisoning I. Microanalysis of erythrocyte protoporphyrin levels by spectrofluorometry in the detection of chronic lead intoxication on the subclinical range. Biochem. Med. **8**, 135 – 148 (1973b)

Sassa, S., Granick, S., Bickers, D.R., Bradlow, H.L., Kappas, A.: Studies in porphyria III. A microassay for uroporphyrinogen I synthetase, one of the three abnormal enzyme activities in acute intermittent porphyria, and its application to the study of the genetics of this disease. Proc. nat. Acad. Sci. (Wash.) **71**, 732 – 736 (1974)

Sassa, S., Granick, S., Bickers, D.R., Levere, R.D., Kappas, A.: Studies on the inheritance of human erythrocyte δ-aminolevulinate dehydratase and uroporphyrinogen synthetase. Enzyme **16**, 326 – 333 (1973a)

Sassa, S., Granick, S., Kappas, A.: Effect of lead and genetic factors on heme biosynthesis in the human red cell. Ann. N.Y. Acad. Sci. **244**, 419 – 440 (1975)

Sawada, H., Takeshita, M., Sugita, Y., Yoneyama, Y.: Effect of lipid on protoheme ferrolyase. Biochim. biophys. Acta **178**, 145 – 155 (1969)

Sawinsky, A., Durzt, J., Pasztor, G.: Leukozytenschädigung by Bleiexposition. Z. ges. Hyg. **17**, 239 – 240 (1971)

Schoomaker, E.B., Prasad, A., Oclshlcgel, F.J., Ortego, J., Brewer, G.J.: Role of zinc in sickle cell disease. I. Zinc deficiency through hemolysis. Clin. Res. **21**, 834 (1973)

Schwartz, S.: Clinical aspects of porphyrin metabolism. V.A. Admin. Techn. Bull. TB 10 – 94, Washington, D.C. (1953)

Scoppa, P., Roumengous, M., Penning, W.: Hepatic drug metabolizing activity in lead-poisoned rats. Experientia (Basel) **29**, 970 – 972 (1973)

Seppelainen, A.M.: Peripheral nervous system in lead exposed workers. In: Behavioral Toxicology. Early Detection of Occupational Hazards. U.S. DHEW, PHS, CDC, NIOSH, HEW Publ. No. (NIOSH) 74 – 126, 1974

Shanley, B.C., Neethling, A.C., Percy, V.A.: Neurochemical aspects of porphyria. S. Afr. med. J. **49**, 576 – 580 (1975)

Shemin, D.: Structure and function of δ-aminolevulinic acid dehydratase. "Porphyrins in Human Diseases", 1st International Porphyrin Meeting, p. 15, Freiburg, Germany 1975

Shemin, D., London, I.M., Rittenberg, D.: The in vitro synthesis of heme from glycine by the nucleated red blood cell. J. biol. Chem. **173**, 799 – 800 (1948)

Shetty, A.S., Miller, G.W.: Purification and general properties of δ-aminolaevulinate dehydratase from Nicotiana tabacum L. Biochem. J. **114**, 331 – 337 (1969)

Shiraishi, A.: Concentration of reduced glutathione in the blood of lead-poisoned persons. Nisshin Igaku **39**, 478 – 483 (1952)

Silverstein, E.: Inhibition of certain mitochondrial oxidative enzymes by porphyrins and metalloporphyrins. Biochem. Pharmacol. **11**, 431 – 444 (1962)

Simpson, C.F., Damron, B.L., Harms, R.H.: Abnormality of erythrocytes and renal tubules of chicks poisoned with lead. Amer. J. vet. Res. **31**, 515 – 523 (1970)

Six, K.M., Goyer, R.A.: Experimental enhancement of lead toxicity by low dietary calcium. J. Lab. clin. Med. **76**, 933 – 940 (1970)

Six, K.M., Goyer, R.A.: The influence of iron deficiency on tissue content and toxicity of ingested lead in the rat. J. Lab. clin. Med. **79,** 128–136 (1972)

Skaar, H., Ophus, E., Gullväg, B.M.: Lead accumulation within nuclei of moss leaf cells. Nature (Lond.) **241,** 215–216 (1973)

Spector, M.J., Guinee, V.F., Davidow, B.: The unsuitability of random urinary delta-aminolevulinic acid samples as a screening test for lead poisoning. J. Pediat. **79,** 799–804 (1971)

Steiger, M.: Die Bedeutung von Blei bei hereditären Erythrozytenanomalien. Schw. Zschr. f. Unfallmedizin und Berufskrankheiten **61,** 199–221 (1968)

Stetson, C.A., Jr.: Pica: Its relationship to lead poisoning in children. J. Maine med. Ass. **38,** 10–12 (1947)

Stevens, E., Frydman, R.B., Frydman, B.: Separation of porphobilinogen deaminase and uroporphyrinogen III cosynthetase from human erythrocytes. Biochim. biophys. Acta **158,** 496–498 (1968)

Strand, L.J. Manning, J., Marver, H.S.: The induction of δ-aminolevulinic acid synthetase in cultured liver cells: The effect of end product and inhibitors of heme biosynthesis. J. biol. Chem. **247,** 2820–2827 (1972a)

Strand, L.J., Meyer, U.A., Felscher, B.F., Redeker, A.G., Marver, H.S.: Decreased red cell uroporphyrinogen I synthetase in intermittent acute porphyria. J. clin. Invest. **51,** 2530–2536 (1972b)

Stuik, E.J.: Biological response of male and female volunteers to inorganic lead. Int. Arch. Arbeitsmed. **33,** 83–97 (1974)

Sutherland, D.A., Eisentraut, A.M.: The direct Coombs test in lead poisoning. Blood **11,** 1024–1031 (1956).

Tephly, T.R., Hasegawa, E., Baron, J.: Effect of drugs on heme synthesis in the liver. Metabolism **20,** 200–214 (1971)

Teras, L.E., Kakhn, K.A.: Oxidative processes and phosphorylation in liver in lead intoxication. Vop. med. khim. **12,** 40–45 (1967)

Thomas, P.K., Lascelles, R.G.: The pathology of diabetic neuropathy. Quart. J. Med. **35,** 489–509 (1966)

Thomas, P.K., Lascelles, R.G.: Hypertrophic neuropathy. Quart. J. Med. **36,** 223–238 (1967)

Tice, L.W.: Lead-adenosine triphosphate complexes in adenosine triphosphatase histochemistry, J. Histochem. Cytochem. **17,** 85–94 (1969)

Tokunaga, R., Sano, S.: Comparative studies on nonenzymic and enzymic protoheme formation. Biochim. biophys. Acta **264,** 263–271 (1972)

Tomio, J.M., Tuzman, V., Grinstein, M.: δ-Aminolevulinate dehydratase from rat Harderian gland. Purification and properties. Europ. J. Biochem. **6,** 84–87 (1968)

Tomokuni, K.: New method for determination of aminolaevulinate dehydratase activity of human erythrocytes as an index of lead exposure. Clin. Chem. **20,** 1280–1291 (1974)

Tomokuni, K., Kawanishi, T.: Relationship between activation of delta-aminolevulinic acid dehydratase by heating and blood lead level. Arch. Toxicol. **34,** 253–258 (1975)

Traketeller, A.C., Hemle, E.W., Montjar, M., Axelrod, A.E., Jensen, W.N.: Studies on rat reticulocyte polysomes during in vitro maturation. Arch. Biochem. **112,** 89–97 (1965)

Tuttle, A.H., Fitch, C.: Alteration in the electrophoretic characteristics of hemoglobin in paint eaters". Amer. J. Dis. Child. **96,** 503 (1958)

Ulmer, D.D., Vallee, B.L.: Trace substances in environmental health. II. Proceedings Univ. Missouri Ann. Conf. Trace Substances. Environm. Health, 2nd ed., D.D. Hemphill, 7. Columbia: Univ. Missouri 1969

Valentine, W.N., Fink, K., Paglia, D.E., Harris, S.R., Adams, W.S.: Hereditary hemolytic anemia with human erythrocyte pyrimidine 5′-nucleotidase deficiency. J. clin. Invest. **54,** 866–879 (1974)

Van Esch, G.J., Van Genderen, H., Vink, H.H.: The induction of renal tumours by feeding of basic lead acetate to rats. Brit. J. Cancer **16,** 289–297 (1962)

Vasiliu, A., Stavri, G., Freund, S.: Value of reduced glutathione determinations in workers exposed to lead. Revista Iasi **73,** 647–652 (1962)

Vergnano, C., Cartasegna, C., Bonsignore, D.: Livelli di glutatione ridotto nella intossicazione sperimentale da piombo. Boll. Soc. ital. Biol. sper. **43,** 1099–1102 (1967)

Vincent, P.C., Blackburn, C.R.B.: Effects of heavy metal ions on the human erythrocyte I. Comparison of the action of several heavy metals. Aust. J. exp. Biol. med. Sci. **36**, 471 – 479 (1958a)

Vincent, P.C., Blackburn, C.R.B.: Effects of heavy metal ions on the human erythrocyte: II. Effects of lead and mercury. Aust. J. exp. Biol. med. Sci. **36**, 589 – 601 (1958b)

Vitale, L.F., Joselow, M.M., Wedeen, R.P., Pawlow, M.: Blood lead – an inadequate measure of occupational exposure. J. occup. Med. **17**, 155 – 156 (1975)

Wachstein, M.: Studies on inclusion bodies: I. Acid-fastness of nuclear inclusion bodies that are induced by ingestion of lead and bismuth. Amer. J. clin. Path. **19**, 608 – 614 (1949).

Wada, O., Toyokawa, K., Suzuki, T., Suzuki, S., Yano, Y., Nakao, K.: Response to low concentration of mercury vapor. Arch. environ. Hlth. **19**, 485 – 488 (1969)

Wada, O., Yano, Y., Toyokawa, K., Suzuki, T., Suzuki, S., Katsunuma, H.: Human response to lead: In special references to porhyrin metabolism in bone marrow erythroid cells and clinical and laboratory study. Industr. Hlth. **10**, 84 – 92 (1972)

Waldron, H.A.: The anemia of lead poisoning: A review. Brit. J. industr. Med. **23**, 83 – 100 (1966)

Watrach, A.M.: Degeneration of mitochondria in lead poisoning. J. Ultrastruct. Res. **10**, 177 – 181 (1964)

Watson, R.J., Decker, E., Lichtman, H.C.: Hematologic studies in children with lead poisoning. Pediatrics **21**, 40 – 46 (1958)

Waxman, H.S., Rabinovitz, M.: Control of reticulocyte polyribosome content and hemoglobin synthesis by heme. Biochim. biophys. Acta **129**, 369 – 379 (1966)

Weed, R.I., Eber, J., Rothstein, A.: Interaction of mercury with human embryos. J. gen. Physiol. **45**, 395 – 410 (1962)

Weippl, G.: Anemia with geophagia in early childhood. Z. Kinderheilk. **160**, 142 (1959)

Weissberg, J.N. Lipschutz, F., Oski, F.A.: δ-Aminolevulinic acid dehydratase activity in circulating blood cells. A sensitive laboratory test for the detection of childhood lead poisoning. New Engl. J. Med. **284**, 565 – 569 (1971)

Weissberg, J.B., Voytek, P.E.: Liver and red cell porphobilinogen synthetase in the adult and fetal guinea pig. Biochim. biophys. Acta **364**, 304 – 319 (1974)

White, J.M., Harvey, D.R.: Defective synthesis of α and β globin chains in lead poisoning. Nature (Lond.) **236**, 71 – 73 (1972)

Whitfield, C.L., Ch'ien, L.T., Whitehead, J.D.: Lead encephalopathy in adults. Amer. J. Med. **52**, 289 – 298 (1972)

Whiting, M., Granick, S.: δ-Aminolevulinic acid synthetase from chick embryo liver mitochondria. II. Immunochemical correlation between synthesis and activity in induction and repression. J. biol. Chem. **251**, 1347 – 1353 (1976)

Wilson, E.L., Burger, P.E., Dowdle, E.B.: Beef-liver 5-aminolevulinic avid dehydratase. Europ. J. Biochem. **29**, 563 – 571 (1972)

Wilson, V.K., Thompson, M.L., Dent, C.E.: Aminoaciduria in lead poisoning. Lancet **1953 ii**, 66 – 68

Wintrobe, M.M.: Factors and mechanisms in the production of red blood corpuscles. Harvey Lect. **45**, 87 – 126 (1949 – 1950)

Yoneyama, Y., Sawada, H., Takeshita, M., Sugita, Y.: The role of lipids in heme synthesis. Lipids **4**, 321 – 326 (1969)

Yoshikawa, H.: Tolerance to lethal doses of metals in mice pretreated with their low doses. Industr. Hlth. **6**, 88 – 89 (1968)

Zollinger, H.U.: Durch chronische Bleivergiftung erzeugte Nierenadenome und Carcinome bei Ratten und ihre Beziehungen zu den entsprechenden Neubildungen des Menschen. Virchows Arch. path. Anat. **323**, 694 – 710 (1953)

Author Index

Page numbers in *italics* indicate References

Abbott, D.C., Collins, G.B., Goulding, R. 161, *193*

Abboud, M.M., Jordan, P.M., Akhtar, M. 8, *35*

Abboud, M.M., see Zaman, Z. 8, 21, *48*

Abbritti, G., De Matteis, F. 102, 120, *121*, 132, 134, 135, 138, 139, 142, *150*, 204, 205, 226, *233*

Abdulla, M., Haeger-Aronsen, B. 338, *361*

Abdulla, M., see Haeger-Aronsen, B. 337, *365*

Abou-El-Makarem, M.M., Bock, K.W. 149, *151*

Abramsky, T., see Shemin, D. 258, *270*

Abritti, G., see De Matteis, F. 12, 23, 31, 37, 84, *92*, 132, 134–141, 143–149, *151*, 224, *233*

Ackermann, E., Heinrich, I. 57, *70*

Acocella, G., Billing, B.H. 291, *309*

Acocella, G., Nicolis, F.B., Tenconi, L.T. 291, *309*

Adachi, Y., Yamamoto, T. 295, *309*

Adams, W.S., see Valentine, W.N. 348, *370*

Adlard, B.P.F., Lathe, G.H. 301, *309*

Adlercreutz, H., Tenhunen, R. 304, *309*

Admirand, W.H., see Stiehl, A. 305, 306, *329*

Ahn, K., see Machinist, J.M. 293, *322*

Aitio, A., see Hanninen, O. 295, 299, *317*

Akera, T., see Brody, T.M. 304, *312*

Åkeson, Å., Ehrenstein, G. v., Hevesy, G., Theorell, H. 5, *35*

Akhtar, M., see Abboud, M.M. 8, *35*

Akhtar, M., see Zaman, Z. 8, 21, *48*

Albahary, C. 349, *361*

Albert, A.D., see Gear, A.R.L. 68, 69, *73*

Albin, R., see Aschenbrenner, V. 5, *36*

Aldrich, R.A., see Talman, E.L. 201, 217, 219, *237*

Alexanderson, E., Price Evans, D.A., Sjöqvist, F. 61, 62, *70*

Ali, M.A.M., see White, J.M. 30, *48*

Alison, F., see Ploussard, J.P. 305, *325*

Allan, D.J., see McIntyre, N. 241, *253*

Alme, B., Nystrom, E. 99, *121*

Alpert, S., Mosher, M., Shanske, A., Arias, I.M. 280, *309*

Alpert, S., see Gutstein, S. 280, *316*

Altshuler, T., see Lascelles, J. 11, *42*

Alvares, A.P., Anderson, K.E., Conney, A.H., Kappas, A. 63, *70*

Alvares, A.P., Bickers, D.R., Kappas, A. 177–179, *193*

Alvares, A.P., Kapelner, S., Sassa, S., Kappas, A. 82, *92*, 352, *361*

Alvares, A.P., Leigh, S., Cohn, J., Kappas, A. 352, *361*

Alvares, A.P., Schilling, G., Levin, W., Kuntzman, R. 59, *70*

Alvares, A.P., Schilling, G., Levin, W., Kuntzman, R., Brand, L., Mark, L.C. 57, *70*

Alvares, A.P., Siekevitz, P. 59, *70*

Alvares, A.P., see Kappas, A. 351, *366*

Alvarez, A.P., see Anderson, K.E. 249, 251, *252*

Alving, A.S., see Beutler, E. 340, *362*

Alving, A.S., see Derni, R.J. 282, *314*

Alving, A.S.P., see Kellermeyer, R.W. 282, *319*

Amrutavalli, J., see Rajamanickam, C. 170, 177, 178, 180, 185, *198*

Anders, W., see Maines, M.D. 119, *124*

Andersen, E.M., see Frydman, R.B. 15, *39*

Anderson, D.H., see Silverman, W.A. 288, *328*

Anderson, K.E., Alvarez, A.P., Sassa, S., Kappas, A. 249, 251, *252*

Anderson, K.E., see Alvares, A.P. 63, *70*

Anderson, R.C., see Owen, N.V. 65, *77*

Anderson, S.M., see Hansch, C. 220, 221, *234*

Anderson, W.A.D., see Gunn, S.A. 357, *365*

Anderson, W.B., Schneider, A.B., Emmer, M., Perlman, R.L., Pastan, I. 258, *267*

Anderson, W.B., see Nissley, S.P. 258, *269*

Angle, C.R., McIntyre, M.S. 341, *361*

Angle, C.R., see McIntyre, M.S. 340, *367*

Aoki, Y., Urata, G., Wada, O., Takaku, F. 11, 12, 28, *35*

Aoki, Y., Wada, O., Urata, G., Takaku, F., Nakao, K. 10, 12, 30, *35*

Applebaum, I.L., see Bleiberg, J. 157, 174, 175, *194*

Applemen, D., see Heim, W.G. 82, *92*

Arditti, R.R., Eron, L., Zubay, G., Tocchini-Valentini, G., Connaway, S., Beckwith, J. 258, *267*

Ardoino, V., see Bonsignore, B. 340, *362*

Argyris, T.S., Layman, D.L. 65, *70*

Argyris, T.S., Magnus, D. 65, 66, *70*

Arias, I.M. 277–279, 291–293, 295, 296, 304, *309*

Arias, I.M., Doyle, D., Schimke, R.T. 59, *70*

Arias, I.M., Gartner, L.M. 301, *309*

Arias, I.M., Gartner, L.M., Cohen, M., Ben Ezzer, J., Levi, A.J. 279, 296, *310*

Arias, I.M., Gartner, L., Furman, M., Wolfson, S. 298, 299, *310*

Arias, I.M., Gartner, L.M. Seifter, S., Furman, M. 301, *310*

Arias, I.M., Jansen, P. 291, 292, *310*

Arias, I.M., Johnson, L., Wolfson, S. *310*

Arias, I.M., see Alpert, S. 280, *309*

Arias, I.M., see Bernstein, L.H. 277–279, *310*

Arias, I.M., see Cornelius, C.E. 277, 291, *313*

Arias, I.M., see Deleon, A.L. 279, 295, 296, 306, *314*

Arias, I.M., see Fleischner, G. 68, *73*, 278, 292, 293, *315*

Arias, I.M., see Goldfischer, S. 304, *315*

Arias, I.M., see Gutstein, S. 280, *316*

Arias, I.M., see Habig, W.H. 64, *74*, 292, *316*

Arias, I.M., see Kamisaka, K. 277, 289, 292, *319*

Arias, I.M., see Kirsch, R. 292, 293, *320*

Arias, I.M., see Levi, A.J. 277, 278, 292, 293, *321*

Arias, I.M., see Levine, R.I. 278, *321*

Arias, I.M., see Litwack, G. 278, 292, *321*

Arias, I.M., see Mishkin, S. 292, *323*

Arias, I.M., see Mowat, A.P. 27, *44*

Arias, I.M., see Reyes, H. 278, 293, *326*

Arimura, K., see Kawasaki, H. 292, *319*

Arnstein, H.R.V., see Denton, M.J. 28, *38*

Aronow, L., see Goldstein, A. 51, *73*

Arrenius, E., see Smuckler, E.A. 109, *126*

Arrowsmith, W.A., Payne, R.B., Littlewood, J.M. 301, 305, *310*

Arroyo, F.L., see Landow, S.A. 349, *366*

Asbury, A.K., see Sweeny, V.P. 11, *47*

Aschenbrenner, V., Druyan, R., Albin, R., Rabinowitz, M. 5, *36*

Ascher, K., see Windorfer, A. 305, *331*

Aschoff, L. 274, *310*

Ashbrook, J.D., Spector, A.A., Santos, E.C., Fletcher, J.E. 277, *310*

Ashbrook, J.D., see Spector, A.A. 288, *328*

Ashenbrucker, G.E., see Goldberg, A. 341, *364*

Ashmore, S.A., see Cameron, G.R. 159, *194*

Athanassopoulos, S., see Reiner, O. 111, *126*

Atkins, C., see Salvador, R.A. 67, 68, *78*

Atsmon, A. 231, *233*

Atsmon, A., Blum, I. 231, *233*

Atsmon, A., see Blum, I. 231, *233*

Attardi, B., see Attardi, C. 50, *70*

Attardi, C., Parnas, H., Hwang, M.T.H., Attardi, B. 50, *70*

Augsburg, G., see Grassl, M. 4, *39*

Aust, D., see Ippen, H. 170, 171, *196*

Aust, J.B., see Lottsfeldt, F.I. 305, *321*

Aust, S.D., see Pederson, T.C. 113, *125*

Aust, S.D., see Welton, A.F. 5, *48*

Awruch, J., see Frydman, R.B. 15, *39*

Axelrod, A.E., see Traketeller, A.C. 347, *370*

Axelrod, J., see Inscoe, J.K. 63, *74*, 299, *318*

Axelrod, J., see Quinn, G.P. 62, *78*

Axelrod, J., see Schmid, R. 278, 279, *328*

Azarnoff, D.L., Tucker, D.R., Barr, G.A. 67, *70*

Azarnoff, D., see Reddy, J. 65, 68, *78*

Azzi, A., see Fleischer, S. 66, *73*

Bacchin, P., see Raisfeld, J. 83, *93*

Bach, G.G., see Goresky, C.A. 280, 302, *316*

Bach, P.H., Taljaard, J.J.F., Joubert, S.M., Shanley, B.C. 171, *193*

Bacon, P.A., see Scott, C.L. 283, *328*

Badawy, A.A.B., Evans, M. 52, 53, *70*, 142, *151*

Bain, E., see Medline, A. 177, 178, 187, 188, *197*

Baird, M.B., Samis, H.V., Massie, H.R., Zimmermann, J.A., Sfeir, G.A. 142, *151*

Baker, A., see Farber, T.M. 177, *195*

Baker, H., see Ramsay, C.A. 158, 191, *198*

Baker, H., see Turnbull, A. 158, 191, *199*

Baker, K.J., see Macarol, V. 302, *322*

Baker-Cohen, K.F., see Nandi, D.L. 333, *367*

Bakken, A.F., Thaler, M.M., Schmid, R. 24, *36*, 117, 118, *121*, 287, *310*

Bakkeren, J.A.J.M., see Vanleusden, H.A.J.M 279, *330*

Baldas, J., see Battersby, A.R. 21, *36*

Baliah, T., see Yaffe, S.J. 296, *331*

Balkow, K., Mizuno, S., Rabinovitz, M. 30, *36*

Balliano, M., see Beloff-Chain, A. 113, *122*

Baloh, R.W. 358, *361*

Bannerman, R.M., see Grinstein, M. 341, *365*

Baptista de Almeide, J.A.P., Kenner, G.W., Smith, K.M., Sutton, M.J. 170, *193*

Baranafi, L., see Espinoza, J. 305, *315*

Barbuto, A.J., see Kushner, J.P. 158, 184, 189, *196*

Barka, T., Popper, H. 65, *71*

Barltrop, D. 358, *362*

Barltrop, D., Smith, A 347, *362*

Barnes, J.M., see Bond, E.J. 105, *122*

Barnes, R., Connelly, J.L., Jones, O.T.G. 22, *36*

Barnes, R., Jones, M.S., Jones, O.T.G., Porra, R.J. 9, 22, 23, *36*

Barnhart, J.L., Clarenburg, R. 291, *310*

Baron, J., Tephly, T.R. 31, *36*, 82, 83, 86, 89, *92*, 109, *121*, 284, *310*

Baron, J., see Tephly, T.R. 84, *94*, 284, 286, *329*, 335, *370*

Bartok, I., Varga, L., Varga, G. 304, *310*

Barr, G.A., see Azarnoff, D.L. 67, *70*

Barr, P.S., see Freedman, A.L. 283, *315*

Barrett, M.B., see Chisolm, J.J., Jr. 335, 342, 344, *362*

Baskin, S.I., see Brody, T.M. 304, *312*

Bass, R.K., see Muirhead, E.E. *323*

Bast, R.C., Jr., see Gelboin, H.V. 61, *73*

Batlle, A.M., del C., Benson, A., Rimington, C. 20, *36*

Batlle, A.M. del C., Ferramola, A.M., Grinstein, M. 14, *36*

Batlle, A.M. del C., Grinstein, M. 18, *36*, 181, *194*

Batlle, A.M. del C., see Llambias, E.B.C. 15, 16, 18, *43*

Batlle, A.M.C., see Sancovich, H.A. 15, *45*

Batolska, A., Marinova, H. 340, *362*

Batt, A.M., Ziegler, J.M., Siest, G. 299, *310*

Battersby, A.R., Baldas, J., Collins, J., Grayson, D.H., James, K.J., McDonald, E. 21, *36*

Battersby, A.R., Hunt, E., McDonald, E. 17, *36*

Battistini, V., Morrow, J.J., Ginsburg, D., Thompson, G., Moore, M.R., Goldberg, A. 341, *362*

Battistini, V., see Millar, J.A. 337, *367*

Battistini, V., see Moore, M.R. 172, *197*, 224, 231, *235*

Baucum, R., see Brazda, F.G. 56, *71*

Bauer, K., see Callahan, E.W., Jr. 308, *313*

Baum, S. 335, *362*

Beale, D., see Ketterer, B. 23, *42*

Beale, S.I., Gaugh, S.P., Granick, S. 258, *267*

Beattie, A.D., Moore, M.R., Goldberg, A., Ward, R.L. 251, *252*

Beattie, A.D., see Goldberg, A. 266, *267*

Beattie, A.D., see McIntyre, N. 241, *253*

Beattie, A.D., see Moore, M.R. 158, 172, 185, *197*, 224, 231, *235*, 265, 266, *269*

Beattie, A.D., see Paxton, J.W. 265, 266, *269*

Beattie, D.S., Patton, G.M., Rubin, E. 32, *36*

Beattie, D.S., see Patton, G.M. 9, 11, 32, 34, *44*, 149, 150, *153*

Beaven, G.H., Chen, S.H., D'Albis, A., Gratzer, W.B. 277, *310*

Beaven, G.H., D'Albis, A., Gratzer, W.B. 277, *310*

Beaver, D.L. 354, *362*

Beaver, D.L., see Bracken, E.C. 354, *362*

Beck, W.T., Bellantone, R.A., Canellakis, E.S. 260, *267*

Becker, B.A., Plaa, G.L. 285, *310*

Becker, B.A., see Machinist, J.M. 293, *322*

Becker, D., Viljoen, D., Kramer, S. 353, *362*

Beckett, R.B., Weiss, R., Stitzel, R.E., Cenedella, R.J. 65, 68, *71*

Beckwith, J., see Arditti, R.R. 258, *267*

Beckwith, J., see Zubay, G. 258, *271*

Beckwith, J.R., see Epstein, W. 50, *72*

Bednarek, J.M., see Gear, A.R.L. 68, 69, *73*

Beems, R.B., see Vos, J.G. 172, *200*

Belcher, R.B., see Jackson, A.H. 21, *41*

Belfi, K.J., see Nelson, E.B. 58, *71*

Bellantone, R.A., see Beck, W.T. 260, *267*

Bellet, H., Raynaud, A. 296, *310*

Beloff-Chain, A., Serlupi-Crescenzi, G., Catanzaro, R., Venettacci, D., Balliano, M. 113, *122*

Ben-Bassat, I., Mozel, M., Ramot, B. 30, *36*

Ben Ezzer, J., see Arias, I.M. 279, 296, *310*

Ben Ezzer, J., see Bernstein, L.H. 277–279, *310*

Ben Ezzer, J., see Cornelius, C.E. 277, 291, *313*

Ben Ezzer, J., see Shani, M. 305, *328*

Benedict, W.F., see Nebert, D.W. 62, *76*

Benhamou, J.R., see Dhumeaux, D. 302, *314*

Benhamou, J.P., see Edmond, M. 300, *314*

Benjamin, W., see Gellhorn,
   A. 66, *73*
Benko, B., see Rein, H. 135,
   154
Benson, A., see Batlle, A.M.
   del. C. 20, *36*
Benson, A.M., Talalay, P.,
   Keen, J.H., Jakoby, W.B.
   64, *71*
Bentley, D., see Hansch, C.
   220, 221, *234*
Ber, R., Valero, A. 358, *362*
Bergan, J.G., see Kokatnur,
   M.G. 113, *124*
Berger, D., see Sausville,
   J.W. 307, 308, *327*
Bergeron, J.J.M., see Farqu-
   har, M.G. 66, *73*
Bergman, H., see Goldstein,
   J.A. 157, 175, 180, 187,
   188, *195*
Bergstrand, A., see Högberg,
   J. 113, *123*
Bergstrand, A., see Sottocasa,
   L. 66, *79*
Berk, P., see Stein, J.A. 263,
   270
Berk, P.D. 297, *310*
Berk, P.D., Blaschke, T. 297,
   310
Berk, P.D., Bloomer, J.R.,
   Howe, R.B., Berlin, N.I.
   293, *310*
Berk, P.D., Howe, R.B., Ber-
   lin, N.I. 1, 5, *36,* 297,
   310
Berk, P.D., Howe, R.B., Bloo-
   mer, J.R., Berlin, H.I. 277,
   278, 291, *310*
Berk, P.D., Rodkey, F.L.,
   Blaschke, T.F., Collison,
   H.A., Waggoner, J.G. 5, 7,
   36
Berk, P.D., Tschudy, D.P.,
   Shepley, L.A., Waggoner,
   J.G., Berlin, N.I. 349, *362*
Berk, P.D., see Blaschke,
   T.F. 284, 285, 293,
   295–297, 306, *311*
Berk, P.D., see Bloomer, J.R.
   277, 283, *311, 312*
Berk, P.D., see Gisselbrecht,
   C. 284, 285, *315*
Berk, P.D., see Martini, J.F.
   293, *322*
Berk, P.D., see Scharschmidt,
   B.F. 277, 292, 293, *327*

Berko, G., see Simon, N.
   169, 170, 180, 188, *198*
Berlin, C.M., Schimke, R.T.
   51, 52, *71*
Berlin, C.M., see Schimke,
   R.T. 50–52, *79,* 142, *154*
Berlin, N.I., see Berk, P.D. 1,
   5, *36,* 277, 278, 291, 293,
   297, *310, 362*
Berlin, N.I., see Bloomer,
   J.R. 277, 283, *311, 312*
Berlin, N.I., see Jones, E.A.
   6, *41,* 283, 285, *319*
Bernado, D., see Moore,
   M.R. 158, 185, *197*
Bernard, B., see Druyan, B.
   50, *72*
Bernard, B.De, see Druyan,
   R. 4, 5, *38*
Bernstein, L.H., Ben Ezzer, J.,
   Gartner, L., Arias, I.M.
   277–279, *310*
Berry, C.S., see Ostrow, J.D.
   308, *325*
Berthelot, P. 274, *311*
Berthelot, P., Billing, B.H.
   291, *311*
Berthelot, P., Erlinger, S.,
   Dhumeaux, D., Preaux,
   A.M. 300, *311*
Berthelot, P., see Capelle, P.
   291, *313*
Berthelot, P., see Dhumeaux,
   D. 293, *314*
Berthelot, P., see Duvaldestin,
   P. 27, *38*
Berthelot, P., see Edmond,
   M. 300, *314*
Berthelot, P., see Erlinger, S.
   302, *314*
Berthelot, P., see Franco, D.
   26, *38*
Bertinchamps, A.J., Miller,
   S.T., Cotzias, G.C. 88,
   92
Bessis, M., Breton-Gorius, J.,
   Thiery, J.P. 275, *311*
Bessis, M.C., Breton-Gorius,
   J. 348, *362*
Bessis, M.C., Jensen, W.N.
   348, 354, 357, *362*
Bessis, M.C., see Jensen,
   W.N. 347, *366*
Bessman, S.P., see Hammel,
   C.L. 30, *40*
Best, M.M., Duncan, C.H.
   67, *71*

Betheil, J.J., see Kamisaka,
   K. 277, *319*
Betke, L., see Frick, P.G.
   282, *315*
Beutler, E. 281, 282, *311*
Beutler, E., Dern, R.J., Flana-
   gan, C.L., Alving, A.S.
   340, *362*
Beutler, E., see Fairbanks,
   V.F. 358, *363*
Beuzard, Y., London, I.M.
   31, *36*
Bevan, B.R., Holton, J.B.
   301, *311*
Bianco, G., see Prato, V. 282,
   326
Bickers, D.R., see Alvares,
   A.P. 177–179, *193*
Bickers, D.R., see Sassa, S.
   16, *45,* 334, 339, 340, 353,
   369
Billing, B., see Gollan, J.L.
   296, *315*
Billing, B.H., Cole, P.G., La-
   the, G.H. 26, *36,* 278, *311*
Billing, B.H., Maggiore, Q.,
   Cartter, M.A. 278, 291,
   311
Billing, B.H., Williams, R., Ri-
   chards, T.G. 277, 278, 293,
   311
Billing, B.H., see Acocella,
   G. 291, *309*
Billing, B.H., see Berthelot,
   P. 291, *311*
Billing, B.H., see Black, M.
   278, 295–297, *311*
Billing, B.H., see Cole, P.G.
   278, *313*
Billing, B.H., see Jansen,
   F.H. 26, *41,* 278, *319*
Billing, B.H., see Weinbren,
   K. 279, *330*
Billing, B.H., see Whelton,
   M.J. 296, *331*
Billing, H.B., Black, M. 274,
   311
Bismuth, H., see Franco, D.
   26, *38*
Bissell, D.M., Guzelian, P.S.,
   Hammaker, L.E., Schmidt,
   R. 117, 118, 120, *122*
Bissell, D.M., Hammaker,
   L.E. 119, *122,* 140, *151*
Bissell, D.M., Hammaker, L.,
   Schmid, R. 24, *36,* 117,
   122, 276, *311*

Bixler, T.J., see Rudman, D. 288, *327*

Black, M., Billing, B.H. 296, *311*

Black, M., Billing, B.II., Ilcirwegh, K.P.M. 278, *311*

Black, M., Fevery, J., Parker, D., Jacobson, J., Billing, B.H., Carson, E.R. 295, 296, 297, *311*

Black, M., Perret, R.D., Carter, A.E. 295, 297, *311*

Black, M., Sherlock, S. 296, 297, *311*

Black, M., see Billing, H.B. 274, *311*

Blackburn, C.R.B., see Vincent, P.C. 350, *371*

Blackburn, M.G., Orzalesi, M.M., Pigram, P. 308, *311*

Blackburn, N.R., see Oelboin, H.V. 56, *73*

Blackman, S.S., Jr. 356, *362*

Blades, E.J., see Mann, F.C. 274, *322*

Blake, D.A., see Weiner, M. 117, *127*

Blanc, W.A., see Johnson, L. 288, 289, *319*

Blanc, W.A., see Silverman, W.A. 288, *328*

Blaschke, T., see Berk, P.D. 297, *310*

Blaschke, T.F., Berk, P.D. 297, *311*

Blaschke, T.F., Berk, P.D., Rodkey, F.L., Scharschmidt, B.F., Collison, H.A., Waggoner, J.G. 284, 285, 295, 296, 297, *311*

Blaschke, T.F., Berk, P.D., Scharschmidt, B.F., Guyther, J.R., Vergalla, J.M., Waggoner, J.G. 293, 296, 306, *311*

Blaschke, T.F., see Berk, P.D. 5, 7, *36*

Blattel, R.A., see Krupa, V. 226—228, *235*

Blattel, R.A., see Marks, G.S. 204, 206, 208, 209, *235*

Bleiberg, J., Wallen, M., Brodkin, R., Applebaum, I.L. 157, 174, 175, *194*

Blekkenhorst, G., see Pimstone, N.R. 23, *44*, 158, *197*

Blodgett, F.M., see Kammholz, L.P. 359, *366*

Blondheim, S.H., see Kapitulnik, J. 290, *319*

Bloomer, J.R., Beik, P.D., Berlin, N.I. 277, *311*

Bloomer, J.R., Berk, P.D., Bonkowsky, H.L., Stein, J.A., Berlin, N.I., Tschudy, D.P. 283, *312*

Bloomer, J.R, Boyer, J.L. 305, *312*

Bloomer, J.R., Boyer, J.L., Klatskin, G. 303, *312*

Bloomer, J.R., see Berk, P.D. 277, 278, 291, 293, *310*

Bloomer, J.R., see Bonkowsky, H.L. 342, *362*

Bloomer, J.R., see Jones, E.A. 6, *41*, 283, 285, *319*

Blum, D., Etienne, J. 305, *312*

Blum, I., Schoenfeld, N., Atsmon, A. 231, *233*

Blum, I., see Atsmon, A. 231, *233*

Blumberg, W., see Fischbein, A. 344, *364*

Blumberg, W.E., Eisinger, J., Lamola, A.A., Zuckerman, D.M. 344, 359, *362*

Blumenschein, S.D., Kallen, R.J., Storcy, D., Natzschka, J., Odell, G.B., Childs, B. 305, *312*

Bock, K.W. 294, *312*

Bock, K.W., Clausbruch, U.C. v., Josting, D., Ottenwälder, H. 64, *71*

Bock, K.W., Fröhling, W., Remmer, H. 62, *71*, 111, *122*

Bock, K.W., Fröhling, W., Remmer, H., Rexer, B. 27, *36*, 62, 63, *71*, 294, 295, 299, *312*

Bock, K.W., Krauss, E., Fröhling, W. 10, 12, *36*, 60, *71*

Bock, K.W., Siekevitz, P. 50, 67, *71*, 283, *312*

Bock, K.W., Weiner, R., Fröhling, W. 143, *151*, 252

Bock, K.W., White, I.N.H. 294, 295, 299, 301, *312*

Bock, K.W., see Abou-El-Makarem, M.M. 149, *151*

Bock, K.W., see Matern, S. 65, *76*

Boggs, T.R., see Johnson, L. 308, *319*

Bogorad, L. 15, *36*, *37*, *362*

Boivin, P., see Hakim, J. 298, *316*

Bolen, J.L., see Odell, G.B. 305, *324*

Bolender, R.P., Weibel, E.R. 65, 66, *71*

Bollman, J.L., see Hunton, D.B. 280, 291, *318*

Bollman, J.L., see Mann, F.C. 274, *322*

Bollman, J.L., see Schoenfield, L.J. 279, *328*

Bolt, R.J., Dillon, R.S., Pollard, H.M. 291, *312*

Bolze, H., see Windorfer, A. 305, *331*

Bond, E.J., Butler, W.H., De Matteis, F., Barnes, J.M. 105, *122*

Bond, E.J., De Matteis, F. 105, 108, 109, *122*

Bonkowsky, H.I., Bloomer, J.R., Ebert, P.S., Mahoney, M.J. 342, *362*

Bonkowsky, H.L., Collins, A., Doherty, J.M., Tschudy, D.P. 90, *92*, 260—262, *267*

Bonkowsky, H.L., see Bloomer, J.R. 283, *312*

Bonkowsky, H.L., see Song, C.S. · 233, *236*, 249, 251, *254*

Bonkowski, H.L., see Tschudy, D.P. 130, *154*, 157, *199*, 244, *254*

Bonnett, R., Stewart, J.C.M. 307, *312*

Bonsignore, B., Cartasegna, C., Ardoino, V., Vergnano, C. 340, *362*

Bonsignore, D., Calissano, P., Cartasegna, C. 338, *362*

Bonsignore, D., see Calissano, P. 334, 339, *362*

Bonsignore, D., see Vergnano, C. 340, *370*

Bonura, F., see Waltman, R. 299, *330*

Bonzanino, A., see Pisani, W. 34, *45*

Borová, J., Ponka, P., Neuwirt, J. 348, *362*

Borová, J., see Neuwirt, J.
  30, *44*
Borová, J., see Poňka, P. 30,
  45
Borst, P., see Zuyderhoudt,
  F.M.J. 9, *48*, 149, *155*
Boscherini, B., see Girotti, F.
  305, *315*
Bossenmaier, I., see Dhar,
  G.J. 243, *253*
Bossenmaier, I., see Miyagi,
  K. 16, *44*, 353, *367*
Bothwell, T.H., see Zail, S.S.
  282, *332*
Botterweg, P.F., see Vos,
  J.G. 200, 222, *237*
Bottomley, S.S. 23, *37*
Bottomley, S.S., Smithee,
  G.A. 30, *37*
Bottomley, S.S., Tanaka, M.,
  Everett, M.A. 342, *362*
Bottomley, S.S., see Tanaka,
  M. 12, *47*
Boucherot, J., see Hakim, J.
  298, *316*
Bourke, E., Milne, M.D., Sto-
  kes, G.S. 280, *312*
Bousquer, W.F., see Hoog-
  land, D.R. 56, *74*
Bousquet, W.F., see Hadley,
  W.M. 88, *92*, 115, *123*
Bousquet, W.F., see Piper,
  W.N. 145, *153*
Boveris, A., Chance, B. 4, *37*
Bowen, W.R., see Waters,
  W.J. 300, *330*
Boyd, D.W., see MacGibbon,
  B.H. 283, *322*
Boyd, G., Grimwade, A.,
  Lawson, M. *71*
Boyer, J.L., Klatskin, G. 302,
  312
Boyer, J.L., see Bloomer,
  J.R. 303, 305, *312*
Bozian, R.C., see Vilter,
  R.W. 86, 87, *94*
Bracci, R., see Gross, R.T.
  281, *316*
Bracken, E.C., Beaver, D.L.,
  Randall, C.C. 354, *362*
Bradley, S.E., see Macarol,
  V. 302, *322*
Bradlow, H.L., Gillette, P.N.,
  Gallagher, T.F., Kappas,
  A. 266, *267*
Bradlow, H.L., see Kappas,
  A. 266, *268*

Bradlow, H.L., see Sassa, S.
  16, *45*, 334, 353, *369*
Bradshaw, J.J., see Ivanetich,
  K.M. 103, *123*
Brady, M.N., Siyali, D.S.
  161, *194*
Brain, M.C., see White, J.M.
  30, *48*, 282, *331*
Brammar, W.J., see Clarke,
  P.H. 256, *267*
Branch, R.A., Shand, D.G.,
  Wilkinson, G.R., Nies,
  A.S. 293, *312*
Branch, S., see Strand, L.J.
  10, 12, *46*
Brand, L., see Alvares, A.P.
  57, *70*
Brand, L., see Kuntzman, R.
  57, *75*
Branham, R.V., see Ostrow,
  J.D. 307, *325*
Bratlid, D. 289, *312*
Bratlid, D., see Rugstad,
  H.E. 291, *327*
Brauer, R.W., Leong, G.F.,
  Holloway, R.J. 280, *312*
Brauser, B., see Sies, H. 64,
  79
Bray, H.G., Humphris, B.G.,
  Thorpe, W.V., White, K.,
  Wood, P.B. 89, *92*
Brayley, A., see Matthews,
  M.B. 22, 31, *43*
Brazda, F.G., Baucum, R.
  56, *71*
Brdiczka, D., see Reith, A.
  69, *78*
Breckenridge, A., see Orme,
  M.L.E. 295, 297, *324*
Breton-Gorius, J., see Bessis,
  M. 275, *311*, 348, *362*
Brewer, G.J., see Kellermeyer,
  R.W. 282, *319*
Brewer, G.J., see Schoomaker,
  E.B. 357, *369*
Brewer, J.G., Dern, P.J. 281,
  312
Breyer, U. 56, *71*
Broad, R.D., see Tropham,
  J.C. 306, *329*
Brodersen, R. 289, *312*
Brodersen, R., Hermann,
  L.S. 280, *312*
Brodersen, R., see Thiessen,
  H. 289, *329*
Brodie, B.B., Cosmides, G.J.,
  Rall, D.P. 228, *233*

Brodie, B.B., Gillette, J.R. *70*
Brodie, B.B., see Gillette,
  J.R. 54, *73*
Brodie, B.B., see Mitchell,
  J.R. 85, *93*
Brodie, B.B., see Potter, W.Z.
  85, *93*
Brodie, B.B., see Quinn, G.P.
  62, *78*
Brodina-Persson, G., see
  Schersten, T. 302, *327*
Brodkin, R., see Bleiberg, J.
  157, 174, 175, *194*
Brody, E.A., see Freedman,
  A.L. 283, *315*
Brody, T.M., Akera, T., Bas-
  kin, S.I., Gubitz, R., Lee,
  C.Y. 304, *312*
Brook, S.K., see Murty,
  H.S. 14, *44*
Brooks, F.P., see Fritz, M.E.
  302, *315*
Broughton, P.M.G., Rossiter,
  E., Jr., Warren, C.B.M.,
  Goulis, G., Lord, P.S. 306,
  308, *312*
Brown, A.K. 308, *312*
Brown, A.K., Henning, G.
  301, *313*
Brown, A.K., Zuelzer, W.W.
  278, *313*
Brown, B.W., see Robinson,
  S.H. 275, *327*
Brown, D.H., see Chisolm,
  J.J., Jr. 342, *363*
Brown, D.V.L., see Hass,
  G.M. 354, *365*
Brown, R.S., see Kopelman,
  A.E. 308, *320*
Brown, R.S., see Odell, G.B.
  308, *324*
Brown, W.R., Grodsky, G.M.,
  Carbone, J. 277, 278, *313*
Brubaker, P.E., see Lucier,
  G.W. 115, 116, *124*
Bruckner, J.V., Khanna, K.L.,
  Cornish, H.H. 57, 71, *194*
Bryan, S., see Muirhead, E.E.
  350, 351, *367*
Bubbar, G.L., see Hirsch,
  G.H. 203, *234*
Bubbar, G.L., see Schneck,
  D.W. 203, 209, *236*
Buchan, J.L., see Cameron,
  G.R. 159, *194*
Bucher, H., see Preisig, R.
  302, *326*

Buchet, J.P., see Lauwerys, R. 341, *366*

Buchet, J.P., see Roels, H.A. 337, 340, 341, 358, *368*

Buck, W.B., see Hemphill, F.E. 351, *365*

Büch, H., see Heymann, E. 203, *234*

Buege, J.A., see Pederson, T.C. 113, *125*

Bürgi, M., see Michot, F. 56, *76*

Büttner, J., see Michot, F. 56, *76*

Bugany, H., Flothe, L., Weser, U. 22, 23, *37*

Bunyaratvej, S., see Reddy, J. 68, *78*

Burch, H.B., Siegel, A.L. 339, *362*

Burchell, B. 295, *313*

Burchell, B., see Dutton, G.J. 64, *72*

Burger, P.E., see Wilson, E.L. 13, *48*, 333, 334, 339, 341, *371*

Burkhalter, A., see Howland, R.D. 279, *318*

Burnett, J., Pathak, M. 169, *194*

Burnham, B.F., Lascelles, J. 132, *151*, 333, *362*

Burnham, B.F., see Warnick, G.R. 10, *48*

Burns, J.J., see Chen, W. 56, 57, *71*

Burns, J.J., see Conney, A.H. 56, 63, *70–72*

Burns, J.J., see Cucinell, S.A. 57, *72*

Burse, V.M., Kimbrough, R.D., Villeneuva, E.C., Jennins, R.W., Linder, R.E., Sovocool, G.W. 187, *194*

Burse, V.W., see Poland, A. 176, *197*

Burse, V.M., see Villeneuva, E.C. 160, *199*

Butcher, R.W., see Robison, G.A. 263, *270*

Buterbaugh, G.G., see Weiner, M. 117, *127*

Butler, T.C. 110, *122*

Butler, W.H., see Bond, E.J. 105, *122*

Butler, W.H., see Jones, G. 188, *196*

Butler, W.H., see Magos, L. 105, *124*

Buu-Hoi, N.P., Hien, D., Scint-Ruf, G., Servoin-Sidoine, J. 57, *71*

Buzello, W., see Heymann, E. 203, *234*

Caasi, P.I., see Murty, H.S. 14, *44*

Cahlin, E., see Schersten, T. 302, *327*

Calissano, P., Bonsignore, D., Cartasegna, C. 334, 339, *362*

Calissano, P., Cartasegna, C., Matteini, M. 14, *37*

Calissano, P., see Bonsignore, D. 338, *362*

Call, N.B., Fisher, C.C. 305, *313*

Callahan, E.W., Jr., Thaler, M.M., Karon, M., Bauer, K., Schmid, R. 308, *313*

Callahan, E.W., Jr., see Landaw, S.A. 5, *42*, 102, *124*, 135, 140–142, *152*, 284, 286, 287, *320*

Cam, C. 162, 164, *194*

Cam, C., Nigogosyan, G. 163, 164, 166, *194*

Cam, J., see Hargreaves, T. 301, *317*

Cam, S., see Peters, H.A. 162–164, 168, *197*

Cameron, G.R., Karunaratne, W.E. 109, *122*

Cameron, G.R., Thomas, J.C., Ashmore, S.A., Buchan, J.L., Warren, E.H., Hughes, A.W. 159, *194*

Campbell, J.A.H. 169, 177, 182, 187, *194*

Campbell, M., see Watson, C.J. 280, *330*

Canellakis, E.S., see Beck, W.T. 260, *267*

Cantrell, E., see Kellermann, G. 62, *75*

Capelle, P., Dhumeaux, D., Mora, M., Feldman, G., Berthelot, P. 291, *313*

Capizzo, F., Roberts, R.J. 285, *313*

Capuano, A., see Pinelli, A. 260, 261, *270*

Carbone, J., see Brown, W.R. 277, 278, *313*

Carbone, J.V., see Grodsky, G.M. 278, 300, *316*

Cardinal, R., see Dhar, G.J. 243, *253*

Cardinal, R., see Miyagi, K. 16, *44*, 353, *367*

Cardinal, R.A., see Feldman, D.S. 353, *363*

Cardona, E., see Lessler, M.A. 357, *366*

Careddu, P., Marini, A. 301, *313*

Careddu, P., Picenisereni, L., Guinta, A., Sereni, F. 298, *313*

Carella, M., see Maxwell, J.D. 295, 296, *323*

Carey, J.B., see Lottsfeldt, F.I. 305, *321*

Carey, M.C., Small, D.M. 280, *313*

Carlander, O. 358, *362*

Carlson, G.P., see Shah, H.C. 110, *126*

Carluccio, A., see Okolicsanyi, L. 298, 302, *324*

Carpenter, J.T., Jr., see McLaren, G.D. 342, *367*

Carpenter, M., see Shotton, D. 291, *328*

Carpenter, S.J., see Ferm, V.H. 355, 357, *364*

Carpio, N., see Felsher, B.F. 295, 296, *315*

Carson, E.R., see Black, M. 295–297, *311*

Carson, P.E., see Degowin, R.L. 282, *314*

Carson, P.E., see Kellermeyer, R.W. 282, *319*

Carswell, F., see Millar, J.A. 337, *367*

Cartasegna, C., see Bonsignore, B. 338, 340, *362*

Cartasegna, C., see Calissano, P. 14, *37*, 334, 339, *362*

Cartasegna, C., see Vergnano, C. 340, *370*

Cartei, G., see Okolicsanyi, L. 299, *324*

Carter, A.E., see Black, M. 295, 297, *311*

Cartter, M.A., see Billing, B.H. 271, 291, *311*

Cartwright, G.E., Deiss, A. 348, *362*

Cartwright, G.E., see Goldberg, A. 341, *364*

Cartwright, G.E., see Lee, G.R. 86, *93*

Cartwright, G.E., see Lewis, M. 10, *43*

Casida, J.E., see Vinopal, J.N. 162, *200*

Castro, J.A., see De Toranzo, E.G.D. 109, 110, *123*

Castro, J.A., see Sasame, H.A. 109, *126*

Cataldi, L., see Romagnoli, G. 305, *327*

Catanzaro, R., see Beloff-Chain, A. 113, *122*

Catignani, G.L., Neal, R.A. 106, 109, *122*

Catz, C., Yaffe, S.J. 295, 297, *313*

Catz, C.S., see Yaffe, S.J. 297, *331*

Cavaleiro, J.A.S., Kenner, G.W., Smith, K.M. 20, *37*

Cavallin-Stahl, E., see Lundh, B. 286, *321*

Cenedella, R.J., see Beckett, R.B. 65, 68, *71*

Cetingil, A.I., Özen, M.A. 163, 164, *194*

Chabner, B.A., Stein, J.A., Tschudy, D.P. 263, *267*

Chaix, P., see Labbe, P. 341, *366*

Chan, G., Shiff, D., Stern, L. 289, *313*

Chan, G., see Schiff, D. 289, *327*

Chan, T.-H., see Gordon, E.R. 27, *39*

Chance, B., see Boveris, A. 5, *37*

Chance, B., see Fleischer, S. 66, *73*

Chanmougan, D., see Swanson, M.A. 283, *329*

Charache, S., Weatherall, D.J. 348, *362*

Charles, H.P., see Powell, K.A. 137, *153*

Charlton, R.W., see Zail, S.S. 282, *332*

Chee, P.Y., see Ip, M.M. 4, 5, *41*

Cheh, A., Neilands, J.B. 13, *37*

Chen, S.H., see Beaven, G.H. 277, *310*

Chen, W., Vrindten, P.A., Dayton, P.G., Burns, J.J. 56, 57, *71*

Cheng, L.C., see Weissman, E.B. 265, *270*

Cheripko, J.A., see Coutinho, C.B. 289, *313*

Ch'ien, L.T., see Whitfield, C.L. 352, *371*

Chiesara, E., see Kato, R. 56, 75, 147, *152*

Chiga, M., see Reddy, J. 68, *78*

Chignell, C.F., Starkweather, D.K. 288, *313*

Chignell, C.F., Vessell, E.S., Starkweather, D.K. 290, *313*

Childs, B., see Blumenschein, S.D. 305, *312*

Childs, B., see Zinkham, W.H. 282, *332*

Chirigos, M.A., see Ebert, P.S. 10, *38*

Chisolm, J.J., Jr., Barrett, M.B., Mettits, E.D. 335, 342, 344, *362*

Chisolm, J.J., Jr., Brown, D.H. 342, *363*

Choie, D.D., Richter, G.W. 356, *363*

Choudhry, J.N., see Ebert, P.S. 10, *38*

Chrabas, M.F., see Isselbacher, K.J. 279, *318*

Christianse, K., see De Goeiji, A.F.P.M. 342, *363*

Christoffersen, T., see Jervell, K.F. 257, *268*

Christoforov, B., see Ploussard, J.P. 305, *325*

Chu, E.J.-H., see Chu, T.C. 164, 165, *194*

Chu, T.C., Chu, E.J.-H. 164, 165, *194*

Chvapil, M., Ryan, J.N., Elias, S.L., Peng, Y.M. 112, *122*

Chytil, F., see Moses, H.L. 145, *153*

Cinti, D.L., see Moldeus, P.W. 64, *76*

Cinti, D.L., see Schenkman, J.B. 54, *79*

Clarenburg, R., Kao, L. 303, *313*

Clarenburg, R., see Barnhart, J.L. 291, *310*

Clark, M.L., see Villeneuve, D.C. 57, *80*

Clarke, P.H., Brammar, W.J. 256, *267*

Clarkson, T.W., Kench, J.E. 346, 347, *363*

Clarkson, T.W., see Passow, H. 350, *368*

Classen, H.G., see Solymoss, B. 56, *79*

Clausbruch, U.C. v., see Bock, K.W. 64, *71*

Clayton, J.M., see Hansch, C. 206, 207, *234*

Clegg, D.J., see Villeneuve, D.C. 57, *80*

Clemens, M.J., Henshaw, E.C., Rahamimoff, H., London, I.M. 347, *363*

Clement-Metral, J., see Fanica-Gaignier, M. 8, *38*

Cobrun, R.F. 284, *313*

Cockrill, B.L., see Platt, D.S. 65, *77*

Cohen, G., see Riely, C.A. 112, *126*

Cohen, G.J., see Gutelius, M.F. 358, *365*

Cohen, M., see Arias, I.M. 279, 296, *310*

Cohen, M.I., see Nathenson, G. 289, 299, *323, 324*

Cohen, S.N., see Odell, G.B. 289 – 291, *324*

Cohn, J., see Alvares, A.P. 352, *361*

Cole, P.G., Lathe, G.H., Billing, B.H. 278, *313*

Cole, P.G., see Billing, B.H. 26, *36*, 278, *311*

Coleman, D.L. 13, 14, *37*, 334, 339, 340, *363*

Coleman, D.L., see Levin, E.Y. 15, *43*

Coleman, D.L., see Russell, R.L. 340, *369*

Colleran, E., O'Carra, P. 25, *37*

Colleran, E., see O'Carra, P. 26, *44*, 118, *125*

Collier, H.B. 339, *363*

Collins, A., see Bonkowsky, H.L. 90, *92*, 260–262, *267*

Collins, A., see Marver, H.S.
9−12, *43*, 132, 134, *153*,
256, 257, 259, 261, 264, *269*,
287, *322*
Collins, A., see Stein, J.A. 9,
13, 32, *46*, 263, *270*
Collins, A., see Tschudy,
D.P. 9, 11, 14, 35, *47*, 82,
94, 256, 265, *270*
Collins, A., see Waxman,
A.D. 265, *270*
Collins, A., see Welland,
F.H. 256, *271*
Collins, G.B., see Abbott,
D.C. 161, *193*
Collins, J., see Battersby,
A.R. 21, *36*
Collison, H.A., see Berk,
P.D. 5, 6, *36*
Collison, H.A., see Blaschke,
T.F. 284, 285, 295−297,
311
Comai, J., Gaylor, J.L. 59, *71*
Comai, K., Gaylor, J.L. 4,
37, 85, *92*
Combs, G.F., Jr., see Scott,
M.L. 115, *126*
Comi, P., see Giglioni, B. 31,
39
Committee on Biologic Effects
of Atm. Poll. 346, 359,
363
Compernolle, F., Hees, G.P.
van Fevery, F., Heirwegh,
K.P.M. *21*, *37*
Compernolle, F., Jansen, F.H.,
Heirwegh, K.P.M. 26, *37*
Compernolle, F., see Fevery,
J. 27, *38*
Condie, L.W., see Piper,
W.N. 89, 90, *93*
Conklin, J., see Visintine,
R.E. 305, *330*
Connaway, S., see Arditti,
R.R. 258, *267*
Connelly, J.L., see Barnes, R.
22, *36*
Conney, A.H. 58, 61−63, *70*,
71, 177−179, *194*, 245, *252*,
284, 286, 295, *313*
Conney, A.H., Burns, J.J. *70*
Conney, A.H., Davison, C.,
Gastel, R., Burns, J.J. 56,
63, *71*
Conney, A.H., Kapitulnik, J.,
Levin, W., Dansette, P., Je-
rina, D. 61, *71*

Conney, A.H., Kuntzman, R.
53, 54, *71*
Conney, A.H., Levin, W., Ja-
cobson, M., Kuntzmann,
R. 295, *313*
Conney, A.H., Lu, A.Y.H.,
Levin, W., Smogys, A.,
West, S., Jacobson, M.,
Ryan, D., Kuntzman, R.
59, *71*
Conney, A.H., Michaelson,
I.A., Burns, J.J. 56, *72*
Conney, A.H., Miller, E.C.,
Miller, J.A. 55, 56, *72*
Conney, A.H., see Alvares,
A.P. 63, *70*
Conney, A.H., see Cucinell,
S.A. 57, *72*
Conney, A.H., see Holder, G.
59, *74*
Conney, A.H., see Jacobson,
M.M. 63, *74*
Conney, A.H., see Kuntzman,
R. 57, *75*
Conney, A.H., see Lu,
A.Y.H. 58, 59, *76*
Conolly, R.B., see Jaeger,
R.J. 112, *124*
Coon, M.J., see Haugen,
D.A. 59, 61, *74*
Coon, M.J., see Hoeven, T.A.
van der 54, *80*
Coon, M.J., see Radtke, H.E.
114, *125*
Coon, M.J., see Strobel,
H.W. 54, *80*
Cooper, D.Y., see Estabrook,
R.W. 351, *363*
Cooper, D.Y., see Omura, T.
77
Cooper, D.Y., see Remmer,
H. 54, *78*
Cooper, D.Y., see Tenhunen,
R. 23−25, *47*, 275, 276, *329*
Cooper, H.L., see Preisig, R.
302, *326*
Cooper, J.M., Thomas, P. 4,
37
Copp, D.H., see Greenberg,
D.M. 88, *92*
Corchs, J.L., Serrani, R.E.,
Rodriguez Garay, E. 291,
313
Corchs, J.L., see Serrani,
R.E. 291, *328*
Corcoran, D., see Strittmatter,
P. 66, *79*

Corcoran, L.P., see Stein,
J.A. 263, *270*
Corcoran, P.L., see Stein,
J.A. 9, 13, 32, *46*
Cornelius, C.E., Ben Ezzer, J.,
Arias, I.M. 277, 291, *313*
Cornelius, C.E., see Mia,
A.S. 293, *323*
Cornelius, C.E., see Upson,
D.W. 303, *330*
Cornford, P. 18, 19, *37*
Cornish, H.H., see Bruckner,
J.V. 57, *71*, *194*
Cornu, F., see Schmid, K. 56,
79
Cornwall, C.C., see Richter,
G.W. 354, *368*
Correia, A.M., see Meyer,
U.A. 250, *253*
Correira, M.A., Mannering,
G.J. 67, *72*
Correira, M.A., Meyer, U.A.
60, *72*, 145, *151*, 250, *252*
Corsi, G.C., see Galzigna, L.
337, *364*
Cortelazzo, S., see Okolic-
sanyi, L. 298, 302, *324*
Coscia, G.C., see Pisani, W.
34, *45*
Coscia, G.C., see Rubino,
G.F. 340, *369*
Cosmides, G.J., see Brodie,
B.B. 228, *233*
Cotzias, G.C., see Dollin-
champs, A.J. 88, *92*
Cotzias, G.C., see Maynard,
L.S. 88, *93*
Cotzias, G.C., see Papavasi-
liou, P.S. 88, *93*
Couch, P., see Jackson, A.H.
21, *41*
Coutinho, C.B., Lucek, R.W.,
Cheripko, J.A., Kuntzman,
R. 289, *313*
Cowger, M.L., Labbe, R.F.
231, 232, *233*
Cowger, M.L., Labbe, R.F.,
Sewell, M. 32, *37*
Cowger, M.L., see Lee, J.J.
288, *320*
Cox, R., see Powell, K.A.
137, *153*
Coy, U., see Grassl, M. 4, *39*
Craig, J.R., see Felsher, B.F.
295, 296, *315*
Craig, W.A., see Kunin,
C.M. 292, *320*

Cramer, J.W., Miller, J.A., Miller, E.C. 56, *72*
Cramér, K. 357, *363*
Crandall, D.C., see Lightner, D.A. 307, *321*
Cranston, W.I., see Wheeler, H.O. 280, *331*
Craske, S., see McIntyre, N. 241, *253*
Creighton, J.C., see Krupa, V. 222, *235*
Creighton, J.C., see Marks, G.S. 148, *153*
Creighton, J.M., Marks, G.S. 219, 222, 224—226, 228, *233*
Creighton, J.M., Racz, W.J., Tyrrell, D.L.J., Schneck, D.W., Marks, G.S. 133, *151*
Cremer, J.E. 355, *363*
Cremer, R.J., Perryman, P.W., Richards, D.H. 306, 308, *314*
Crigler, J.F., Jr., Gold, N.I. 296, *314*
Cripps, D.J., see Rimington, C. 242, *254*
Crow, K.D. 174, 175, *194*
Croy, R.G., see Selkirk, J.K. 59, *79*
Crozier, D.N., see Silverman, W.A. 288, *328*
Cucinell, S.A., Conney, A.H., Sansur, M., Burns, J.J. 57, *72*
Cucinell, S.A., Odessky, L., Weiss, M., Dayton, P.G. *72*
Cukier, J.O., see Odell, G.B. 291, 305, *324*
Cumming, R.L.C., see Millar, J.A. 337, *367*
Cunningham, A.G., Szenberg, A. 351, *363*
Cuthbertson, E.M., see Greenberg, D.M. 88, *92*

Dacie, J.V. 282, 283, *314*
Dadoun, M., see Gordon, E.R. 27, *39*
Dagg, J.H., Goldberg, A., Lochhead, A., Smith, J.A. 243, *253*, 353, *363*
Dagg, J.H., see Lockhead, A.C. 137, *152*
Dahlgren, J.G., see Paghia, D.E. 341, 348, *368*

Dahm, P.A., see Nakatsugawa, T. 107, *125*
Dailey, H.A., Lascelles, J. 22, *37*
D'Albis, A., see Beaven, G.H. 277, *310*
Dallner, G., Siekevitz, P., Palade, G.E. 60, 62, *72*
Dallner, G., see Orrenius, S. 113, *125*
Dalvi, R.R., Hunter, A.L., Neal, R.A. 107, 108, *122*
Dalvi, R.R., Poore, R.E., Neal, R.A. 106, 107, *122*
Daly, J. 103, *122*
Daly, J., see Oesch, F. 63, *77*
Daly, J.S.F., Little, J.M., Troxler, R.F., Lester, R. 4, 5, *37*
Daly, J.W., see Nebert, D.W. 62, *76*
Daly, J.W., see Oesch, F. 64, *77*
Damme, B. van, see Fevery, J. 27, *38*
Damron, B.L., see Simpson, C.F. 354, *369*
Dancewicz, A.M., see Kowalski, E. 34, *42*
Daniel, M., see Dingle, J.T. 87, *92*
Danielsson, H., see Mitropoulos, K.A. 62, *76*
Dansette, P., see Conney, A.H. 61, *71*
Dansette, P., see Holder, G. 59, *74*
Dashman, T., see Feigelson, P. 6, *38*
Davidow, B., see Spector, M.J. 359, *370*
Davidson, J.N., see Skea, B.R. 33, *46*
Davies, D.S., Thorgeirsson, S.S. 58, *72*
Davies, D.R., see Yeary, R.A. 289, *331*
Davies, L., see Orme, M.L.E. 295, 297, *324*
Davies, R.C., Gorchein, A., Neuberger, A., Sandy, J.D., Tait, G.H. 11, 17, 21, *37*
Davies, R.C., Neuberger, A. 15, 16, *37*
Davies, R.E., Keohane, S.J. 307, *314*

Davis, D.C., see Mitchell, J.R. 85, *93*
Davis, D.C., see Potter, W.Z. 85, *93*
Davison, A.N. 105, *122*
Davison, C., see Conney, A.H. 56, 63, *71*
Davison, S.C., Wills, E.D. 63, *72*
Dawber, N.H., see Thaler, M.M. 308, *329*
Dawber, N.H., see Troxler, R.F. 280, *330*
Dawes, E., see Goudy, B. 335, *364*
Day, R., see Johnson, L. 288, 289, *319*
Dayton, P.G., see Chen, W. 56, 57, *71*
Dayton, P.G., see Cucinell, S.A. 56, *72*
Dean, G. 163, 164, *194*, 232, *233*, 243, *253*
De Bruin, A., Hoolboom, H. 337, *363*
De Crombrugghe, B., Perlman, R.L., Varmus, H.E., Pastan, I. 258, *267*
De Dueve, C., see Lazarow, P.B. 142, *152*
De Goeiji, A.F.P.M., Christianse, K., Van Steveninck, J. 342, *363*
De Groote, J., see Fevery, J. 278, 279, *315*
De Leeuw, N.K.M. 281, *323*
De Matteis, F. 31, 32, *37*, 97—99, 101—104, 106—108, 110—112, 116, 118, 119, *122*, 132, 134, 135, 138—141, 143—149, *151*, 157, 175, 192, *194*, 203—205, 209, 221, 225—227, 230—232, *233*, 245, 246, 249, 251, 252, *253*, 256, *267*, 287, *314*
De Matteis, F., Abbritti, G., Gibbs, A. 12, 23, 31, *37*, 84, *92*, 136, 137, 148, *151*, 224, *233*
De Matteis, F., Gibbs, A.H. 31, 32, *37*, 60, *72*, 86, 88, *92*, 115, 116, 120, *122*, 132, 136, 138, 139, 143, 144, 145, 148, 150, *151*, 246, 251, *253*

De Matteis, F., Prior, B.E.,
Rimington, C. 162, 167,
168, 169, 170, 171, 179, 181,
184, 188, *194*
De Matteis, F., Rimington, C.
142, *151*
De Matteis, F., Seawright,
A.A.S. 105–107, *122*
De Matteis, F., Sparks, R.G.
111, *122*, 192, *194*, 264,
267
De Matteis, F., Unseld, A.
102, 104, 120, *123*
De Matteis, F., see Abbritti,
G. 102, 120, *121*, 132, 134,
135, 138, 139, 142, *150*, 204,
205, 226, *233*
De Matteis, F., see Bond,
E.J. 105, 108, 109, *122*
De Matteis, F., see Greig,
I.R. 57, 61, *73*, 177, 179, *195*
De Matteis, F., see Seawright,
A.A. 107, *126*
De Matteis, F., see Unseld,
A. 98–102, 104, *127*
De Toranzo, E.G.D., Diaz
Gomez, M.I., Castro, J.A.
109, 110, *123*
De Turris, P., see Romagnoli,
G. 305, *327*
De Vos, R.H., see Vos, J.G.
200
Decker, E., see Watson, R.J.
349, *371*
Decker, P., see Stich, W. 138,
154, 225, 226, *231*, *236*
Defranchis, R., see Ideo, G.
298, 299, *318*
Defreitas, A.S.W., see Hutzin-
ger, O. 159, 161, *195*
Degowin, R.L., Eppes, R.B.,
Powell, R.D., Carson, P.E.
282, *314*
Dehlinger, P.J., Schimke,
R.T. 59, *72*
Deiss, A., see Cartwright,
G.E. 348, *362*
Del C. Battle, A.M., see Llam-
bias, E.B.C. 334, 345, *366*
Del Favero, A., Gamulin, S.,
Gray, C.H., Norman,
M.R. 145, *151*
Del Favero, A., see Water-
field, M.D. 97, *127*, 134,
154
Del Ninno, E., see Ideo, G.
298, 299, *318*

Del Rio, A.E., see Rudman,
D. 288, *327*
Deleon, A.L., Gartner, M.,
Arias, I.M. 279, 295, 296,
306, *314*
Dent, C.E., see Wilson, V.K.
355, *371*
Denton, M.J., Spencer, N.,
Arnstein, H.R.V. 28, *38*
Deppe, W.M., see Taljaard,
J.J.F. 19, *47*, 165, 169, 170,
171, 180, 182, 184, 185, 186,
189, 192, *199*
Derepentigny, L., see Traiger,
G.J. 286, *329*
Dern, P.J., see Brewer, J.G.
281, *312*
Dern, R.J., Beutler, E., Al-
ving, A.S. 282, *314*
Dern, R.J., see Beutler, E.
340, *362*
Desalu, O., see Lodish, H.F.
31, *43*
Desforges, J., see Silverberg,
M. 300, *328*
Detwiler, P., see Halac, E.
28, *40*
Deutsch, H.F., see Hartz,
J.W. 4, *40*
Dewalz, A.T., see Noir, B.A.
279, *324*
Dhar, G.J., Bossenmaier, I.,
Petryka, Z.J., Cardinal, R.,
Watson, C.J. 243, *253*
Dhumeaux, D., Berthelot, P.
293, *314*
Dhumeaux, D., Erlinger, S.,
Benhamou, J.P., Fauvert,
R. 302, *314*
Dhumeaux, D., see Berthelot,
P. 300, *311*
Dhumeaux, D., see Capelle,
P. 291, *313*
Dhumeaux, D., see Erlinger,
S. 302, *314*
Diamond, I. 288, *314*
Diaz Gomez, M.I., see De To-
ranzo, E.G.D. 109, 110,
123
Diehl, H., see Ullrich, V. 67,
80
Dillon, R.S., see Bolt, R.J.
291, *312*
Dimant, E., Landerg, E., Lon-
don, I.M. 340, *363*
Dinamarca, M.L., see Wagner,
G.S. 84, 86–88, *94*

Dingell, J.V., see Heath, E.C.
299, *317*
Dingle, J.T., Heath, J.C.,
Webb, M., Daniel, M. 87,
92
Dioguardi, N., see Ideo, G.
298, 299, *318*
Dipiazza, M., see Halac, E.
28, *40*
Dixon, R.L., see Woods, J.S.
12, 34, *48*, 147, *155*, 226,
237
Dobozy, A., see Simon, N.
169, 170, 180, 188, *198*
Dobrschansky, M. 243, *253*
Doedens, D.J. 103, *123*
Dogramaci, I., Kenanoglu, A.,
Muftu, Y., Ergene, T.,
Wray, J.D. 163, *194*
Dogramaci, I., Tinaztepe, B.,
Gunalp, A. 163, *194*
Dogramaci, I., Wray, J.D., Er-
gene, T., Sezer, V., Muftu,
Y. 163, *194*
Dogramaci, I., see Wray,
J.D. 162, 163, *200*
Doherty, J.M., see Bonkow-
sky, H.L. 90, *92*, 260–262,
267
Dolle, W., see Doss, M. 165,
194
Done, A.K. 274, 288, 289,
314
Doss, M. 132, *151*
Doss, M., Kaltepoth, B. 210,
233
Doss, M., Meinhof, W., Look,
D., Henning, H., Nawrocki,
P., Dolle, W., Strohmeyer,
G., Filippini, L. 165, *194*
Doss, M., Schermuly, E.,
Koss, G. 169, *194*
Doss, M., see Meyer, U.A.
233, 235, 241, *253*
Douglas, J.F., Ludwig, B.J.,
Smith, N. 56, *72*
Dowben, R.M., see Hsia,
D.Y. 300, 301, *318*
Dowben, R.M., see Lokietz,
H. 300, *321*
Dowdle, E., Goldswain, P.,
Spong, N., Eales, L. 165,
194
Dowdle, E., see Hickman, R.
33, *40*, 259, *268*
Dowdle, E.B., Mustard, P.,
Eales, L. 256, *267*

Dowdle, E.B., see Ginsburg, A.D. 142, *152*
Dowdle, E.B., see Wilson, E.L. 13, *48*, 333, 334, 339, 341, *371*
Downie, E.D., see Skea, B.R. 33, *46*
Doyle, D. 13, *38*
Doyle, D., Schimke, R.T. 13, 14, 16, *38*, 334, *363*
Doyle, D., see Arias, I.M. 59, 70
Doyle, D., see Schimke, R.T. 4, *46*, 50, 51, 59, *70, 79*
Drabkin, D.L. 283, *314*
Draper, D.A., see Maurer, H.M. 305, *322*
Draper, H.H., see Kokatnur, M.G. 113, *124*
Dreher, W., see Freundt, K.J. 105, *123*
Dresel, E.I.B., Falk, J.D. 333, 341, *363*
Druyan, R., Bernard, B. de, Rabinowitz, M. 4, 5, *38*, 50, *72*
Druyan, R., Jakovicic, S., Rabinowitz, M. 67, *72*
Druyan, R., Kelly, A. 23, 28, 31, *38*, 60, *72*, 132, *151*
Druyan, R., see Aschenbrenner, V. 6, *36*
Druyan, R., see McKay, R. 9, 11, 22, *44*, 149, *153*
Dublin, C.C., see Gutelius, M.F. 358, *365*
Dumont, M., see Erlinger, S. 302, *314*
Duncan, C.H., see Best, M.M. 67, *71*
Dunham, R., see Waters, W.J. 300, *330*
Dunn, W.J., see Hansch, C. 206, 207, *234*
Durzt, J., see Sawinsky, A. 351, *369*
Dutton, G.J. 274, 278, 279, 294, 301, *314*
Dutton, G.J., Burchell, B. 64, *72*
Dutton, G.J., see Winsnes, A. 294, 295, *331*
Duvaldestin, P., Mahu, J.-L., Berthelot, P. 27, *38*
Duve, C. de, see Lazarow, P.B. 5, 23, *42*, 67, 68, 75

Duve, C. de, see Leighton, F. 67, *75*
Duve, C. de, see Poole, B. 50, 67, *78*
Dybing, E. 301, *314*
Dybing, E., Rugstad, H.E. 300, 301, *314*
Dybing, E., see Rugstad, H.E. 300, *327*
Dyck, W.P., see Waitman, A.M. 302, *330*

Eales, L. 219, 230, 231, 232, *233*, 244, *253*
Eales, L., see Dowdle, E. 165, *194*, 256, *267*
Eales, L., see Hickman, R. 33, *40*, 259, *268*
Eales, L., see Pimstone, N.R. 23, *44*, 158, *197*
Eber, J., see Weed, R.I. 350, *371*
Ebert, P.S., Tschudy, D.P., Choudhry, J.N., Chirigos, M.A. 10, *38*
Ebert, P.S., see Bonkowsky, H.L. 342, *362*
Ecobichon, D.J., see Hansell, M.M. 187, *195*
Ecobichon, D.J., see Johnstone, G.J. 177–179, *196*
Edmond, M., Erlinger, S., Berthelot, P., Benhamon, J.P., Fauvert, R. 300, *314*
Edwards, A.M., Elliott, W.H. 222, 223, 224, *234*
Edwards, M., Elliot, W.H. 259, 260, *267*
Ehrenstein, G.v., see Åkeson, Å. 5, *35*
Eilon, L., see Hershko, Ch. 187, *195*
Eisalo, A., see Koskelo, P. 219, *235*
Eisenklam, E., see Ulstrom, R.A. 305, *330*
Eisenstein, R., see Hass, G.M. 354, *365*
Eisentraut, A.M., see Sutherland, D.A. 350, *370*
Eisinger, J., see Blumberg, W.E. 344, 359, *362*
Eisinger, J., see Fischbein, A. 344, *364*
Eisner, M., see Eliakim, M. 285, *314*

Elder, G., Gray, C.H., Nicholson, D.C. 280, *314*
Elder, G.H. 166, 169, 170, 184, 188, *195*
Elder, G.H., Evans, J.O., Matlin, S. 170, 181–184, 190, *195*
Elder, G.H., Gray, C.H., Nicholson, D.C. 240, *253*
Elder, G.H., Nicholson, D.C., Gray, C.H. 157, 184, *195*
Elder, G.H., see Jackson, A.H. 19, *41*, 170, 181, *196*
Elder, G.H., see Stoll, M.S. 19, *46*, 170, *199*
Eliakim, M., Eisner, M., Ungar, H. 285, *314*
Elias, S.L., see Chvapil, M. 112, *122*
Elkins, D., see Leo, A. 206, 221, *235*
Ellin, A., Orrenius, S. 115, *123*
Elliott, W.B., see Nicholls, P. 6, *44*
Elliott, W.H., see Edwards, A.M. 222–224, *234*, 259, 260, *267*
Elliott, W.H., see Irving, E.A. 10, 11, *41*, 150, *152*
Elliott, W.H., see Whiting, M.J. 9, 12, *48*, 148, 149, *155*
Elton, W., see Gralnick, H.R. 283, *316*
Emerman, S., see Javitt, N.B. 304, *319*
Emmer, M., see Anderson, W.B. 258, *267*
Enerback, L., see Lundvall, O. 174, *197*
Eng, G., see Leiken, S. 349, *366*
Eng, M., see Kjellström, T. 344, *366*
Engel, P., see Pimstone, N.R. 24, *45*, 118, *125*, 276, *325*
Engstrom, J., Hellstrom, K., Posse, N., Sjovall, J. 306, *314*
Eppes, R.B., see Degowin, R.L. 282, *314*
Epps, H.M.R., Gale, E.F. 256, *267*
Epstein, S.S., Mantel, N. 355, *363*

Epstein, W., Beckwith, J.R. 50, *72*

Erenberg, G., Rinsler, S.S., Fish, B.G. 357, *363*

Ergene, T., see Dogramaci, I. 163, *194*

Ergene, T., see Peters, H.A. 162–164, 168, *197*

Eriksson, L.C. 63, *72*

Erlinger, S. 280, *314*

Erlinger, S., Dhumeaux, D., Berthelot, P., Dumont, M. 302, *314*

Erlinger, S., Dumont, M. 302, *314*

Erlinger, S., see Berthelot, P. 300, *311*

Erlinger, S., see Dhumeaux, D. 302, *314*

Erlinger, S., see Edmond, M. 300, *314*

Ernster, L., Orrenius, S. 59, 60, 63, *72*

Ernster, L., see Nilsson, R. 113, *125*

Ernster, L., see Orrenius, S. 113, *125*

Ernster, L., see Sottocasa, L. 66, *79*

Ernster, L., see Zeidenberg, P. 63, *80*, 279, 295, 301, *332*

Eron, L., see Arditti, R.R. 258, *267*

Ertel, I.J., Newton, W.A. 296, 298, *315*

Ertel, I.J., see Levy, G. 300, *321*

Espinoza, J., Baranafi, L., Schnaidt, E. 305, *315*

Essner, E., see Goldfischer, S. 304, *315*

Estabrook, R.W. 53, 55, *72*

Estabrook, R.W., Hildebrandt, A., Remmer, H., Schenkman, J.B., Rosenthal, O., Cooper, D.Y. 351, *363*

Estabrook, R.W., see Hildebrandt, A. 59, 67, *74*

Estabrook, R.W., see Nishibayashi, H. 111, *125*

Estabrook, R.W., see Omura, T. *77*

Estabrook, R.W., see Remmer, H. 54, *78*

Estabrook, R.W., see Schenkman, J.B. 62, *79*

Etienne, J., see Blum, D. 305, *312*

Etienne, J.P., see Ploussard, J.P. 305, *325*

Evans, J.O., see Elder, G.H. 170, 181–184, 190, *195*

Evans, M., see Badawy, A.A.B. 52, 53, *70*, 142, *151*

Evans, N., see Jackson, A.H. 19, *41*, 170, 181, *196*

Everett, M.A., see Bottomley, S.S. 342, *362*

Faeder, E., see Lucier, G.W. 177, *196*

Fairbanks, V.F., Beutler, E. 358, *363*

Falk, J.D., see Dresel, E.I.B. 333, 341, *363*

Falk, J.E. 2, 3, 15, *38*, 101, *123*, 335, *363*

Falk, J.E., see Lemberg, R. 101, *124*

Falk, J.E., see Porra, R.J. 20, 21, *45*

Falk, J.F. 68, *73*

Fanica-Gaignier, M., Clement-Metral, J. 8, *38*

Farber, T.M., Baker, A. 177, *195*

Farquhar, M.G., Bergeron, J.J.M., Palade, G.E. 66, *73*

Farr, R.S., see Pinckard, R.N. 287, *325*

Fauvert, R., see Dhumeaux, D. 302, *314*

Fauvert, R., see Edmond, M. 300, *314*

Feigelson, P., Dashman, T., Margolis, F. 5, *38*

Feigelson, P., Greengard, O. 52, *73*

Feinstein, G., see Frydman, R.B. 15, 16, *38*

Feldman, D.S., Levere, R.D., Lieberman, J.S., Cardinal, R.A., Watson, C.J. 353, *363*

Feldman, G., see Capelle, P. 291, *313*

Feldmann, G., see Hakim, J. 298, *316*

Felsher, B.F., Craig, J.R., Carpio, N. 295, 296, *315*

Felsher, B.F., Redeker, A.G. 256, *267*

Felsher, B.F., see Strand, J.L. 241, *254*

Felsher, B.F., see Strand, L.J. 11, 12, 16, *46*, 334, 353, *370*

Ferguson, J.H., Keaton, A.G. 358, *364*

Ferm, V.H. 355, *364*

Ferm, V.H., Carpenter, S.J. 355, 357, *364*

Ferramola, A.M., see Batlle, A.M. del C. 14, *36*

Ferramola, A.M., see Jackson, A.H. 19, *41*, 170, 181, *196*

Ferramola, A.M., see San Martin de Viale, L.C. 181, 185, *198*

Ferrand, C.F., Jr., see Mooty, J. 358, *367*

Ferreiro, M., see Lucey, J.F. 307, *322*

Fevery, F., see Compernolle, F. 27, *37*

Fevery, J., Damme, B. van, Michiels, R., Groote, J. de, Heirwegh, K.P.M. 27, *38*, 278, 279, *315*

Fevery, J., Ilees, G.P. van, Leroy, P., Compernolle, F., Heirwegh, K.P.M. 27, *38*

Fevery, J., Leroy, P., Heirwegh, K.P.M. 27, *38*

Fevery, J., Leroy, P., Vijver, M. van de, Heirwegh, K.P.M. 27, *38*

Fevery, J., see Black, M. 295–297, *311*

Fevery, J., see Heirwegh, K.P.M. 27, *40*, 279, 294, *317*

Fevery, J., see Kutz, K. 296, 298, *320*

Figen, J.F., see Schmid, R. 142, *154*

Figueroa, E., see Johnson, L. 288, 289, *319*

Filippini, L., see Doss, M. 165, *194*

Filipson, M., see Schersten, T. 302, *327*

Finelli, V.N., Klauder, D.S., Karaffa, M.A., Petering, H.G. 338, 357, *364*

Finelli, V.N., Murthy, L., Peirano, W.B., Petering, H.G. 13, *38*, 334, 338, 357, *364*

Fink, K., see Valentine, W.N. 348, *370*

Finkelstein, R.A. 220, *234*
Finocchi, G., see Girotti, F. 305, *315*
Fiorina, L., see Rubino, G.F. 349, *369*
Fischbein, A., Sassa, S., Eisinger, J., Blumberg, W. 344, *364*
Fischer, H., Orth, H. 274, *315*
Fischer, P.W.F., Morgan, R.O., Krupa, V., Marks, G.S. 210, 211, *234*
Fischer, P.W.F., see Morgan, R.O. 211, 223, 229, *235*
Fish, B.G., see Erenberg, G. 357, *363*
Fishbein, L. 159, *195*
Fitch, C., see Tuttle, A.H. 347, 348, *370*
Fitzhugh, O.G., Nelson, A.A. 65, 66, *73*
Fitzpatrick, T.B., see Kalivas, J.T. 169, 171, *196*
Flanagan, C.L., see Beutler, E. 340, *362*
Fleischer, B., see Fleischer, S. 66, *73*
Fleischer, S., Fleischer, B., Azzi, A., Chance, B. 66, *73*
Fleischmann, R., Mattenheimer, H., Holmes, A.W., Remmer, H. 67, *38*
Fleischmann, R.A., see Remmer, H. 56, 58, *78*
Fleischmann, R.A., see Schoene, B. 58, *79*
Fleischner, G., Kamisaka, K., Habig, W., Jakoby, W., Arias, J.M. 292, 293, *315*
Fleischner, G., Meijer, D.K.F., Levine, W.G., Gatmaitan, Z., Gluck, R., Arias, I.M. 68, *73, 293, 315*
Fleischner, G., Robbins, J., Arias, I.M. 293, *315*
Fleischner, G., Robbins, J., Reyes, H., Levi, A.J., Arias, I.M. 278, *315*
Fleischner, G., see Habig, W.H. 64, *74, 292, 316*
Fleischner, G., see Kirsch, R. 292, 293, *320*
Fleischner, G., see Mishkin, S. 292, *323*

Fletcher, J.E., see Ashbrook, J.D. 277, *310*
Fletcher, J.E., see Spector, A.A. 288, *328*
Fletcher, M.J., Sanadi, D.R. 283, *315*
Flock, E.V., see Robinson, S.H. 275, *327*
Flothe, L., see Bugany, H. 22, 23, *37*
Flyger, V., see Levin, E.Y. 15, *43*
Foadi, M., see Robinson, M.G. 283, *326*
Foliot, A., see Ploussard, J.P. 305, *325*
Fong, K., McKay, P.B., Poyer, J.L., Keele, B.B., Misra, H. 111, *123*
Forbes, A., see Schmid, R. 305, *328*
Forbes, G.B., Reino, J.C. 353, *364*
Foreman, R.L., Maynert, E.W. 103, *123*
Foschini, M., see Romagnoli, G. 305, *327*
Foulk, W.T., see Metge, W.R. 296, 306, *323*
Fouts, J.R., see Gram, T.E. 279, *316*
Fouts, J.R., see Hart, L.G. 56, *74*
Fowler, B.A., see Lucier, G.W. 177, *196*
Fowler, J.S.L. 110, *123*
Franco, D., Preaux, A.-M., Bismuth, H., Berthelot, P. 26, *38*
Fratianne, R.B., Griggs, R.C., Harris, J.W. 350, *364*
Freedman, A.L., Barr, P.S., Brody, E.A. 283, *315*
Freedman, M.L., Geraghty, M., Rosman, J. 30, *38*
Freeman, M., see Krupa, V. 222, *235*
Frei, J., see Okolicsanyi, L. 295, 296, 305, *324*
French, S.W., Todoroff, T. 357, *364*
Frenzel, J., see Reinicke, C. 298, *326*
Freshney, R.I., Paul, J. 10, 12, 14, 23, *38*
Freund, S., see Vasiliu, A. 340, *370*

Freundt, K.J., Dreher, W. 105, *123*
Frey, I., see Schenkman, J.B. 62, *79*
Frick, P.G., Hitzig, W.II., Betke, L. 282, *315*
Fristedt, B.I., see Haeger-Aronsen, B. 337, *365*
Fritz, M.E., Brooks, F.P. 302, *315*
Fröhling, W., see Bock, K.W. 10, 12, 27, *36*, 60, 62, 63, *71*, 143, *151*
Fröhling, W., see Matern, S. 65, *76*
Frohling, W., see Bock, K.W. 111, *122, 252*, 294, 295, 299, *312, 252*
Fromke, V.L., Miller, D. 286, *315*
Frommer, U., Ullrich, V., Staudinger, H., Orrenius, S. 58, *73*
Frontino, G., see Kato, R. 147, *152*
Frydman, B., see Frydman, R.B. 15, 18, 35, *38, 39*
Frydman, B., see Stevens, E. 15, *46*, 345, *370*
Frydman, B., see Tomaro, M.L. 15, 35, *42, 47*
Frydman, R.B., Feinstein, G. 15, 16, *38*
Frydman, R.B., Tomaro, M.L., Frydman, B., Wanschelbaum, A. 35, *38*
Frydman, R.B., Tomaro, M.L., Wanschelbaum, A., Andersen, E.M., Awruch, J., Friedman, B. 15, *39*
Frydman, R.B., Valasinas, A., Frydman, B. 18, *39*
Frydman, R.B., see Stevens, E. 15, *46*, 345, *370*
Fuhr, J.E., see Grayzel, A.I. 30, *40*
Fujimoto, J.M., see Smith, D.S. 303, *328*
Fukanama, G., see Visintine, R.E. 305, *330*
Fullerton, M. 349, *364*
Funakoshi, S., see Hartz, J.W. 4, *40*
Furman, M., see Arias, I.M. 298, 299, 301, *310*
Furst, P., see Josephson, B. 289, *319*

Gaddis, E.M., see Welland,
  F.H. 256, *271*
Gaines, T.B., see Kimbrough,
  R.D. 177, 178, 187, 188,
  196
Gajdos, A., Gajdos-Török,
  M. 1, 2, 32, *39*, 162,
  168–170, *195*, 261, *267*, 345,
  364
Gajdos-Török, M., see Gaj-
  dos, A. 1, 2, 32, *39*, 162,
  168–170, *195*, 261, *267*, 345,
  364
Galambos, J.T., see Raymond,
  G.D. 278, *326*
Gale, E.F., see Epps, H.M.R.
  256, *267*
Gallagher, T.F., see Bradlow,
  H.L. 266, *267*
Gallagher, T.F., see Kappas,
  A. 266, *268*
Gallo, E., see Prato, V. 282,
  326
Galzigna, L., Corsi, G.C.,
  Saia, B., Rizzoli, A.A. 337,
  364
Games, D.E., see Jackson,
  A.H. 19, 21, *41*, 170, 181,
  196
Games, D.E., see Stoll, M.S.
  19, *46*, 170, *199*
Gamulin, S., see Del Favero,
  A. 145, *151*
Ganote, C.E., see Rosenthal,
  A.S. 337, *368*
Gansinger, G., see Haurowitz,
  F. 113, *123*
Ganther, H.E., see Rotruck,
  J.T. 115, *126*
Garcia, D.C., San Martin de
  Viale, L.L., Tomio, J.M.,
  Grinstein, M. 181, *195*
Garcia, M.L., see Johnson,
  L. 288, 289, *319*
Garcia, R.C., San Martin de
  Viale, L.C., Tomio, J.M.,
  Grinstein, M. 18, *39*
Garcia, R.C., see San Martin
  de Viale, L.C. 18, *45*
Garcia, R.C., see Tomio,
  J.M. 18, *47*, 181, *199*
Gardner, F.H., see Gorshein,
  D. 30, *39*, 265, *268*
Garner, R.C., McLean,
  A.E.M. 110, *123*, 283, *315*
Garrick, M.D., see Mohler,
  D.N. 281, *323*

Garro, F., see Pentschew, A.
  352, *368*
Garrod, A.E. 239, *253*
Gartner, L., see Arias, I.M.
  298, 299, *310*
Gartner, L., see Bernstein,
  L.H. 277–279, *310*
Gartner, L.M., see Arias,
  I.M. 279, 296, 301, *309*,
  310
Gartner, L.M., see Vaisman,
  S.L. 295, *330*
Gartner, M., see Deleon,
  A.L. 279, 295, 296, 306,
  314
Gastel, van, C., see Schlesin-
  ger, F.G. 231, *236*
Gastel, R., see Conney, A.H.
  56, 63, *71*
Gatmaitan, Z., see Fleischner,
  G. 68, *73*, 293, *315*
Gatmaitan, Z., see Habig,
  W.H. 64, *74*, 292, *316*
Gatmaitan, Z., see Kamisaka,
  K. 292, *319*
Gatmaitan, Z., see Levi, A.J.
  277, 278, 292, 293, *321*
Gatmaitan, Z., see Levine,
  R.I. 278, *321*
Gatmaitan, Z., see Mishkin,
  S. 292, *323*
Gatmaitan, Z., see Reyes, H.
  278, 293, *326*
Gaugh, S.P., see Beale, S.I.
  258
Gayathri, A.K., Rao, M.R.S.,
  Padmanaban, G. 9, 33, 34,
  39, 149, *151*
Gaylor, J.L., see Comai, K.
  5, *37*, 59, *71*, 85, *92*
Gear, A.R.L., Albert, A.D.,
  Bednarek, J.M. 68, 69,
  73
Geary, D., see Morley, A.
  167, *197*
Gehring, P.J., see Piper,
  W.N. 162, *197*
Gelboin, H.V. 59, *73*
Gelboin, H.V., Blackburn,
  N.R. 56, *73*
Gelboin, H.V., Okuda, T., Sel-
  kirk, J., Nemoto, Yang,
  S.K., Wiebel, F.J., Whit-
  lock, J.P., Jr., Rapp, H.J.,
  Bast, R.C., Jr. 61, *73*
Gelboin, H.V., Wortham, J.S.,
  Wilson, R.G. 145, *152*

Gelboin, H.V., see Nebert,
  D.W. 58, *76*, 212, *235*
Gelboin, H.V., see Nemoto,
  N. 64, *77*
Gelboin, H.V., see Selkirk,
  J.K. 59, *79*
Gelboin, H.V., see Whitlock,
  J.P., Jr. 58, 60, *80*
Geller, E., see Yuwiler, A.
  257, 259, *271*
Gellhorn, A., Benjamin, W.
  66, *73*
Gellis, S., see Silverberg, M.
  300, *328*
Geraghty, M., see Freedman,
  M.L. 30, *38*
Gertler, S., see Lightner,
  D.A. 307, *321*
Getz, G.S., see McKay, R. 9,
  11, 22, *44*, 149, *153*
Ghazal, A., Koransky, W.,
  Portig, J., Vohland, H.W.,
  Klempau, I. 56, *73*
Ghazarian, J.G., Jefcoate,
  C.R., Knutson, J.C., Orme-
  Johnson, W.H., Luca, H.F.
  de 4, *39*
Giacoia, G.P., see Krasner, J.
  290, *320*
Gianni, A.M., see Giglioni,
  B. 31, *39*
Gibbs, A.H., see De Matteis,
  F. 12, 23, 31, 32, *37*, 60,
  72, 84, 86, 88, *92*, 115, 116,
  120, *122*, 132, 136–138,
  139, 143–145, 148, 150,
  151, 224, *233*, 246, 251, *253*
Gibson, K.D., Laver, W.G.,
  Neuberger, A. 333, *364*
Gibson, K.D., Matthew, M.,
  Newberger, A., Thait,
  G.H. 258, *267*
Gibson, K.D., Neuberger, A.,
  Scott, J.J. 13, 14, *39*, 333,
  334, 337, *364*
Gibson, S.L.M., Goldberg,
  A. 13, 23, *39*
Gibson, S.L.M., MacKenzie,
  G.C., Goldberg, A. 346,
  364
Gibson, S.M., Goldberg, A.
  337, 341, 353, *364*
Gibson, W.R., see Owen,
  N.V. 65, *77*
Gielen, J.E., Goujon, F.M.,
  Nebert, D.W. 60–62,
  73

Gielen, J.E., see Nebert, D.W. 58, 60, 62, *76*

Gielen, J.E., see Oesch, F. 64, 77

Giglioni, B., Gianni, A.M., Comi, P., Ottolenghi, S., Rungger 31, *39*

Gilder, H., see Granick, S. *39*

Gillette, J., see Remmer, H. 54, *78*

Gillette, J.R. *70*

Gillette, J.R., Mitchell, J.R., Brodie, B.B. 54, *73*

Gillette, J.R., Stripp, B. 62, *73*

Gillette, J.R., see Brodie, B.B. *70*

Gillette, J.R., see Greene, F.E. 109, *123*

Gillette, J.R., see Kato, R. 62, *75*

Gillette, J.R., see Mitchell, J.R. 85, *93*

Gillette, J.R., see Potter, W.Z. 85, *93*

Gillette, J.R., see Sasame, H.A. 109, *126*

Gillette, P.N., see Bradlow, H.L. 266, *267*

Gillette, P.N., see Kappas, A. 266, *268*

Gillette, P.N., see Rifkind, A.B. 218, 219, 222, 223, 231, 232, *236*, 249, *254*

Gillis, J.D., see Hirsch, G.H. 205, 226, 231, *234*

Ginsburg, A.D., Dowdle, E.B. 142, *152*

Ginsburg, D., see Battistini, V. 341, *362*

Girotti, F., Finocchi, G., Sartori, L., Boscherini, B. 305, *315*

Gisselbrecht, C., Berk, P.D. 284, 285, *315*

Glader, B.E. 281, *315*

Glass, J., Yannoni, C.Z., Robinson, S.H. 275, *315*

Glaumann, H. 85, *92*, 279, *315*

Glazener, L., see Harvey, D.J. 103, *123*

Glende, E.A., Jr., see Recknagel, R.O. 110, *126*

Glover, E., see Poland, A. 57, 58, 61, 66, *77*, *78*, 157, 174, *197*, 220, *236*

Gluck, R., see Fleischner, G. 68, *73*, 293, *315*

Goerz, G., see Ippen, H. 170, *196*

Gold, N.I., see Crigler, J.F., Jr. 296, *314*

Goldberg, A. 82, 84, 87, *92*, 225, 231, *234*, 244, 246, *253*, 353, *364*

Goldberg, A., Ashenbrucker, G.E., Cartwright, G.E., Wintrobe, M.M. 341, *364*

Goldberg, A., McGillion, F.B. 353, *364*

Goldberg, A., Moore, M.R., Beattie, A.D., Hall, P.E., McCallum, J., Grant, J.K. 266, *267*

Goldberg, A., Paton, W.D.M., Thompson, J.W. 353, *364*

Goldberg, A., Rimington, C. 138, *152*, 222, *234*

Goldberg, A., see Battistini, V. 341, *362*

Goldberg, A., see Beattie, A.D. 251, *252*

Goldberg, A., see Dagg, J.H. 243, *253*, 353, *363*

Goldberg, A., see Gibson, S.L.M. 13, 23, *39*, 337, 341, 346, 353, *364*

Goldberg, A., see Lochhead, A.C. 87, *93*

Goldberg, A., see Lockhead, A.C. 137, *152*

Goldberg, A., see McIntyre, N. 241, *253*

Goldberg, A., see Meredith, P.A. 338, *367*

Goldberg, A., see Millar, J.A. 337, *367*

Goldberg, A., see Moore, M.R. 12, *44*, 158, 172, 185, *197*, 224, 231, *235*, 265, 266, 269

Goldberg, A., see Morrow, J.J. 345, *367*

Goldberg, A., see Paxton, J.W. 265, 266, 269

Goldberg, A.L., Howell, E.M., Li, J.B., Martel, S.B., Prouty, W.F. 3, *39*

Goldenberg, G.J., see Israel, L.G. 24, *41*

Goldenberg, G.J., see Israels, L.G. 276, *318*

Goldenberg, J., see Vessey, D.A. 27, 47, 279, 294, 301, *330*

Goldenberg, J., see Zakim, D. 296, *332*

Goldfischer, S., Arias, I.M., Essner, E., Novikoff, A.B. 304, *315*

Goldstein, A., Aronow, L., Kalman, S.M. 51, *73*

Goldstein, J., see Poland, A. 176, *197*

Goldstein, J.A., Hickman, P., Bergman, H., Vos, J.G. 157, 175, 180, 187, 188, *195*

Goldstein, J.A., Hickman, P., Jue, D.L. 177, 178, 180, 183, 192, *195*

Goldstein, J.A., Taurog, A. 299, *315*

Goldswain, P., see Dowdle, E. 165, *194*

Gollan, J.L., Huang, S.N., Billing, B., Sherlock, S. 296, *315*

Gombos, B., Pechanova, A., Koziak, B., Moscovicova, E. 167, *195*

Gommi, B.W., see Salvador, R.A. 67, 68, *78*

González, M., see González-Cadavid, N.F. 23, *39*

González-Cadavid, N.F., Ortega, J.P., Gonzaléz, M. 23, *39*

Good, T.A., see Kammholz, L.P. 359, *366*

Goodman, D.S. 277, *315*

Goodman, H., see Porto, S.O. 308, *325*

Gorchein, A., see Davies, R.C. 11, 17, 21, *37*

Gordon, A.S., Zanjani, E.D., Levere, R.D., Kappas, A. 30, *39*, 265, *267*

Gordon, E.R., Dadoun, M., Goresky, C.A., Chan, T.-H., Perlin, A.S. 27, *39*

Goresky, C.A. 277, 279, *315*

Goresky, C.A., Haddad, H.H., Kluger, W.S., Nadeau, B.E., Bach, G.G. 280, 302, *316*

Goresky, C.A., Kluger, S.W. 303, *316*

Goresky, C.A., see Gordon, E.R. 27, *39*

Gorshein, D., Gardner, F.H. 30, *39*, 265, *268*

Gottesman, M.E., see Nissley, S.P. 258, *269*

Goudy, B., Dawes, E., Wilkinson, A.E., Wills, E.D. 335, *364*

Goujon, F.M., see Gielen, J.E. 60, 61, 62, *73*

Gould, T.C., see Gunn, S.A. 357, *365*

Goulding, R., see Abbott, D.C. 161, *193*

Goulis, G., see Broughton, P.M.G. 306, 308, *312*

Goyer, R.A. 354, 355, 357, *364*

Goyer, R.A., Leonard, D., Moore, J.F., Rhyne, B., Krigman, M.R. 354, 356, *364*

Goyer, R.A., see Six, K.M. 358, *369*

Grafflin, A.L. 335, *364*

Gralnick, H.R., McGinness, M., Elton, W., McCurdy, P. 283, *316*

Gram, T.E., Hansen, A.R., Fouts, J.R. 279, *316*

Gram, T.E., Rogers, L.A., Fouts, J.R. 279, *316*

Granick, J.L., Sassa, S., Granick, S., Levere, R.D., Kappas, A. 13, *39*

Granick, J.L., see Granick, S. 335, 342, *365*

Granick, J.L., see Sassa, S 342, 343, 344, 359, *369*

Granick, S. 4, 9, 30, *39*, 60, *73*, 132, 133, 143, 145, 148, *152*, 189, *195*, 201, 202, 209, 210, 212, 213, 215, 217, 218, 231, *234*, 249, *253*, 260, 264, *268*, 284, 287, *316*, 333, *364*

Granick, S., Gilder, H. *39*

Granick, S., Kappas, A. 202, *234*

Granick, S., Mauzerall, D. 3, *39*, 334, *365*

Granick, S., Sassa, S., Granick, J.L., Levere, R.D., Kappas, A. 335, 337, 339, 342, 359, *365*

Granick, S., Sano, S. 21, *39*

Granick, S., Sassa, S. 1, 8, 35, *39*, 130, *152*, 202, 208–210, *234*

Granick, S., Sinclair, P., Sassa, S., Grieninger, G. 140, 152, 211, *234*

Granick, S., Urata, G. 10, *39*, 132, *152*, 256, *268*

Granick, S., see Beale, S.I. 258, *267*

Granick, S., see Sassa, S. 9, 16, 33, *45*, 149, 154, 213–217, 236, 241, *254*, 336, 338 340, 344, 353, *369*

Granick, S., see Sinclair, P.R. 144, *154*, 189, 190, 192, *198*, 209, 210, *236*, 246, *254*

Granick, S., see Urata, G. 10, *47*

Granick, S., see Whiting, M.J. 9, *48*, 150, 155, 345, *371*

Grant, D., see Kuiper-Goodman, T. 177, 178, *196*

Grant, D.L., Iverson, F., Hatina, G.V., Villeneuve, D.C. 160, 170, 172, 177–179, 187, *195*

Grant, D.L., see Villeneuve, D.C. 57, *80*, 160, *199*

Grant, J.K., see Goldberg, A. 266, *267*

Granzoni, A., Rhomberg, F. 340, *365*

Grassl, M., Augsburg, G., Coy, U., Lynen, F. 4, *39*

Grassl, M., Coy, U., Seyffert, R., Lynen, F. 34, *39*

Gratzer, W.B., see Beaven, G.H. 277, *310*

Gray, C.H. 280, *316*

Gray, C.H., Neuberger, A., Sneath, P.H.A. 5, *40*, 275, *316*

Gray, C.H., see Del Favero, A. 145, *151*

Gray, C.H., see Elder, G.H. 157, 184, *195*, 240, *253*, 280, 314

Gray, C.H., see Waterfield, M.D. 97, *127*, 134, *154*

Gray, D.W.G., Mowat, A.P. 301, *316*

Grayson, D.H., see Battersby, A.R. 21, *36*

Grayzel, A.I., Fuhr, J.E., London, I.M. 30, *40*

Green, R.S., see Turner, J.C. 177, *199*

Greenbaum, D., Richardson, P.C., Salmon, M.V., Urich, H. 354, *365*

Greenberg, D.M., Copp, D.H., Cuthbertson, E.M. 88, *92*

Greenberg, M.S., see Harris, J.W. 350, *365*

Greene, F.E., Stripp, B., Gillette, J.R. 109, *123*

Greengard, O., see Feigelson, P. 52, *73*

Greenwood, D.T., Stevenson, I.H. 299, *316*

Greer, M., Schotland, D. 357, *365*

Gregory, D.H. II, Strickland, R.D. 28, *40*, 279, 294, *316*

Greig, J.B. 177, 179, *195*

Greig, J.B., De Matteis, F. 57, 61, *73*, 177, 179, *195*

Greim, H. *73*

Greim, H., Schenkman, J.B., Klotzbücher, M., Remmer, H. 50, 62, 67, *74*, 283, *316*

Greiner, I., see Remmer, H. 61, *78*

Grieninger, G., see Granick, S. 140, *152*, 211, *234*

Griffing, W.J., see Owen, N.V. 65, *77*

Grigarzik, H., Passow, H. 350, *365*

Griggs, R.C. 349, 357, 358, *365*

Griggs, R.C., Harris, J.W. 350, *365*

Griggs, R.C., see Fratianne, R.B. 350, *364*

Grimwade, A., see Boyd, G. *71*

Grinstein, M., Bannerman, R.M., Moore, C.V. 341, *365*

Grinstein, M., see Batlle, A.M. del C. 14, 18, *36*, 181, *194*

Grinstein, M., see Garcia, R.C. 18, *39*, 181, *195*

Grinstein, M., see Kreimer-Birnbaum, M. 346, *366*

Grinstein, M., see Sancovich, H.A. 15, *45*

Grinstein, M., see San Martin de Viale, L.C. 18, *45*, 165, 169, 170, 181, 184, 187, *198*

Grinstein, M., see Tomio, J.M. 18, *47*, 181, 199, 334, *370*

Grodsky, G.M., Carbone, J.V. 278, 300, *316*

Grodsky, G.M., see Brown, W.R. 277, 278, *313*

Groh, M., see Haurowitz, F. 113, *123*

Gronwall, R.R., see Mia, A.S. 293, *323*

Gronwall, R.R., see Upson, D.W. 303, *330*

Groote, J. de, see Fevery, J. 27, *38*

Gross, M. 30, *40*

Gross, M., Rabinovitz, M. 30, *40*

Gross, R.T., Bracci, R., Rudolph, N., Schroeder, E., Kochen, J.A. 281, *316*

Gross, S.R., Hutton, J.J. 11, 12, *40*, 224, *234*

Gross, S.R., see Hutton, J.J. 14, 16, *41*, 224, *234*

Grossman, M.I., see Jones, R.S. 302, *319*

Grossman, M.I., see Zatepka, S. 302, *332*

Groszmann, R.J., Kotelanski, B., Kendler, J., Zimmerman, H.J. 302, *316*

Groves, M.P., see Muirhead, E.E. 283, *323*, 350, 351, *367*

Gubitz, R., see Brody, T.M. 304, *312*

Guibot, P., see Hakim, J. 298, *316*

Guidotti, G., see Rosenberg, S.A. 347, *368*

Guinee, V.F., see Spector, M.J. 359, *370*

Guinta, A., see Carddu, P. 298, *313*

Gulbenkian, A., see Tabachnick, I.T.A. 262, *270*

Gullväg, B.M., see Skaar, H. 354, *370*

Gumusio, J.J., Valdivieso, V.D. 304, *316*

Gunalp, A., see Dogramaci, I. 163, *194*

Gunn, S.A., Gould, T.C., Anderson, W.A.D. 357, *365*

Gunsalus, I.C., see Yu, C.A. 95, *127*

Gurba, P.E., Sennett, R.E., Kobes, R.D. 12, 13, *40*, 334, 338, *365*

Gustafsson, J., see Hrycay, E.G. 115, *123*

Gutelius, M.F., Millican, F.K., Layman, E.M., Cohen, G.J., Dublin, C.C. 358, *365*

Gutstein, S., Alpert, S., Arias, I.M. 280, *316*

Guttman, D.E., see Meyer, M.C. 288, *323*

Guy, R., see Muirhead, E.E. *323*

Guyda, H., see Israels, L.G. 275, *318*

Guyther, J.R., see Blaschke, T.F. 293, 296, 306, *311*

Guzelian, P.S., see Bissell, D.M. 117, 118, 120, *122*

Gydell, K. 286, *316*

Haber, S., see Salvador, R.A. 67, 68, *78*

Haberman, H.F., see Medline, A. 177, 178, 187, 188, *197*

Habig, W., see Fleischner, G. 292, 293, *315*

Habig, W.H., Papst, M.J., Fleischner, G., Gatmaitan, Z., Arias, I.M., Jacoby, W.B. 64, *74*, 292, *316*

Haddad, H.H., see Goresky, C.A. 280, 302, *316*

Hadley, W.M., Miya, T.S., Bousquet, W.F. 88, *92*, 115, *123*

Haeger-Aronsen, B. 142, 152, 346, *365*

Haeger-Aronsen, B., Abdulla, M., Fristedt, B.I. 337, *365*

Haeger-Aronsen, B., see Abdulla, M. 338, *361*

Hafeman, D.F., Hoekstra, W.F. 112, 115, *123*

Hafeman, D.G., see Rotruck, J.T. 115, *126*

Hakim, J., Feldmann, G., Boivin, P., Troube, H., Boucherot, J., Penaud, J., Guibot, P., Kreis, B. 298, *316*

Halac, E., Dipiazza, M., Detwiler, P. 28, *40*

Halac, E., Reff, A. 294, *316*

Halac, E., Sicignano, C. 295, 297, *317*

Halden, E.R., see Muirhead, E.E. 283, *323*

Hall, P.E., see Goldberg, A. 266, *267*

Hammaker, L., Schmid, R. 291, 299, *317*

Hammaker, L., see Bissell, D.M. 24, *36*, 117–120, *122*, 140, *151*, 276, *311*

Hammaker, L., see Lester, R. 305, *320*

Hammaker, L., see Schmid, R. 275, 278, 279, 283–286, 306, *328*

Hammaker, L.E., see Scholnick, P.L. 8–10, 12, *46*, 89, *94*, 149, *154*

Hammel, C.L., Bessman, S.P. 30, *40*

Hamrick, M., see Stripp, B. 56, *79*

Hanawa, Y., see Labbe, R.F. 135, *152*

Hanninen, O. 301, *317*

Hanninen, O., Aitio, A. 295, 299, *317*

Hanninen, O., see Laitinen, M. 299, *320*

Hansch, C. 206, *234*

Hansch, C., Clayton, J.M. 206, 207, *234*

Hansch, C., Dunn, W.J. 206, 207, *234*

Hansch, C., Steward, A.R., Anderson, S.M., Bentley, D. 220, 221, *234*

Hansch, C., see Leo, A. 206, 221, *235*

Hansell, M.M., Ecobichon, D.J. 187, *195*

Hansen, A.R., see Gram, T.E. 279, *316*

Hansen, W., see Scholz, R. 64, *79*

Hara, T., Minakami, S. 67, *74*

Harben, F., see Morley, A. 167, *197*

Harber, L., see Lamola, A.A. 344, 345, *366*

Harber, L.C., see Piomelli, S. 344, *368*

Harbison, R.D., Spratt, J.L. 300, *317*

Harding, B.W., Wong, S.H., Nelson, D.H. 4, *40*

Hardy, J.B., Mellits, E.D. 299, *317*

Hargreaves, T. 300, 301, 304, 317

Hargreaves, T., Holton, J.B. 300, 317

Hargreaves, T., Lathe, G.H. 300, 301, 317

Hargreaves, T., Piper, R.F., Trickey, R. 300, 301, 317

Harms, R.H., see Simpson, C.F. 354, 369

Harpur, E.R., see Khanna, N.N. 289, 298, 319

Harris, D.F., see Song, C.S. 226, 236

Harris, E.J., see Parr, D.R. 354, 368

Harris, F., see Moosa, A. 349, 367

Harris, H. 50, 74

Harris, J.W. 283, 317

Harris, J.W., Greenburg, M.S. 350, 365

Harris, J.W., Kellermeyer, R.W. 336, 349, 365

Harris, J.W., see Fratianne, R.B. 350, 364

Harris, J.W., see Griggs, R.C. 350, 365

Harris, P., see Mooty, J. 358, 367

Harris, R.C., Lucey, J.F., McLean, J.R. 288, 317

Harris, S.R., see Valentine, W.N. 348, 370

Hart, L.G., Fouts, J.R. 74

Hart, L.G., Shultice, R.W., Fouts, J.R. 56, 74

Hartley, R.W., Jr., see Price, V.E. 51, 78, 142, 153

Hartz, J.W., Funakoshi, S., Deutsch, H.F. 4, 40

Harvey, D.J., Glazener, L., Stratton, C., Johnson, D.B., Mill, R.M., Horning, E.C., Horning, M.G. 103, 123

Harvey, D.R., see White, J.M. 30, 48, 344, 347, 371

Hasan, J., Vihko, V., Hernberg, S. 350, 365

Hasegawa, A.T., see Roerig, D.L. 295, 327

Hasegawa, E., Smith, C., Tephly, T.R. 22, 40

Hasegawa, E., see Tephly, T.R. 84–86, 89, 94, 115, 127, 284, 286, 329, 335, 370

Hasegawa, T., see Sanai, G.H. 352, 356, 369

Hashimoto, C., Imai, Y. 59, 74

Hass, G.M., Brown, D.V.L., Eisenstein, R., Hemmens, A. 354, 365

Hatina, G.V., see Grant, D.L. 160, 170, 172, 177–179, 187, 195

Hatina, G.V., see Villeneuve, D.C. 160, 199

Haugen, D.A., Coon, M.J. 59, 74

Haugen, D.A., Coon, M.J., Nebert, D.W. 61, 74

Haugen, D.A., see Hoeven, T.A. van der 54, 80

Haurowitz, F., Groh, M., Gausinger, G. 113, 123

Havel, R.J., Kane, J.P. 68, 69, 70, 74

Hawkins, D., see Pinckard, R.N. 278, 325

Hayaishi, O. 54, 74

Hayasaka, S., Tuboi, S. 11, 40

Hayashi, N., Kurashima, Y., Kikuchi, G. 9, 33, 40, 216, 217, 234

Hayashi, N., Yoda, B., Kikuchi, G. 9, 10, 33, 40

Hayashi, N., see Kurashima, Y. 260, 268

Heath, E.C., Dingell, J.V. 299, 317

Heath, H., see Hoare, D.S. 15, 40

Heath, J.C., see Dingle, J.T. 87, 92

Hees, G.P. van, see Compernolle, F. 27, 37

Hees, G.P. van, see Fevery, J. 27, 38

Hees, G.P. van, see Heirwegh, K.P.M. 26, 40

Hegman, S., see Howland, R.D. 279, 318

Heidema, J., see Strobel, H.W. 54, 80

Heikel, T., Lockwood, W.H., Rimington, C. 189, 195

Heikel, T.A.J., Lathe, G.H. 302, 304, 317

Heim, W.G., Applemen, D., Pyfrom, H.T. 82, 92

Heinrich, I., see Ackermann, E. 57, 70

Heirwegh, K.P.M., Hees, G.P. van, Leroy, P., Roy, F.P. van, Jansen, F.H. 26, 40

Heirwegh, K.P.M., Meuwissen, J.A.T.P., Fevery, J. 279, 294, 317

Heirwegh, K.P.M., Van de Vijver, M., Fevery, J. 294, 317

Heirwegh, K.P.M., Vanhees, G.P., Leroy, P., Vanroy, F.P., Jansen, F.H. 279, 317

Heirwegh, K.P.M., Vijer, M. van de, Fevery, J. 27, 40

Heirwegh, K.P.M., see Black, M. 278, 311

Heirwegh, K.P.M., see Compernolle, F. 26, 27, 37

Heirwegh, K.P.M., see Fevery, J. 27, 38, 278, 279, 315

Heirwegh, K.P.M., see Vanroy, F.P. 278, 279, 330

Hellman, E., see Tschudy, D.P. 35, 47

Hellman, E.S., see Rose, J.A. 255, 270

Hellman, E.S., see Welland, F.H. 256, 271

Hellmer, K.H., see Reiner, O. 111, 126

Hellmer, K.H., see Uehleke, H. 110, 127

Hellstrom, K., see Engstrom, J. 306, 314

Hemle, E.W., see Traketeller, A.C. 347, 370

Hemmens, A., see Hass, G.M. 354, 365

Hemphill, F.E., Kaeberle, M.L., Buck, W.B. 351, 365

Henderson, P.Th., see Jansen, P.L.M. 27, 41, 295, 296, 306, 319

Henning, G., see Brown, A.K. 301, 313

Henning, H., see Doss, M. 165, 194

Henshaw, E.C., see Clemens, M.J. 347, 363

Hermann, L.S., see Brodersen, R. 280, 312

Hernberg, S., Nikkanen, G. 337, 365

Hernberg, S., see Hasan, J. 350, 365

Hershko, Ch., Eilon, L. 187, 195

Hess, C.E., see Mohler, D.N. 281, *323*

Hess, E.V., see Vilter, R.W. 86, 87, *94*

Hess, R., Stäubli, W., Riess, W. 67, 68, *74*

Hess, R., see Stäubli, W. 65, 79

Hertz, H. 289, *317*

Heubel, F. 298, *318*

Heubel, F., Muhlberger, G. 298, *318*

Hevesy, G., see Åkeson, Å. 5, 35

Hewitt, J., see Lucey, J.F. 307, *322*

Heymann, E., Krisch, K., Büch, H., Buzello, W. 203, *234*

Hiatt, H.H., see Revel, M. 50, *78*

Hibbeln, P., see Tephly, T.R. 84, 85, *94*, 115, *127*

Hickman, P., see Goldstein, J.A. 157, 175, 177, 178, 180, 183, 187, 188, 192, *195*

Hickman, P., see Poland, A. 176, *197*

Hickman, R., Saunders, S.J., Dowdle, E., Eales, L. 33, *40*, 259, *268*

Hien, D., see Buu-Hoi, N.P. 57, *71*

Hietanen, E., see Vainio, H. 295, 296, 306, *330*

Higashi, T., see Kawamata, F. 142, *152*

Higashi, T., see Tateishi, N. 112, *127*

Hildebrandt, A., Estabrook, R.W. 67, *74*

Hildebrandt, A., Remmer, H., Estabrook, R.W. 59, *74*

Hildebrandt, A., see Estabrook, R.W. 351, *363*

Hinderakter, P.H., see Sudilovsky, O. 257, 259, *270*

Hinkel, G.K., see Kintzel, H.W. 301, *319*

Hinkel, G.K., see Schwarze, R. 301, *328*

Hirayama, C., see Kawasaki, H. 292, *319*

Hirsch, G.H., Bubbar, G.L., Marks, G.S. 203, *234*

Hirsch,G.H.,Gillis,J.D.,Marks, G.S. 205, 226, 231, *234*

Hirsch, G.H., see Schneck, D.W. 203, 209, *236*

Hirschman, J., see Remmer, H. 61, *78*

Hitzig, W.H., see Frick, P.G. 282, *315*

Hoare, D.S., Heath, H. 15, *40*

Hodgman, J.E., Schwartz, A. 307, *318*

Högberg, J. 112, *123*

Högberg, J., Bergstrand, A., Jakobsson, S.V. 113, *123*

Högberg, J., Orrenius, S., Larson, R.E. 112, *123*

Hoehne, K., see Windorfer, A. 305, *331*

Hoekstra, W.F., see Hafeman, D.F. 112, 115, *123*

Hoekstra, W.G., see Rotruck, J.T. 115, *126*

Hoeven, T.A. van der, Coon, M.J. 54, *80*

Hoeven, T.A. van der, Haugen, D.A., Coon, M.J. 54, *80*

Hoffbrand, A.V., see White, J.M. 30, *48*

Hoffman, D.G., see Owen, N.V. 65, *77*

Hoffman, H.N., see Metge, W.R. 296, 306, *323*

Hoffman, H.N., see Schoenfield, L.J. 279, *328*

Hoffman, H.N.H., see Hunton, D.B. 280, 291, *318*

Holder, G., Yagi, H., Dansette, P., Jerina, D.M., Levin, W., Lu, A.Y.H., Conney, A.H. 59, *74*

Hollman, S., Touster, O. 301, *318*

Holloway, P.W., Peluffo, P., Wakil, S.J. 66, *74*

Holloway, R.J., see Brauer, R.W. 280, *312*

Holmes, A.W., see Fleischmann, R. 6, *38*

Holton, J.B., see Bevan, B.R. 301, *311*

Holton, J.B., see Hargreaves, T. 300, *317*

Holtzmann, N.A., see Odell, G.B. 308, *324*

Holzer, H. 3, *40*

Hoogeveen, J.T. 350, *365*

Hoogland, D.R., Miya, T.S., Bousquer, W.F. 56, *74*

Hook, G.E.R., see Lucier, G.W. 177, *196*

Hoolboom, H., see De Bruin, A. 337, *363*

Hooper, C.W., see Whipple, G.H. 274, *331*

Hornef, W. 65, *74*

Horner-Mibashan, R., see Kapitulnik, J. 290, *319*

Horning, E.C., see Harvey, D.J. 103, *123*

Horning, M.G., see Harvey, D.J. 103, *123*

Hossaini, A.A., see Maurer, H.M. 305, *322*

Hourihane, D.O., see MacGibbon, B.H. 283, *322*

Housset, L., see Ploussard, J.P. 305, *325*

Howe, R.B., see Berk, P.D. 1, 5, *36*, 277, 278, 291, 293, 297, *310*

Howell, E.M., see Goldberg, A.L. 4, *39*

Howland, R.D., Burkhalter, A., Trevor, A.J., Hegman, S., Shirachi, D.Y. 279, *318*

Hrdlicka, J., see Seawright, A.A. 107, *126*

Hruskewycz, A.M., see Recknagel, R.O. 110, *126*

Hrycay, E.G., Gustafsson, J., Ingelman-Sundberg, M., Ernster, L. 115, *123*

Hrycay, E.G., O'Brien, P.J. 113−115, *123*

Hsia, D.Y., Dowben, R.M., Riabov, S. 300, 301, *318*

Hsia, D.Y., see Lokietz, H. 300, *321*

HSMHA 359, *365*

Hsu, W.P., Miller, G.W. 20, *41*

Huang, M.-T., West, S.B., Lu, A.Y.H. 59, *74*

Huang, S.N., see Gollan, J.L. 296, *315*

Hubbard, N., see Labbe, R.F. 22, *42*, 84, 88, *93*, 335, *366*

Hudson, L.D., see Lakshminarayan, S. 283, *320*

Hüttenhain, S., see Ippen, H. 171, *196*

Hughes, A.W., see Cameron, G.R. 159, *194*

Huijing, J., see Zuyderhoudt, F.M.J. 9, *48*, 149, *155*

Hultin, T., see Smuckler, E.A. 109, *126*

Humphris, B.G., see Bray, H.G. 89, *92*

Humphries, W.R., see Quaterman, J. 358, *368*

Hunt, E., see Battersby, A.R. 17, *36*

Hunt, T., see Mathews, M.B. 22, 31, *43*

Hunter, A., Neal, R.A. 108, *123*

Hunter, A.L., see Dalvi, R.R. 106, 107, *122*

Hunter, E.G., see Marks, G.S. 138, *153*, 218, 228, *235*

Hunter, G., Jr., see Tschudy, D.P. 11, 14, *47*, 256, *270*

Hunter, G.W., Jr., see Welland, F.H. 256, *271*

Hunter, J., Thompson, R.P.H , Rake, M.O., Williams, R. 296, *318*

Hunter, J., see Maxwell, J.D. 295, 296, *323*

Hunter, J., see Williams, R. 298, *331*

Hunter, M.J., see Woolley, P.V. 289, *331*

Hunton, D.B., Bollman, J.L., Hoffman, H.N H. 280, 291, *318*

Hupka, A.L., Karler, R. 117, *123*, 286, *318*

Huse, T., see Nagai, T. 340, *367*

Hutchinson, D.W., Johnson, B., Knell, A.J. 26, *41*

Hutterer, F., Schaffner, F., Klion, F.M., Popper, H. 178, *195*

Hutterer, F., see Raisfeld, J. 83, *93*

Hutton, J.J., Gross, S.R. 14, 16, *41*, 224, *234*

Hutton, J.J., see Gross, S.R. 11, 12, *40*, 224, 234

Hutzinger, O., Nash, D.M., Safe, S., Defreitas, A.S.W., Norstrom, R.J., Wildish, D.J., Zitko, V. 159, 161, *195*

Hutzinger, O., see Johnstone, G.J. 177, 178, 179, *196*

Hwang, M.I.H., see Attardi, C. 50, *70*

Ibayashi, H., see Kawasaki, H. 292, *319*

Ibrahim, G.W., Schwartz, S., Watson, C.J. 275, *318*

Icen, A. 341, *365*

Ideo, G., Defranchis, R., Del Ninno, E., Dioguardi, N. 298, 299, *318*

Ikeda, K., see Schwartz, S. 98, 100, 104, *126*, 287, *328*

Imai, J., Sato, R. 54, *74*

Imai, Y., see Hashimoto, C. 59, *74*

Imai, Y., see Oshino, N. 66, *77*

Imhof, P., see Schmid, K. 56, *79*

Incefy, G.S., Kappas, A. 35, *41*

Incefy, G.S., Rifkind, A.B., Kappas, A. 35, *41*

Indacochea-Redmond, N., Plaa, G.L. 285, *318*

Indacochea-Redmond, N., Witschi, H.P., Plaa, G.L. 285, *318*

Ingelman-Sundberg, M., see Hrycay, E.G. 115, *123*

Inscoe, J.K., Axelrod, J. 63, *74*, 299, *318*

Ip, M.M., Chee, P.Y., Swick, R.W. 4, 5, *41*

Ippen, H., Aust, D. 171, *196*

Ippen, H., Aust, D., Goerz, G. 170, *196*

Ippen, H., Hüttenhain, S., Aust, D. 171, *196*

Irisa, T., see Kawasaki, H. 292, *319*

Irving, E.A., Elliott, W.H. 10, 11, *41*, 150, *152*

Israel, L.G., see Levitt, M. 6, *43*

Israels, L.G. 355, *365*

Israels, L.G., Schacter, B.A., Yoda, B., Goldenberg, G.J. 24, *41*, 276, *318*

Israels, L.G., Skanderbeg, J., Guyda, H., Zingg, W., Zipursky, A. 275, *318*

Israels, L.G., Yamamoto, T., Skanderbeg, J., Zipursky, A. 275, 283, *318*

Israels, L.G., see Levitt, M. 275, 283–286, *321*

Israels, L.G., see Yamamoto, T. 5, *48*, 275, 283, 331

Isaels, L.G., see Yoda, B. 23, *48*

Isselbacher, K.J., Chrabas, M.F., Quinn, R.C. 279, *318*

Isselbacher, K.J., McCarthy, E.A. 278, 279, *318*

Isselbacher, K.J., see Ockner, R.K. 292, *318*

Ito, A., see Sato, R. *78*

Ivanetich, K.M., Marsh, J.A., Bradshaw, J.J., Kaminski, L.S. 103, *123*

Iverson, F., see Grant, D.L. 160, 170, 172, 177–179, 187, *195*

Jackson, A.H., Games, D.E., Couch, P., Jackson, J.R., Belcher, R.B., Smith, S.G. 21, *41*

Jackson, A.H., Jackson, J.R. 120, *123*

Jackson, A.H., Sancovich, H.A., Ferramola, A.M., Evans, N., Games, D.E., Matlin, S.A., Elder, G.H., Smith, S.G. 19, *41*, 170, *181*, 196

Jackson, A.H., see Kennedy, G.Y. 20, *42*

Jackson, A.H., see Kondo, T. 25, *42*

Jackson, A.H., see Stoll, M.S. 19, *46*, 170, *199*

Jackson, J.R., see Jackson, A.H. 21, *41*, 120, *123*

Jacob, F., Monod, J. 50, *74*

Jacob, S.T., Scharf, M.B., Vessel, E.S. 59, *74*, *152*

Jacobsen, C. *318*

Jacobsen, J. 277, 278, 288, *318*, *319*

Jacobsen, J., see Black, M. 295–297, *311*

Jacobsen, J., see Lund, H.T. 308, *322*

Jacobsen, J., see Nelson, T. 291, *324*

Jacobsen, J., see Thiessen, H. 289, *329*

Jacobson, M., see Conney, A.H. 59, 71, 295, *313*

Jacobson, M., see Kuntzman, R. 57, *75*

Jacobson, M., see Levin, W.
98, 103, 104, 109, 111, 113,
124, 134, 147, *152*, 287, *321*
Jacobson, M., see Lu,
A.Y.H. 58, 59, *76*
Jacobson, M.M., Levin, W.,
Conney, A.H. 63, *74*
Jacoby, W.B., see Habig,
W.H. 64, *74*
Jaeger, R.J., Conolly, R.B.,
Murphy, S.D. 112, *124*
Jänig, G.-R., see Rein, H.
135, *154*
Jaffe, J.S., see MacDonald,
M.G. 57, *76*
Jakob, F., Monod, J. 212,
235
Jakobsson, S.V., see Högberg,
J. 113, *123*
Jakoby, W., see Fleischner,
G. 292, 293, *315*
Jakoby, W.B., see Benson,
A.M. 64, *71*
Jakoby, W.B., see Habig,
W.H. 292, *316*
Jakovicic, S., see Druyan, R.
67, *72*
Jalling, B., see Rane, A. 290,
326
James, K.J., see Battersby,
A.R. 21, *36*
Jandl, J.H. 351, *365*
Janigan, D., see Sweeney,
G.D. 134, *154*, 160, 167,
177, 178, 180, 182,
187–189, 192, *199*
Janoušek, V., see Maines,
M.D. 142, *152*
Janowitz, H.D., see Waitman,
A.M. 302, *330*
Jansen, F.H., Billing, B.H.
26, *41*, 278, *319*
Jansen, F.H., Stoll, M.S. 26,
41
Jansen, F.H., see Compernolle,
F. 26, *37*
Jansen, F.H., see Heirwegh,
K.P.M. 26, *40*, 279, *317*
Jansen, P., see Arias, I.M.
291, 292, *310*
Jansen, P.L., Henderson, P.T.
295, 296, 306, *319*
Jansen, P.L.M. 28, *41*
Jansen, P.L.M., Henderson,
P.Th. 27, *41*
Jarret, A., Rimington, C., Wil-
loughby, D.A. 353, *366*

Javitt, N.B., Emerman, S.
304, *319*
Javitt, N.B., Rifkind, A., Kap-
pas, A. *268*
Javitt, N.B., see Kaplowitz,
N. 292, *319*
Jefcoate, C.R., see Ghazarian,
J.G. 4, *39*
Jennings, R.W., see Villeneu-
va, E.C. 160, *199*
Jennins, R.W., see Burse,
V.M. 187, *194*
Jensen, N.M., see Kumaki,
K. 64, *75*
Jensen, S., Sundstrom, G.
162, *196*
Jensen, W.N., Moreno, G.D.,
Bessis, M.C. 347, *366*
Jensen, W.N., see Bessis,
M.C. 348, 354, 257, *362*
Jensen, W.N., see Lessler,
M.A. 357, *366*
Jensen, W.N., see Traketeller,
A.C. 347, *370*
Jerina, D., see Conney, A.H.
61, *71*
Jerina, D.M., see Holder, G.
59, *74*
Jerina, D.M., see Oesch, F.
77
Jervell, K.F., Christoffersen,
T., Mörland, J. 257, *268*
Jick, H., Shuster, L. 59, *74*
Jick, H., Shuster, L. 59, *74*
Jirásek, L., Kalensky, J., Ku-
bec, K. 174, *196*
Jirásek, L., Kalensky, J., Ku-
bec, K., Pazderová, J., Lu-
káš, E. 174, 175, *196*
Jirsa, M., Vecerek, B. 279,
319
Johnson, A., Jones, O.T.G.
22, *41*
Johnson, B., see Hutchinson,
D.W. 26, *41*
Johnson, D.B., see Harvey,
D.J. 103, *123*
Johnson, E.F., Muller-Eber-
hard, U. 59, *75*
Johnson, L., Boggs, T.R. 308,
319
Johnson, L., Garcia, M.L., Fi-
gueroa, E., Sarmiento, F.
288, 289, *319*
Johnson, L., Sarmiento, F.,
Blanc, W.A., Day, R. 288,
289, *319*

Johnson, L., see Arias, I.M.
310
Johnson, S.A.M., see Peters,
H.A. 162–164, 168, *197*
Johnston, R.E., Miya, T.S.,
Schnell, R.C. 88, *92*
Johnstone, G.J., Ecobichon,
D.J., Hutzinger, O.
177–179, *196*
Jollow, D.J., see Mitchell,
J.R. 85, *93*
Jollow, D.J., see Potter, W.Z.
85, *93*
Jones, B. 301, *319*
Jones, E.A., Bloomer, J.R.,
Berlin, N.I. 6, 41, 283, 285,
319
Jones, G., Butler, W.H. 188,
196
Jones, M.S., Jones, O.T.G.
11, 22, 23, *41*, 84, *92*, 149,
152
Jones, M.S., see Barnes, R. 9,
22, 23, *36*
Jones, O.T.G. 335, *366*
Jones, O.T.G., see Barnes, R.
9, 22, 23, *36*
Jones, O.T.G., see Johnson,
A. 22, *41*
Jones, O.T.G., see Jones,
M.S. 11, 22, 23, *41*, 84, *92*,
149, *152*
Jones, O.T.G., see Porra,
R.J. 22, 45, 84, *93*, 335,
341, *368*
Jones, R.S., Grossman, M.I.
302, *319*
Jordan, P.M., Shemin, D. 8,
10, 12, *41*, 334, 345, *366*
Jordan, P.M., see Abboud,
M.M. 8, *35*
Jose, P.J., Slater, T.F., Saw-
yer, B.C. 115, *124*
Joselow, M., see Lamola,
A.A. 344, 358, *366*
Joselow, M.M., see Vitale,
L.F. 359, *371*
Josephson, B., Furst, P. 289,
319
Josting, D., see Bock, K.W.
64, *71*
Joubert, S.M., Taljaard, J.J.F.,
Shanley, B.C. 182, 183, *196*
Joubert, S.M., see Bach, P.H.
171, *193*
Joubert, S.M., see Shanley,
B.C. 20, *46*, 191, *198*

Joubert, S.M., see Taljaard, J.J.F. 19, *47*, 165, 169, 170, 171, 180, 182, 184–186, 189, 191, 192, *199*

Joubert, S.M., see Timme, A.H. 177, 187, 188, *199*

Joyce, C.R.B., Moore, H.L., Weatherall, M. 350, *366*

Juchau, M.R., see Krasner, J. 294, 295, 297, *320*

Jue, D.L., see Goldstein, J.A. 177, 178, 180, 183, 192, *195*

Kadlubar, F.F., Morton, K.C., Ziegler, D.M. 115, *124*

Kaeberle, M.L., see Hemphill, F.E. 351, *365*

Kärki, N.T., see Pelkonen, O. 58, *77*

Karatos, F.C., Reich, J. 50, *75*

Kagawa, Y., Minakami, S., Yoneyama, Y. 341, *366*

Kakhn, K.A., see Teras, L.E. 357, *370*

Kalensky, J., see Jirásek, L. 174, 175, *196*

Kalivas, J. 189, *196*

Kalivas, J.T., Pathak, M.A., Fitzpatrick, T.B. 169, 171, 196

Kallen, R.J., see Blumen-schein, S.D. 305, *312*

Kalman, S.M., see Goldstein, A. 51, *73*

Kaltepoth, B., see Doss, M. 210, *233*

Kaltiala, E.H., see Pelkonen, O. 58, *77*

Kamataki, T., Kitagawa, H. 113, *124*

Kamin, H., see White-Stevens, R.H. 67, *80*

Kaminski, L.S., see Ivanetich, K.M. 103, *123*

Kamisaka, K., Listowsky, I., Arias, I.M. 289, 292, *319*

Kamisaka, K., Listowsky, I., Betheil, J.J., Arias, I.M. 277, *319*

Kamisaka, K., Listowsky, I., Gatmaitan, Z., Arias, I.M. 292, *319*

Kamisaka, K., see Fleischner, G. 292, 293, *315*

Kamisaka, K., see Kirsch, R. 292, 293, *320*

Kammholz, L.P., Thatcher, L.G., Blodgett, F.M., Good, T.A. 342, 359, *366*

Kanai, Y., Sugimura, T., Matsushima, T., Kawamura, A. 4, 5, *41*

Kandler, H., see Kutz, K. 296, 298, *320*

Kane, J.P., see Havel, R.J. 68, 69, *70*, *74*

Kantemir, I. 162, *196*

Kao, L., see Clarenburg, R. 303, *313*

Kapelner, S., see Alvares, A.P. 82, *92*, 352, *361*

Kapitulnik, J., Horner-Miba-shan, R., Blondheim, S.H., Kaufmann, N.A., Russell, A. 290, *319*

Kapitulnik, J., see Conney, A.H. 61, *71*

Kaplan, B.H. 9, 11, 12, *41*, 149, *152*

Kaplowitz, N., Percy-Robb, I.W., Javitt, N.B. 292, *319*

Kappas, A., Alvares, A.P. 351, *366*

Kappas, A., Bradlow, H.L., Gillette, P.N., Gallagher, T.F. 266, *268*

Kappas, A., Bradlow, H.L., Gillette, P.N., Levere, R.D., Gallagher, T.F. 266, *268*

Kappas, A., Granick, S. 202, *235*, 261, 265, *268*

Kappas, A., Levere, R.D., Granick, S. 261, 266, *268*

Kappas, A., Song, C.S., Levere, R.D., Sachson, R.A., Granick, S. 220, 224, *235*, 265, *268*

Kappas, A., see Alvares, A.P. 63, *70*, 82, *92*, 177–179, *193*, 352, *361*

Kappas, A., see Anderson, K.E. 249, 251, *252*

Kappas, A., see Bradlow, H.L. 266, *267*

Kappas, A., see Gordon, A.S. 30, *39*, 265, *267*

Kappas, A., see Granick, J.L. 13, 29, *39*, *43*, 202, *234*, 265, *268*, 335, 337, 339, 342, 359, *365*

Kappas, A., see Incefy, G.S. 35, *41*

Kappas, A., see Javitt, N.B. 268

Kappas, A., see Levere, R.D. 265, *269*

Kappas, A., see Maines, M.D. 24, *43*, 85, *93*, 115, 116, 118–120, *124*, 142, *153*, 276, *322*, 345, 346, *367*

Kappas, A., see Rifkind, A.B. 218, 219, 222, 223, 231, 232, *236*, 249, *253*

Kappas, A., see Sassa, S. 16, *45*, 334, 336, 338–340, 342–344, 353, 359, *369*

Kappas, A., see Song, C.S. 226, *236*

Karaffa, M.A., see Finelli, V.N. 338, 357, *364*

Karlblän, D., London, I.M. 30, *41*, 333, *366*

Karler, R., see Hupka, A.L. 117, *123*, 286, *318*

Karnovsky, M.J., see Strum, J.M. 83, *94*

Karon, M., see Callahan, E.W., Jr. 308, *313*

Karunaratne, W.E., see Cameron, G.R. 109, *122*

Kassenaar, A., Morell, H., London, I.M. 347, *366*

Kassner, R.J., Walchak, H. 22, *41*

Kato, K., see Nawata, H. 145, *153*

Kato, R. 82, *92*

Kato, R., Chiesara, E., Vasanelli, P. 56, *75*

Kato, R., Gillette, J.R. 62, *75*

Kato, R., Takahashi, A. 62, *75*

Kato, R., Vasanelli, P. 56, *75*

Kato, R., Vassanelli, P., Frontino, G., Chiesara, E. 147, *152*

Katsunuma, H., see Wada, O. 341, *371*

Kaufman, L., Marver, H.S. 23, *41*

Kaufman, L., Swanson, A.L., Marver, H.S. 35, *42*, 148, *152*, 251, 252, *253*

Kaufmann, N.A., see Kapitulnik, J. 290, *319*

Kawalek, J., see Thomas, P.E. 59, *80*

Kawalek, J.C., Lu, A.Y.H. 85, *92*

Kawamata, F., Sakurai, T., Higashi, T. 142, *152*

Kawamura, A., see Kanai, Y. 4, 5, *41*

Kawanishi, T., see Tomokuni, K. 338, *370*

Kawasaki, H., Sakaguchi, S., Arimura, K., Irisa, T., Tominaga, K., Hirayama, C., Ibayashi, H. 292, *319*

Kay, C.M., see Ketterer, B. 23, *42*

Keaton, A.G., see Ferguson, J.H. 358, *364*

Keberle, H., see Schmid, K. 56, *79*

Keele, B.B., see Fong, K.K. 111, *123*

Keen, J.H., see Benson, A.M. 64, *71*

Kehoe, R.A. 359, *366*

Keller, H.H., see Sutherland, J.M. 300, *329*

Kellermann, G., Cantrell, E., Shaw, C.R. 62, *75*

Kellermann, G., Shaw, C.R., Luyten-Kellermann, M. 62, *75*

Kellermeyer, R.W., Tarlov, A.R., Brewer, G.J., Carson, P.E., Alving, A.S.P. 282, *319*

Kellermeyer, R.W., see Harris, J.W. 336, 349, *365*

Kelly, A., see Druyan, R. 23, 28, 31, *38*, 60, *72*, 132, *151*

Kelly, P.C., see Odell, G.B. 289 − 291, *324*

Kenanoglu, A., see Dogramaci, I. 163, *194*

Kench, J.E., see Clarkson, T.W. 346, 347, *363*

Kende, A.S., see Poland, A. 61, *77*

Kendler, J., see Groszmann, R.J. 302, *316*

Kennedy, G.Y., Jackson, A.H., Kenner, G.W., Suckling, C.J. 20, *42*

Kenner, G.W., see Baptista de Almeide, J.A.P. 170, *193*

Kenner, G.W., see Cavaleiro, J.A.S. 20, *37*

Kenner, G.W., see Kennedy, G.Y. 20, *42*

Kenner, G.W., see Kondo, T. 25, *42*

Kenney, F.T., see Wicks, W.D. 259, *271*

Kenwright, S., Levi, A.J. 289, 291, 292, *319*

Keohane, S.J., see Davies, R.E. 307, *314*

Ketterer, B., Tipping, E., Beale, D., Meuwissen, J., Kay, C.M. 23, *42*

Ketterer, B., see Litwack, G. 278, 292, *321*

Khanna, K.L., see Bruckner, J.V. 57, *71*, *194*

Khanna, N.N., Harpur, E.R., Stern, L. 289, 298, *319*

Kielley, R.K., Schneider, W.C. 89, *92*

Kiese, M., Kurz, H., Thofern, E. 3, *42*

Kikuchi, G., Kumar, A., Talmage, P., Shemin, D. 8, *42*

Kikuchi, G., see Hayashi, N. 9, 10, 33, *40*, 216, 217, *234*

Kikuchi, G., see Kim, H.J. 259, 260, 262, 263, *268*

Kikuchi, G., see Matsuoka, T. 264, *269*

Kikuchi, G., see Narisawa, K. 13, *44*, 264, *269*, 333, *367*

Kikuchi, G., see Ohashi, A. 216, 217, *235*

Kikuchi, G., see Tomita, Y. 33, *47*, 145, *154*, 213 − 217, *237*

Kikuchi, G., see Yoshida, T. 25, *48*, 118, *127*, 276, 287, *331*

Kim, H.J., Kikuchi, G. 259, 260, 262, 263, *268*

Kimbrough, R.D. 159, 161, 162, 172, *196*

Kimbrough, R.D., Linder, R.E., Gaines, T.B. 177, 178, 187, 188, *196*

Kimbrough, R.D., see Burse, V.M. 187, *194*

Kimbrough, R.D., see Villeneuva, E.C. 160, *199*

King, M.A.R., Wiltshire, B.G., Lehmann, H., Morimoto, H. 282, *319*

Kinsell, L.W., see Visintine, R.E. 305, *330*

Kintzel, H.W., Hinkel, G.K., Schwarze, R. 301, *319*

Kintzel, H.W., see Schwarze, R. 301, *328*

Kirsch, R., Fleischner, G., Kamisaka, K., Arias, I.M. 292, 293, *320*

Kitagawa, H., see Kamataki, T. 113, *124*

Kitamura, T., see Nakao, K. 23, *44*, 256, *269*

Kiuchi, G., see Kurashima, Y. 260, *268*

Kjellström, T., Eng, M. 344, *366*

Klaassen, C.D. 293, 303, *320*

Klatskin, G. 274, 300, 304, *320*

Klatskin, G., see Bloomer, J.R. 303, *312*

Klatskin, G., see Boyer, J.L. 302, *312*

Klauder, D.S., see Finelli, V.N. 338, 357, *364*

Klein, P.D., see Lester, R. 280, *320*

Klein, R., see Lucier, G.W. 115, 116, *124*

Klempau, I., see Ghazal, A. 56, *73*

Klempau, I., see Koransky, W. 56, *75*

Klinger, W., see Reinicke, C. 298, *326*

Klion, F.M., see Hutterer, F. 178, *195*

Klotzbücher, M., see Greim, H. 50, 62, 67, *74*, 283, *316*

Klugen, W.S., see Goresky, C.A. 280, 302, 303, *316*

Knell, A.J., see Hutchinson, D.W. 26, *41*

Kniffen, F., see Tephly, T.R. 84 − 86, *94*, 115, *127*

Knox, W.E. 52, *75*

Knox, W.E., Piras, M.M. 50, *75*

Knutson, J.C., see Ghazarian, J.G. 4, *39*

Kobes, R.D., see Gurba, P.E. 12, 13, *40*, 334, 338, *365*

Kochen, J.A., see Gross, R.T. 281, *316*

Koeman, J.H., Noever de Brauw, M.C., Vos, R.H. 161, *196*

Koeman, J.H., see Strik, J.J.T.W.A. 157, 175, *199*

Koeman, J.H., see Vos, J.G. 157, *200*, 222, *237*

Koeppel, E., see Robinson, S.H. 275, *326*

Kokatnur, M.G., Bergan, J.G., Draper, H.H. 113, *124*

Koller, L.D., Kovacic, S. 351, *366*

Komai, H., Neilands, J.B. 334, *366*

Kon, H., see Nebert, D.W. 58, 59, *76*

Kondo, T., Nicholson, D.C., Jackson, A.H., Kenner, G.W. 25, *42*

Kopelman, A.E., Brown, R.S., Odell, G.B. 308, *320*

Koransky, W., Magour, S., Merker, H.J., Schlicht, I., Schulte-Hermann, R. 65, *75*

Koransky, W., Portig, J., Vohland, H.W., Klempau, I. 56, *75*

Koransky, W., see Ghazal, A. 56, *73*

Koransky, W., see Schlicht, I. 65, 66, *79*

Koransky, W., see Schulte-Hermann, R. 65, *79*

Korinek, J., Moses, H.L. 12, *42*, 59, 260, 261, *268*

Korinek, J., see Moses, H.L. 145, *153*

Kornguth, M., see Kunin, C.M. 292, *320*

Korsrod, G., see Kuiper-Goodman, T. 177, 178, *196*

Koskelo, P., Eisalo, A., Toivonen, I. 219, *235*

Koss, G. 160, 161, 190, *196*

Koss, G., see Doss, M. 169, *194*

Kostial, K., McMailovic, B. 353, *366*

Koszo, F., see Simon, N. 188, 190, *198*

Kotelanski, B., see Groszmann, R.J. 302, *316*

Kovacic, S., see Koller, L.D. 351, *366*

Kowalsky, E., Dancewicz, A.M., Szot, Z., Lipinski, B., Rosiek, O. 34, *42*

Koziak, B., see Gombos, B. 167, *195*

Kraines, R., see Paumgartner, G. 291, *325*

Kramer, S., see Becker, D. 353, *362*

Kraschnitz, R., see Schenkman, J.B. 54, *79*

Krasner, J., Giacoia, G.P., Yaffe, S.J. 290, *320*

Krasner, J., Juchau, M.R., Yaffe, S.J. 294, 295, 297, *320*

Krasner, J., see Thaler, M.M. 308, *329*

Krauss, E., see Bock, K.W. 10, 12, *36*, 60, *71*

Krauss, P., see Witmer, C. 59, *80*

Kreek, M.J., Sleisenger, M.H. 296, 306, *320*

Kreimer-Birnbaum, M., Grinstein, M. 346, *366*

Kreis, B., see Hakim, J. 298, *316*

Kress, Y., see Richter, G.W. 354, *368*

Krigman, M.R., see Goyer, R.A. 354, 356, *364*

Krisch, K. 203, *235*

Krisch, K., see Heymann, E. 203, *234*

Krishnakantha, T.P., Kurup, C.K.R. 6, *42*

Krivit, W., see Lottsfeldt, F.I. 305, *321*

Krupa, V., Blattel, R.A., Marks, G.S. 226, 227, 228, *235*

Krupa, V., Creighton, J.C., Freeman, M., Marks, G.S. 222, *235*

Krupa, V., see Fischer, P.W.F. 210, 211, *234*

Krupa, V., see Marks, G.S. 148, *153*, 204–206, 208, 209, 223, 226, *235*

Krupa, V., see Murphy, F.R. 143, 148, *153*, 204–208, 226, 227, 229, *235*

Krupa, V., see Taub, H. 225, 226, 228, *237*

Krustev, L.P., see Whelton, M.J. 296, *331*

Kubec, K., see Jirásek, L. 174, 175, *196*

Kuenzle, C.C. 26, 27, *42*, 279, *320*

Kuiper-Goodman, T., Grant, D., Korsrod, G., Moodie, C.A., Munro, I.C. 177, 178, *196*

Kuksis, A., see O'Doherty, P.J.A. 292, *324*

Kumaki, K., Jensen, N.M., Shire, J.G.M., Nebert, D.W. 64, *75*

Kumar, A., see Kikuchi, G. 8, *42*

Kunin, C.M., Craig, W.A., Kornguth, M., Monson, R. 292, *320*

Kuntzman, R. 70

Kuntzman, R., Mark, L.C., Brand, L., Jacobson, M., Levin, W., Conney, A.H. 57, *75*

Kuntzman, R., see Alvares, A.P. 57, 59, *70*

Kuntzman, R., see Conney, A.H. 53, 54, 59, *71*, 295, *313*

Kuntzman, R., see Coutinho, C.B. 289, *313*

Kuntzman, R., see Levin, W. 5, *43*, 50, 60, *75*, 98, 103, 104, 109, 111, 113, 115, *124*, 134, 147, *152*, 283, 287, *321*

Kuntzman, R., see Lu, A.Y.H. 58, 59, *76*

Kunz, W., Schaude, G., Schimasseck, H., Schmid, W., Siess, M. 65, *75*

Kunz, W., Schaude, G., Schmid, W., Siess, M. 64, 65, *75*

Kunzer, W., see Windorfer, A. 305, *331*

Kurashima, Y., Hayashi, N., Kiuchi, G. 260, *268*

Kuriyama, Y., Omura, T., Siekevitz, P., Palade, G.E. 50, 59, 67, *75*

Kurashima, Y., see Hayashi, N. 9, 33, *40*, 216, 217, *234*

Kurz, H., see Kiese, M. 3, *42*

Kurumada, T., see Labbe, R.F. 32, *42*

Kurup, C.K.R., see Krishnakantha, T.P. 7, *42*

Kushner, J.P., Barbuto, A.J. 158, 184, 189, *196*

Kushner, J.P., Lee, G.R., Nacht, S. 191, *196*

Kushner, J.P., Steinmuller, D.P., Lee, G.R. 191, *196*, 264, *268*

Kutt, H.W., McDowell, F. 56, *75*

Kutz, K., Loffler, A., Kandler, H., Fevery, J. 296, 298, *320*

Kuwahara, S., see Mannering, G.J. 67, *76*

Kuylenstierna, B., see Sottocasa, L. 66, *79*

Labbe, P., Volland, C., Chaix, P. 341, *366*

Labbe, R.F. 32, *42*

Labbe, R.F., Hanawa, Y., Lottsfeldt, F.I. 135, *152*

Labbe, R.F., Hubbard, N. 22, *42*, 84, 88, *93*, 335, *366*

Labbe, R.F., Kurumada, T., Onisawa, J. 32, *42*

Labbe, R.F., see Cowger, M.L. 32, 37, 231, 232, *233*

Labbe, R.F., see Nishida, G. 84, *93*

Labbe, R.F., see Onisawa, J. 84, *93*, 137, *153*

Labbe, R.F., see Porra, R.J. 22, *45*, 84, *93*

Labbe, R.F., see Talman, E.L. 201, 217, 219, *237*

Lacroix, S., see Rothwell, J.D. 119, 120, *126*, 142, *154*, 286, 287, *327*

Laforet, M.T., Thomas, E.D. 87, *93*

Lage, G.L., Spratt, J.L. 278, *320*

Lai, H., see Sweeney, G.D. 134, *154*, 160, 167, 177, 178, 180, 182, 187–189, 192, *199*

Laitinen, M., Lang, M., Hanninen, O. 299, *320*

Lakshminarayan, S., Sahn, S.A., Hudson, L.D. 283, *320*

Lamar, C., Jr., see Peraino, C. 261, *269*

Lamola, A.A., Joselow, M., Yamane, T. 344, 358, *366*

Lamola, A.A., Piomelli, S., Poh-Fitzpatrick, M., Yamane, T., Harber, L. 344, 345, *366*

Lamola, A.A., Yamane, T. 344, 359, *366*

Lamola, A.A., see Blumberg, W.E. 344, 359, *362*

Lamola, A.A., see Piomelli, S. 344, *368*

Landaw, S.A., Callahan, E.W., Jr., Schmid, R. 5, *42*, 102, *124*, 135, 140–142, *152*, 284, 286, 287, *320*

Landerg, E., see Dimant, E. 340, *363*

Landow, S.A., Schooley, J.C., Arroyo, F.L. 349, *366*

Lang, M., see Laitinen, M. 299, *320*

Langelaan, D.E., Losowsky, M.S., Toothill, C. 23, *42*

Lanzkowsky, P. 358, *366*

Lardinios, R., see Tuilié, M. 290, *330*

Lardy, H.A., see Young, J.W. 259, *271*

Larmi, T.K.I., see Pelkonen, O. 58, *77*

Larson, R.E., see Högberg, J. 112, *123*

Lascelles, J. 22, *42*

Lascelles, J., Altshuler, T. 11, *42*

Lascelles, J., see Burnham, B.F. 132, *151*, 333, *362*

Lascelles, J., see Dailey, H.A. 22, *37*

Lascelles, R.G., see Thomas, P.K. 354, *370*

Laster, L., see Singleton, J.W. 25, *46*

Lathe, G.H. 1, 26, 27, *42*

Lathe, G.H., Lord, P., Toothill, C. 307, *320*

Lathe, G.H., Walker, M. 278, 299, *320*

Lathe, G.H., see Adlard, B.P.F. 301, *309*

Lathe, G.H., see Billing, B.H. 26, *36*, 278, *311*

Lathe, G.H., see Cole, P.G. 278, *313*

Lathe, G.H., see Hargreaves, T. 300, 301, *317*

Lathe, G.H., see Heikel, T.A.J. 302, 304, *317*

Lauwerys, R., Bachet, J.P. 341, *366*

Lauwerys, R.R., see Roels, H.A. 337, 340, 341, 358, *368*

Laver, W.G., see Gibson, K.D. 333, *364*

Lawson, M., see Boyd, G. *71*

Layman, D.L., see Argyris, T.S. 65, *70*

Layman, E.M., see Gutelius, M.F. 358, *365*

Lazarow, P.B., De Dueve, C. 4, 23, *42*, 67, 68, *75*, 142, *152*

Lazarow, P.B., see Leighton, F. 67, *75*

Lee, C.Y., see Brody, T.M. 304, *312*

Lee, G.R., Cartwright, G.E., Wintrobe, M.M. 86, *93*

Lee, G.R., see Kushner, J.P. 191, *196*, 264, *268*

Lee, G.R., see Lewis, M. 10, *43*

Lee, J.J., Cowger, M.L. 288, *320*

Lee, K.L., see Wicks, W.D. 259, *271*

Lee, K.S., see Vaisman, S.L. 295, *330*

Leevy, C.M., see Paumgartner, G. 291, *325*

Lehmann, H., see King, M.A.R. 282, *319*

Lehmann, H., see Prato, V. 282, *326*

Lehmann, H., see White, J.M. 282, *331*

Leigh, S., see Alvares, A.P. 352, *361*

Leighton, F., Poole, B., Lazarow, P.B., Duve, C. de 67, *75*

Leighton, F., see Poole, B. 50, 67, *78*

Leiken, S., Eng, G. 349, *366*

Lemberg, R., Falk, J.E. 101, *124*

Lemberg, R., Wyndham, R.A. 25, *42*

Lenaghan, R., see Sardesai, V.M. 12, *45*

Leo, A., Hansch, C., Elkins, D. 206, 221, *235*

Leonard, D., see Goyer, R.A. 354, 356, *364*

Leong, G.F., see Brauer, R.W. 280, *312*

Leong, J.L., see Wattenberg, L.W. 56, 57, *80*

Leroy, P., see Fevery, J. 27, 38

Leroy, P., see Heirwegh, K.P.M. 26, 40, 279, 317

Lessler, M.A., Cardona, E., Padilla, F., Jensen, W.N. 357, 366

Lester, R., Hammaker, L., Schmid, R. 305, 320

Lester, R., Klein, P.D. 280, 320

Lester, R., Schmid, R. 280, 320, 321

Lester, R., Schumer, W., Schmid, R. 280, 321

Lester, R., see Daly, J.S.F. 4, 5, 37

Lester, R., see Levy, M. 280, 321

Lester, R., see Schmid, R. 305, 328

Lester, R., see Stumpf, W.E. 280, 329

Lester, R., see Troxler, R.F. 280, 330

Lester, R., see Wolf, M. 190, 200

Levere, R.D., Granick, S. 29, 42, 43, 265, 269

Levere, R.D., Kappas, A., Granick, S. 29, 43, 265, 269

Levere, R.D., see Feldman, D.S. 353, 363

Levere, R.D., see Gordon, A.S. 30, 39, 265, 267

Levere, R.D., see Granick, J.L. 13, 39, 335, 337, 339, 342, 359, 365

Levere, R.D., see Kappas, A. 220, 224, 235, 261, 265, 266, 268

Levere, R.D., see Sassa, S. 339, 340, 342–344, 359, 369

Levere, R.D., see Song, C.S. 226, 236

Levey, M., see Saunders, S.J. 190, 198

Levi, A.J., Gatmaitan, Z., Arias, I.M. 277, 278, 292, 293, 321

Levi, A.J., see Arias, I.M. 279, 296, 310

Levi, A.J., see Fleischner, G. 278, 315

Levi, A.J., see Kenwright, S. 289, 291, 292, 319

Levi, A.J., see Levine, R.I. 278, 321

Levi, A.J., see Reyes, H. 278, 293, 326

Levin, E.Y. 15, 16, 43

Levin, E.Y., Coleman, D.L. 15, 43

Levin, E.Y., Flyger, V. 15, 43

Levin, E.Y., see Romeo, G. 181, 190, 198

Levin, W., Jacobson, M., Kuntzman, R. 98, 109, 124, 287, 321

Levin, W., Jacobson, M., Sernatinger, E., Kuntzman, R. 103, 124, 134, 147, 152, 287, 321

Levin, W., Kuntzman, R. 5, 43, 50, 60, 75, 115, 124, 283, 321

Levin, W., Lu, A.Y.H., Jacobson, M., Kuntzman, R., Poyer, J.L., McCay, P.B. 104, 111, 113, 124

Levin, W., Sernatinger, E., Jacobson, M., Kuntzman, R. 103, 124

Levin, W., see Alvares, A.P. 57, 59, 70

Levin, W., see Conney, A.H. 59, 61, 71, 295, 313

Levin, W., see Holder, G. 59, 74

Levin, W., see Jacobson, M.M. 63, 74

Levin, W., see Kuntzman, R. 57, 75

Levin, W., see Lu, A.Y.H. 4, 43, 58, 59, 76

Levin, E.Y., see Romeo, G. 15, 18, 19, 45

Levin, W., see Ryan, D. 179, 198

Levine, B.B. 283, 321

Levine, R.I., Reyes, H., Levi, A.J., Gatmaitan, Z., Arias, I.M. 278, 321

Levine, W.G., see Fleischner, G. 68, 73, 293, 315

Levinsky, N.G., see Levy, M. 280, 321

Levison, F., see Levy, H. 87, 93

Levitt, M., Schacter, B.A., Zipursky, A., Israels, L.G. 5, 43, 275, 283, 284, 285, 286, 321

Levy, G., Ertel, I.J. 300, 321

Levy, G., see Yaffe, S.J. 296, 297, 331

Levy, H., Levison, F., Schade, A.L. 87, 93

Levy, M., Lester, R., Levinsky, N.G. 280, 321

Lewin, W., see Thomas, P.E. 59, 80

Lewis, M., Lee, G.R., Cartwright, G.E., Wintrobe, M.M. 10, 43

Li, J.B., see Goldberg, A.L. 4, 39

Lichtenberger, F., see Staudt, H. 67, 79

Lichtman, H.C., see Watson, R.J. 349, 371

Lieber, C.S., see Rubin, E. 298, 327

Liebermann, J.S., see Feldman, D.S. 353, 363

Liebermann, M., see Riely, C.A. 112, 126

Liem, H.H., Muller-Eberhard, U. 135, 140, 141, 152

Lightner, D.A. 307, 321

Lightner, D.A., Crandall, D.C. 307, 321

Lightner, D.A., Crandall, D.C., Gertler, S., Quistad, G.B. 307, 321

Lightner, D.A., Quistad, G.B. 307, 321

Linberg, L.G., Norden, A. 283, 321

Linder, R.E., see Burse, V.M. 187, 194

Linder, R.E., see Kimbrough, R.D. 177, 178, 187, 188, 196

Lin-Fu, J.S. 353, 366

Linhart, P. 299, 321

Lipinski, B., see Kowalski, E. 34, 42

Lipschutz, F., see Weissberg, J.N. 338, 359, 371

Listowsky, I., see Kamisaka, K. 277, 289, 292, 319

Litt, I.F., see Nathenson, G. 299, 323

Little, C., O'Brien, P.J. 115, 124

Little, J.M., see Daly, J.S.F. 4, 5, 37

Littlewood, J.M., see Arrowsmith, W.A. 301, 305, 310

Litwack, G., Ketterer, B., Arias, I.M. 278, 292, *321*

Llambias, E.B.C., Del C. Battle, A.M. 15, 16, 18, *43* 334, 345, *366*

Locher, J.T., see Öhnhaus, E.E. 293, *324*

Lochhead, A., see Dagg, J.H. 243, *253*

Lochhead, A.C., Goldberg, A. 87, *93*

Lockhead, A., see Dagg, J.H. 353, *363*

Lockhead, A.C., Dagg, J.H., Goldberg, A. 137, *152*

Lockwood, W.H., see Heikel, T. 189, *195*

Lodish, H.F., Desalu, O. 31, *43*

Loffler, A., see Kutz, K. 296, 298, *320*

Lokietz, H., Dowben, R.M., Hsia, D.Y. 300, *321*

Lombardi, B., see Recknagel, R.O. 109, *126*

London, I.M. 5, *43*

London, I.M., West, R., Shemin, D., Rittenberg, D. 5, *43*, 275, *321*

London, I.M., see Becczard, Y. 31, *36*

London, I.M., see Clemens, M.J. 347, *363*

London, I.M., see Dimant, E. 340, *363*

London, I.M., see Grayzel, A.I. 30, *40*

London, I.M., see Karibian, D. 30, *41*, 333, *366*

London, I.M., s. Kassenaar, A. 347, *366*

London, I.M., sec Shemin, D. 333, *369*

Look, D., see Doss, M. 165, *194*

Lord, P., see Lathe, G.H. 307, *320*

Lord, P.S., see Broughton, P.M.G. 306, 308, *312*

Lorkin, P.A., see White, J.M. 282, *331*

Losowsky, M.S., see Langelaan, D.E. 23, *42*

Lottsfeldt, F.I., Krivit, W., R.F. 135, *152*

Lottsfeldt, F.I., see Labbe, Aust, J.B., Carey, J.B. 305, *321*

Loughbridge, L.W., see MacGibbon, B.H. 283, *322*

Lowry, P.T., see Watson, C.J. 280, *330*

Lu, A.Y.H., Kuntzman, R., West, S., Jacobson, M., Conney, A.H. 58, *76*

Lu, A.Y.H., Levin, W., West, S.B., Jacobson, M., Ryan, D., Kuntzman, R., Conney, A.H. 58, 59, *76*

Lu, A.Y.H., West, S.B., Vore, M., Ryan, D., Levin, W. 4, *43*

Lu, A.Y.H., see Conney, A.H. 59, *71*

Lu, A.Y.H., see Holder, G. 59, *74*

Lu, A.Y.H., see Huang, M.-T. 59, *74*

Lu, A.Y.H., see Kawalek, J.C. 85, *92*

Lu, A.Y.H., see Levin, W. 104, 111, 113, *124*

Lu, A.Y.H., see Ryan, D. 179, *198*

Lu, A.Y.H., see Strobel, H.W. 54, *80*

Lu, A.Y.H., see Thomas, P.E. 59, *80*

Luca, H.F., see Ghazarian, J.G. 4, *39*

Lucek, R.W., see Coutinho, C.B. 289, *313*

Lucey, J.F. 307, 308, *322*

Lucey, J.F., Ferreiro, M., Hewitt, J. 307, *322*

Lucey, J.F., see Harris, R.C. 288, *317*

Lucier, G.W., Matthews, H.B. Brubaker, P.E., Klein, R., McDaniel, O.S. 115, 116, *124*

Lucier, G.W., McDaniel, O.S. 299, 305, *322*

Lucier, G.W., McDaniel, O.S., Hook, G.E.R., Fowler, B.A., Sonawane, B.R., Faeder, E. 177, *196*

Luders, D. 306, *322*

Ludwig, B.J., see Douglas, J.F. 56, *72*

Lui, H., Sampson, R., Sweeney, G.D. 161, 190, *197*

Lui, H., Sweeney, G.D. 161, 190, *197*

Lukáš, E., see Jirásek, L. 174, 175, *196*

Lund, H.T., Jacobsen, J. 308, *322*

Lunde, P.K.M., see Rane, A. 290, *326*

Lundh, B., Cavallin-Stahl, E., Mercke, C. 286, *322*

Lundvall, O. 158, 191, *197*

Lundvall, O., Enerback, L. 174, *197*

Lussana, S., see Saita, G. 340, *369*

Lynen, F., see Grassl, M. 4, *39*

Luyten-Kellermann, M., see Kellermann, G. 62, *75*

Maak, B., see Reinicke, C. 298, *326*

Macarol, V., Morris, T.Q., Baker, K.J., Bradley, S.E. 302, *322*

MacDonald, M.G., Robinson, D.S., Jaffe, J.S., Sylvester, D. 57, *76*

MacGibbon, B.H., Loughbridge, L.W., Hourihane, D.O., Boyd, D.W. 283, *322*

Machinist, J.M., Ahn, K., Becker, B.A. 293, *322*

MacKenzie, G.C., see Gibson, S.L.M. 346, *364*

Magasanik, B. 258, *269*

Magasanik, B., see Nakada, D. 256, *269*

Magasanik, B., see Neidhardt, F.C. 256, 258, *269*

Maggiore, Q., see Billing, B.H. 278, 291, *311*

Maglalang, A.C., see Odell, G.B. 291, *324*

Magnenat, P., see Okolicsanyi, L. 295, 296, 305, *324*

Magnus, D., see Argyris, T.S. 65, 66, *70*

Magnus, I.A., see Moore, M.R. 158, 185, *197*

Magnus, I.A., see Ramsay, C.A. 158, 191, *198*

Magnus, I.A., see Rimington, C. 242, *254*

Magnus, I.A., see Turnbull, A. 158, 191, *199*

Magos, L., Butler, W.H. 105, *124*

Magour, S., see Koransky, W. 65, *75*

Magour, S., see Schlicht, I. 65, 66, 79

Mahoney, M.J., see Bonkowsky, H.L. 342, 362

Mahu, J.-L., see Duvalestin, P. 27, 38

Maines, M.D., Anders, M.W., Muller-Eberhard, U. 119, 124

Maines, M.D., Janoušek, V., Tomio, J.M., Kappas, A. 142, 152

Maines, M D., Kappas, A. 24, 43, 85, 93, 115, 116, 118–120, 124, 142, 153, 276, 322, 345, 346, 367

Maisels, M.J. 297, 322

Majerus, P.W., see Mohler, D.N. 281, 323

Malathi, K., see Padmanaban, G. 31, 33, 44, 144, 145, 147, 149, 153, 250, 253

Malathi, K., see Satayanarayana Rao, M.R. 135, 154

Malkinson, F.D., see Pearson, R.W., 168, 169, 170, 171, 197

Mann, F.C., Sheard, C., Bollman, J.L., Blades, E.J. 274, 322

Mannering, G.J. 300, 322

Mannering, G.J., Kuwahara, S., Omura, T. 67, 76

Mannering, G.J., see Correira, M.A. 67, 72

Mannering, G.J., see Sladek, N.E. 58, 59, 79

Mannering, G.J., see Tephly, T.R. 82, 94

Manning, J., see Strand, L.J. 10, 12, 46, 144, 149, 154, 210, 213, 214, 216, 236, 241, 246, 254, 341, 345, 370

Mantel, N., see Epstein, S.S. 355, 363

Margoliash, E., Novogrodsky, A. 82, 93

Margolis, F., see Feigelson, P. 6, 38

Margolis, F.L. 12, 43

Maricic, S., see Rein, H. 135, 154

Marini, A., see Careddu, P. 301, 313

Marini, A., see Sereni, F. 298, 328

Marinova, H., see Batolska, A. 340, 362

Mark, L.C., see Alvares, A.P. 57, 70

Mark, L.C., see Kuntzman, R. 57, 75

Marks, G.S. 1, 3, 15, 43, 231, 232, 235

Marks, G.S., Hunter, E.G., Terner, U.K., Schneck, D. 138, 153, 218, 228, 235

Marks, G.S., Krupa, V., Creighton, J.C., Roomi, W.M. 148, 153

Marks, G.S., Krupa, V., Murphy, F., Taub, H., Blattel, R.A. 204, 206, 208, 209, 235

Marks, G.S., Krupa, V., Roomi, M.W. 204, 205, 223, 226, 235

Marks, G.S., see Creighton, J.M. 133, 151, 219, 222, 224–226, 228, 233

Marks, G.S., see Fischer, P.W.F. 210, 211, 234

Marks, G.S., see Hirsch, G.H. 203, 205, 226, 231, 234

Marks, G.S., see Krupa, V. 222, 226–228, 235

Marks, G.S., see Morgan, R.O. 211, 223, 229, 235

Marks, G.S., see Murphy, F.R. 143, 148, 153, 204, 208, 226, 227, 235

Marks, G.S., see Racz, W.J. 143, 148, 153, 203, 218–220, 223, 224, 231, 232, 236

Marks, G.S., see Schneck, D.W. 203, 209, 216, 236

Marks, G.S., see Taub, H. 221, 225, 226, 228, 232, 237

Marks, G.S., see Tyrrell, D.L.J. 33, 47, 145, 149, 154, 212–214, 216, 217, 237

Marniemi, J. 294, 299, 322

Marsh, J.A., see Ivanetich, K.M. 103, 123

Marshall, J.W., McLean, A.E.M. 62, 63, 76

Martel, S.B., see Goldberg, A.L. 4, 39

Martin, J.F., Vierling, J.M., Wolkoff, A.W., Scharschmidt, B.F., Vergalla, J., Waggoner, J.G., Berk, P.D. 293, 322

Marver, H.S. 60, 76, 133, 153, 261, 269, 284, 286, 322

Marver, H.S., Collins, A., Tschudy, D.P. 259, 269

Marver, H.S., Collins, A., Tschudy, D.P., Rechcigl, J., Jr. 287, 322

Marver, H.S., Collins, A., Tschudy, D.P., Rechcigl, M., Jr. 9, 43, 132, 134, 153, 256, 259, 264, 269, 333, 367

Marver, H.S., Schmid, R. 1, 5, 32, 43, 60, 76, 157, 158, 163, 197

Marver, H.S., Schmid, R., Schutzel, H. 284, 286, 322

Marver, H.S., Tschudy, D.P., Perlroth, M.G. 53, 76

Marver, H.S., Tschudy, D.P., Perlroth, M.G., Collins, A. 10–12, 43, 257, 261, 269, 333, 367

Marver, H.S., see Kaufman, L. 23, 35, 41, 42, 148, 152, 251, 252, 253

Marver, H.S., see Meyer, U.A. 5, 44, 98, 125, 186, 197, 233, 235, 241, 245, 253, 283, 287, 323

Marver, H.S., see Perlroth, M.G. 264, 269

Marver, H.S., see Pimstone, N.R. 24, 45, 118, 125, 276, 325

Marver, H.S., see Schacter, B.A. 23, 46, 104, 111, 126, 275, 276, 286, 327

Marver, H.S., see Schmid, R. 275, 283–286, 328

Marver, H.S., see Scholnick, P.L. 8, 9, 10, 12, 46, 89, 94, 149, 154

Marver, H.S., see Strand, L.J. 10–12, 16, 46, 144, 149, 154, 210, 213, 214, 216, 236, 241, 246, 254, 334, 341, 345, 353, 370

Marver, H.S., see Tenhunen, R. 23, 24, 25, 47, 275, 276, 286, 329

Marver, H.S., see Tschudy, D.P. 9, 11, 14, 47, 256, 270

Marver, H.S., see Wetterberg, L. 12, 48

Mason, H.S., North, J.C., Vanneste, M. 54, 76

Mason, J.I., see Schacter,
B.A. 286, 287, *327*
Mason, S., see Murakami, K.
119, *125*
Mason, T.L., see Schatz, G.
68, *78*
Massie, H.R., see Baird,
M.B. 142, *151*
Masters, B.S.S., Schacter,
B.A. 276, *322*
Masters, B.S.S., see Nelson,
E.B. 58, *77*
Masters, B.S.S., see Schacter,
B.A. 23, *46*, 275, 276, 286,
327
Mastrangelo, R., see Roma-
gnoli, G. 305, *327*
Matern, S., Fröhling, W.,
Bock, K.W. 65, *76*
Mathews, M.B., Hunt, T.,
Brayley, A. 22, 31, *43*
Matlin, S., see Elder, G.H.
170, 181 – 184, 190,
Matlin, S.A., see Jackson,
A.H. 19, *41*, 170, 181,
196
Matsuda, I., Shirahata, T.
301, *322*
Matsuoka, T., Yoda, B., Ki-
kuchi, G. 264, *269*
Matsushima, T., see Kanai,
Y. 4, 5, *41*
Matsuzawa, T., see Yaffe,
S.J. 296, *331*
Matteini, M., see Calissano,
P. 14, *37*
Mattenheimer, H., see Fleisch-
mann, R. 7, *38*
Matthew, M., see Gibson,
K.D. 258, *267*
Matthews, H.B., see Lucier,
G.W. 115, 116, *124*
Maurer, H.M., Shumway,
C.N., Draper, D.A., Hossai-
ni, A.A. 305, *322*
Mauzerall, D. 333, *367*
Mauzerall, D., Granick, S. 3,
18, 19, *44*, 181, 182, *197*,
334, *367*
Mauzerall, D., see Granick,
S. 4, *39*, 334, *365*
Maxwell, J.D., Hunter, J., Stew-
art, D.A., Carella, M.,
Williams, R. 295, 296, *323*
Maxwell, J.D., Meyer, U.A.
130, 137, 144, 148, *153*, 246,
248, 250, 251, *253*

Maxwell, J.D., see Meyer,
U.A. 82, 84, 85, *93*
Maxwell, J.D., see Williams,
R. 298, *331*
May, G. 174, 175, *197*
Mayaman, D., see Sweeney,
G.D. 134, *154*
Mayman, D., see Sweeney,
G.D. 134, *154*, 160, 167,
177, 178, 180, 182, 187, 188,
189, 192, *199*
Maynard, L.S., Cotzias, G.C.
88, *93*
Maynert, E.W., see Foreman,
R.L. 103, *123*
Mazanowska, A.M., Neuber-
ger, A., Tait, G.H. 22, *44*
Mazza, H., see Prato, V. 282,
326
McCallum, J., see Goldberg,
A. 266, *267*
McCarthy, E.A., see Isselba-
cher, K.J. 278, 279, *318*
McCay, P.B., Pfeifer, P.M.,
Stipe, W.H. 112, *124*
McCay, P.B., see Levin, W.
104, 111, 113, *124*
McConville, M., see Powell,
K.A. 137, *153*
McCurdy, P., see Gralnick,
H.R. 283, *316*
McDaniel, O.S., see Lucier,
G.W. 115, 116, *124*, 177,
196, 299, 305, *322*
McDonagh, A.F. 307, 308,
323
McDonagh, A.F., Pospisil, R.,
Meyer, U.A. 100, 104, *124*
McDonagh, A.F., see Schmid,
R. 104, 118, *126*, 140, *154*
McDonald, F., see Battersby,
A.R. 17, 21, *36*
McDowell, F., see Kutt,
H.W. 56, *75*
McGillion, F.B., see Goldberg,
A. 353, *364*
McGinness, M., see Gralnick,
H.R. 283, *316*
McIntire, M.S., Angle, C.R.
340, *367*
McIntyre, M.S., see Angle,
C.R. 341, *361*
McIntyre, N., Pearson, A.J.G.,
Allan, D.J., Craske, S.,
West, G.M.L., Moore,
M.R., Paxton, J., Beattie,
A.D., Goldberg, A. 241, *253*

McKay, P.B., see Fong, K.
111, *123*
McKay, R., Druyan, R., Getz,
G.S., Rabinowitz, M. 9,
11, 22, *44*, 149, *153*
McLaren, G.D., Carpenter,
J.T., Jr., Nino, H.V. 342,
367
McLean, A.E.M. 110, *125*
McLean, A.E.M., McLean,
E.K. 110, *125*, 257, *269*
McLean, A.E.M., see Garner,
R.C. 110, *123*, 283, *315*
McLean, A.E.M., see Mar-
shall, J.W. 62, 63, *76*
McLean, A.E.M., see Sea-
wright, A.A. 110, *126*
McLean, A.E.M., see Thomp-
son, R.P.H. 298, *329*
McLean, E.K., see McLean,
A.E.M. 110, *125*, 257, *269*
McLean, J.R., see Harris,
R.C. 288, *317*
McMcilovic, B., see Kostial,
K. 353, *366*
McMillan, W.O., see Young,
D.L. 63, *80*
McMillin, J.M., see Zimmer-
man, T.S. 265, *271*
McNamara,H., see Nathenson,
G. 289, 299, *323*, *324*
McNee, N.W. 274, *323*
Medline, A., Bain, E., Menon,
A.I., Haberman, H.F. 177,
178, 187, 188, *197*
Meier, P.J., see Meyer, U.A.
250, *253*
Meigs, R.A., Ryan, K.J. 4,
44
Meijer, D.K.F., see Fleischner,
G. 68, *73*, 293, *315*
Meinhof, W., see Doss, M.
165, *194*
Melichar, V., see Polacek, K.
290, *325*
Mellits, E.D., see Hardy, J.B.
299, *317*
Meltzer, J.I., see Wheeler,
H.O. 280, *331*
Mendoza, C.E., see Villeneuve,
D.C. 160, *199*
Menon, A.I., see Medline, A.
177, 178, 187, 188, *197*
Mercke, C., see Lundh, B.
286, *322*
Meredith, P.A., Moore, M.R.,
Goldberg, A. 338, *367*

Merker, H.J., see Koransky, W. 65, *75*

Merker, H.-J., see Remmer, H. 56, 63, 67, *78*

Merker, J., see Remmer, H. 288, *326*

Metge, W.R., Owen, C.A., Foulk, W.T., Hoffman, H.N. 296, 306, *323*

Metter, G., see Poland, A.P. 157, 174, *198*

Mettits, E.D., see Chisolm, J.J., Jr. 335, 342, 344, *362*

Meuwissen, J., see Ketterer, B. *42*

Meuwissen, J.A.T.P., see Heirwegh, K.P.M. 279, 294, *317*

Meyer, M.C., Guttman, D.E. 288, *323*

Meyer, U.A. 240, 243, *253*

Meyer, U.A., Marver, H.S. 5, *44*, 98, *125*, 186, *197*, 245, *253*, 283, 287, *323*

Meyer, U.A., Maxwell, J.D. 82, 84, 85, *93*

Meyer, U.A., Meier, P.J., Correia, A.M. 250, *253*

Meyer, U.A., Schmid, R. 32, *44*, 130, *153*, 243, 244, 250, 252, *253*, 353, *367*

Meyer, U.A., Strand, L.J., Doss, M., Rees, A.C., Marver, H.S. 233, *235*, 241, *253*

Meyer, U.A., see Correira, M.A. 60, *72*, 145, *151*, 250, *252*

Meyer, U.A., see Maxwell, J.D. 130, 137, 144, 148, *153*, 246, 248, 250, 251, *253*

Meyer, U.A., see McDonagh, A.F. 100, 104, *124*

Meyer, U.A., see Schacter, B.A. 104, 111, *126*

Meyer, U.A., see Strand, L.J. 12, 16, *46*, 334, 353, *370*

Mia, A.S., Gronwall, R.R., Cornelius, C.E. 293, *323*

Miani, N., Viterbo, B. 349 *367*

Michaels, G.D., see Visintine, R.E. 305, *330*

Michaelson, I.A., see Conney, A.H. 56, *72*

Michiels, R., see Fevery, J. 27, *38*, 278, 279, *315*

Michot, F., Bürgi, M., Büttner, J. 56, *76*

Mijnlieff, P.F., see Verschure, J.C.M. 280, *330*

Mill, R.M., see Harvey, D.J. 103, 123

Millar, J., Peloquin, R., DeLeeuw, N.K.M. 281, *323*

Millar, J.A., Battistini, V., Cumming, R.L.C., Carswell, F., Goldberg, A. 337, *367*

Miller, D., see Fromke, V.L. 286, *315*

Miller, E.C., see Conney, A.H. 55, 56, *72*

Miller, E.C., see Cramer, J.W. 56, *72*

Miller, G.W., see Hsu, W.P. 20, *41*

Miller, G.W., see Shetty, A.S. 334, *369*

Miller, J.A., see Cramer, J.W. 56, *72*

Miller, J.A., see Conney, A.H. 55, 56, *72*

Miller, S.T., see Bertinchamps, A.J. 88, *92*

Miller, S.T., see Papavasiliou, P.S. 88, *93*

Millican, F.K., see Gutelius, M.F. 358, *365*

Millington, D.S., see Stoll, M.S. 19, *46*, 170, *199*

Milne, M.D., see Bourke, E. 280, *312*

Milne, M.H. 174, *197*

Minakami, S., see Hara, T. 67, *74*

Minakami, S., see Kagawa, Y. 341, *366*

Minakami, S., see Nakamura, M. 86, 88, *93*, 115, *125*

Minakami, S., see Yasukochi, Y. 87, *94*

Minnich, V., see Mohler, D.N. 281, *323*

Mishkin, S., Stein, L., Fleischner, G., Gatmaitan, Z., Arias, I.M. 292, *323*

Misra, H., see Fong, K. 111, *123*

Mitchell, J.R., Jollow, D.J., Potter, W.Z., Davis, D.C., Gillette, J.R., Brodie, B.B. 85, *93*

Mitchell, J.R., see Gillette, J.R. 54, *73*

Mitchell, J.R., see Potter, W.Z. 85, *93*

Mitropoulos, K.A., Suzuki, M., Myant, N.B., Danielsson, H. 62, *76*

Miya, R.S., see Hadley, W.M. 115, *123*

Miya, T.A., see Phillips, B.M. 56, *77*

Miya, T.S., see Hadley, W.M. 88, *92*

Miya, T.S., see Hoogland, D.R. 56, *74*

Miya, T.S., see Johnston, R.E. 88, *92*

Miyagi, K., Cardinal R., Bossenmaier, I., Watson, C.J. 16, *44*, 353, *367*

Mizuno, S., see Balkow, K. 30, *36*

Mörland, J., see Jervell, K.F. 257, *268*

Moffat, J.A., see Racz, W.J 223, *236*

Mohler, D.N., Majerus, P.W., Minnich, V., Hess, C.E., Garrick, M.D. 281, *323*

Moldeus, P.W., Young-Nam, C., Cinti, D.L., Schenkman, J.B. 64, *76*

Moldeus, P., see Schenkman, J.B. 54, *79*

Moller, J. 305, 306, *323*

Monod, J. 256, *269*

Monod, J., see Jacob, F. 50, 74, 212, *235*

Monson, R., see Kunin, C.M. 292, *320*

Montjar, M., see Trakatellar, A.C. 347, *370*

Moodie, C.A., see Kuiper-Goodman, T. 177, 178, *196*

Moore, C.V., see Grinstein, M. 341, *365*

Moore, H.L., see Joyce, C.R.B. 350, *366*

Moore, J.F., see Goyer, R.A. 354, 356, *364*

Moore, M.R. 357, *367*

Moore, M.R., Battistini, V., Beattie, A.D., Goldberg, A. 172, *197*, 224, 231, *235*

Moore, M.R., Goldberg, A. 12, *44*

Moore, M.R., Paxton, J.W., Beattie, A.D., Goldberg, A. 265, 266, *269*

Moore, M.R., Turnbull, A.L.,
  Bernado, D., Beattie, A.D.,
  Magnus, I.A., Goldberg,
  A. 158, 185, 197
Moore, M.R., see Battistini,
  V. 341, 362
Moore, M.R., see Beattie,
  A.D. 251, 252
Moore, M.R., see Goldberg,
  A. 266, 267
Moore, M.R., see McIntyre,
  N. 241, 253
Moore, M.R., see Meredith,
  P.A. 338, 367
Moore, M.R., see Paxton,
  J.W. 265, 266, 269
Moore, M.R., see Skea, B.R.
  33, 46
Moosa, A., Harris, F. 349,
  367
Mooty, J., Ferrand, C.F., Jr.,
  Harris, P. 358, 367
Mora, M., see Capelle, P.
  291, 313
Moreno, G.D., see Jensen,
  W.N. 347, 366
Morell, H., see Kassenaar, A.
  347, 366
Morgan, E.H., see Nosslin,
  B. 291, 324
Morgan, R.O., Fischer,
  P.W.F., Marks, G.S. 211,
  223, 229, 235
Morgan, R.O., Fischer,
  P.W.F., Stephens, J.K.,
  Marks, G.S. 211, 229, 235
Morgan, R.O., see Fischer,
  P.W.F. 210, 211, 234
Morimoto, H., see King,
  M.A.R. 282, 319
Morley, A., Geary, D., Har-
  ben, F. 167, 197
Morris, N., see Oesch, F. 64,
  77
Morris, T.Q. 302, 323
Morris, T.Q., see Macarol,
  V. 302, 322
Morrison, J.N., see Quater-
  man, J. 358, 368
Morrow, J.J., Urata, G.,
  Goldberg, A. 345, 367
Morrow, J.J., see Battistini,
  V. 341, 362
Morton, K.C., see Kadlubar,
  F.F. 115, 124
Moscovicova, E., see Gombos,
  B. 167, 195

Moses, H.L., Spelsberg, T.C.,
  Korinek, J., Chytil, F. 145,
  153
Moses, H.L., see Korinek, J.
  12, 42, 259—261, 268
Moses, H.L., see Rosenthal,
  A.S. 337, 368
Mosher, M., see Alpert, S.
  280, 309
Mosovich, L., see Thaler,
  M.M. 308, 329
Mowat, A.P., Arias, I.M. 27,
  44
Mowat, A.P., see Gray,
  D.W.G. 301, 316
Mozel, M., see Ben-Bassat, I.
  30, 36
Mucci, P., see Perugini, S.
  275, 325
Müftü, Y., see Peters, H.A.
  162—164, 168, 197
Müftü, Y., see Wray, J.D.
  162, 163, 200
Muftu, Y., see Dogramaci, I.
  163, 194
Muhlberger, G., see Heubel,
  F. 298, 318
Muirhead, E.E., Groves, M.,
  Bryan, S. 350, 351, 367
Muirhead, E.E., Groves, M.,
  Guy, R., Halden, E.R.,
  Bass, R.K. 323
Muirhead, E.E., Halden, E.R.,
  Groves, M.P. 283, 323
Mulder, G.J. 27, 44, 63, 76,
  294, 299, 300, 323
Mulder, G.J., Pilon, A.H.E.
  299, 323
Muller-Eberhard, U., see
  Johnson, E.F. 59, 75
Muller-Eberhard, U., see
  Liem, H.H. 135, 140, 141,
  152
Muller-Eberhard, U., see
  Maines, M.D. 119, 124
Munro, I.C., see Kuiper-
  Goodman, T. 177, 178,
  196
Murakami, K., Mason, S.
  119, 125
Murphy, F., see Marks, G.S.
  204, 206, 208, 209, 235
Murphy, F.R., Krupa, V.,
  Marks, G.S. 143, 148, 153,
  204—208, 226, 227, 229, 235
Murphy, N.H., see Ostrow,
  J.D. 26, 44, 278, 325

Murphy, S.D., see Jaeger,
  R.J. 112, 124
Murray, R.E., see Reiner, O.
  111, 126
Murthy, L., see Finelli, V.N.
  13, 38, 334, 338, 357,
  364
Murthy, V.V., Woods, J.S.
  12, 44, 226, 235
Murthy, V.V., see Woods,
  J.S. 10, 12, 34, 48
Murty, H.S., Caasi, P.I.,
  Brook, S.K., Nair, P.P. 14,
  44
Musch, A., see Vos, J.G. 172,
  188, 200
Mustard, P., see Dowdle,
  E.B. 256, 267
Muthukrishnan, S., see Satya-
  naryana Rao, M.R. 13, 46
Muzyka, V.I. 12, 44
Myant, N.B., see Mitropoulos,
  K.A. 62, 76
Myles, A.B., see Scott, C.L.
  283, 328

Naccarato, R., see Okolicsanyi,
  L. 296, 298, 299, 302,
  324
Nacht, S., see Kushner, J.P.
  191, 196
Nacht, S., see San Martin de
  Viale, L.C. 165, 169, 170,
  184, 198
Nadeau, B.E., see Goresky,
  C.A. 280, 302, 316
Nagahashi, M., Oho, T. 356,
  367
Nagai, T., Huse, T., Saikawa,
  S. 340, 367
Nagasawa, S., see Robinson,
  S.H. 295, 296, 306, 327
Nagel, R.L., Ranney, H.M.
  282, 323
Nair, P.P., see Murty, H.S.
  14, 44
Nakada, D., Magasanik, B.
  256, 269
Nakamura, M., Yasukochi, Y.,
  Minakami, S. 86, 88, 93,
  115, 125
Nakamura, M., see Yasuko-
  chi, Y. 87, 94
Nakao, K., Wada, O., Kita-
  mura, T., Uono, K., Urata,
  G. 23, 44, 256, 269

Nakao, K., Wada, O., Taka-
ku, F., Sassa, S., Yano, Y.,
Urata, G. 132, *153*, 171,
197
Nakao, K., Wada, O., Yano,
Y. 337, 341, *367*
Nakao, K., see Aoki, Y. 10,
12, 30, *35*
Nakao, K., see Wada, O. 56,
80, 97, *127*, 134, *154*, 171,
177, 180, *200*, 337, 341, *371*
Nakatsugawa, T., Dahm,
P.A. 10/, *125*
Nakatsugawa, T., Tolman,
N.M., Dahm, P.A. 107,
125
Nandi, D.L., Baker-Cohen,
K.F., Shemin, D. 333, *367*
Nanet, H., see Noir, B.A. 27,
44
Narasimhulu, S 67, *76*
Narasimhulu, S., see Remmer,
H. 54, *78*
Narisawa, K., Kikuchi, G.
13, *44*, 264, *269*, 333, *367*
Naruse, A., see Tateishi, N.
112, *127*
Nash, D.M., see Hutzinger,
O. 159, 161, *195*
Nathenson, G., Cohen, M.I.,
Litt, I.F., McNamara, H.
299, *323*
Nathenson, G., Cohen, M.I.,
McNamara, H. 289, *324*
Natzschka, J., see Blumen-
schein, S.D. 305, *312*
Nawata, H., Kato, K. 145, *153*
Nawrocki, P., see Doss, M.
165, *194*
Neal, R.A. 105, *125*
Neal, R.A., see Catignani,
G.L. 106, 109, *122*
Neal, R.A., see Dalvi, R.R.
107, *122*
Neal, R.A., see Hunter, A.
108, *123*
Neal, R.A., see Poore, R.E.
105, 107, *125*
Neal, R.A., see Ptashne, R.A.
105, *125*
Nebert, D.E., see Poland,
A.P. 57, 61, *78*
Nebert, D.W., Benedict, W.F.,
Gielen, J.E., Oesch, F., Da-
ly, J.W. 62, *76*
Nebert, D.W., Gelboin, H.V.
58, *76*, 212, *235*

Nebert, D.W., Gielen, J.E.
58, 60, *76*
Nebert, D.W., Kon, H. 58,
59, *76*
Nebert, D.W., see Gielen,
J.E. 60–62, *73*
Nebert, D.W., see Haugen,
D.A. 61, *74*
Nebert, D.W., see Kumaki,
K. 64, *75*
Nebert, D.W., see Oesch, F.
64, *77*
Neethling, A.C., see Shanley,
B.C. 353, *369*
Negishi, M., Omura, T. 67,
77
Nehls, R., see Witmer, C. 59,
80
Neidhardt, F.C., Magasanik,
B. 256, 258, *269*
Neilands, J.B., see Cheh, A.
13, *37*
Neilands, J.B., see Komai, H.
334, *366*
Neims, A.H., see Warner, M.
292, *330*
Nelson, A.A., see Fitzhugh,
O.G. 65, 66, *73*
Nelson, D.H., see Harding,
B.W. 4, *40*
Nelson, E.B., Raj, P.P., Belfi,
K.J., Masters, B.S.S. 58,
77
Nelson, E.B., see Schacter,
B.A. 23, *46*, 275, 276, 286,
327
Nelson, T., Jacobsen, J.,
Wennberg, R.P. 291, *324*
Nemoto, N., Gelboin, H.V.
64, *77*
Nemoto, N., see Gelboin,
H.V. 61, *73*
Nenov, P.Z., see Stonard,
M.D. 56, *79*, 160, 177, 178,
199
Neuberger, A. 8, *44*
Neuberger, A., Turner, J.M.
258, *269*
Neuberger, A., see Davies,
R.C. 11, 15–17, 21, *37*
Neuberger, A., see Gibson,
K.D. 13, 14, *39*, 333, 334,
337, *364*
Neuberger, A., see Gray,
C.H. 5, *40*, 275, *316*
Neuberger, A., see Mazanow-
ska, A.M. 22, *44*

Neuberger, J.A., Scott, J.J.
275, *324*
Neuwirt, G., see Poňka, P.
348, *368*
Neuwirt, J., Poňka, P., Boro-
vá, J. 30, *44*
Neuwirt, J., see Borová, J.
348, *362*
Neuwirt, J., see Poňka, P. 30,
45
Newberger, A., see Gibson,
K.D. 258, *267*
Newton, N.A., see Porra,
R.J. 22, *45*, 84, *93*
Newton, W.A., see Ertel, I.J.
296, 298, *315*
Nicholls, P., Elliott, W.B. 5,
44
Nicholson, D.C., see Elder,
G,H. 157, 184, *195*, 240,
253, 280, *314*
Nicholson, D.C., see Kondo,
T. 25, *42*
Nicholson, D.C., see Ostrow,
J.D. 307, *325*
Nicolis, F.B., see Acocella,
G. 291, *309*
Nies, A.S., see Branch, R.A.
293, *312*
Nigogosyan, G., see Cam, C.
163, 164, 166, *194*
Nigrin, G., see Waltman, R.
299, *330*
Nikkanen, G., see Hernberg,
S. 337, *365*
Nilsson, R., Orrenius, S., Ern-
ster, L. 113, *125*
Nilsson, S., see Schersten, T.
302, *327*
Nino, H.V., see McLaren,
G:D. 342, *36/*
NIOSH 359, *367*
Nishibayashi, H., Omura, T.,
Sato, R., Estabrook, R.W.
111, *125*
Nishibayashi, H., see Sato,
R. *78*
Nishida, G., Labbe, R.F. 84,
93
Nissley, S.P., Anderson, W.B.,
Gottesman, M.E., Perlman,
R.L., Pastan, I. 258,
269
Noever de Brauw, M.C., see
Koeman, J.H. 161, *196*
Noguchi, T., see Scott, M.L.
115, *126*

Noir, B.A., Dewalz, A.T., Rod-
riguez-Garay, E.A. 279,
324
Noir, B.A., Nanet, H. 27, *44*
Nolte, J., see Reith, A. 69, *78*
Norden, A., see Linberg,
L.G. 283, *321*
Norman, M.R., see Del Fa-
vero, A. 145; *151*
Norred, W.P., Wade, A.E.
62, *77*
Norstrom, R.J., see Hutzinger,
O. 159, 161, *195*
North, J.C., see Mason, H.S.
54, *76*
Nosslin, B. 278, 291, *324*
Nosslin, B., Morgan, E.H.
291, *324*
Notenboom-Ram, E., see Vos,
J.G. 157, 172, 178, 187,
188, *200*
Novak, M., see Polacek, K.
290, *325*
Novikoff, A.B., see Gold-
fischer, S. 304, *315*
Novogrodsky, A., see Margo-
liash, E. 82, *93*
Nymand, G. 299, *324*
Nystrom, E., see Alme, B. 99,
121

Obes-Polleri, J. 306, *324*
O'Brien, P.J., see Hrycay,
E.G. 113–115, *123*
O'Brien, P.J., see Little, C.
115, *124*
O'Brien, P.J., see Rahimtula,
A.D. 115, *125*
O'Brien, R.D. 105, *125*
O'Carra, P., Colleran, E. 26,
44, 118, *125*
O'Carra, P., Colleran, E. 118,
125
O'Carra, P., see Colleran, E.
25, *37*
Ockner, R.K., Isselbacher,
K.J. 292, *324*
Ockner, R.K., Schmid, R.
162, 165, 167, 169, 170, 179,
184, 185, 187, *197*
Odell, G.B. 289, 290, *324*
Odell, G.B., Bolen, J.L., Po-
land, R.L., Seungdamrong,
S., Cukier, J.O. 305, *324*
Odell, G.B., Brown, R.S.,
Holtzmann, N.A. 308,
324

Odell, G.B., Cohen, S.N., Kel-
ly, P.C. 289, 290, 291,
324
Odell, G.B., Cukier, J.O., Ma-
glalang, A.C. 291, *324*
Odell, G.B., see Blumenschein,
S.D. 305, *312*
Odell, G.B., see Kopelman,
A.E. 308, *320*
Odell, G.B., see Poland, R.L.
305, 306, *325*
Odell, G.B., see Strebel, L.
278, 294, *329*
Odell, W.D., see Perlroth,
M.G. 257, *269*
Odell, W.D., see Waxman, A.
257, *270*
Odessky, L., see Cucinell,
S.A. 72
O'Doherty, P.J.A., Kuksis,
A. 292, *324*
Oelshlegel, F.J., s. Schoo-
maker, E.B. 357, *369*
Oesch, F. 77
Oesch, F., Daly, J. 63, *77*
Oesch, F., Jerina, D.M. Daly,
J. 77
Oesch, F., Morris, N., Daly,
J.W., Gielen, J.E., Nebert,
D.W. 64, *77*
Oesch, F., see Nebert, D.W.
62, *76*
Özen, M.A., see Cetingil, A.I.
163, 164, *194*
O'Hanlon, P., see Stoll, M.S.
19, *46*
Ohashi, A., Kikuchi, G. 216,
217, *235*
Ohashi, A., see Tomita, Y.
33, *47*, 145, *154*, 213–217,
237
Ohnhaus, E.E., Locher, J.T.
293, *324*
O'Honlan, P., see Stoll, M.
170, *199*
Okolicsanyi, L., Cartei, G.,
Naccarato, R. 299, *324*
Okolicsanyi, L., Cortelazzo,
S., Carluccio, A., Naccara-
to, R. 298, 302, *324*
Okolicsanyi, L., Frei, J., Mag-
nenat, P. 295, 305, *324*
Okolicsanyi, L., Frei, J., Mag-
nenat, P., Naccarato, R.
296, *324*
Okuda, T., see Gelboin, H.V.
61, *73*

Oldershausen, H.F., see Schoe-
ne, B. 58, *79*
Omura, T., Sato, R. 57, *77*
Omura, T., Sato, R., Cooper,
D.Y., Rosenthal, O., Esta-
brook, R.W. 77
Omura, T., Siekevitz, P., Pa-
lade, G.E. 51, *77*
Omura, T., see Kuriyama, Y.
50, 59, 67, *75*
Omura, T., see Mannering,
G.J. 67, *76*
Omura, T., see Negishi, M.
67, *77*
Omura, T., see Nishibayashi,
H. 111, *125*
Onisawa, J., Labbe, R.F. 84,
93, 137, *153*
Onisawa, J., see Labbe, R.F.
32, *42*
Ono, T., Wada, O., Nagaha-
shi, M., Yamaguchi, N.,
Toyokawa, K. 356, *367*
Ophus, E., see Skaar, H. 354,
370
Oppelt, W.W., see Ross,
W.E. 117, *126*
Oral, S., see Peters, H.A.
162–164, 168, *197*
Orme, M.L.E., Davies, L.,
Breckenridge, A. 295, 297,
324
Orme-Johnson, W.H., see
Ghazarian, J.G. 4, *39*
Orrenius, S., Dallner, G., Ern-
ster, L. 113, *125*
Orrenius, S., see Ellin, A.
115, *123*
Orrenius, S., see Ernster, L.
59, 60, 63, *72*
Orrenius, S., see Frommer,
U. 58, *73*
Orrenius, S., see Högberg, J.
112, *123*
Orrenius, S., see Nilsson, R.
113, *125*
Orrenius, S., see Schenkman,
J.B. 54, *79*
Orrenius, S., see Zeidenberg,
P. 63, *80*, 279, 295, 301, *332*
Ørskov, S.L. 350, *368*
Ortega, J.P., see González-Ca-
david, N.F. 23, *39*
Ortego, J., see Schoomaker,
E.B. 357, *369*
Orten, J.M., see Weisman,
E.B. 265, *270*

Orth, H., see Fischer, H. 274, *315*

Orzalesi, M.M., see Blackburn, M.G. 308, *311*

Oshino, N., Imai, Y., Sato, R 66, *77*

Oski, F.A., see Weissberg, J.B. 338, 359, *371*

Ostrow, J.D. 274, 297, 307, 308, 309, *324, 325*

Ostrow, J.D., Berry, C.S. 308, *325*

Ostrow, J.D., Branham, R.V. 307, *325*

Ostrow, J.D., Murphy, N.H. 26, *44*, 278, *325*

Ostrow, J.D., Nicholson, D.C., Stoll, M.S. 307, *325*

Ottenwälder, H., see Bock, K.W. 64, *71*

Ottolonghi, S., see Giglloni, B. 31, *39*

Owen, C.A., see Metge, W.R. 296, 306, *323*

Owen, C.A., Jr., see Robinson, S.H. 275, *327*

Owen, N.V., Griffing, W.J., Hoffman, D.G., Gibson, W.R., Anderson, R.C. 65, *77*

Owens, I.S. 64, *77*

Oyama, H., Sugita, Y., Yoneyama, Y., Yoshikawa, H. 335, *368*

Pabst, M.J., see Habig, W.H. 292, *316*

Padilla, F., see Lessler, M.A. 357, *366*

Padmanaban, G., Rao, M.R.S., Malathi, K. 250, *253*

Padmanaban, G., Satyanarayana Rao, M.R., Malathi, K. 31, 33, *44*, 144, 145, 147, 149, *153*

Padmanaban, G., see Gayathri, A.K. 9, 33, 34, *39*, 149, *151*

Padmanaban, G., see Rajumanickan, C. 31, *45*, 145, *153*, 170, 177, 178, 180, 185, *198*, 250, *253*

Padmanaban, G., see Sardana, M.K. 135, 145, *154*

Padmanaban, G., see Satyanarayana Rao, M.R. 13, *46*, 146, *154*

Page, J.G., see Vesell, E.S. 62, *80*

Page, M.A., see Wattenberg, L.W. 57, *80*

Paglia, D.E., Valentine, W.N. 341, 348, *368, 370*

Paglia, D.E., Valentine, W.N., Dahlgren, J.G. 341, 348, *368*

Palade, G.E., see Dallner, G. 60, 62, *72*

Palade, G.E., see Farquhar, M.G. 66, *73*

Palade, G.E., see Kuriyama, Y. 50, 59, 67, *75*

Palade, G.E., see Omura, T. 51, *77*

Panopio, L.G., see Villeneuve, D.C. 160, *199*

Papavasiliou, P.S., Miller, S.T., Cotzias G.C. 88, *93*

Papst, M.J., see Habig, W.H. 64, *74*

Parigi, A., see Rubino, G.F. 340, 349, *369*

Parke, D.V., Rahman, H. 57, *77*

Parke, D.V., Williams, R.T. 160, 161, *197*

Parker, D., see Black, M. 295–297, *311*

Parks, R.E., see Tephly, T.R. 82, *94*

Parnas, H., see Attardi, C. 50, *70*

Parr, D.R., Harris, E.J. 354, *368*

Passow, H. 350, 359, *368*

Passow, H., Rothstein, A., Clarkson, T.W. 350, *368*

Passow, H., Tillman, K. 350, *368*

Passow, H., see Grigarzik, H. 350, *365*

Pastan, I., see Anderson, W.B. 258, *267*

Pastan, I., see De Crombrugghe, B. 258

Pastan, I., see Nissley, S.P. 258, *269*

Pastan, I., see Varmus, H.E. 258, *270*

Pasztor, G., see Sarwinsky, A. 351, *369*

Pathak, M., see Burnett, J. 169, *194*

Pathak, M.A., see Kalivas, J.T. 169, 171, *196*

Pathak, M.A., see Sweeney, V.P. 11, *47*

Paton, W.D.M., see Goldberg, A. 353, *364*

Patrignani, A., Sternieri, E., Perugini, S. 275, *325*

Patrignani, A., see Perugini, S. 275, *325*

Patton, G.M., Beattie, D.S. 9, 11, 32, 34, *44*, 149, 150, *153*

Patton, G.M., see Beattie, D.S. 32, *36*

Paul, J., see Freshney, R.I. 10, 12, 14, 23, *38*

Paumgartner, G. 291, *325*

Paumgartner, G., Probst, P., Kraines, R., Leevy, C.M. 291, *325*

Pawlow, M., see Vitale, L.F. 359, *371*

Paxton, J., see McIntyre, N. 241, *253*

Paxton, J.W., Moore, M.R., Beattie, A.D., Goldberg, A. 265, 266, *269*

Paxton, J.W., see Moore, M.R. 265, 266, *269*

Payne, R.B., see Arrowsmith, W.A. 301, 305, *310*

Pazderova, J., see Jirásek, L. 174, 175, *196*

Pearson, A.J.G., see McIntyre, N. 241, *253*

Pearson, R.W., Malkinson, F.D. 168, 169, 170, 171, *197*

Pechanova, A., see Gombos, B. 167, *195*

Pederson, T.C., Aust, S.D. 113, *125*

Pederson, T.C., Buege, J.A., Aust, S.D. 113, *125*

Peirano, W.B., see Finelli, V.N. 13, *38*, 334, 338, 357

Peisach, J., see Stern, J.O. 95, *127*

Pelkonen, O., Kaltiala, E.H., Larmi, T.K.I., Kärki, N.T. 58, *77*

Peloquin, R., see Millar, J. 281, *323*

Peluffo, P., see Holloway, P.W. 66, *74*

Penaud, J., see Hakim, J. 298, *316*

Peng, Y.M., see Chvapil, M. 112, *122*

Penning, W., Scoppa, P. 116, *125*

Penning, W., see Scoppa, P. 115, *126*, 352, *369*

Pentschew, A., Garro, F. 352, *368*

Peraino, C., Lamar, C., Jr., Pitot, H.C. 261, *269*

Peraino, C., Pitot, H.C. 256, *269*

Peraino, C., see Pitot, H.C. 256, *270*

Percy, V.A., see Shanley, B.C. 353, *369*

Percy-Robb, I.W., see Kaplowitz, N. 292, *319*

Perez, V., Schaffner, F., Popper, H. 178, 188, *197*, 274, 304, *325*

Perletti, L., see Sereni, F. 298, *328*

Perlin, A.S., see Gordon, E.R. 27, *39*

Perlman, R.I., see Varmus, H.E. 258, *270*

Perlman, R.L., see Anderson, W.B. 258, *267*

Perlman, R.L., see De Crombrugghe, B. 258, *267*

Perlman, R.L., see Nissley, S.P. 258, *269*

Perlroth, M.G., Marver, H.S., Tschudy, D.P. 264, *269*

Perlroth, M.G., Tschudy, D.P., Ratner, A., Spaur, W., Redeker, A. 256, *269*

Perlroth, M.G., Tschudy, D.P., Waxman, A., Odell, W.D. 257, *269*

Perlroth, M.G., see Marver, H.S. 10, 11, 12, *43,* 53, *76,* 257, 261, *269,* 333, *367*

Perlroth, M.G., see Tschudy, D.P. 11, 14, *47*, 256, *270*

Perrelli, G., see Rubino, G.F. 340, *369*

Perret, R.D., see Black, M. 295, 297, *311*

Perrin, E., see Spiegel, E.L. 305, *328*

Perryman, P.W., see Cremer, R.J. 306, 308, *314*

Perugini, S., Patrignani, A., Sternieri, E., Mucci, P. 275, *325*

Perugini, S., see Patrignani, A. 275, *325*

Pestaña, A. 257, 258, 259, *269*

Pestana, A., see Sudilovsky, O. 257, 259, *270*

Petering, H.G., see Finelli, V.N. 13, *38,* 334, 338, 357, *364*

Petering, H.G., see Vilter, R.W. 86, 87, *94*

Peterkofsky, B., Tomkins, G.M. 212, *236*

Peters, H.A., Johnson, S.A.M., Cam, S., Oral, S., Müftü, Y., Ergene, T. 162, 163, 164, 168, *197*

Peters, R.W., see Territo, M.C. 283, *329*

Peterson, R.E., see Roerig, D.L. 295, *327*

Petite, J.P., see Ploussard, J.P. 305, *325*

Petryka, Z.J., see Dhar, G.J. 243, *253*

Pfeifer, P.M., see McCay, P.B. 112, *124*

Phillips, B.M., Miya, T.A., Yim, G.K.W. 56, *77*

Phillips, W.E.J., see Villeneuve, D.C. 57, *80*, 160, *199*

Piceni sereni, L., see Careddu, P. 298, *313*

Pigram, P., see Blackburn, M.G. 308, *311*

Pilcher, C.W.T., see Thompson, R.P.H. 298, *329*

Pildes, R.S., see Porto, S.O. 308, *325*

Pilon, A.H.E., see Mulder, G.J. 299, *323*

Pimstone, N.R., Blekkenhorst, G., Eales, L. 23, *44*, 158, *197*

Pimstone, N.R., Engel, P., Tenhunen, R., Seitz, P.T., Marver, H.S., Schmid, R. 24, *45,* 118, *125,* 276, *325*

Pimstone, N.R., see Tenhunen, R. 23–25, *47*, 275, 276, *329*

Pinckard, R.N., Hawkins, D., Farr, R.S. 287, *325*

Pinelli, A., Capuano, A. 260, 261, *270*

Piomelli, S. 342, 359, *368*

Piomelli, S., Lamola, A.A., Poh-Fitzpatrick, M.B., Seaman, C., Harber, L.C. 344, *368*

Piomelli, S., see Lamola, A.A. 344, 345, *366*

Pipat, C., see Waltman, R. 299, *330*

Piper, R.F., see Hargreaves, T. 300, 301, *317*

Piper, W., see Tephly, T.R. 84—86, 89, *94*, 115, *127*

Piper, W.N., Bousquet, W.F. 145, *153*

Piper, W.N., Condie, L.W., Tephly, T.R. 89, 90, *93*

Piper, W.N., Rose, J.Q., Gehring, P.J. 162, *197*

Piper, W.N., Tephly, T.R. 90, *93, 261, 270, 334, 346, 368*

Piras, M.M., see Knox, W.E. 50, *75*

Pisani, W., Bonzanino, A., Coscia, G.C. 34, *45*

Pisarev, D.K. de, see San Martin de Viale, L.C. 18, *45*

Pitot, H.C., Peraino, C. 256, *270*

Pitot, H.C., see Peraino, C. 256, 261, *269*

Pitot, H.C., see Sudilovsky, O. 257, 259, *270*

Plaa, G.L., see Becker, B.A. 285, *310*

Plaa, G.L., see Indacochea-Redmond, N. 285, *318*

Plaa, G.L., see Roberts, R.J. 285, 293, 302, 303, *325*

Plaa, G.L., see Traiger, G.J. 286, *329*

Platt, D.S., Cockrill, B.L. 65, *77*

Platt, D.S., Thorp, J.M. 67, *77*

Ploussard, J.P., Foliot, A., Christoforov, B., Petite, J.P., Alison, F., Etienne, J.P., Housset, L. 305, *325*

Poh-Fitzpatrick, M., see Lamola, A.A. 344, 345, *366*

Poh-Fitzpatrick, M.B., see Piomelli, S. 344, *368*

Polacek, K., Novak, M., Melichar, V. 290, *325*

Poland, A., Glover, E. 58, 61, 66, *77*, 157, 174, *197*, 220, *236*

Poland, A., Glover, E., Kende, A.S. 61, *77*

Poland, A., Goldstein, J., Hickman, P., Burse, V.W. 176, *197*

Poland, A.P., Glover, E., Robinson, J.R., Nebert, D.E. 57, 61, *78*

Poland, A.P., Smith, D., Metter, G., Possick, P. 157, 174, *198*

Poland, R.L., Odell, G.B. 305, 306, *325*

Poland, R.L., see Odell, G.B. 305, *324*

Polglase, W.J., see Poulson, R. 20, 21, *45*

Polidori, G., see Romagnoli, G. 305, *327*

Pollard, H.M., see Bolt, R.J. 291, *312*

Ponka, P., see Borová, J. 348, *362*

Ponka, P., see Neuwirt, J. 30, *44*

Poňka, P., Neuwirt, J., Borová, J. 30, *45*, 348, *368*

Poole, B. 4, *45*

Poole, B., Leighton, T., Duve, C. de 50, 67, *78*

Poole, B., see Leighton, F. 67, *75*

Poore, R.E., Neal, R.A. 105, 107, *125*

Poore, R.E., see Dalvi, R.R. 107, *122*

Pope, A.L., see Rotruck, J.T. 115, *126*

Popper, H., see Barka, T. 65, *70*

Popper, H., see Hutterer, F. 178, *195*

Popper, H., see Perez, V. 178, 188, *197*, 274, 304, *325*

Porra, R.J., Falk, J.E. 20, 21, *45*

Porra, R.J., Jones, O.T.G. 22, *45*, 84, *93*, 335, 341, *368*

Porra, R.J., Vitols, K.S., Labbe, R.F., Newton, N.A. 22, *45*, 84, *93*

Porra, R.J., see Barnes, R. 9, 22, 23, *36*

Porter, E.G., Waters, W.J. 289, *325*

Porter, S. 342, *368*

Portig, J., see Ghazal, A. 56, *73*

Portig, J., see Koransky, W. 56, *75*

Porto, S.O. 307, *325*

Porto, S.O., Pildes, R.S., Goodman, H. 308, *325*

Pospisil, R., see McDonagh, A.F. 100, 104, *124*

Posse, N., see Engstrom, J. 306, *314*

Possick, P., see Poland, A.P. 157, 174, *198*

Potrepka, R.F., Spratt, J.L. 295, 299, *326*

Potter, W.Z., Davis, D.C., Mitchell, J.R., Jollow, D.J., Gillette, J.R., Brodie, B.B. 85, *93*

Potter, W.Z., see Mitchell, J.R. 85, *93*

Poulson, R., Polglase, W.J. 20, 21, *45*

Powell, C., see Young, D.L. 63, *80*

Powell, K.A., Cox, R., McConville, M., Charles, H.P. 137, *153*

Powell, R.D., see Degowin, R.L. 282, *314*

Poyer, J.L., see Fong, K. 111, *123*

Poyer, J.L., see Levin, W. 104, 111, 113, *124*

Prasad, A., see Schoomaker, E.B. 357, *369*

Prato, V., Gallo, E., Ricco, G., Mazza, U., Bianco, G., Lehmann, H. 282, *326*

Prato, V., see Rubino, G.F. 349, *369*

Preaux, A.M., see Berthelot, P. 300, *311*

Preaux, A.-M., see Franco, D. 26, *38*

Preisig, R., Bucher, H., Stirnemann, H., Tauber, J. 302, *326*

Preisig, R., Cooper, H.L., Wheeler, H.O. 302, *326*

Price, D.C., see Raffin, S.B. 276, *326*

Price, V.E., Sterlin, W.R., Tarantola, V.A., Hartley, R.W., Jr., Rechcigl, M., Jr. 51, *78*, 142, *153*

Price Evans, D.A., see Alexanderson, E. 61, 62, *70*

Prior, B.E., see De Matteis, F. 162, 167–171, 179, 181, 184, 188, *194*

Probst, P., see Paumgartner, G. 291, *325*

Prouty, W.F., see Goldberg, A.L. 4, *39*

Ptashne, K.A., Wolcott, R.M., Neal, R.A. 105, *125*

Pyfrom, H.T., see Heim, W.G. 82, *92*

Quaterman, J., Morrison, J.N., Humphries, W.R. 358, *368*

Quinn, G.P., Axelrod, J., Brodie, B.B. 62, *78*

Quinn, R.C., see Isselbacher, K.J. 279, *318*

Quistad, G.B., see Lightner, D.A. 307, *321*

Rabinowitz, M., see Aschenbrenner, V. 5, *36*

Rabinovitz, M., see Balkow, K. 30, *36*

Rabinovitz, M., see Gross, M 30, *40*

Rabinowitz, M., see Waxman, H.S. 347, *371*

Rabinowitz, M., see Druyan, R. 4, 6, *38*, 50, 67, *72*

Rabinowitz, M., see McKay, R. 9, 11, 22, *44*, 149, *153*

Racz, W.J., Marks, G.S. 143, 148, *153*, 203, 218–220, 223, 224, 231, 232, *236*

Racz, W.J., Moffat, J.A. 223, *236*

Racz, W.J., see Creighton, J.M. 133, *151*

Racz, W.J., see Schneck, D.W. 203, 209, *236*

Radtke, H.E., Coon, M.J. 114, *125*

Radzialowski, F.M. 299, *326*

Raffin, S.B., Woo, C.H., Roost, K.T., Price, D.C., Schmid, R. 276, *326*

Rahamimoff, H., see Clemens, M.J. 347, *363*

Rahimtula, A.D., O'Brien, P.J. 115, *125*

Rahman, H., see Parke, D.V. 57, *77*

Raisfeld, I., Bacchin, P., Hutterer, F., Schaffner, F. 83, *93*

Raj, P.P., see Nelson, E.B. 58, *77*

Rajamanickam, C., Amrutavalli, J., Rao, M.R.S., Padmanaban, G. 170, 177, 178, 180, 185, *198*

Rajamanickam, C., see Sardana, M.K. 135, 145, *154*

Rajamanickam, C., Satyanarayana Rao, M.R., Padmanaban, G. 31, *45*, 145 *153*

Rajamanickam, C., Rao, M.R.S., Padmanaban, G. 250, *253*

Rake, M.O., see Hunter, J. 296, *318*

Rall, D.P., see Brodie, B.B. 228, *233*

Ram, E., see Vos, J.G. 172, 188, *200*

Ramos, A., Silverberg, M., Stern, L. 301, *326*

Ramot, B., see Ben-Bassat, I. 30, *36*

Ramsay, C.A., Magnus, I.A., Turnbull, A., Baker, H. 158, 191, *198*

Randall, C.C., see Bracken, E.C. 354, *362*

Rane, A., Lunde, P.K.M., Jalling, B., Yaffe, S.J., Sjoqvist, F. 290, *326*

Ranney, H.M., see Nagel, R.L. 282, *323*

Rao, M.R.S., see Gayathri, A.K. 9, 33, 34, *39*

Rao, M.R.S., see Padmanaban, G. 250, *253*

Rao, M.R.S., see Rajamanickam, C. 170, 177, 178, 180, 185, *198*, 250, *253*

Rapp, H.J., see Gelboin, H.V. 61, *73*

Rasmussen, L.F., see Wennberg, R.P. 291, *331*

Ratner, A., see Perlroth, M.G. 256, *269*

Raymond, G.D., Galambos, J.T. 278, *326*

Raynaud, A., see Bellet, H. 296, *310*

Rechcigl, J., Jr., see Marver, H.S. 287, *322*

Rechcigl, M., Jr., see Marver, H.S. 9, *43*, 132, 134, *153*, 333, *367*

Rechcigl, M., Jr., see Price, V.E. 51, *78*, 142, *153*

Rechcigl, M., Jr., see Tschudy, D.P. 11, 14, 35, *47*, 256, *270*

Rechcigl, N., Jr., see Marver, H.S. 256, 259, 264, *269*

Recknagel, R.O. 110, *126*

Recknagel, R.O., Glende, E.A., Jr., Hruszkewycz, A.M. 110, *126*

Recknagel, R.O., Lombardi, B. 109, *126*

Reddy, J., Chiga, M., Bunyaratvej, S., Svoboda, D. 68, *78*

Reddy, J., Svoboda, D., Azarnoff, D. 65, 68, *78*

Redeker, A., see Perlroth, M.G. 256, *269*

Redeker, A.G., see Felsher, B.F. 256, *267*

Redeker, A.G., see Strand, L.J. 11, 12, 16, *46*, 241, *254*, 334, 353, *370*

Redline, R., see Strittmatter, P. 66, *79*

Rees, A.C., see Meyer, U.A. 233, *235*, 241, *253*

Reff, A., see Halac, E. 294, *316*

Reich, J., see Kafatos, F.C. 50, *75*

Rein, H., Maricic, S., Jänig, G.-R., Vuc-Pavlovic, S., Benko, B., Ristan, O., Ruckpaul, K. 135, *154*

Reiner, O., Athanassopoulos, S., Hellmer, K.H., Murray, R.E., Uehleke, H. 111, *126*

Reiner, O., Uehleke, H. 110, *126*

Reinicke, C., Rogner, G., Frenzel, J., Maak, B., Klinger, W. 298, *326*

Reino, J.C., see Forbes, G.B. 353, *364*

Reith, A., Brdiczka, D., Nolte, J., Staudte, H.W. 69, *78*

Remmer, H. 55, 56, 58, 62, *70*, *78*, 257, *270*

Remmer, H., Hirschmann, J., Greiner, I. 61, *78*

Remmer, H., Merker, H.-J. 63, 67, *78*

Remmer, H., Merker, J. 284, *326*

Remmer, H., Schenkman, J., Estabrook, R.W., Sasame, H., Gillette, J., Narasimhulu, S., Cooper, D.Y., Rosenthal, O. 54, *78*

Remmer, H., Schoene, B., Fleischmann, R.A. 56, 58, *78*

Remmer, H., Siegert, M., Merker, H.-J. 56, *78*

Remmer, H., see Bock, K.W. 27, *36*, 62, 63, *71*, 111, *122*, 294, 295, 299, *312*

Remmer, H., see Estabrook, R.W. 351, *363*

Remmer, H., see Fleischmann, R. 6, *38*

Remmer, H., see Greim, H. 50, 62, 67, *74*, 283, *316*

Remmer, H., see Hildebrandt, A. 59, *74*

Remmer, H., see Schenkman, J.B. 62, *79*

Remmer, H., see Schoene, B. 58, *79*

Remmer, H., see Witmer, C. 59, *80*

Revel, M., Hiatt, H.H. 50, *78*

Rexer, B., see Bock, K.W. 27, *36*, 62, 63, *71*, 294, 295, 299, *312*

Reyes, H., Levi, A.J., Gatmaitan, Z., Arias, I.M. 278, 293, *326*

Reyes, H., see Fleischner, G. 278, *315*

Reyes, H., see Levine, R.I. 278, *321*

Rhomberg, F., see Granzoni, A. 340, *365*

Rhyne, B., see Goyer, R.A. 354, 356, *364*

Riabov, S., see Hsia, D.Y. 300, 301, *318*

Ricco, G., see Prato, V. 282, *326*

Rich, A.R. 274, *326*

Richards, D.H., see Cremer, R.J. 306, 308, *314*

Richards, K.E., see Wu, W.H. 13, *48*

Richards, T.G., see Billing, B.H. 277, 278, 293, *311*

Richardson, P.C., see Greenbaum, D. 354, *365*

Richert, D.A., see Westerfeld, W.R. 68, 69, *80*

Richter, G.W., Kress, Y., Cornwall, C.C. 354, *368*

Richter, G.W., see Choie, D.D. 356, *362*

Ridley, A. 242, *254*

Riely, C.A., Cohen, G., Liebermann, M. 112, *126*

Riess, W., see Hess, R. 67, 68, *74*

Rifkind, A., see Javitt, N.B. *268*

Rifkind, A.B., Gillette, P.N., Song, C.S., Kappas, A. 218, 219, 222, 223, 231, 232, *236*, 249, *254*

Rifkind, A.B., see Incety, G.S. 35, *41*

Rimington, C. 189, *198*

Rimington, C., Magnus, I.A., Ryan, E.A., Cripps, D.J. 242, *253*

Rimington, C., Ziegler, G. 175, 176, *198*

Rimington, C., see Batlle, A.M. del C. 20, *36*

Rimington, C., see De Matteis, F. 142, *151*, 162, 167–171, 179, 181, 184, 188, *194*

Rimington, C., see Goldberg, A. 138, *152*, 222, *234*

Rimington, C., see Heikel, T. 189, *195*

Rimington, C., see Jarrett, A. 353, *366*

Rinehart, W.B., see Shotton, D. 291, *328*

Rinsler, S.S., see Erenberg, G. 357, *363*

Rios de Molina, M. del C., see San Martin de Viale, L.C. 170, 181, 187, *198*

Ristau, O., see Rein, H. 135, *154*

Rittenberg, D., see London, I.M. 5, *43*, 275, *321*

Rittenberg, D., see Shemin, D. 333, *369*

Rizzoli, A.A., see Galzigna, L. 337, *364*

Robbins, J., see Fleischner, G. 278, 293, *315*

Roberts, R.J., Plaa, G.L. 285, 293, 302, 303, *325*

Roberts, R.J., see Capizzo, F. 285, *313*

Robertson, D.H.H. 282, *326*

Robinson, D.S., see MacDonald, M.G. 57, *76*

Robinson, J., see Thompson, R.P.H. 298, *329*

Robinson, J.R., see Poland, A.P. 57, 61, *78*

Robinson, M.G., Foadi, M. 283, *326*

Robinson, S.H. 275, 284, 285, 296, 306, *326*

Robinson, S.H., Koeppel, E. 275, *326*

Robinson, S.H., Owen, C.A., Jr., Flock, E.V., Schmid, B. 275, *327*

Robinson, S.H., Rugstad, H.E., Yannoni, C., Tashijian, A.H., Jr. 275, *327*

Robinson, S.H., Tsong, M. 275, *327*

Robinson, S.H., Tsong, M., Brown, B.W., Schmid, R. 275, *327*

Robinson, S.H., Yannoni, C., Nagasawa, S. 295, 296, 306, *327*

Robinson, S.H., see Glass, J. 275, *315*

Robinson, S.H., see Snyder, A.L. 279, *328*

Robison, G.A., Butcher, R.W., Sutherland, E.W. 263, *270*

Robison, G.A., see Sutherland, E.W. 262, *270*

Rodkey, F.L., see Berk, P.D. 5, 6, *36*

Rodkey, F.L., see Blaschke, T.F. 284, 285, 295–297, *311*

Rodriguez-Garay, E., see Corchs, J.L. 291, *313*

Rodriguez-Garay, E.A., see Noir, B.A. 279, *324*

Rodriguez-Garay, E.A., see Serrani, R.E. 291, *328*

Roels, H.A., Buchet, J.P., Lauwerys, R.R., Sonnett, J. 337, 340, 341, *368*

Roels, H.A., Lauwerys, R.R., Buchet, J.P., Vrelust, M.T.H. 358, *368*

Roerig, D.L., Hasegawa, A.T., Peterson, R.E., Wang, R.I.H. 295, *327*

Rogers, L.A., see Gram, T.E. 279, *316*

Rogers, M.J., Strittmatter, P. 54, *78*

Rogers, M.J., see Strittmatter, P. 66, *79*

Rogner, G., see Reinicke, C. 298, *326*

Roller, P.P., see Selkirk, J.K. 59, *79*

Romagnoli, G., Polidori, G., Foschini, M., Cataldi, L., DeTurris, P., Tortorolo, G., Mastrangelo, R. 305, *327*

Romeo, G., Levin, E.Y. 15, 18, 19, *45*, 181, 190, *198*

Roomi, W.M., see Marks, G.S. 148, *153*, 204, 205, 223, 226, 235

Roost, K.T., see Raffin, S.B. 276, *326*

Rose, J., see Tschudy, D.P. 35, *47*

Rose, J.A., Hellman, E.S., Tschudy, D.P. 255, *270*

Rose, J.Q., see Piper, W.N. 162, *197*

Rosen, J.F., Zarate-Salvador, C., Trinidad, E.E. 347, *368*

Rosenberg, J.C., see Sardesai, V.M. 12, *45*

Rosenberg, S.A., Guidotti, G. 347, *368*

Rosenthal, A.S., Moses, H.L., Tice, L., Ganote, C.E. 337, *368*

Rosenthal, I.M., see Schmid, R. 305, *328*

Rosenthal, O., see Estabrook, R.W. 351, *363*

Rosenthal, O., see Omura, T. *77*

Rosenthal, O., see Remmer, H. 54, *78*

Rosher, M.L., see White, P. 275, *331*

Rosiek, O., see Kowalski, E. 34, *42*

Rosman, J., see Freedman, M.L. 30, *38*

Ross, M., see Tenhunen, R. 276, *329*

Ross, M.E., see Tenhunen, R. 25, *47*

Ross, W.E., Simrell, C., Oppelt, W.W. 117, *126*

Rossiter, E., Jr., see Broughton, P.M.G. 306, 308, *312*

Rothstein, A., see Passow, II. 350, *368*

Rothstein, A., see Weed, R.I. 350, *371*

Rothwell, J.D., Lacroix, S., Sweeney, G.D. 119, 120, *126*, 142, *154*, 286, 287, *327*

Rotruck, J.T., Pope, A.L., Ganther, H.E., Swanson, A.B., Hafeman, D.G., Hoekstra, W.G. 115, *126*

Roumengous, M., see Scoppa, P. 115, *126*, 352, *369*

Roy, F.P., van, see Heirwegh, K.P.M. 26, *40*

Rubin, E., see Beattie, D.S. 32, *36*

Rubin, F., Lieber, C.S. 298, *327*

Rubino, G.F., Coscia, G.C., Perrelli, G., Parigi, A. 340, *369*

Rubino, G.F., Prato, V., Fiorina, L. 349, *369*

Rubio, E., see Zelson, C. 299, *332*

Ruckpaul, K., see Rein, H. 135, *154*

Rudman, D., Bixler, T.J., Del Rio, A.E. 288, *327*

Rudolph, N., see Gross, R.T. 281, *316*

Ruegamer, W.R., see Westerfeld, W.R. 68, 69, *80*

Rugstad, H.E., Bratlid, D. 291, *327*

Rugstad, H.E., Dybing, E. 300, *327*

Rugstad, H.E., see Dybing, E. 300, 301, *314*

Rugstad, H.E., see Robinson, S.H. 275, *327*

Rungger, D., see Giglioni, B. 31, *39*

Russell, A., see Kapitulnik, J. 290, *319*

Russel, C.S., see Shemin, D. 258, *270*

Russell, C.S., see Yuan, M. 15, *48*

Russell, R.L., Coleman, D.L. 340, *369*

Russo, M.C., see San Martin de Viale, L.C. 170, 187, *198*

Ryan, D., Lu, A.Y.H., West, S., Levin, W. 179, *198*

Ryan, D., see Conney, A.H. 59, *71*

Ryan, D., see Lu, A.Y.H. 5, *43*, 58, 59, *76*

Ryan, D., see Thomas, P.E. 59, *80*

Ryan, E.A., see Rimington, C. 242, *254*

Ryan, J.N., see Chvapil, M. 112, *122*

Ryan, K.J., see Meigs, R.A. 5, *44*

Sachson, R.A., see Kappas, A. 220, 224, *235*

Sachson, R.D., see Kappas, A. 265, *268*

Safe, S., see Hutzinger, O. 159, 161, *195*

Sahn, S.A., see Lakshminarayan, S. 283, *320*

Saia, B., see Galzigna, L. 337, *364*

Saikawa, S., see Nagai, T. 340, *367*

Saint-Ruf, G., see Buu-Hoi, N.P. 57, *71*

Saita, G., Lussana, S. 340, *369*

Sakaguchi, S., see Kawasaki, H. 292, *319*

Sakamoto, Y., see Tateishi, N. 112, *127*

Sakurai, T., see Kawamata, F. 142, *152*

Salmon, M.V., see Greenbaum, D. 354, *365*

Salvador, R.A., Haber, S., Atkins, C., Gommi, B.W., Welch, R.M. 67, 68, *78*

Samis, H.V., see Baird, M.B. 142, *151*

Sampson, R., see Lui, H. 161, 190, *197*

Sanadi, D.R., see Fletcher, M.J. 283, *315*

Sanai, G.H., Hasegawa, T., Yoshikawa, H. 352, 356, *369*

Sanchez, E., Tephly, T.R. 300, *327*

Sancovich, H.A., Batlle, A.M.C., Grinstein, M. 15, *45*

Sancovich, H.A., see Jackson, A.H. 19, *41*, 170, 181, *196*

Sancovich, H.A., see San Martin de Viale, L.C. 181, 185, *198*

Sandy, J.D., see Davies, R.C. 11, 17, 21, *37*

San Martin de Viale, L.C., Garcia, R.C., Pisarev, D.K., de, Tomio, J.M., Grinstein, M. 18, *45*

San Martin de Viale, L.C., Grinstein, M. 18, *45*, 181, *198*

San Martin de Viale, L.C., Rios de Molina, M. del C., Wainstock, de Calmanovici, R., Tomio, J.M. 181, *198*

San Martin de Viale, L.C., Russo, M.C., Rios de Molina, M. del C., Grinstein, M. 170, 187, *198*

San Martin de Viale, L.C., Tomio, J.M., Ferramola, A.M., Sancovich, H.A., Tigier, H.A. 181, 185, *198*

San Martin de Viale, L.C., Viale, A.A., Nacht, S., Grinstein, M. 165, 169, 170, 184, *198*

San Martin de Viale, L.C., see Garcia, R.C. 18, *39*

San Martin de Viale, L.C., see Tomio, J.M. 18, *47*, 181, *199*

San Martin de Viale, L.L., see Garcia, D.C. 181, *195*

Sano, S. 21, *45*, 335, 348, 349, *369*

Sano, S., Granick, S. 20, 21, *45*, 335, 346, *369*

Sano, S., see Granick, S. 21, *39*

Sano, S., see Tokunaga, R. 335, *370*

Sansur, M., see Cucinell, S.A. 57, *72*

Santos, E.C., see Ashbrook, J.D. 277, *310*

Santos, E.C., see Spector, A.A. 288, *328*

Sardana, M.K., Rajamanickam, C., Padmanaban, G. 135, 145, *154*

Sardana, M.K., Satyanarayana Rao, M.R., Padmanaban, G. 135, 145, *154*

Sardesai, V.M., Lenaghan, R., Rosenberg, J.C. 12, *45*

Sarma, P.S., see Satyanarayana Rao, M.R. 13, *46*

Sarmiento, F., see Johnson, L. 288, 289, *319*

Sartori, L., see Girotti, F. 305, *315*

Sasame, H., see Remmer, H. 54, *78*

Sasame, H.A., Castro, J.A., Gillette, J.R. 109, *126*

Sassa, S. 346

Sassa, S., Granick, J.L., Granick, S., Kappas, A., Levere, R.D. 342–344, 359, *369*

Sassa, S., Granick, S. 9, 33, *45*, 149, *154*, 213–217, *236*, 241, *254*

Sassa, S., Granick, S., Bickers, D.R., Bradlow, H.L., Kappas, A. 16, *45*, 334, 353, *369*

Sassa, S., Granick, S., Bickers, D.R., Levere, R.D., Kappas, A. 339, 340, *369*

Sassa, S., Granick, S., Kappas, A. 336, 338, 339, 340, 344, 353, *369*

Sassa, S., see Anderson, K.E. 249, 251, *252*

Sassa, S., see Alvares, A.P. 82, *92*, 352, *361*

Sassa, S., see Fischbein, A. 344, *364*

Sassa, S., see Granick, J.L. 1, 8, 13, 35, *39*, 130, 140, *152*, 202, 208–211, *234*, 335, 337, 339, 342, 359, *365*

Sassa, S., see Nakao, K. 132, *153*, 171, *197*

Sato, R., Nishibayashi, H., Ito, A. *78*

Sato, R., see Imai, J. 54, *74*

Sato, R., see Nishibayashi, H. 111, *125*

Sato, R., see Omura, T. 57, *77*

Sato, R., see Oshino, N. 66, *77*

Satterlee, W., see Snyder, A.L. 279, *328*

Satyanarayana Rao, M.R., Malathi, K., Padmanaban, G. 146, *154*

Satyanarayana Rao, M.R., Padmanaban, G., Muthukrishnan, S., Sarma, P.S. 13, *46*

Satyanarayana Rao, M.R., see Padmanaban, G. 31, 33, *44*, 144, 145, 147, 149, *153*

Satyanarayana Rao, M.R., see Rajamanickam, C. 31, *45*, 145, *153*

Satyanarayana Rao, M.R., see Sardana, M.K. 135, 145, *154*

Saunders, S.J., Williams, J., Levey, M. 190, *198*

Saunders, S.J., see Hickman, R. 33, *40*, 259, *268*

Sausville, J.W., Sisson, T.R.C., Berger, D. 307, 308, *327*

Sawada, H., Takeshita, M., Sugita, Y., Yoneyama, Y. 22, *46*, 341, *369*

Sawada, H., see Yoneyama, Y. 341, *371*

Sawinsky, A., Durzt, J., Pasztor, G. 351, *369*

Sawyer, B.C., see Jose, P.J. 115, *124*

Sawyer, B.C., see Slater, T.F. 110, *126*

Schacter, D., Taggart, J.V. 89, *93*

Schacter, B.A. 276, *327*

Schacter, B.A., Marver, H.S., Meyer, U.A. 104, 111, *126*

Schacter, B.A., Mason, J.I. 286, 287, *327*

Schacter, B.A., Nelson, E.B., Marver, H.S., Masters, B.S.S. 23, *46*, 275, 276, 286, *327*

Schacter, B.A., Waterman, M.R. 24, *46*, 120, *126*, 276, *327*

Schacter, B.A., see Israel, L.G. 24, *41*

Schacter, B.A., see Israels, L.G. 276, *318*

Schacter, B.A., see Levitt, M. 5, *43*, 275, 283–286, *321*

Schacter, B.A., see Masters, B.S.S. 276, *322*

Schade, A.L., see Levy, H. 87, *93*

Schaffner, F., see Hutterer, F. 178, *195*

Schaffner, F., see Perez, V. 178, 188, *197*, 274, 304, *325*

Schaffner, F., see Raisfeld, J. 83, *93*

Schalch, D.S., see Waxman, A. 257, *270*

Schalm, L., see Weber, A.P. 278, *330*

Scharf, M.B., see Jacob, S.T. 59, *74*, 152

Scharschmidt, B.F., Waggoner, J.G., Berk, P.D. 277, 292, 293, *327*

Scharschmidt, B.F., see Blaschke, T.F. 284, 285, 293, 295–297, 306, *311*

Scharschmidt, B.F., see Martin, J.F. 293, *322*

Schatz, G., Mason, T.L. 68, *78*

Schaude, G. 66, *78*

Schaude, G., see Kunz, W. 64, 65, *75*

Schenkman, J.B., Cinti, D.L., Orrenius, S., Moldeus, P., Kraschnitz, R. 54, *79*

Schenkman, J.B., Frey, I., Remmer, H., Estabrook, R.W. 62, *79*

Schenkman, J.B., see Estabrook, R.W. 351, *363*

Schenkman, J.B., see Greim, H. 50, 62, 67, *74*, 283, *316*

Schenkman, J., see Remmer, H. 54, *78*

Schenkman, J.B., see Moldeus, P.W. 64, *76*

Schermuly, E., see Doss, M. 169, *194*

Schersten, T., Nilsson, S., Cahlin, E., Filipson, M., Brodina-Persson, G. 302, *327*

Schiff, D., Chan, G., Stern, L. 289, *327*

Schiff, L., see Spiegel, E.L. 305, *328*

Schilling, G., see Alvares, A.P. 57, 59, *70*

Schimasseck, H., see Kunz, W. 65, *75*

Schimke, R.T. 3, 4, *46*

Schimke, R.T., Doyle, D. 3, *46*, 50, 51, 59, *70, 79*

Schimke, R.T., Sweeney, F.W., Berlin, C.M. 50, 51, 52, 79, 142, 154
Schimke, R.T., see Arias, I.M. 59, 70
Schimke, R.T., see Berlin, C.M. 51, 52, 71
Schimke, R.T., see Dehlinger, P.J. 59, 72
Schimke, R.T., see Doyle, D. 13, 14, 16, 38, 334, 363
Schlesinger, F.G., Gastel, van, C. 231, 236
Schlicht, I., Koransky, W., Magour, S., Schulte-Hermann, R. 65, 66, 79
Schlicht, I., see Koransky, W. 65, 75
Schlicht, I., see Schulte-Hermann, R. 65, 79
Schmid, K., Cornu, F., Imhof, P., Keberle, H. 56, 79
Schmid, R. 1, 44, 157, 162–164, 198, 251, 254, 277, 278, 327, 328
Schmid, R., Axelrod, J., Hammaker, L., Swarm, R.L. 278, 279, 328
Schmid, R., Figen, J.F., Schwartz, S. 142, 154
Schmid, R., Forbes, A., Rosenthal, I.M., Lester, R. 305, 328
Schmid, R., Hammaker, L. 306, 328
Schmid, R., Hammaker, L., Axelrod, J. 278, 328
Schmid, R., Marver, H.S., Hammaker, L. 275, 283, 284–286, 328
Schmid, R., McDonagh, A.F. 104, 118, 126, 140, 154
Schmid, R., Schwartz, S. 201, 236
Schmid, R., see Bakken, A.F. 24, 36, 117, 118, 121, 287, 310
Schmid, R., see Bissell, D.M. 24, 36, 117, 118, 120, 122, 276, 311
Schmid, R., see Callahan, E.W., Jr. 308, 313
Schmid, R., see Hammaker, L. 291, 299, 317
Schmid, R., see Landaw, S.A. 5, 42, 102, 124, 135, 140–142, 152, 284, 286, 287, 320

Schmid, R., see Lester, R. 280, 305, 320, 321
Schmid, R., see Marver, H.S. 1, 6, 32, 43, 60, 76, 157, 158, 163, 197, 284, 286, 322
Schmid, R., see Meyer, U.A. 32, 44, 130, 153, 239, 240, 241, 243, 244, 250, 252, 253, 353, 367
Schmid, R., see Ockner, R.K. 162, 165, 167, 169, 170, 179, 184, 185, 187, 197
Schmid, R., see Pimstone, N.R. 24, 45, 118, 125, 276, 325
Schmid, R., see Raffin, S.B. 276, 326
Schmid, R., see Robinson, S.H. 275, 327
Schmid, R., see Snyder, A. 140, 154
Schmid, R., see Snyder, A.L. 279, 328
Schmid, R., see Tenhunen, R. 23–25, 47, 275, 276, 286, 328, 329
Schmid, R., see Wolf, M. 190, 200
Schmid, W., see Kunz, W. 64, 65, 75
Schnaidt, E., see Espinoza, J. 305, 315
Schneck, D., see Marks, G.S. 138, 153, 218, 228, 235
Schneck, D.W., Marks, G.S. 216, 236
Schneck, D.W., Racz, W.J., Hirsch, G.H., Bubbar, G.L., Marks, G.S. 203, 209, 236
Schneck, D.W., see Creighton, J.M. 133, 151
Schneider, A.B., see Anderson, W.B. 258, 267
Schneider, W.C. 6, 46
Schneider, W.C., see Kielley, R.K. 89, 92
Schnell, R.C., see Johnston, R.E. 88, 92
Schoene, B., Fleischmann, R.A., Remmer, H., Oldershausen, H.F. v. 58, 79
Schoene, B., see Remmer, H. 56, 58, 78
Schoenfeld, N., see Blum, I. 231, 233
Schoenfield, L.J., Bollman, J.L., Hoffman, H.N. 279, 328

Schoenheimer, R. 50, 79
Scholnick, P.L., Hammaker, L.E., Marver, H.S. 8, 9, 10, 12, 46, 89, 94, 149, 154
Scholz, R., Hansen, W., Thurman, R.G. 64, 79
Scholz, R., see Thurman, R.G. 64, 80
Schooley, J.C., see Landow, S.A. 349, 366
Schoomaker, E.B., Prasad, A., Oelshlegel, F.J., Ortego, J., Brewer, G.J. 357, 369
Schotland, D., see Greer, M. 357, 365
Schroeder, E., see Gross, R.T. 281, 316
Schubert, W., see Spiegel, E.L. 305, 328
Schulte-Hermann, R. 65, 70, 79
Schulte-Hermann, R., Thom, R., Schlicht, I., Koransky, W. 65, 79
Schulte-Hermann, R., see Koransky, W. 65, 75
Schulte-Herman, R., see Schlicht, I. 65, 66, 79
Schumer, W., see Lester, R. 280, 321
Schutzel, H., see Marver, H.S. 284, 286, 322
Schwartz, A., see Hodgman, J.E. 307, 318
Schwartz, D., see Zubay, G. 258, 271
Schwartz, H., see Tabachnick, I.T.A. 262, 270
Schwartz, R.S., see Swanson, M.A. 283, 329
Schwartz, S. 335, 369
Schwartz, S., Ikeda, K. 98, 100, 104, 126, 287, 328
Schwartz, S., see Ibrahim, G.W. 275, 318
Schwartz, S., see Schmid, R. 142, 154, 201, 236
Schwarze, R., Kintzel, H.W., Hinkel, G.K. 301, 328
Schwarze, R., see Kintzel, H.W. 301, 319
Scoppa, P., Roumengous, M., Penning, W. 115, 126, 352, 369
Scoppa, P., see Penning, W. 116, 125

Scott, C.L., Myles, A.B., Bacon, P.A. 283, *328*

Scott, J.J. 132, *154*

Scott, J.J., see Gibson, K.D. 13, 14, *39*, 333, 334, 337, *364*

Scott, J.J., see Neuberger, J.A. 275, *324*

Scott, M.L., Noguchi, T., Combs, G.F., Jr. 115, *126*

Seaman, C., see Piomelli, S. 344, *368*

Seawright, A.A., Hrdlicka, J., De Matteis, F. 107, *126*

Seawright, A.A., McLean, A.E.M. 110, *126*

Seawright, A.A.S., see De Matteis, F. 105–107, *122*

Seidman, F., see Tabachnick, I.I.A. 262, *270*

Scifter, S., see Arias, I.M. 301, *310*

Seitz, P.T., see Pimstone, N.R. 24, *45*, 118, *125*, 276, *325*

Seligsohn, U., see Shani, M. 305, *328*

Selkirk, J., see Gelboin, H.V. 61, *73*

Selkirk, J.G., Croy, R.G., Roller, P.P., Gelboin, H.V. 59, *79*

Sennett, R.E., see Gurba, P.E. 12, 13, *40*, 334, 338, *365*

Seppelainen, A.M. 359, *369*

Sereni, F., Perletti, L., Marini, A. 298, *328*

Sereni, F., see Careddu, P. 298, *313*

Serlupi-Crescenzi, G., see Beloff-Chain, A. 113, *122*

Sernatinger, E., see Levin, W. 103, *124*, 134, 147, *152*, 287, *321*

Serrani, R.E., Corchs, J.L., Rodriguez Garay, E.A. 291, *328*

Serrani, R.E., see Corchs, J.L. 291, *313*

Servoin-Sidoine, J., see Buu-Hoi, N.P. 57, *71*

Setlow, B., see Strittmatter, P. 66, *79*

Seungdamrong, S., see Odell, G.B. 305, *324*

Sewell, M., see Cowger, M.L. 32, *37*

Seyffert, R., see Grassl, M. 4, *39*

Sezer, V., see Dogramaci, I. 163, *194*

Sfeir, G.A., see Baird, M.B. 142, *151*

Shafer, B.C., see White, P. 275, *331*

Shafrir, E., see Starinsky, R. 289, *328*

Shah, H.C., Carlson, G.P. 110, *126*

Shand, D.G., see Branch, R.A. 293, *312*

Shani, M., Seligsohn, U., Ben Ezzer, J. 305, *328*

Shanley, B.C., Neethhing, A.C., Percy, V.A. 353, *369*

Shanley, B.C., Zail, S.S., Joubert, S.M. 20, *46*, 191, *198*

Shanley, B.C., see Bach, P.H. 171, *193*

Shanley, B.C., see Joubert, S.M. 182, 183, *196*

Shanley, B.C., see Taljaard, J.J.F. 19, *47*, 165, 169, 170, 171, 180, 181, 182, 184–186, 189, 191, 192, *199*

Shanley, B.C., see Timme, A.H. 177, 187, 188, *199*

Shanske, A., see Alport, S. 280, *309*

Sharma, D.C., 14, *46*

Shaw, C.R., see Kellermann, G. 62, *75*

Sheard, C., see Mann, F.C. 274, *322*

Shemin, D. 12, 13, *46*, 334, *369*

Shemin, D., London, I.M., Rittenberg, D. 333, *369*

Shemin, D., Russel, C.S., Abramsky, T. 258, *270*

Shemin, D., see Jordan, P.M. 8, 10, 12, *41*, 334, 345, *366*

Shemin, D., see Kikuchi, G. 8, *42*

Shemin, D., see London, I.M. 5, *43*, 275, *321*

Shemin, D., see Nandi, D.L. 333, *367*

Shemin, D., see Wu, W.H. 13, *48*

Shepley, L.A., see Berk, P.D. 349, *362*

Sherlock, S., see Black, M. 296, 297, *311*

Sherlock, S., see Gollan, J.L. 296, *315*

Shetty, A.S., Miller, G.W. 334, *369*

Shiff, D., see Chan, G. 289, *313*

Shinya, S., see Tateishi, N. 112, *127*

Shirachi, D.Y., see Howland, R.D. 279, *318*

Shirahata, T., see Matsuda, I. 301, *322*

Shiraishi, A. 340, *369*

Shire, J.G.M., see Kumaki, K. 64, *75*

Shrago, E., see Young, J.W. 259, *271*

Shotton, D., Carpenter, M., Rinehart, W.B. 291, *328*

Shultice, R.W., see Hart, L.G. 56, *74*

Shumway, C.N., see Maurer, H.M. 305, *322*

Shuster, L., see Jick, H. 59, *74*

Sicignano, C., see Halac, E. 295, 297, *317*

Siegel, A.L., see Burch, H.B. 339, *362*

Siegert, M., see Remmer, H. 56, *78*

Siekevitz, P., see Alvares, A.P. 59, *70*

Siekevitz, P., see Bock, K.W. 50, 67, *71*, 283, *312*

Siekevitz, P., see Dallner, G. 60, 62, *72*

Siekevitz, P., see Kuriyama, Y. 50, 59, 67, *75*

Siekevitz, P., see Omura, T. 51, *77*

Sies, H., Brauser, B. 64, *79*

Siess, M., see Kunz, W. 64, 65, *75*

Siest, G., see Batt, A.M. 299, *310*

Siklosi, C., see Simon, N. 188, 190, *198*

Silverberg, M., see Ramos, A. 301, *326*

Silvers, A.A., see White, P. 275, *331*

Silverstein, E. 348, *369*

Simon, N., Dobozy, A., Berko, G. 169, 170, 180, 188, *198*

Simon, N., Siklosi, C. *198*
Simon, N., Siklosi, C., Koszo,
 F. 188, 190, *198*
Simons, J. 259, *270*
Simpson, C.F., Damron, B.L.,
 Harms, R.H. 354, *369*
Simrell, C., see Ross, W.E.
 117, *126*
Sinclair, P., see Granick, S.
 140, *152*, 211, *234*
Sinclair, P.R., Granick, S.
 144, *154*, 189, 190, 192, *198*,
 209, 210, *236*, 246, *254*
Singer, J.W., see Song, C.S.
 226, *236*
Singleton, J.W., Laster, L.
 25, *46*
Silverberg, M., Desforges, J.,
 Gellis, S. 300, *328*
Silverman, W.A., Anderson,
 D.H., Blanc, W.A., Crozier,
 D.N. 288, *328*
Sisson, T.R.C., see Sausville,
 J.W. 307, 308, *327*
Six, K.M., Goyer, R.A. 358,
 369
Siyali, D.S. 167, *198*
Siyali, D.S., see Brady, M.N.
 161, *194*
Sjöqvist, F., see Alexanderson,
 E. 61, 62, *70*
Sjoqvist, F., see Rane, A.
 290, *326*
Sjovall, J., see Engstrom, J.
 306, *314*
Skaar, H., Ophus, E., Gullväg,
 B.M. 354, *370*
Skanderbeg, J., see Israels,
 L.G. 275, 283, *318*
Skanderbeg, J., see Yamamo-
 to, T. 5, *48*, 275, 283, *331*
Skea, B.R., Downie, E.D.,
 Moore, M.R., Davidson,
 J.N. 33, *46*
Sladek, N.E., Mannering,
 G.J. 58, 59, *79*
Slater, T.F. 110, *126*
Slater, T.F., Sawyer, B.C.
 110, *126*
Slater, T.F., Ziegler, G. 189,
 198
Slater, T.F., see Jose, P.J.
 115, *124*
Sleisenger, M.H., see Kreek,
 M.J. 296, 306, *320*
Small, D.M., see Carey, M.C.
 280, *313*

Smith, A., see Barltrop, D.
 347, *362*
Smith, C., see Hasegawa, E.
 22, *40*
Smith, D., see Poland, A.P.
 157, 174, *198*
Smith, D.S., Fujimoto, J.M.
 303, *328*
Smith, J.A., see Dagg, J.H.
 243, *253*, 353, *363*
Smith, K.M., see Baptista de
 Almeide, J.A.P. 170, *193*
 193
Smith, K.M., see Cavaleiro,
 J.A.S. 20, *37*
Smith, M., see White, J.M.
 282, *331*
Smith, N., see Douglas, J.F.
 56, *72*
Smith, S.G., see Jackson,
 A.H. 19, 21, *41*, 170, 181,
 196
Smithee, G.A., see Bottomley,
 S.S. 30, *37*
Smogys, A., see Conney,
 A.H. 59, *71*
Smuckler, E.A., Arrenius, E.,
 Hultin, T. 109, *126*
Sneath, P.H.A., see Gray,
 C.H. 5, *40*, 275, *316*
Snyder, A., Schmid, R. 140,
 154
Snyder, A.L., Satterlee, W.,
 Robinson, S.H., Schmid,
 R. 279, *328*
Snyder, R., see Witmer, C.
 59, *80*
Solomon, H.M. 277, *328*
Solymoss, B., Classen, H.G.,
 Varga, S. 56, *79*
Solymoss, B., Werringloer, J.,
 Toth, S. 56, *79*
Solymoss, B., Zsigmond, G.
 299, 302, 303, *328*
Sonawane, B.R., see Lucier,
 G.W. 177, *196*
Song, C.S., Bonkowsky, H.L.,
 Tschudy, D.P. 233, *236*,
 249, 251, *254*
Song, C.S., Singer, J.W., Le-
 vere, R.D., Harris, D.F.,
 Kappas, A. 226, *236*
Song, C.S., see Kappas, A.
 220, 224, *235*, 265, *268*
Song, C.S., see Rifkind, A.B.
 218, 219, 222, 223, 231, 232,
 236, 249, *253*

Sonnett, J., see Roels, H.A.
 337, 340, 341, *368*
Sottocasa, L., Kuylenstierna,
 B., Ernster, L., Bergstrand,
 A. 66, *79*
Sovocool, G.W., see Burse,
 V.M. 187, *194*
Sparks, R.G., see De Matteis,
 F. 111, *122*, 192, *194*, 264,
 267
Spatz, L., Strittmatter, P. 66,
 79
Spatz, L., see Strittmatter, P.
 66, *79*
Spaur, W., see Perlroth,
 M.G. 256, *269*
Spector, A.A., Santos, E.C.,
 Ashbrook, J.D., Fletcher,
 J.E. 288, *328*
Spector, A.A., see Ashbrook,
 J.D. 277, *310*
Spector, M.J., Guinee, V.F.,
 Davidow, B. 359, *370*
Spelsberg, T.C., see Moses,
 H.L. 145, *153*
Spencer, N., see Denton,
 M.J. 28, *38*
Sperber, I. 280, *328*
Spiegel, E.L., Schubert, W.,
 Perrin, E., Schiff, L. 305,
 328
Spong, N., see Dowdle, E.
 165, *194*
Spratt, J.L., see Harbison,
 R.D. 300, *317*
Spratt, J.L., see Lage, G.L.
 278, *320*
Spratt, J.L., see Potrepka,
 R.F. 295, 299, *326*
Stäubli, W., Hess, R., Weibel,
 E.R. 65, *79*
Stäubli, W., see Hess, R. 67,
 68, *74*
Starinsky, R., Shafrir, E. 289,
 328
Starkweather, D.K., see Chig-
 nell, C.F. 288, 290, *313*
Stathers, G.M., see Thomp-
 son, R.P.H. 298, *329*
Staudinger, H., see Frommer,
 U. 58, *73*
Staudt, H., Lichtenberger, F.,
 Ullrich, V. 67, *79*
Staudte, H.W., see Reith, A.
 69, *78*
Stavri, G., see Vasiliu, A.
 340, *370*

Steiger, M. 340, *370*
Stein, J.A., Berk, P., Tschudy, D.P. 263, *270*
Stein, J.A., Tschudy, D.P. 244, *254*, 256, *270*
Stein, J.A., Tschudy, D.P., Corcoran, P.L., Collins, A. 9, 13, 32, *46*, 263, *270*
Stein, J.A., see Bloomer, J.R. 283, *312*
Stein, J.A., see Chabner, B.A. 263, *267*
Stein, L., see Mishkin, S. 292, *323*
Steinmuller, D.P., see Kushner, J.P. 191, *196*, 264, *268*
Stephens, J.K., see Morgan, R.O. 211, 229, *235*
Sterlin, W.R., see Price, V.E. 51, *78*
Sterling, W.R., see Price, V.E. 142, *153*
Stern, J.O., Peisach, J. 95, *121*
Stern, L. 289, *328*
Stern, L., see Chan, G. 289, *313*
Stern, L., see Khanna, N.N. 289, 298, *319*
Stern, L., see Ramos, A. 301, *326*
Stern, L., see Schiff, D. 289, *327*
Stern, L., see Valle, S.J. 291, *331*
Sternieri, E., see Patrignani, A. 275, *325*
Sternieri, E., see Perugini, S. 275, *325*
Stetson, C.A., Jr. 358, *370*
Stevens, E., Frydman, R.B., Frydman, B. 15, *46*, 345, *370*
Stevenson, I.H., see Greenwood, D.T. 299, *316*
Steward, A.R., see Hansch, C. 220, 221, *234*
Stewart, D.A., see Maxwell, J.D. 295, 296, *323*
Stewart, J.C.M., see Bonnett, R. 307, *312*
Stich, W., Decker, P. 138, *154*, 225, 226, 231, *236*
Stiehl, A., Thaler, M.M., Admirand, W.H. 305, 306, *329*
Stipe, W.H., see McCay, P.B. 112, *124*

Stirnemann, H., see Preisig, R. 302, *326*
Stitzel, R.E., see Beckett, R.B. 65, 68, *71*
Stokes, G.S., see Bourke, E. 280, *312*
Stoll, M.S., Elder, G.H., Games, D.E., O'Hanlon, P., Millington, D.S., Jackson, A.H. 19, *46*, 170, *199*
Stoll, M.S., see Jansen, F.H. 26, *41*
Stoll, M.S., see Ostrow, J.D. 307, *325*
Stolte, L.A.M., see Vanleusden, H.A.I.M. 279, *330*
Stonard, M.D. 169, 170, 171, 178–180, 185, 187, 188, *199*
Stonard, M.D., Nenov, P.Z. 56, *79*, 160, 177, 178, *199*
Storev, B., see Blumenschein, S.D. 305, *312*
Strand, L.J., Felsher, B.F., Redeker, A.G., Marver, H.S. 11, *46*, 241, *254*
Strand, L.J., Manning, J., Marver, H.S. 144, 149, *154*, 210, 213, 214, 216, *236*, 241, 246, *254*, 341, 345, *370*
Strand, L.J., Meyer, U.A., Felsher, B.F., Redeker, A.G., Marver, H.S. 12, 16, *46*, 334, 353, *370*
Strand, L.J., Swanson, A.L., Manning, J. Branch, S., Marver, H.S. 10, 12, *46*
Strand, L.J., see Meyer, U.A. 233, *235*
Strand, L.T., see Meyer, U.A. 241, *253*
Stratton, C., see Harvey, D.J. 103, *123*
Strebel, L., Odell, G.B. 278, 294, *329*
Strickland, R.D., see Gregory, D.H. II 28, *40*, 279, 294, *316*
Strik, J.J.T.W.A. 157, 159, 172, 177, 179, 180, 187, 188, *199*, 222, 224, *236*
Strik, J.J.T.W.A., Koeman, J.H. 157, 175, *199*
Strik, J.J.T.W.A., Wit, J.G. 171, *199*, 222, 224, *236*
Strik, J.J.T.W.A., see Vos, J.G. 200, 222, *237*

Stripp, B., Hamrick, M., Zampaglione, N. 56, *79*
Stripp, B., see Greene, F.E. 109, *123*
Stripp, B., see Gillette, J.R. 62, *73*
Strittmatter, C.F., Umberger, F.T. 221, *236*
Strittmatter, P., Spatz, L., Corcoran, D., Rogers, M.J., Setlow, B., Redline, R. 66, *79*
Strittmatter, P., see Rogers, M.J. 54, *78*
Strittmatter, P., see Spatz, L. 66, *79*
Strobel, H.W., Lu, A.Y.H., Heidema, J., Coon, M.J. 54, *80*
Strohmeyer, G., see Doss, M. 165, *194*
Strum, J.M., Karnovsky, M.J. 83, *94*
Stuik, E.J. 358, *370*
Stumpf, W.E., Lester, R. 280, *329*
Suckling, C.J., see Kennedy, G.Y. 20, *42*
Sudilovsky, O., Pestana, A., Hinderaker, P.H., Pitot, H.C. 257, 259, *270*
Sugimura, T., see Kanai, Y. 4, 5, *41*
Sugita, Y., see Oyama, H. 335, *368*
Sugita, Y., see Sawada, H. 22, *46*, 341, *369*
Sugita, Y., see Takeshita, M. 22, *47*
Sugita, Y., see Yoneyama, Y. 341, *371*
Sundstrom, G., see Jensen, S. 162, *196*
Sutherland, D.A., Eisentraut, A.M. 350, *370*
Sutherland, E.W., Robison, G.A. 262, *270*
Sutherland, E.W., see Robison, G.A. 263, *270*
Sutherland, J.M., Keller, H.H. 300, *329*
Sutton, M.J., see Baptista de Almeide, J.A.P. 170, *193*
Suzuki, M., see Mitropoulos, K.A. 62, *76*
Suzuki, S., see Wada, O. 337, 341, *371*

Suzuki, T., see Wada, O. 337, 341, *371*

Svoboda, D., see Reddy, J. 65, 68, *78*

Swanson, A.B., see Rotruck, J.T. 115, *126*

Swanson, A.L., see Kaufman, L. 35, *42*, 148, *152*, 251, 252, *253*

Swanson, A.L., see Strand, L.J. 10, 12, *46*

Swanson, A.L., see Wetterberg, L. 12, *48*

Swanson, M.A., Chanmougan, D., Schwartz, R.S. 283, *329*

Swarm, R.L., see Schmid, R. 278, 279, *328*

Sweeney, E.W., see Schimke, R.T. 142, *154*

Sweeney, F.W., see Schimke, R.T. 50 – 52, *79*

Sweeney, G.D. 88, *94*, 146, *154*, 179, *199*

Sweeney, G.D., Janigan, D., Mayaman, D., Lai, H. 134, *154*, 160, 167, 177, 178, 180, 182, 187, 189, 192, *199*

Sweeney, G.D., see Lui, H. 161, 190, *197*

Sweeney, G.D., see Rothwell, J.D. 119, 120, *126*, 142, *154*, 286, 287, *327*

Sweeney, V.P., Pathak, M.A., Asbury, A.K. 11, *47*

Swick, R.W., see Ip, M.M. 4, 5, *41*

Sylvester, D., see MacDonald, M.G. 57, *76*

Szenberg, A., see Cunningham, A.G. 351, *363*

Szof, Z., see Kowalski, E. 34, *42*

Tabachnick, I.T.A., Gulbenkian, A., Seidman, F. 262, *270*

Tabachnick, I.A., Schwartz, H. 262, *270*

Tabarelli, S., see Uehleke, H. 110, *127*

Taddeini, L., Watson, C.J. 241, *254*

Taggart, J.V., see Schacter, D. 89, *93*

Tait, G.H. 3, 10, 11, 20, 21, *47*

Tait, G.H., see Davies, R.C. 11, 17, 21, *37*

Tait, G.H., see Mazanowska, A.M. 22, *44*

Takaku, F., see Aoki, Y. 10 – 12, 28, 30, *35*

Takahashi, A., see Kato, R. 62, *75*, 276, 287, *331*

Takashi, S., see Yoshida, T. 25, *48*, 118, *127*

Takaku, F., see Nakao, K. 132, *153*, 171, *197*

Takemori, A.E. *329*

Takeshita, M., Sugita, Y., Yoneyama, Y. 22, *47*

Takeshita, M., see Sawada, H. 22, *46*, 341, *369*

Takeshita, M., see Yoneyama, Y. 341, *371*

Talafant, E. 278, *329*

Talalay, P., see Benson, A.M. 64, *71*

Taljaard, J.J.F., Shanley, B.C., Deppe, W.M., Joubert, S.M. 19, *47*, 165, 169 – 171, 180, 182, 184 – 186, 189, 192, *199*

Taljaard, J.J.F., Shanley, B.C., Joubert, S.M. 169, 171, 180 – 182, 191, *199*

Taljaard, J.J.F., see Bach, P.H. 171, *193*

Taljaard, J.J.F., see Joubert, S.M. 182, 183, *196*

Taljaard, J.J.F., see Timme, A.H. 177, 187, 188, *199*

Talmage, P., see Kikuchi, G. 8, *42*

Talman, E.L., Labbe, R.F., Aldrich, R.A. 201, 217, 219, *237*

Tanaka, K.P., see Territo, M.C. 283, *329*

Tanaka, M., Bottomley, S.S. 12, *47*

Tanaka, M., see Bottomley, S.S. 342, *362*

Tappel, A.L. 112, 113, 115, *127*

Tarantola, V.A., see Price, V.E. 51, *78*, 142, *153*

Tarchanoff, J.F. 274, *329*

Tarlov, A.R., see Kellermeyer, R.W. 282, *319*

Tashijian, A.H., Jr., see Robinson, S.H. 275, *327*

Tateishi, N., Higashi, T., Shinya, S., Naruse, A., Sakamoto, Y. 112, *127*

Taub, H. 219, 221, 222, 225, 231, 232, *237*

Taub, H., Krupa, V., Marks, G.S. 225, 226, 228, *237*

Taub, H., Marks, G.S. 221, 232, *237*

Taub, H., see Marks, G.S. 204, 206, 208, 209, *235*

Tauber, J., see Preisig, R. 302, *326*

Taurog, A., see Goldstein, J.A. 299, *315*

Tenconi, L.T., see Acocella, G. 291, *309*

Tenhunen, R. 279, *329*

Tenhunen, R., Marver, H.S., Pimstone, N.R., Trager, W.F., Cooper, D.Y., Schmid, R. 23 – 25, *47*, 275, 276, *329*

Tenhunen, R., Marver, H.S., Schmid, R. 23, 24, *47*, 275, 276, 286, *329*

Tenhunen, R., Ross, M., Marver, H.S. 276, *329*

Tenhunen, R., Ross, M.E., Marver, H.S., Schmid, R. 25, *47*

Tenhunen, R., see Adlercreutz, H. 304, *309*

Tenhunen, R., see Pimstone, N.R. 24, *45*, 118, *125*, 276, *325*

Ten Noever de Brauw, M.C., see Vos, J.G. *200*

Tephly, T.R., Hasegawa, E., Baron, J. 84, *94*, 284, 286, *329*, 335, *370*

Tephly, T.R., Hibbeln, P. 84, 85, *94*, 115, *127*

Tephly, T.R., Mannering, G.J., Parks, R.E. 82, *94*

Tephly, T.R., Webb, D., Trussler, P., Kniffen, F., Hasegawa, E., Piper, W. 84 – 86, 89, *94*, 115, *127*

Tephly, T.R., see Baron, J. 31, *36*, 82, 83, 86, 89, *92*, 109, 284, *310*

Tephly, T.R., see Hasegawa, E. 22, *40*

Tephly, T.R., see Piper, W.N. 89, 90, *93*, 261, *270*, 334, 346, *368*

Tephly, T.R., see Sanchez, E. 300, *327*

Tephly, T.R., see Wagner, G.S. 84, 86–88, *94*

Teras, L.E., Kakhn, K.A. 357, *370*

Terner, U.K., see Marks, G.S. 138, *153*, 218, 228, *235*

Territo, M.C., Peters, R.W., Tanaka, K.P. 283, *329*

Tettenborn, D. 56, *80*

Thait, G.H., see Gibson, K.D. 258, *267*

Thaler, M.M. 297, *329*

Thaler, M.M., Dawber, N.H., Krasner, J., Mosovich, L., Yaffe, S. 308, *329*

Thaler, M.M., see Bakken, A.F. 24, *36*, 117, 118, *121*, 287, *310*

Thaler, M.M., see Callahan, E.W., Jr. 308, *313*

Thaler, M.M., see Stiehl, A. 305, 306, *329*

Thatcher, L.G., see Kammholz, L.P. 359, *366*

Theorell, H., see Åkeson, Å. 5, *35*

Thiery, J.P., see Bessis, M. 275, *311*

Thiessen, H., Jacobsen, J., Brodersen, R. 289, *329*

Thofern, F., see Kiese, M. 3, *42*

Thom, R., see Schulte-Hermann, R. 65, *79*

Thomas, E.D., see Laforet, M.T. 87, *93*

Thomas, J.C., see Cameron, G.R. 159, *194*

Thomas, P., see Cooper, J.M. 5, *37*

Thomas, P.E., Lu, A.Y.H., Ryan, D., West, S.B., Kawalek, J., Lewin, W. 59, *80*

Thomas, P.K., Lascelles, R.G. 354, *370*

Thompson, G., see Battistini, V. 341, *362*

Thompson, J.W., see Goldberg, A. 353, *364*

Thompson, M.L., see Wilson, V.K. 355, *371*

Thompson, R.P.H., Stathers, G.M., Pilcher, C.W.T., McLean, A.E.M., Robinson, J., Williams, R. 298, *329*

Thompson, R.P.H., see Hunter, J. 296, *318*

Thorgeirsson, S.S., see Davies, D.S. 58, *72*

Thorp, J.M., see Platt, D.S. 67, *77*

Thorpe, W.V., see Bray, H.G. 89, *92*

Thurman, R.G., Scholz, R. 64, *80*

Tice, L., see Rosenthal, A.S. 337, *368*

Tice, L.W. 337, *370*

Tigier, H.A., see San Martin de Viale, L.C. 181, 185, *198*

Tillman, K., see Passow, H. 350, *368*

Timme, A.H., Taljaard, J.J.F., Shanley, B.C., Joubert, S.M. 177, 187, 188, *199*

Tinaztepe, B., see Dogramaci, I. 163, *194*

Tipping, E., see Ketterer, B. 23, *42*

Tisher, C.C., see Call, N.B. 305, *313*

Tocchini-Valentini, G., see Arditti, R.R. 258, *267*

Todoroff, T., see French, S.W. 357, *364*

Toivonen, I., see Koskelo, P. 219, *235*

Tokunaga, R., Sano, S. 335, *370*

Tolman, N.M., see Nakatsugawa, T. 107, *125*

Tomaro, M.L., Frydman, R.B., Frydman, B. 15, 35, *47*

Tomaro, M.L., see Frydman, R.B. 15, 35, *38*, *39*

Tominaga, K., see Kawasaki, H. 292, *319*

Tomio, J.M., Garcia, R.C., San Martin de Viale, L.C., Grinstein, M. 18, *47*, 181, *199*

Tomio, J.M., Tuzman, V., Grinstein, M. 334, *370*

Tomio, J.M., see Garcia, R.C. 18, *39*, 181, *195*

Tomio, J.M., see Maines, M.D. 142, *152*

Tomio, J.M., see San Martin de Viale, L.C. 18, *45*, 181, 185, *198*

Tomita, Y., Ohashi, A., Kikuchi, G. 33, *47*, 145, *154*, 213–217, *237*

Tomkins, G.M., see Peterkofsky, B. 212, *236*

Tomlinson, G.A., Yaffe, S.J. 300, *329*

Tomokuni, K. 339, *370*

Tomokuni, K., Kawanishi, T. 338, *370*

Toothill, C., see Langelaan, D.E. 23, *42*

Toothill, C., see Lathe, G.H. 307, *320*

Tortorolo, G., see Romagnoli, G. 305, *327*

Toth, S., see Solymoss, B. 56, *79*

Touster, O., see Hollman, S. 301, *318*

Toyokawa, K., see Ono, T. 356, *367*

Toyokawa, K., see Wada, O. 337, 341, *371*

Trager, W.F., see Tenhunen, R. 23–25, *47*, 275, 276, *329*

Traiger, G.J., Derpentigny, L., Plaa, G.L. 286, *329*

Traketeller, A.C., Hemle, E.W., Montjar, M., Axelrod, A.E., Jensen, W.N. 347, *370*

Trevor, A.J., see Howland, R.D. 279, *318*

Trickey, R., see Hargreaves, T. 300, 301, *317*

Trinidad, E.E., see Rosen, J.F. 347, *368*

Tropham, J.C., Broad, R.D. 306, *329*

Troube, H., see Hakim, J. 298, *316*

Troxler, R.F., Dawber, N.H., Lester, R. 280, *330*

Troxler, R.F., see Daly, J.S.F. 4, 5, *37*

Trussler, P., see Tephly, T.R. 84–86, 89, *94*, 115, *127*

Tschudy, D.P. 1, *47*, 257, 264, *270*

Tschudy, D.P., Bonkowski, H.L. 130, *154*, 157, *199*, 244, *254*

Tschudy, D.P., Collins, A. 82, *94*

Tschudy, D.P., Marver, H.S., Collins, A. 9, *47*

Tschudy, D.P., Perlroth, M.G., Marver, H.S., Collins, A., Hunter, G., Jr., Rechcigl, M., Jr. 11, 14, 47, 256, 270

Tschudy, D.P., Rose, J., Hellman, E., Collins, A., Rechcigl, M., Jr. 35, 47

Tschudy, D.P., Waxman, A.D., Collins, A. 265, 270

Tschudy, D.P., Welland, F.H., Collins, A., Hunter, G.W., Jr. 256, 270

Tschudy, D.P., see Berk, P.D. 349, 362

Tschudy, D.R., see Bonkowsky, H.L. 90, 92, 260, 261, 262, 267

Tschudy, D.P., see Bloomer, J.R. 283, 312

Tschudy, D.P., see Chabner, B.A. 263, 267

Tschudy, D.P., see Ebert, P.S. 10, 38

Tschudy, D.P., see Marver, H.S. 9, 10–12, 43, 53, 76, 132, 134, 153, 256, 257, 259, 261, 264, 269, 287, 322, 333, 367

Tschudy, D.P., see Perlroth, M.G. 256, 257, 264, 269

Tschudy, D.P., see Rose, J.A. 255, 270

Tschudy, D.P., see Song, C.S. 233, 236, 249, 251, 254

Tschudy, D.P., see Stein, J.A. 9, 13, 32, 46, 244, 254, 256, 263, 270

Tschudy, D.P., see Waxman, A. 257, 265, 270

Tschudy, D.P., see Welland, F.H. 256, 271

Tsong, M., see Robinson, S.H. 275, 327

Tuboi, S., see Hayasaka, S. 11, 40

Tucker, D.R., see Azarnoff, D.L. 67, 70

Tuilié, M., Lardinios, R. 290, 330

Turnbull, A., Baker, H., Vernon-Roberts, B., Magnus, I.A. 158, 191, 199

Turnbull, A., see Ramsay, C.A. 158, 191, 198

Turnbull, A.L., see Moore, M.R. 158, 185, 197

Turner, J.C., Green, R.S. 177, 199

Turner, J. M., see Neuberger, A. 258, 269

Tuttle, A.H., Fitch, C. 347, 348, 370

Tuzman, V., see Tomio, J.M. 334, 370

Tyrrell, D.L.J., Marks, G.S. 33, 47, 145, 149, 154, 212–214, 216, 217, 237

Tyrrell, D.L.J., see Creighton, J.M. 133, 151

Uehleke, H., Hellmer, K.H. 110, 127

Uehleke, H., Hellmer, K.H., Tabarelli, S. 110, 127

Uehleke, H., see Reiner, O. 110, 111, 126

Ullrich, V., Diehl, H. 67, 80

Ullrich, V., see Frommer, U. 58, 73

Ullrich, V., see Staudt, H. 67, 79

Ulmer, D.D., Vallee, B.L. 356, 370

Ulstrom, R.A., Eisenklam, E. 305, 330

Umberger, F.T., see Strittmatter, C.F. 221, 236

Ungar, H., see Eliakim, M. 285, 314

Unseld, A., De Matteis, F. 98–102, 104, 127

Unseld, A., see De Matteis, F. 102, 104, 120, 123

Uono, K., see Nakao, K. 256, 269

Upson, D.W., Gronwall, R.R., Cornelius, C.E. 303, 330

Urata, G., Granick, S. 10, 47

Urata, G., see Aoki, Y. 10–12, 28, 30, 35

Urata, G., see Granick, S. 10, 39, 132, 152, 256, 268

Urata, G., see Morrow, J.J. 345, 367

Urata, G., see Nakao, K. 23, 44, 132, 153, 171, 197, 256, 269

Urata, G., see Wada, O. 56, 80, 97, 127, 134, 154, 171, 177, 180, 200

Urich, H., see Greenbaum, D. 354, 365

Vainio, H. 119, 127, 299, 330

Vainio, H., Hietanen, E. 295, 296, 306, 330

Vaisman, S.L., Lee, K.S., Gartner, L.M. 295, 330

Valasinas, A., see Frydman, R.B. 18, 39

Valdivieso, V.D., see Gumusio, J.J. 304, 316

Valentine, W.N., Fink, K., Paglia, D.E., Harris, S.R., Adams, W.S. 348, 370

Valentine, W.N., see Paglia, D.E. 348, 368

Valero, A., see Ber, R. 358, 362

Vallee, B.L., see Ulmer, D.D. 356, 370

Van Damme, B., see Fevery, J. 278, 279, 315

Van Esch, G.J., Van Genderen, H., Vink, H.H. 355, 370

Van de Vijver, M., see Heirwegh, K.P.M. 294, 317

Van der Maas, H.L., see Vos, J.G. 172, 188, 200

Van Genderen, H., see Van Esch, G.J. 355, 370

Vanhees, G.P., see Heirwegh, K.P.M. 279, 317

Van Leusden, H.A.I.M., Bakkeren, J.A.J.M., Zilliken, F., Stolte, L.A.M. 279, 330

Vanneste, M., see Mason, H.S. 54, 76

Vanroy, F.P., Heirwegh, K.P.M. 278, 279, 330

Vanroy, F.P., see Heirwegh, K.P.M. 279, 317

Van Steveninck, J., see DeGoeiji, A.F.P.M. 342, 363

Varga, G., see Bartok, I. 304, 310

Varga, L., Bartok, I. 304, 310

Varga, S., see Solymoss, B. 56, 79

Varmus, H.E., Perlman, R.I., Pastan, I. 258, 270

Varmus, H.E., see De Crombrugghe, B. 258, 267

Vasanelli, P., see Kato, R. 56, 75, 147, 152

Vasiliu, A., Stavri, G., Freund, S. 340, 370

Vecerek, B., see Jirsa, M. 279, *319*

Vergalla, J.M., see Blaschke, T.F. 293, 296, 306, *311*

Vergalla, J., see Martin, J.F. 293, *322*

Vergnano, C., Cartasegna, C., Bonsignore, D. 340, *370*

Vergnano, C., see Bonsignore, B. 340, *362*

Vernon-Roberts, B., see Turnbull, A. 158, 191, *199*

Verschure, J.C.M., Mijnlieff, P.F. 280, *330*

Venettacci, D., see Beloff-Chain, A. 113, *122*

Vesell, E.S. 62, *80*, 239, 252, *254*

Vesell, E.S., Page, J.G. 62, *80*

Vessel, E.S., see Jacob, S.T. 59, *74, 152*

Vessell, E.S., see Chignell, C.F. 290, *313*

Vessey, D.A., Goldenberg, J., Zakim, D. 27, *47*, 279, 294, 301, *330*

Vessey, D.A., Zakim, D. 294, *330*

Vessey, D.A., see Zakim, D. 294, 296, *332*

Viale, A.A., see San Martin de Viale, L.C. 165, 169, 170, 184, *198*

Vierling, J.M., see Martin, J.F. 293, *322*

Vihko, V., see Hasan, J. 350, *365*

Vijver, M., see Fevery, J. 27, *38*

Vijver, M. van de, see Heirwegh, K.P.M. 27, *40*

Viljoen, D., see Becker, D. 353, *362*

Villeneuva, E.C., Jennings, R.W., Burse, V.M., Kimbrough, R.D. 160, *199*

Villeneuva, E.C., see Burse, V.M. 187, *194*

Villeneuve, D.C. 160, 161, 169, *199*

Villeneuve, D.C., Grant, D.L., Phillips, W.E.J., Clark, M.L., Clegg, D.J. 57, *80*

Villeneuve, D.C., Phillips, W.E.J., Panopio, L.G., Mendoza, C.E., Hatina, G.V., Grant, D.L. 160, *199*

Villeneuve, D.C., see Grant, D.L. 160, 170, 172, 177-179, 187, *195*

Vilter, R.W., Bozian, R.C., Hess, E.V., Zellner, D.C., Petering, H.G. 86, 87, *94*

Vincent, P.C., Blackburn, C.R.B. 350, *371*

Vink, H.H., see Van Esch, G.J. 355, *370*

Vinopal, J.N., Casida, J.E. 162, *200*

Virchow, R. 274, *330*

Visintine, R.E., Michaels, G.D., Fukanama, G., Conklin, J., Kinsell, L.W. 305, *330*

Vitale, L.F., Joselow, M.M., Wedeen, R.P., Pawlow, M. 359, *371*

Viterbo, B., see Miani, N. 349, *367*

Vitols, K.S., see Porra, R.J. 22, 45, 84, *93*

Vohland, H.W., see Ghazal, A. 56, *73*

Vohland, H.W., see Koransky, W. 56, *75*

Volland, C., see Labbe, P. 341, *366*

Vono, K., see Nakao, K. 23, *44*

Vore, M., see Lu, A.Y.H. 4, *43*

Vos, J.G., Beems, R.B. 172, *200*

Vos, J.G., Botterweg, P.F., Strik, J.J.T.W.A., Koeman, J.H. 200, 222, 237

Vos, J.G., Koeman, J.H. 157, *200*

Vos, J.G., Koeman, J.H., Van der Maas, H.L., Ten Noever de Brauw, M.C., De Vos, R.H. *200*

Vos, J.G., Notenboom-Ram, E. 157, 172, 178, 187, 188, *200*

Vos, J.G., Van der Maas, H.L., Musch, A., Ram, E. 172, 188, *200*

Vos, J.G., see Goldstein, J.A. 157, 175, 180, 187, 188, *195*

Vos, R.H., see Koeman, J.H. 161, *196*

Voytek, P.E., see Weissberg, J.B. 13, 14, *48*, 333, *371*

Vrelust, M.T.H., see Roels, H.A. 358, *368*

Vrindten, P.A., see Chen, W. 56, 57, *71*

Vuc-Pavlovic, S., see Rein, H. 135, *154*

Wachstein, M. 356, *371*

Wada, O., Toyokawa, K., Suzuki, T., Suzuki, S., Yano, Y., Nakao, K. 337, 341, *371*

Wada, O., Yano, Y., Toyokawa, K., Suzuki, T., Suzuki, S., Katsunuma, H. 341, *371*

Wada, O., Yano, Y., Urata, G., Nakao, K. 56, *80*, 97, *127*, 134, *154*, 171, 177, 180, *200*

Wada, O., see Aoki, Y. 10-12, 28, 30, *35*

Wada, O., see Nakao, K. 23, 44, 132, *153*, 171, *197*, 256, *269*, 337, 341, *367*

Wada, O., see Ono, T. 356, *367*

Wade, A.E., see Norred, W.P. 62, *77*

Waggoner, J.D., see Berk, P.D. 349, *362*

Waggoner, J.G., see Berk, P.D. 5, 7, *36*

Waggoner, J.G., see Blaschke, T.F. 284, 285, 293, 295-297, 306, *311*

Waggoner, J.G., see Martin, J.F. 293, *322*

Waggoner, J.G., see Scharschmidt, B.F. 277, 292, 293, *327*

Wagner, G.S., Dinamarca, M.L., Tephly, T.R. 84, 86-88, *94*

Wagner, G.S., Tephly, T.R. 84, 86, 88, *94*

Wainstock de Calmanovici, R., see San Martin de Viale, L.C. 181, *198*

Wainwright, L.K., see Wainwright, S.D. 29, *47, 48*

Wainwright, S.D., Wainwright, L.K. 29, *47, 48*

Waitman, A.M., Dyck, W.P., Janowitz, H.D. 302, *330*

Wakil, S.J., see Holloway, P.W. 66, *74*

Walchak, H., see Kassner, R.J. 22, *41*
Waldenstrom, J. *254*
Waldron, H.A. 346, 349, 350, *371*
Walker, M., see Lathe, G.H. 278, 299, *320*
Wallen, M., see Bleiberg, J. 157, 174, 175, *194*
Waller, H.D. 281, *330*
Waltman, R., Bonura, F., Nigrin, G., Pipat, C. 299, *330*
Wang, R.I.H., see Roerig, D.L. 295, *327*
Wanschelbaum, A., see Frydman, R.B. 15, 35, 38, *39*
Ward, R.L., see Beattie, A.D. 251, *252*
Warner, M., Neims, A.H. 292, *330*
Warnick, G.R., Burnham, B.F. 10, *48*
Warren, C.B.M., see Broughton, P.M.G. 306, 308, *312*
Warren, E.H., see Cameron, G.R. 159, *194*
Wasserman, E., see Zelson, C. 299, *332*
Waterfield, M.D., Del Favero, A., Gray, C.H. 97, *127*, 134, *154*
Waterman, M.R., see Schacter, B.A. 24, *46*, 120, *126*, 276, *327*
Waters, W.J., Dunham, R., Bowen, W.R. 300, *330*
Waters, W.J., see Porter, E.G. 289, *325*
Watrach, A.M. 354, 357, *371*
Watson, C.J. 164–166, *200*, 218, 230, 231, *237*, 280, *330*
Watson, C.J., Campbell, M., Lowry, P.T. 280, *330*
Watson, C.J., see Dhar, G.J. 243, *253*
Watson, C.J., see Feldman, D.S. 353, *363*
Watson, C.J., see Ibrahim, G.W. 275, *318*
Watson, C.J., see Miyagi, K. 16, *44*, 353, *367*
Watson, C.J., see Taddeini, L. 241, *254*
Watson, C.J., see Zimmerman, T.S. 265, *271*
Watson, C.T. 243, *254*

Watson, R.J., Decker, E., Lichtman, H.C. 349, *371*
Wattenberg, L.W., Leong, J.L. 56, *80*
Wattenberg, L.W., Page, M.A., Leong, J.L. 57, *80*
Waxman, A., Schalch, D.S., Odell, W.D., Tschudy, D.P. 257, *270*
Waxman, A., see Perlroth, M.G. 257, *269*
Waxman, A.D., Collins, A., Tschudy, D.P. 265, *270*
Waxman, A.D., see Tschudy, D.P. 265, *270*
Waxman, H.S., Rabinovitz, M. 347, *371*
Weatherall, D.J., see Charache, S. 348, *362*
Weatherall, M., see Joyce, C.R.B. 350, *366*
Webb, C., see Tephly, T.R. 115, *127*
Webb, D., see Tephly, T.R. 84–86, 89, *94*
Webb, J.L. 262, *270*
Webb, M., see Dingle, J.T. 87, *92*
Weber, A.P., Schalm, L., Witmans, J. 278, *330*
Wedeen, R.P., see Vitale, L.F. 359, *371*
Weed, R.I., Eber, J., Rothstein, A. 350, *371*
Weibel, E.R., see Bolender, R.P. 65, 66, *71*
Weibel, E.R., see Stäubli, W. 65, *79*
Weinbren, K., Billing, B.H. 279, *330*
Weiner, M., Buterbaugh, G.G., Blake, D.A. 117, *127*
Weiner, R., see Bock, K.W. 143, *151, 252*
Weippl, G. 358, *371*
Weiss, M., see Cucinell, S.A. *72*
Weiss, R., see Beckett, R.B. 65, 68, *71*
Weissberg, J.B., Voytek, P.E. 13, 14, *48*, 333, *371*
Weissberg, J.N., Lipschutz, F., Oski, F.A. 338, 359, *371*
Weissman, E.B., Cheng, L.C., Orten, J.M. 265, *270*
Welch, R.M., see Salvador, R.A. 67, 68, *78*

Welland, F.H., Hellman, E.S., Gaddis, E.M., Collins, A., Hunter, G.W., Jr., Tschudy, D.P. 256, *271*
Welland, F.H., see Tschudy, D.P. 256, *270*
Welton, A.F., Aust, S.D. 4, *48*
Wennberg, R.P., Rasmussen, L.F. 291, *331*
Wennberg, R.P., see Nelson, T. 291, *324*
Werringloer, J., see Solymoss, B. 56, *79*
Weser, U., see Bugany, H. 22, 23, *37*
West, G.M.L., see McIntyre, N. 241, *253*
West, R., see London, I.M. 5, *43*, 275, *321*
West, S., see Conney, A.H. 59, *71*
West, S., see Lu, A.Y.H. 58, *76*
West, S., see Ryan, D. 179, *198*
West, S.B., see Huang, M.-T. 59, *74*
West, S.B., see Lu, A.Y.H. 4, 43, 58, 59, *76*
West, S.B., see Thomas, P.E. 59, *80*
Westerfeld, W.R., Richert, D.A., Ruegamer, W.R. 68, 69, *80*
Wetterberg, L. 130, *155*
Wetterberg, L., Marver, H.S., Swanson, A.L. 12, *48*
Wetterberg, L., see Yuwiler, A. 257, 259, *271*
Wheeler, H.O. 280, *331*
Wheeler, H.O., Cranston, W.I., Meltzer, J.I. 280, *331*
Wheeler, H.O., see Preisig, R. 302, *326*
Whelton, M.J., Krustev, L.P., Billing, B.H. 296, *331*
Whipple, G.H., Hooper, C.W. 274, *331*
White, I.N.H., see Bock, K.W. 294, 295, 301, *312*
White, J.M., Brain, M.C., Ali, M.A.M. 30, *48*
White, J.M., Brain, M.C., Lorkin, P.A., Lehmann, H., Smith, M. 282, *331*

White, J.M., Harvey, D.R. 30, 48, 344, 347, 371
White, J.M., Hoffbrand, A.V. 30, 48
White, K., see Bray, H.G. 89, 92
White, P., Silvers, A.A., Rosher, M.L., Shafer, B.C., Williams, W.J. 275, 331
Whitehead, J.D., see Whitfield, C.L. 352, 371
White-Stevens, R.H., Kamin, H. 67, 80
Whitfield, C.L., Ch'ien, L.T., Whitehead, J.D. 352, 371
Whiting, M., Granick, S. 345, 371
Whiting, M.J., Elliott, W.H. 9, 12, 48, 148, 149, 155
Whiting, M.J., Granick, S. 9, 48, 150, 155
Whitlock, J.P., Jr., Gelboin, H.V. 58, 60, 80
Whitlock, J.P., Jr., see Gelboin, H.V. 61, 73
Wicks, W.D. 259, 271
Wicks, W.D., Kenney, F.T., Lee, K.L. 259, 271
Wiebel, F.J., see Gelboin, H.V. 61, 73
Wilcken, F., see Windorfer, A. 305, 331
Wildish, D.J., see Hutzinger, O. 159, 161, 195
Wilkinson, G.R., see Branch, R.A. 293, 312
Williams, J., see Saunders, S.J. 190, 198
Williams, R., Maxwell, J.D., Hunter, J. 298, 331
Williams, R.T. 107, 127
Williams, R., see Billing, B.H. 277, 278, 293, 311
Williams, R., see Hunter, J. 296, 318
Williams, R., see Thompson, R.P.H. 298, 329
Williams, R., see Maxwell, J.D. 295, 296, 323
Williams, R.T., see Parke, D.V. 160, 161, 197
Williams, R.C., see Wu, W.H. 13, 48
Williams, W.J., see White, P. 275, 331
Willoughby, D.A., see Jarrett, A. 353, 366

Wills, E.D. 112, 113, 127
Wills, E.D., see Davison, S.C. 63, 72
Wills, E.D., see Goudy, B. 335, 364
Wilkinson, A.E., see Goudy, B. 335, 364
Wilson, E.L., Burger, P.E., Dowdle, E.B. 13, 48, 333, 334, 339, 341, 371
Wilson, J.T. 297, 331
Wilson, R.G., see Gelboin, H.V. 145, 152
Wilson, V.K., Thompson, M.L., Dent, C.E. 355, 371
Wiltshire, B.G., see King, M.A.R. 282, 319
Windorfer, A., Kunzer, W., Bolze, H., Ascher, K., Wilkken, F., Hoehne, K. 305, 331
Winsnes, A. 294, 295, 331
Winsnes, A., Dutton, G.J. 294, 295, 331
Wintrobe, M.M. 335, 371
Wintrobe, M.M., see Lee, G.R. 86, 93
Wintrobe, M.M., see Lewis, M. 10, 43
Wintrobe, M.M., see Goldberg, A. 341, 364
Wit, J.G., see Strik, J.J.T.W.A. 171, 199, 222, 224, 236
With, T.K. 243, 254
Witmans, J., see Weber, A.P. 278, 330
Witmer, C., Remmer, H., Nehls, R., Krauss, P., Smyder, R. 59, 80
Witschi, H.P., see Indacochea-Redmond, N. 285, 318
Wolcott, R.M., see Ptashne, K.A. 105, 125
Wolf, M., Lester, R., Schmid, R. 190, 200
Wolfson, S., see Arias, I.M. 298, 299, 310
Wolkoff, A.W., see Martin, J.F. 293, 322
Wong, K. 27, 48
Wong, K.P. 279, 295, 331
Wong, S.H., see Harding, B.W. 4, 40
Woo, C.H., see Raffin, S.B. 276, 326

Wood, P.B., see Bray, H.G. 89, 92
Woods, J.S. 9, 34, 48, 83, 94, 200
Woods, J.S., Dixon, R.L. 12, 34, 48, 147, 155, 226, 237
Woods, J.S., Murthy, V.V. 10, 12, 34, 48
Woods, J.S., see Murthy, V.V. 12, 44, 226, 235
Woolley, P.V., Hunter, M.J. 289, 331
Worlledge, S. 282, 283, 331
Wortham, J.S., see Gelboin, H.V. 145, 152
Wosilait, W.D. 288, 331
Wranne, L. 305, 331
Wray, J.D., Müftü, Y., Dogramaci, I. 162, 163, 200
Wray, J.D., see Dogramaci, I. 163, 194
Wu, W.H., Shemin, D., Richards, K.E., Williams, R.C. 13, 48
Wyndham, R.A., see Lemberg, R. 25, 42

Yaffe, S., see Thaler, M.M. 308, 329
Yaffe, S.J., Catz, C.S., Stern, L., Levy, G. 297, 331
Yaffe, S.J., Levy, G., Matsuzawa, T., Baliah, T. 296, 331
Yaffe, S.J., see Catz, C. 295, 297, 313
Yaffe, S.J., see Krasner, J. 290, 294, 295, 297, 320
Yaffe, S.J., see Rane, A. 290, 326
Yaffe, S.J., see Tomlinson, G.A. 300, 329
Yagi, H., see Holder, G. 59, 74
Yamaguchi, N., see Ono, T. 356, 367
Yamamoto, T., Skanderberg, J., Zipursky, A., Israels, L.G. 5, 48, 275, 283, 331
Yamamoto, T., see Adachi, Y. 295, 309
Yamamoto, T., see Israels, L.G. 275, 283, 318
Yamane, T., see Lamola, A.A. 344, 345, 358, 359, 366

Yang, C.S. 54, *80*
Yang, S.K., see Gelboin,
  H.V. 61, *73*
Yannoni, C.Z., see Glass, J.
  275, *315*
Yannoni, C., see Robinson,
  S.H. 275, 295, 296, 306,
  327
Yano, Y., see Nakao, K.
  132,
  153, 171, *197*, 337, 341, *367*
Yano, Y., see Wada, O. 56,
  80, 97, *127*, 134, *154*, 171,
  177, 180, *200*, 337, 341, *371*
Yasukochi, Y., Nakamura,
  M., Minakami, S. 87, *94*
Yasukochi, Y., see Nakamura,
  M. 86, 88, *93*, 115, *125*
Yeary, R.A., Davies, D.R.
  289, *331*
Yim, G.K.W., see Phillips,
  B.M. 56, *77*
Yoda, B., Israels, L.G. 23, *48*
Yoda, B., see Hayashi, N. 9,
  10, 33, *40*
Yoda, B., see Israel, L.G. 24,
  41
Yoda, B., see Israels, L.G.
  276, *318*
Yoda, B., see Matsuoka, T.
  264, *269*
Yoneyama, Y., Sawada, H.,
  Takeshita, M., Sugita, Y.
  341, *371*
Yoneyama, Y., see Kagawa,
  Y. 341, *366*
Yoneyama, Y., see Oyama,
  H. 335, *368*
Yoneyama, Y., see Sawada,
  H. 22, *46*
Yoneyama, Y., see Sawada,
  H. 341, *369*
Yoneyama, Y., see Takeshita,
  M. 22, *47*
Yoneyama, Y., see Yoshika-
  wa, H. 22, *48*
Yoshida, T., Kikuchi, G. 25,
  48

Yoshida, T., Takashi, S., Ki-
  kuchi, G. 25, *48*, 118, *127*,
  276, 287, *331*
Yoshikawa, H. 352, 356, *371*
Yoshikawa, H., Yoneyama,
  Y. 22, *48*
Yoshikawa, H., see Oyama,
  H. 335, *368*
Yoshikawa, H., see Sanai,
  G.H. 352, 356, *369*
Young, D.L., Powell, C.,
  McMillan, W.O. 63, *80*
Young, J.W., Shrago, E., Lar-
  dy, H.A. 257, *271*
Young-Nam, C., see Moldeus,
  P.W. 64, *76*
Yu, C.A., Gunsalus, I.C. 95,
  127
Yuan, M., Russell, C.S. 15,
  48
Yuwiler, A., Wetterberg, L.,
  Geller, E. 257, 259, *271*

Zail, S.S., Charlton, R.W.,
  Bothwell, T.H. 282, *332*
Zail, S.S., see Shanley, B.C.
  20, *46*, 191, *198*
Zakim, D., Goldenberg, J.,
  Vessey, D.A. 296, *332*
Zakim, D., Vessey, D.A. 294,
  332
Zakim, D., see Vessey, D.A.
  27, *47*, 279, 294, 301, *330*
Zaman, Z., Abboud, M.M.,
  Akhtar, M. 8, 21, *48*
Zampaglione, N., see Stripp,
  B. 56, *79*
Zanjani, E.D., see Gordon,
  A.S. 30, *39*, 265, *267*
Zarafonetis, C.J.D. 90, *94*
Zarate-Salvador, C., see Ro-
  sen, J.F. 347, *368*
Zatepka, S., Grossman, M.I.
  302, *332*
Zeidenberg, P., Orrenius, S.,
  Ernster, L. 63, *80*, 279,
  295, 301, *332*

Zellner, D.C., see Vilter,
  R.W. 86, 87, *94*
Zelson, C., Rubio, E., Wasser-
  man, E. 299, *332*
Ziegler, D.M., see Kadlubar,
  F.F. 115, *124*
Ziegler, G., see Rimington,
  C. 175, 176, *198*
Ziegler, G., see Slater, T.F.
  189, *198*
Ziegler, J.M., see Batt, A.M.
  299, *310*
Zilliken, F., see Vanleusden,
  H.A.I.M. 279, *330*
Zimmerman, H.J., see Grosz-
  mann, R.J. 302, *316*
Zimmermann, J.A., see Baird,
  M.B. 142, *151*
Zimmerman, T.S., McMillin,
  J.M., Watson, C.J. 265,
  271
Zingg, W., see Israels, L.G.
  275, *318*
Zinkham, W.H. 282, 300, *332*
Zinkham, W.H., Childs, B.
  282, *332*
Zipursky, A., see Israels,
  L.G. 275, 283, *318*
Zipursky, A., see Levitt, M.
  5, *43*, 275, 283—286, *321*
Zipursky, A., see Yamamoto,
  T. 5, *48*, 275, 283, *331*
Zitko, V., see Hutzinger, O.
  159, 161, *195*
Zollinger, H.U. 355, *371*
Zsigmond, G., see Solymoss,
  B. 299, 302, 303, *328*
Zubay, G., Schwartz, D.,
  Beckwith, J. 258, *271*
Zubay, G., see Arditti, R.R.
  258, *267*
Zuckerman, D.M., see Blum-
  berg, W.E. 344, 359, *362*
Zuelzer, W.W., see Brown,
  A.K. 278, *313*
Zuyderhoudt, F.M.J., Borst,
  P., Huijing, J. 9, *48*, 149,
  155

Subject Index

Acetanilide 203, 282
Acetate
  inhibition of ALA-S induction 261
  effect on heme biosynthesis 90
Acetazolamide
  displacement of bilirubin by 288, 290
Acetophenetidin (*see* Phenacetin)
Acetoxycycloheximide
  inhibition of ALA-S induction in
    cell cultures 214
Acetylcholine esterase
  inhibition by lead in membranes 337
Acetylsalicylic acid
  and G6PD deficiency 282
  acetylation of albumin by 288
  displacement of bilirubin by 289, 290
Acid phosphatase
  increased in cholestasis 304
Acne (*see* Chloracne)
Actinomycin D
  inhibition of
    induction of ALA-S by 212–216, 220
    induction of heme oxygenase by 276
    5β-H steroid-induced Hb synthesis
      by 30
Acute Intermittent Porphyria (AIP)
  239, 241, 246
  abnormalities of carbohydrate metabolism
    in 257
  ALA-S activity in 32, 249, 252
  defect in
    heme synthesis 246, 249, 250
    PBG deaminase 32, 241, 353
  early labelled bilirubin in 6, 283
  excretion of
    ALA and PBG in 240, 241, 250
    steroids in 266
  glucose effect in 256
  impaired metabolism of antipyrine and sa-
    licylamide in 249, 251
  inappropriate relase of growth hormone
    in 257
  neuropsychiatric disturbances in 241,
    353
  production of 5β-H steroid metabolites
    in 266

sex hormones and porphyrin metabolism
  in 264, 265
Adrenalectomy
  and induction of enzymes 259, 260
  and mixed-function oxidase activity 62
Agar
  effect on bilirubin metabolism 305
AIA-epoxide
  formula 103
AIA-glycol
  formula 103
AIA-glycol-lactone 103
Alanine transaminase
  and glucose effect 257
  induction by tryptophan 258
Albumin
  binding with
    bilirubin 276, 277, 288
    drugs 288
    fatty acids 277
    heme 277
    hormones 277
  effect on porphyrin formation in cell cul-
    ture 211, 212
  liver synthesis and phenobarbital 65
Alcohol (ethanol)
  and lead toxicity 356, 357
  and PCT 158, 171, 242
  precipitation of acute attacks of porphyria
    by 244
  stimulation of drug metabolism by 298
Aldrin
  inducer of cytochrome P-450 56
Allobarbital 287
Allyl acetamides 97, 102, 134, 139, 204
Allyl barbiturates
  and loss of cytochrome P-450 97, 102,
    103, 134, 139, 287
  effect on catalase 142
  increase in ALA-S caused by 132, 133,
    139
Allylisopropylacetamide (AIA)
  decrease in heme oxygenase caused
    by 287
  destruction of liver heme by 98–102,
    104, 134, 135, 139–141, 147, 287

Allylisopropylacetamide (AIA) drug
  interactions 144, 246, 247, 259, 260
  effect on
    catalase 142
    succinyl CoA synthetase 32
    tryptophan pyrrolase 53, 142
  formula 131
  increase in
    cytochrome P-450 in chick embryo 222
    hepatic ligandin 293
    liver synthesis of m-RNA 145
  loss of cytochrome P-450 caused by 31,
    96—98, 108, 133, 134, 139, 245
  metabolism to an epoxide 103
  stimulation of ALA-S
    in chicken embryo 213—217, 226, 227
    in rodents 89, 132—135, 137, 139,
      146—148, 226, 227, 245
Allylisopropylacetamide porphyria
  comparison with other experimental por-
    phyrias 132, 176
  effect of diet on 255, 256
  species differences 148, 224
Allylisopropylacetylurea (see Sedormid)
Amaranth
  biliary excretion of 303
Amides
  porphyrin-inducing activity and lipophil-
    icity 206—208
Aminoacetone synthetase 10
Aminoaciduria
  in lead poisoning 354, 355, 360
p-Aminobenzoic acid (PABA)
  effect on cytochrome P-450 89
  possible treatment for hepatic por-
    phyria 90
  reversal of DDC porphyria by 89, 90
α-Amino-β-ketoadipic acid 8, 9
5-Aminolevulinate (ALA)
  alternative pathways of metabolism 34,
    35
  amount made by normal liver 5
  as a precursor of bilirubin 275
  excretion of
    after lead and phenobarbital 247, 248
    in HCB or PCB porphyria 167, 171,
      173
    in human hereditary
      porphyrias 240—242
    in lead poisoning 336, 345, 354, 355,
      360
  formula 7
  possible role in acute attacks of por-
    phyria 243
  production and utilisation in HCB por-
    phyria 185, 186
5-Aminolevulinate dehydratase

(ALA-dehydratase) 12—14, 23
  activity in different tissues 13, 14
  activity in screening for lead poison-
    ing 338, 359
  combined effect of lead and alcohol
    on 357
  genetic variations 340
  in HCB porphyria 180, 185
  in lead poisoning 340, 344, 352, 353,
    355
  inhibition by
    aminotriazole 82, 83, 84
    cadmium 337, 341
    chelating agents 334
    heme 339
    lead 82, 115, 333, 334, 336—341, 345,
      360
    mercury 334, 337, 341
    sulfhydryl reagents 334, 337
  properties of 13, 334
  role of zinc in activity of 13, 334, 338,
    357, 360
5-Aminolevulinate synthetase (ALA-S)
    8—12, 23
  and regulation of heme metabolism
    28—35, 140, 141
  distribution 11, 12
  effect of cobalt 85, 88, 150
  in human hepatic porphyrias 28, 32, 144,
    158, 240, 241, 256
  inhibition by heme 12, 30, 149
  properties 9, 10
  regulation by heme 29, 31—34, 133, 135,
    244
  stimulation of
    and drug interactions 143, 144, 246,
      247, 263
    by erythropoietin 30
  comparison in different systems
    222—229
  effect of acetate on 90
  effect of inhibitors of protein synthesis
    on 34, 146
  glucose effect on 90, 91, 256, 259,
    260—263
  impaired in experimental diabetes 262
  in chick embryo systems by drugs 35,
    157, 174, 175, 189, 203, 209, 210, 212,
    213, 217—220, 222, 249, 265, 266
  in the liver of rodents by
    AIA 89 132—135, 137, 139,
      146—148, 245
    allyl-containing barbiturates 132,
      133, 138
    aminotriazole 82—84
    DDC 89, 132, 133, 135—137, 139,
      143, 146

stimulation of
  in the liver of rodents by
    griseofulvin   132, 133, 135, 136, 138,
      139
    HCB   180, 185, 186
    iron   111
    PCB   180, 183
    phenobarbital   60, 89, 284
    starvation   12, 111
    tryptophan   257
  inhibition by protoheme   212, 215—217
  mechanism   133—142, 143—150,
    212—217, 249—252
  permissive effect of cAMP and hydro-
    cortisone on   259—261
o-Aminophenol   300
Aminopyrine
  N-demethylation of   177, 222
  inducer of cytochrome P-450   56
  substrate for mixed function oxidase sys-
    tem   59, 64
  type I difference spectrum   54
p-Aminosalicylic acid   283
3-Amino-1,3,4-triazole (aminotriazole)
  goitrogenic effect of   83
  inhibitor of heme and hemoprotein syn-
    thesis   82—84, 89
Amitriptyline   251
Amobarbital   221, 225, 230
5β-Androstan-3,17-dione   222
Androstenediol
  effect on ALA-S   265
Androstenedione
  effect on ALA-S   265
Androsterone
  excretion of in AIP   266
Anemia
  due to lead poisoning   349, 350
Aniline
  type II difference spectrum   54, 179
  N hydroxylation of   177
Aniline hydroxylase
  inhibition by lead   352, 360
Anthranilic acid   300
Antibody formation
  decreased by lead   351, 360
Antipyrine
  effect on ALA-S potentiated by lead   246
  induction of bilirubin GT by   297
  metabolism in lead poisoning   352
  metabolism in AIP   249, 251
Apocytochrome P-450 (see Cytochrome
  P-450 apoprotein)
Aprobarbital
  decrease in cytochrome P-450 caused
    by   287
  induction of ALA-S by   219, 221, 225

Arginase
  increase due to cortisone   51, 52
Aroclors (see also Polychlorinated
  biphenyls)
  effects on drug-metabolising systems   178
  hepatic porphyria caused by   173
  structural changes in liver due to   187, 188
  production of uroporphyrin in cell cul-
    ture   189, 190
Arsine
  hemolytic effect of   281
Aryl hydrocarbon hydroxylase   58,
  59, 61, 64
Ascorbic acid
  and ferrochelatase   86, 87
Aspartic acid
  treatment of hyperbilirubinemia with   301
Aspartate transaminase
  glucose effect and   257
  induction by tryptophan   258
Aspirin
  considered safe in hereditary hepatic por-
    phyria   251
Atropine
  considered safe in hereditary hepatic por-
    phyria   251
ATP
  and glucose effect in ALA-S induction
    261, 262
  fall in hepatic concentration in experimen-
    tal porphyria   32
ATPase
  and bile secretion   302
  decreased in cholestasis   303
  inhibition by
    lead   337, 350
    phenothiazines   304
    substituted estrogens   304

Barbiturates
  and reversibility of induction   65
  effect on supply of UDP-glucuronic
    acid   301
  induction of ALA-S in
    chick embryo systems   219, 249
    rats   224, 225
  induction of cytochromes P-450 by   56
  precipitation of acute attacks of porphyria
    by   32, 130, 218, 219, 230, 243, 244
Bemegride
  effect on porphyrin formation in chick
    embryos   218, 223
Benzodiazepines
  effect on ALA-S in chick embryo   219
3,4-Benzpyrene
  effect on serum bilirubin in Gunn
    rats   306

3,4-Benzpyrene
    increase in hepatic ligandin 293
    induction of
        bilirubin GT by 299
        cytochrome P-450 by 56
        liver enzymes by 82
Benzpyrene hydroxylase 60 – 62, 177
Benzylhydrazine
    interference with glucuronidation 300
Benzylpenicillin
    displacement of bilirubin by 289, 290
Bethanidine
    considered safe in hereditary hepatic por-
        phyria 251
Bile acid secretion
    relation to bilirubin excretion 302,
        303
Bile canaliculus
    transport of bilirubin into 279, 280
Bile flow
    drugs affecting 302, 303
    relation to bilirubin excretion 303
Bile secretion
    two mechanisms 302
Bilichrysins
    products of bilirubin degradation 307
Bilirubin (IXα)
    binding to
        albumin 276, 277
            during phototherapy 308
            displacement by drugs 288 – 290
            Y and Z proteins 291, 292
    conversion of heme into, decreased by
        AIA 140, 141
    determination of 26
    early labelled 275, 283
    effect of
        AIA 287
        CCl$_4$ 284
        hydrocortisone 284
        lead poisoning 349
        phenobarbital 284 – 286
    formation from biliverdin 6, 276
    formula 7
    hepatic clearance of 291 – 293
    hepatocellular uptake of 277
        increase after phenobarbital 293
    incorporation of heme precursors into 5
    intestinal fate of 280
    photodegradation products of 306, 307
Bilirubin conjugates 26 – 28, 278, 279
    chromatographic separation of 26
Bilirubin excretion 279, 280
    alternative pathways of 306
    effect of drugs 302 – 305
    relation to bile acid formation 302, 303
    relation to bile flow 303

Bilirubin glucuronyl transferase
    (Bilirubin GT) 28
    evidence for specific enzyme 279
    in Crigler-Najjar syndrome 273, 296, 297
    in Gilbert's syndrome 273, 296, 297
    in Gunn rats 273
    induction by drugs 295 – 299, 303
    inhibition by drugs 300
Bilirubin metabolism
    definition of abnormalities of 273
    drug-induced alterations in 274,
        280 – 309
    effect of hormones on 300
    influence of ethanol and cigarette smoking
        on neonates 298, 299
    normal 274 – 280
Bilirubin production
    normal sources 274, 275
    from erythrocyte destruction 280 – 283
    effect of drugs 284 – 286
    effect of cobalt 116
Biliverdin (IXα)
    formation from heme breakdown
        23 – 25, 275, 276
    formula 7
    photooxidation of 307
    substrate for biliverdin reductase 25, 26,
        276
Biliverdin (isomers other than IXα)
    as substrates for biliverdin reductase 26
Biliverdin reductase
    activity in different tissues 25
substrates for 25, 26
Biphenyl
    hydroxylation of 177
Bis-(p-nitrophenyl)phosphate (BNPP)
    inhibition of liver carboxylesterase
        by 203 – 209, 221, 232
Borneol
    inhibitor of bilirubin GT 300
Bromophenol blue
    binding to albumin 289
BSP (sulfobromophthalein)
    biliary excretion of 280
        effect of novobiocin 303
    binding to Y and Z proteins 292
    hepatic clearance of 291, 292
    hepatic uptake of 278
        increased by phenobarbital 293
    interference with glucuronidation 300
    reduction of bile flow caused by 302
    retention in cholestasis 304
Bunamiodyl
    binding to Z protein 292
    effect on hepatocellular handling of biliru-
        bin 291
    interference with glucuronidation 300

n-Butanol
    cytochrome P-450 spectral changes 54

Cadmium
    induction of metallothionein by 356
    inhibition of
        ALA-dehydratase by 337, 341
        glutathione reductase by 341
        mixed function oxidase by 88, 89
    loss of cytochrome P-450 caused by 89,
        115
    stimulation of heme oxygenase by 116
    teratogenic and carcinogenic effects of
        355, 357
Calcium
    levels in diet and lead toxicity 358
Camphenol 203
Camphor 203
Carbamazepine
    displacement of bilirubin by 289, 290
Carbohydrates
    dietary intake and
        AIA porphyria 255
        human porphyria 256
Carbon disulphide (CS₂)
    liver lesions caused by 105, 108
    loss of cytochrome P-450 caused by 96,
        97, 104–109
    oxidative desulphuration of 105–107
Carbon monoxide
    increased blood level after nicotinic
        acid 286
    production
        after AIA administration 102
        during heme degradation 23,
            117, 275
        during lipid peroxidation 111
        effect of diphenylhydantoin 284
        effect of phenobarbital 284, 285
Carbon tetrachloride (CCl₄)
    effect on HCB distribution 160
    ethane exhalation after treatment with
        112
    increase in early labelled bilirubin 284
    liver damage caused by 109
    loss of cytochrome P-450 caused by 96,
        97, 109, 110
    mechanism of toxicity 110
Carbutamide
    inducer of cytochrome P-450 56
Cardiac glycosides
    excretion of into bile 280
Catalase
    activity of in HCB porphyria 179
    and regulatory heme 141, 142, 146
    apoprotein of 23, 67, 142
    biosynthesis of 67, 68

induction by drugs 49, 50, 67, 68
inhibition by aminotriazole 82
location in the hepatocyte and half life 4,
    50
loss of activity caused by
    cobalt 87, 88
    manganese 88
    porphyrogenic compounds 135, 142, 146
Cephaloridine
    hemolysis caused by 283
Cephalothin
    hemolysis caused by 283
Charcoal
    lower serum bilirubin in normal neonates
        caused by 305
Chick embryo
    liver cells in culture
        effect of lead on 341, 345
        porphyrin induction by drugs 201–217,
            222, 223, 230–232, 246
        use in screening drugs for human por-
            phyrics 201, 249
    porphyrin induction by drugs in liver of
        217, 222, 223, 230–232
Chloracne 157, 167, 173, 174, 220
Chloral hydrate
    considered safe in porphyric patients 230
    effect on ALA-S potentiated by lead 246
    inducer of cytochrome P-450 56
    induction of ALA-S and porphyrins in
        chick embryo 219, 221
Chloramphenicol
    activity in chick embryo compared with
        cell culture 223
    bilirubin displacement by 289, 290
    considered safe in porphyric patients 230,
        231
    interference with glucuronidation 300
Chlorcyclizine
    inducer of cytochrome P-450 56
Chlordane
    inducer of cytochrome P-450 56
    induction of glucuronyl transferases by
        299
    inhibition of hepatic β-glucuronidase by
        305
Chlordiazepoxide
    effect on ALA-S 219, 232
    inducer of cytochrome P-450 56
    use in porphyric patients 230, 232
Chloretene
    increased UDP-glucuronic acid supply
        caused by 301
Chlorinated dibenzodioxins 159,
    160, 174, 175
Chlorinated dibenzofurans 159, 160
Chlorinated naphthalenes 160, 175

Chlormadinone acetate 220
Chlorobenzenes (other than HCB)
    160, 161, 174, 175
    induction of porphyria by 175, 176
Chlorophenols 157, 159, 174
2-(4-chlorophenyl)thiazo-4-yl
    acetic acid
    effect on serum bilirubin in Gunn rats 306
Chlorophyll 2
Chloroquine
    effect on bilirubin GT in neonatal rats
    298, 299
Chlorpromazine
    considered safe in porphyric patients 230,
    231, 251
    effect on ANIT-induced cholestasis and
        hyperbilirubinemia 285
    hemolysis caused by 283
    inducer of cytochrome P-450 56
    interference with glucuronidation 300
Cholestasis
    decreased canalicular ATPase in 303
    drug-induced 285, 303, 304
    increased acid phosphatase in 304
Cholestasis
    treatment with phenobarbital 305
Cholesterol-7α-hydroxylation
    catalysed by cytochrome P-450 54
Cholesterol-11β-hydroxylation
    catalysed by cytochrome P-450 54
Cholestyramine
    acceptor for bilirubin 289
    effect in cholestatic liver disorders 305
    effect in Gunn rats 305
Cinchophen
    increased UDP-glucuronic acid supply by
    301
Clofibrate
    increase in
        catalase due to 50, 68
        liver mitochondria caused by 68, 69
        liver Z protein caused by 293
    proliferation of hepatic peroxisomes
        caused by 67, 68
Clotrimazole
    inducer of cytochrome P-450 56
Cobalt
    effect on ALA-S 85, 88, 150
    inhibition of
        ferrochelatase by 86, 87, 88
        heme by 84—88, 89
    induction of heme oxygenase by 85,
        116—121, 276
    loss of cytochrome P-450 caused by 84,
        85, 115, 276
    substrate for porphyrin-metal chelatase
        335, 336, 341

Cobalt protoporphyrin 119, 150
    induction of heme oxygenase by 120
Codeine
    considered safe in porphyric patients 230,
    231
Coenzyme A 90, 91
Collidine
    lack of porphyrin-inducing effect in cell
        culture 209
Coombs' test
    positive in lead poisoning 350
Copper
    and ferrochelatase 86, 87
    loss of cytochrome P-450 caused by 115
    stimulation of heme oxygenase by 116
Coprohemin I
    substrate for heme oxygenase 24
Coproporphyrin
    excretion of in
        HCP porphyria 164—172, 184—186
        human prophyrias 240—242
        lead poisoning 336, 355
        PCB porphyria 173
    isomers of 2
    production of in cell culture 210
Coproporphyrinogen III 19—21
    formula 7
Coproporphyrinogen (isomers other
    than III) 20, 21
Coproporphyrinogen oxidase
    (coproporphyrinogen decarboxylase)
    6, 19—21
    activity in HCB porphyria 180, 183—185,
    188
    deficiency in hereditary coproporphyria
    241
    distribution of 20
    inhibition by lead 346
    mechanism of enzyme reaction 20, 21
    possible inhibition by AIA and PIA in cell
        culture 210
    possible role of iron in the reaction 335
Corticosteroids
    induction of tryptophan pyrrolase by 52,
    53
Cortisol (see Hydrocortisone)
Cortisone
    induction of enzymes by 51, 52
Crigler-Najjar syndrome
    definition of 273
    effect of
        cholestyramine on serum bilirubin in
            305
        drugs on bilirubin metabolism in
            296—298, 306
    phototherapy in children with 307
    treatment with aspartic acid 301

Cyclic AMP (*see also* Dibutyryl cyclic AMP)
  increase in
    bile flow caused by 302
    heme oxygenase caused by 117, 287
    "permissive effect" on ALA-S induction
      223, 259
    relationship to glucose effect
      for *E. coli* enzymes 258
      for ALA-S 259, 261, 262
Cycloheximide
  and increased early labelled bilirubin 149,
    283, 284
  inhibition of
    ALA-S induction 146, 148—150,
      212—217, 220, 246, 345
    heme oxygenase induction 276
Cyclopentadecanone 203
Cysteine
  activation of
    ALA-dehydratase by 337
    ferrochelatase by 341
Cytochrome a 3, 50, 68
Cytochrome a₃ 50, 68
Cytochrome b 3, 50, 68
Cytochrome b₅
  function of 66, 67
  increased levels caused by
    HCB and PCBs 177
    phenobarbital 67, 69, 284
  location and half-life 50
Cytochrome b₅ reductase (NADH
  cytochrome-c reductase) 66, 67
Cytochrome c 3, 24, 50, 68
  apoprotein of 23
Cytochrome c₁ 50, 68
Cytochrome P-420 95, 96, 108, 114,
  121
Cytochrome(s) P-450 53—66
  glucose effect and 257
  and regulatory heme 141
  apoprotein of
    and regulation of heme biosynthesis
      33, 135, 145, 147, 149, 150, 250
    increased synthesis in induction of
      cytochrome 250
    preferential damage by CS₂ 109
  cholesterol-7α-hydroxylation catalysed
    by 54
  cholesterol-11β-hydroxylation catalysed
    by 54
  effect of
    acetate on 90
    aminotriazole on 82, 83
    PABA on 89
  factors influencing induction of 61—63
  forms induced by
    phenobarbital 59

3-methylcholanthrene or β-naphtho-
      flavone 59
    HCB and PCB 178, 179
  induction by drugs in the liver of
    chick embryos 221, 222
    rodents 49, 56—60, 139, 140, 145, 146,
      177, 178, 249, 250, 284
  in PCT 158
  location in the hepatocyte and turnover 50
  loss of caused by
    allyl-containing chemicals 96, 97, 102,
      134, 139, 227, 287
    CCl₄ 96, 97, 109, 110
    CS₂ 96, 97, 104—109
    DDC 134
    fluroxene 103
    griseofulvin 134
    lipid peroxidation 110, 111
    metals 84, 85, 88, 89, 115—121, 276,
      352, 360
    phosphorothionates 107
  mechanism of induction 59—61
    mixed-function oxidases dependent on
      53, 54, 63, 66
  mRNA for 149
  possible involvement in heme oxygenase
    reaction 24, 118, 275, 276
  spectral properties 54, 58, 178, 179
  structural properties 4, 95, 96
Cytochrome P-450 reductase (NADPH
  cytochrome c reductase) 66, 103
Cytochrome P₁-450 (or cytochrome
  P-448) 59, 61

Dapsone
  hemolysis caused by 281
DDT (Dicophane)
  decrease in hepatic Z protein 293
  increase in hepatic Y protein caused by
    293
  inducer of mixed function oxidase system
    56, 57, 66, 98, 102
  treatment of Crigler-Najjar syndrome
    with 298
Decanamide
  porphyrin-inducing activity of 204—206
Dehydroepiandrosterone
  effect on ALA-S in rats 265
  excretion of in AIP 266
Dehydroisocoproporphyrinogen
  in HCB porphyria 183, 184, 188, 189
2-Deoxyglucose
  effect on induction of ALA-S 262
Deuterobiliverdin IXα
  substrate for biliverdin reductase 25
Deuterohemin IX
  substrate for heme oxygenase 24

Deuteroporphyrin 22
Diabetes (experimental)
  induction of ALA-S in 262, 263
5,5-Diallylbarbituric acid
  effect on ALA-S and cytochrome P-450 in
    rats 138, 139, 225
  formula 131
Diazepam
  effect on ALA-S in chick embryo 219,
    232
  possible precipitation of acute attacks in
    porphyrics 230, 232
Diazoxide
  induction of hepatic ALA-S 262
Dichloralphenazone 244
2,4-Dichlorophenoxyacetic acid (2,4-D)
  porphyria associated with manufacture
    of 157, 173, 174
Dicloxacillin
  displacement of bilirubin by 290
Dieldrin
  effect on hepatic ligandin and Z
    protein 293
  induction of cytochrome P-450 56
  induction of glucuronyl transferases
    299
  inhibition of β-glucuronidase 305
3,5-Diethoxycarbonyl collidine (DC, also
    OX-DDC) 138, 139
  effect on porphyrin formation in chick
    embryos 210, 211, 218, 223
  formula 131, 202
3,5-Diethoxycarbonyl-1,4-dihydrocollidine
    (DDC) 138
  drug interactions 247, 259
  effect on
    catalase 142
    heme degradation 135
    porphyrin formation in chick em-
      bryo 203, 210, 211, 223
    succinyl CoA synthetase 32
  formula 131
  increase in
    liver synthesis of mRNA 145
  cytochrome P-450 in chick embryo 222
  inhibition of
    aminopyrine demethylase 222
    heme synthesis 135—140
    porphyrin-metal chelatase 31, 84, 87,
      136, 139
  loss of cytochrome P-450 caused by 134
  porphyria caused in rodents 129, 130,
    132, 137, 139
    species differences in 135, 137, 224
  stimulation of ALA-S
    in chick embryo 212, 213, 215—217,
      226

  in rodents 89, 132, 133, 135—137, 139,
    143, 146, 226, 256
3,5-Diethoxycarbonyl-1,4-dihydro-2,6-
    dimethylpyridine 202, 203
1,4-Diethoxycarbonyl-2,3,5,6-
    tetramethylbenzene 218
2-Diethylaminoethyl-3,3-diphenyl-
    propylacetate (see SKF 525-A)
Diethylnicotinamide
  effect on bilirubin metabolism 298
Diethylmaleate 112
Diethylnitrosamine
  induction of glucuronyl transferases by
    299
0,0-Diethyl,0-phenyl phosphorothionate
    (SV_1)
  liver damage caused by 107, 108
Difference spectra
  type I (hexobarbital) 179
  type II (aniline) 179
2,4-Diformyldeuteroporphyrin 101
5,5'-Diformyl-dipyrrylmethane
  product of bilirubin photodegradation
    307
Digitoxin
  effect of novobiocin on biliary excretion
    of 303
Digoxin
  bilirubin displacement by 289, 290
  considered safe in hereditary hepatic por-
    phyria 251
Dihydrocoprostane
  induction of ALA-S by 266
Dimethylbenzene reductase
  glucose effect and 257
2α,17-α-Dimethyldihydrotestosterone
  production of cholestasis by 304
2,4-Dinitrophenol
  accumulation of uroporphyrin in vitro
    caused by 190
γ,δ-Dioxovaleric acid 34
Dioxygenases 52, 54
Diphenhydramine
  considered safe in porphyric patients 230,
    231, 251
  inducer of cytochrome P-450 56
Diphenylhydantoin
  differences in blood levels between pa-
    tients 61
  displacement of bilirubin by 289,
    290
  effect on CO production in man 284
  inducer of cytochrome P-450 56, 58
  induction of ALA-S and porphyrins in
    chick embryo 232
  precipitation of acute attacks of porphyria
    by 230—232

Diphenylsulfone
  hemolysis caused by 282
Dipropylacetamide 207
5,5-Dipropylbarbituric acid 138, 139,
  142
  formula 131
Disulfonate
  biliary excretion of 303
Dithiothreitol (DTT)
  activation of ALA-dehydratase by 339
DNA synthesis
  stimulation by chronic lead exposure 356
Dodecanamide 206
L-Dopa
  hemolysis caused by 283
Drugs
  considered safe in porphyric patients
    230–232, 251
  which displace bilirubin from albumin
    288, 291
  which precipitate acute attacks of porphy-
    ria 219, 230–232, 244
Drug-metabolising enzymes (see Mixed func-
    tion oxidase system)
Drug metabolism
  role of in stimulation of ALA-S by
    drugs 146–150
Dubin-Johnson syndrome
  definition of 273
  treatment with phenobarbitone 305

EDTA
  treatment of
    HCB porphyria with 164
    lead poisoning with 349, 352, 360
Endoplasmic reticulum
  cytochromes of 50, 53–67
  proliferation of membranes of caused by
    phenobarbital 63, 65, 66, 69, 279, 284,
      286
    polyhalogenated hydrocarbons 65, 83,
      177, 178, 188
Endotoxin
  stimulation of heme oxygenase by 117,
    119
Epinephrine
  effect on AIA-induced stimulation of
    ALA-S 263
  stimulation of heme oxygenase by 117,
    287
Epoxide hydrase
  stimulation by phenobarbital and 3-meth-
    ylcholanthrene 63, 64
Erythrocytes
  drug-induced hemolysis associated with
    abnormal hemoglobins 281, 282
  congenital abnormalities in red cell me-
    tabolism 281, 282
  immunohemolytic responses 282,
    283
  effect of lead 346–351
  stippling in lead poisoning 348
Erythropoiesis
  copper deficiency and 86
  in lead-poisoning 349
Erythropoietic porphyria (congenital)
  low uroporphyrinogen cosynthetase ac-
    tivity in 15
Erythropoietic protoporphyria (EPP)
  increased red cell protoporphyrin in 335,
    342
  photosensitivity in 345
Erythropoietin
  effect of testosterone 265
  stimulation of ALA-S by 30
Esters
  porphyrin-inducing activity and lipophili-
    city 208
Estradiol
  effect on porphyrogenic action of HCB in
    male rats 170
  inducer of ALA-S and porphyrins in chick
    embryo 220, 265
  reduction in cytochrome P-450 in male
    rats caused by 62
Estriol
  inhibition of glucuronyl transferases by
    301
Estrogens
  enhancement of HCB porphyria in female
    rats by 170, 193
  precipitation of PCT by 158, 176, 193,
    242
  precipitation of acute attacks of porphyria
    by 244
Estrone
  inducer of porphyrins in chick embryo
    cells 265
Ethacrynic acid 291
  reduction in bile flow caused by 302
Ethchlorvynol
  inducer of porphyrins and ALA-S in chick
    embryo 219, 221
Ethinamate
  inducer of ALA-S and porphyrins in chick
    embryo 219
Ethinylestradiol
  hyperbilirubinemia caused by 304
  reduction of bile flow caused by 304
  stimulation of porphyrins in chick em-
    bryo 265
Ethinylestriol
  inhibition of glucuronyl transferases by
    301

17-α-Ethinyl estrogens
  inhibition of liver ATPase by   304
  reduction of bile flow by   304
17-α-Ethinyl progestogens
  reduction of bile flow by   304
Ethyl benzoate
  inducer of porphyrins in chick embryo
    204, 205, 209
2-Ethylbutyramide
  inducer of porphyrins in chick embryo
    204, 205, 207
Ethylmorphine N-demethylation
  effect of
    acetate 90
    HCB and PCBs   177, 178
    PABA 89
  induction inhibited by aminotriazole   82
  inhibition by lead   352
  relation to cytochrome P-450 concentra-
    tion   85
Etiocholandiol
  inducer of ALA-S in cell culture   266
Etiocholandione
  inducer of ALA-S in chick embryo   220,
    266
Etiocholanolone
  increased excretion in AIP   266
  inducer of ALA-S and porphyrins in chick
    embryo   210, 213, 215, 220
  inducer of ALA-S in rat   265
Evans blue
  binding to ligandin   292

Fatty acids
  bilirubin displacement by   289, 290
Fava beans
  hemolytic effect in patients with G6PD de-
    ficiency   282
Ferrochelatase (see Porphyrin-metal
  chelatase)
Flavaspidic acid
  binding to Y and Z protein   292
  effect on hepatocellular bilirubin   291
  interference with glucuronidation   300
Falvones
  inducers of cytochrome P-450   57
Flurazepam
  induction of ALA-S by   219
5-Fluorouridine deoxyribose
  effect on induction of ALA-S   264
Fluoroxene (2,2,2-trifluoroethyl
  vinyl ether)
  destruction of cytochrome P-450 by   103
Fructose
  glucose effect of   91, 261, 262
Furosemide
  displacement of bilirubin by   289, 290

Galactose
  glucose effect of   262
Gastrin
  increase in bile flow caused by   302
Gilbert's syndrome
  definition of   273
  effect of
    glutethimide on bilirubin metabolism
      and CO formation in   285
    phenobarbital on serum bilirubin level
      in 285, 306
  hepatocellular uptake and binding of bili-
    rubin in   293
Globin synthesis
  control of in erythropoietic cells   29 – 31
  effect of hemin on   30, 31
  in iron-deficiency anemia   30
  inhibitory effect of lead   30, 344, 347
Glucagon
  effect on AIA-induced stimulation of
    ALA-S   262, 263
  effect on cyclic AMP   117, 259
  increase in heme oxygenase due to   117,
    287
Glucocorticoids
  induction of tryptophan pyrrolase by   53
Glucose-6-phosphate dehydrogenase
  (G6PD)
  deficiency in red blood cell and
    increased susceptibility to toxic effect of
      lead   340
    hemolysis caused by drugs   281, 282
    hemolysis during phototherapy in in-
      fants   308
Glucose-6-phosphate isomerase   262
Glucose effect
  in enzyme induction in microorganisms
    256, 258
  in experimental porphyria   255, 256
  in human hepatic porphyria   256, 257
  in the synthesis of ALA-S   90, 91, 252
  mechanism of   257 – 263
Glucuronic acid
  possible role in glucose effect on ALA-S
    261
Glucuronyl transferase(s) (GT) (UDP-
  glucuronyl transferase)   27, 278
  activity in
    Crigler-Najjar syndrome   296, 297
    Gilbert's syndrome   296, 297
    Gunn rats   296, 297
  assay techniques   294
  induction by
    antipyrine   297
    clofibrate   298
    DDT   298
    glutethimide   297

Hyperbilirubinemia
caused by
ANIT 285
novobiocin 300
vitamin K 300
hereditary abnormality in sheep 293
severe unconjugated 288
Hyperbilirubinemia (neonatal)
treatment with
aspartic acid 301
orotic acid 301
phenobarbital 297
phenylbutazone 298
UDP-glucose 301
valium 298
Hypoalbuminemia
in severe unconjugated hyperbilirubinemia 288
Hypophysectomy
effect on mixed function oxidase activity
62

Icterogenin
production of cholestasis by 304
Imipramine
inducer of cytochrome P-450 56
interference with glucuronidation 300
Immunohemolytic anemia
drug-induced 282, 283
Inclusion bodies
formation in kidney in lead poisoning
254, 360
Indocyanine green (ICG)
excretion of by hepatocyte 280
hepatic clearance of 291, 292
interference with glucuronidation 300
binding to Y and Z proteins 292
reduction in bile flow caused by 302
Indomethacin
bilirubin displacement by 289, 290
Insulin
effect on ALA-S induction 262—264
Insulin hypoglycemia
stimulation of bile flow in 302
Iodipamide
binding to liver cell membrane 291
binding to Y and Z protein 292
β-Ionone 203
Iproniazid
interference with glucuronidation 300
Iron
and lipid peroxidation 113
and loss of cytochrome P-450 111
and stimulation of heme oxygenase 116
body stores in PCT 158, 171, 176
effect on
ALA-S 111, 263

HCB porphyria 171
heme degradation 111, 116, 121, 264
Iron deficiency
effect on lead toxicity 358, 361
Iron-deficiency anemia
increased red cell protoporphyrin in 335,
342, 359
pica in 358
synthesis of globin in 30
Zn protoporphyrin in 344, 348
Iron overload
in HCB porphyria 181, 190
in PCT 242, 264
Isocarboxazid
interference with glucuronidation 300
Isocitrate dehydrogenase
inhibition by metalloporphyrins 348
Isocoproporphyrin
excretion in HCB porphyria in the rat 19,
168, 170, 183, 184, 186
excretion in PCT 19
Isocoproporphyrinogen
substrate for UROG-D 182
Isogriseofulvin 138, 139
Isoniazid
hemolysis caused by 283
interference with glucuronidation 300
Isoproterenol
effect on AIA-mediated induction of
ALA-S 263

Jaundice (see Hyperbilirubinemia)

Kanechlors 159, 172
Kernicterus
caused by sulfonamides 288
due to excessive tissue bilirubin in newborn 288
in Crigler-Najjar syndrome 273
α-Ketoglutaraldehyde 258
α-Ketoglutarate
effect on induction of ALA-S 258, 261
11-Ketopregnanolone 220
Δ⁵-3-Ketosteroid isomerase
activity associated with ligandin 64
Kidney
effect of lead on 354

Lactic acid
binding to Z protein 292
Lead
biological defense mechanism against 356
decrease in antibody formation caused by
351, 360
deposition in the bone marrow 349
effect on
ALA-S 246, 345

3-methylcholanthrene 63, 64
phenobarbital 63, 64, 279, 295—297
inhibition by drugs 299—301
substrates (other than bilirubin) for
294—296
β-Glucuronidase (hepatic)
decrease in activity caused by drugs 305
β-Glucuronidase (intestinal)
high activity in newborn 280
L-Glutamate dehydrogenase
inhibition by metalloporphyrins 248
Glutamic-alanine transaminase
increase caused by cortisone 51, 52
Glutathione 281
and ferrochelatase 86, 87
erythrocyte level in lead poisoning 340,
341
role in lipid peroxidation 112, 114
Glutathione peroxidase 281
inactivation of lipid peroxides by 114,
115
Glutathione reductase 281
inhibition by cadmium 241
Glutathione synthetase 281, 240
Glutathione transferase
activity associated with ligandin 64, 292
Glutethimide
effect on bilirubin and CO production
285
inducer of
cytochrome P-450 56
glucuronyl transferase 297
porphyrins in chickens 222, 224
ALA-S and porphyrins in chick embryo 219, 221, 224, 230
precipitation of acute attacks of porphyria
by 218, 230, 232, 244
Glycerol
glucose effect of 91, 261, 262
Glycerolphosphate dehydrogenase
increase caused by clofibrate and nafenopin 68
Glycine
conjugation with bilirubin 279
agents which affect is availability for heme
biosynthesis 89, 90
Glycine acyltransferase
and availability of glycine for heme synthesis 89, 90
Glycogen
and glucose effect 261
Gold
effect on erythrocyte potassium 350
Green pigments
and regulatory heme 140, 141
chromatographic separation of 99—101
conversion of heme into 98—102, 104

production by AIA and allyl barbiturates
5, 98—102, 104, 134, 135, 138, 139, 287
spectral properties of 99—101, 104
Griseofulvin
effect on
catalase 142
porphyrin formation in chick embryo
203, 218, 223
formula 131, 202
2'-β-hydroxyethyl thioether analogue of
(see HET-griseofulvin)
inducer of drug-metabolising enzymes 56
inhibition of
heme synthesis by 135—140
porphyrin-metal chelatase by 31, 136,
138, 139
loss of cytochrome P-450 caused by 134
porphyria caused in rodents by 129, 130,
132, 136, 137, 139
species differences in 136
138, 139
precipitation of acute attacks of porphyria
by 218, 230, 231, 244
stimulation of ALA-S by 132, 133, 135,
136, 138, 139
Growth hormone
effect on AIA-mediated induction of
ALA-S 264
in acute intermittent porphyria 257
Guanethidine
considered safe in hereditary hepatic porphyria 230, 231, 251
Gunn rat
assay for measuring bilirubin displacement
by drugs 288, 290, 291
definition of 273
effect of
drugs on early labelled bilirubin in 284
drugs on serum bilirubin in 305, 306
phototherapy in 308, 309
glucuronyl transferase
effect of phenobarbital 296
effect of glutethimide 297

Halothane 65
Harderoporphyrin 20
Harderoporphyrinogen
a precursor or protoporphyrin 20, 183, 184
Heinz bodies 281
Harmol
interference with glucuronidation 300
Hematinic acid
product of biliverdin photodegradation
307
Hematoporphyrin
displacement of ligandin-bound bilirubin
by 292

Heme (Protoheme IX), *see also* Hemin
  binding to albumin 277
  conversion into green pigments 98—102,
    104, 287
  different components in liver 5
  formula 7
  induction of heme oxygenase by 24, 118,
    119, 120, 276, 286, 287
  inhibition of ALA-dehydratase by 339
  microsomal pool of 60
  regulation of ALA-S by 31—34, 132, 133,
    135, 244
  regulatory pool of 31, 33, 140—142, 145,
    147, 251
Heme-hemopexin complex
  substrate for heme oxygenase 24
Heme a 3, 24
Heme degradation
  during lipid peroxidation 104, 109—115
  effect of
    allyl-containing compounds 134
      138, 147, 227
    DDC 135
    iron 264
  enzymes of 23—35, 275, 276
  to non-bilirubin metabolites 102, 287
Heme oxygenase 23—25, 275, 276
  decrease caused by AIA 142, 287
  distribution 23, 24, 276
  effect of drugs 286—287
  effect of fasting 24, 117, 287
  relation to loss of cytochrome P-450 96,
    115—121
  stimulation by
    cobalt 85, 116, 120, 121
    cobalt-protoporphyrin 120
    endotoxin 117, 119
    heme 24, 118—120, 135, 140, 141,
      276, 286, 287
    lead and other metals 116, 346
  substrates for 24, 276
Heme synthesis
  control of 28—35
  defect in human genetic porphyrias
    239—242, 250
  effect of
    acetate 90, 91
    HCB and polyhalogenated hydrocar-
      bons 171, 176—186, 188, 192
    5β-H steroids 265
  enzymes of 6—23
  influence of nutritional factors on
    255—264
  influence of hormonal factors on
    264—267
  in cytochrome P-450 induction 60
  inhibition by

aminotriazole 82, 83
cobalt 84—88
DDC 135—140
griseofulvin 135—140
lead 84, 246, 249, 250, 336—346, 360,
  361
mercaptomerin 355
Heme synthetase (*see* Porphyrin-metal
  chelatase)
Hemoglobin
  abnormal hemoglobins
    and drug-induced anemias 281, 282
    and toxicity of lead 357, 361
  α and β chains of
    substrates for heme oxygenase 24, 276
  control of formation in erythropoietic
    cells 28—31
Hemoglobin-haptoglobin complex
  substrate for heme oxygenase 24
Hemoglobin Pb (fast hemoglobin)
  in chronic lead poisoning 347—348
Hemolytic anemia
  drug-induced 282
  red cell protoporphyrin in 335
Hemoproteins 3—6
  control of synthesis in the liver 31—35
  effect of polyhalogenated hydrocarbons
    on 177—180, 185, 192
  induction in the liver 49—80
  inhibition of synthesis in the liver 81—91
  location in the hepatocyte 49, 50
  turnover 4, 5, 29, 50
    effect of drugs on 283—287
Hemin (*see also* Heme)
  binding to ligandin 23, 292
  decrease in cytochrome P-450 caused by
    286
  infusion in porphyrics with acute attacks
    243
  inhibition of porphyria in cell cultures by
    211, 212
  inhibition of ALA-S induction by 12, 30,
    33, 215—217, 260, 263
  stimulation of globin synthesis by 30
  stimulation of protein synthesis by 31
Heptacarboxylic porphyrinogen
  as a substrate for UROG-D 181, 184
Heptanamide 206
Hereditary Coproporphyria (HCP) 239, 241
  excretion of porphyrins and porphyrin
    precursors 240, 241
  deficiency of coproporphyrinogen oxidase
    in 241
Hereditary Hepatic Porphyrias (*see
  also* Acute Intermittent Porphyria,
    Hereditary Coproporphyria,
      Variegate Porphyria)

enzyme defects in 240—242
glucose effect in 256, 257
induction of ALA-S in 240, 249—252,
  256
neuropsychiatric disorders in 239—241
porphyrin excretion 240, 241
possible treatment with PABA 90
precipitation of acute attacks by drugs
  129, 130, 219, 230—232, 243, 245
screening of drugs for patients with 201,
  218, 219
HET-griseofulvin 138, 139
  formula 131
Hexabromobiphenyl
  induction of porphyria by 157, 173, 222,
    224
Hexachlorobenzene (HCB)
  absorption and metabolism 160, 161
  effect on drug-metabolising enzymes 56,
    177—179, 186
  formula 158
  liver damage produced by 187—189, 193
  neurotoxic effects 168, 169, 171
  skin lesions in man and rat 163, 164, 168,
    169
HCB porphyria
  effect of estrogens 170, 187, 193
  enzymes of heme biosynthesis in
    180—185
  liver catalase levels in 179
  mechanism of 186—192
  porphyrin accumulation in the liver 168,
    170, 172, 176, 182, 183, 189, 191
  porphyrin excretion 19, 164—172, 176,
    183—185, 191
  role of iron 171, 190—193
  UROG-D activity in 180—184, 186,
    188
2,4,5,2′,4′,5′-Hexachlorobiphenyl
  effect on drug-metabolising enzymes 178
  formula 158
  metabolism to a monohydroxy derivative
    162
  production of
    porphyria by 157, 161, 173
    uroporphyrin in chick embryo
      cells 189
Hexachlorobiphenyls
  components of Aroclors 159, 178
γ-Hexachlorocyclohexane (Lindane)
  effect on ALA-S in chick embryo cells
    214, 215
  inducer of cytochrome P-450 56
  production of uroporphyrin in chick em-
    bryo cells 189
  stimulation of liver growth 65
Hexachloronaphthalene 175

Hexachlorophene
  binding to Z protein 292
Hexanamide 206
Hexobarbital
  hydroxylation of 177
  inducer of porphyrins and ALA-
    embryo 219, 221, 223
  hepatic prophyrin accumulation i.
    ens 222
  metabolism of
    effect of cobalt on 85
    inhibition by cAMP 117
    substrate for mixed function oxidase
      59
  type I difference spectrum 54, 179
Hippurates
  formation during reversal of DDC por-
    phyria with PABA or sodium
      benzoate 89, 90
Histamine
  increase in bile flow due to 302
Histidase 257
Homoserine dehydratase 257
Hormones
  effect on
    bilirubin metabolism 300
    porphyrin and ALA-S formation in
      chick embryo 211, 212, 220
    ALA-S induction in hereditary hepatic
      porphyria 252, 266
    regulation of heme biosynthesis
      264—267
Hydantoins
  precipitation of acute attacks of porphyria
    by 244
Hydrocortisone (Cortisol)
  bilirubin displacement by 289, 290
  effect on AIA-induced stimulation of
    ALA-S 264
  increase in
    bile flow caused by 302, 303
    early labelled bilirubin after 284
  induction of
    porphyrins in chick embryo cells by
      212
    tryptophan pyrrolase by 52, 259
    tyrosine aminotransferase by 259
2-(4′Hydroxybenzeneazo) benzoic acid
  binding to albumin 289
Hydroxybilirubins
  product of bilirubin photodegradation
    307
2-Hydroxy-5-oxoPBG
  formed from PBG by PBG oxygenase
    35
17-Hydroxypregnenolone 265
17-α-Hydroxyprogesterone 170

globin synthesis 30, 344, 247
  the kidney 354
  increase in liver heme turnover caused by
    116, 121
  inhibiton of
    acetylcholine esterase 337
    ALA-dehydratase 82, 333, 334,
      336—341, 344, 345, 352, 353, 360
    erythrocyte ATPase 337, 350
    ferrochelatase 86—88, 341
    heme synthesis 84, 246, 250
    mixed-function oxidases 247, 251, 352
  loss of cytochrome P-450 caused by 115,
    247, 248, 352
  potentiating effect on
    induction of ALA-S by drugs 246, 247
    excretion of ALA caused by phenobar-
      bital 247, 248
  stimulation of heme oxygenase by 116,
    346
  teratogenic and tumorigenic effects 355
Lead poisoning
  amino-aciduria 354, 355
  anemia 349—351
  chelation therapy 343, 352, 360
  diagnosis 358, 359
  encephalopathy 352—354, 357, 360
  erythrocyte protoporphyrin 335, 336, 343,
    344, 358
  erythroid hypoplasia 349
  excretion of porphyrins and porphyrin
    precursors 336, 345, 346, 354, 355, 360
  fast hemoglobin 347
  formation of inclusion bodies in the kid-
    ney 354, 356, 360
  loss of erythrocyte potassium 350, 360
  neuropathy 353, 360
  pica in 358
  positive direct Coombs' test 350
  reduced erythrocyte survival 350
  stippling of erythrocytes 347, 348
  Zn-protoporphyrin accumulation in red
    cell 345, 348, 357
Lead toxicity
  modified by
    alcohol 356, 357
    calcium 358
    iron-deficiency 358, 361
  in patients with sickle cell anemia 357
Ligandin (Y protein)
  binding of hemin to 23
  compounds bound by 291, 292
  glutathione transferase activity of 64, 292
  induction by drugs 64, 68, 293
  Δ^5-3-ketosteroid isomerase activity of 64
  role in uptake and transport of bilirubin
    277, 278

Lindane (see γ-Hexachlorocyclohexane)
Linoleic acid 111
Lipid emulsions
  bilirubin displacement by 289
Lipid peroxidation
  associated degradation of heme 113, 114
  associated loss of cytochrome P-450 104,
    109, 110—116
  evolution of CO during 111
  in CCl_4 toxicity 109, 110
  mechanism of 112—115
  relationship to drug metabolism 113
Lipid-soluble drugs
  exacerbation of acute porphyria by 130
  stimulation of ALA-S by 143, 144, 147,
    221, 249
  stimulation of cytochrome P-450 by 145
Lipophilicity
  correlation with ALA-S induction 143,
    144, 147, 221
  of porphyrin-inducing compounds
    204—209, 220, 245, 249
Lipoxygenase 111
Liver
  uptake of bilirubin by 277, 291—293
Liver damage
  caused by
    CCl_4 109
    CS_2 105, 108
  caused by
    HCB 189, 193
    phosphorothionates 107
    polyhalogenated hydrocarbons
      186—188, 193
    SV_1 107, 108
  in patients with PCT 187, 189, 193
Liver growth
  stimulation of by
    halothane 65
    hexachlorocyclohexanes 65
    nafenopin 65
    phenobarbital 65
Lynestrenol
  reduced bile flow caused by 304
Lysosomal proteases
  increased activity after phenobarbital 65
Lysosomes
  enlargement of after phenobarbital 65

Malondialdehyde
  index of lipid peroxidation 112, 116
Manganese
  decrease in
    catalase caused by 88
    cytochrome P-450 caused by 88,
      115, 116
  inhibitor of ferrochelatase 88

Mefenamic acid
  bilirubin displacement by 289
  hemolysis caused by 283
Melphalan
  considered safe in hereditary hepatic por-
    phyria 230, 231
Menadione sodium diphosphate
  hemolysis in patients with G6PD defi-
    ciency caused by 282
d,l-methanol 203
Menthone
  formula 202
  porphyrin-inducing activity of 203
Meperidine
  considered safe in porphyric patients 230,
    231
Mephenytoin
  precipitation of acute attacks of porphyria
    by 218
  porphyrin accumulation in chick embryo
    224
Meprobamate
  inducer of cytochrome P-450 56
  inducer of porphyrins in cell culture 210,
    232
  precipitation of acute attacks of porphyria
    by 230, 232, 244
Mepyramine
  considered safe in hereditary hepatic por-
    phyria 251
2-Mercaptoethanol
  activation of ferochelatase by 341
Mercaptomerin
  inhibition of heme synthesis by 355
Mercury
  effect on
    ALA-dehydratase 334, 337, 341
    ferrochelatase 87
  efflux of potassium from red blood cells
    caused by 350
  loss of cytochrome P-450 caused by 115
  stimulation of heme oxygenase by 116
Mesobilirubin 25
Mesobiliverdin IX α
  substrate for biliverdin reductase 25
Mesohemin IX
  substrate for heme oxygenase 24
Mesophorphyrin
  substrate for porphyrin-metal chelatase
    22, 136, 137, 335, 336, 341
Mestranol
  hyperbilirubinemia caused by 304
Metallothionein
  produced in response to metals 356
Methandrostenolone
  production of cholestasis by 304
Methaqualone

  inducer of ALA-S and porphyrins in chick
    embryo 219
Methemalbumin
  substrate for heme oxygenase 24, 276
Methemoglobin
  substrate for heme oxygenase 24, 276
Methicillin
  interference with glucuronidation 300
Methohexital
  inducer of ALA-S and porphyrins in chick
    embryo 219, 221
Methsuximide
  inducer of porphyrins in chick embryo
    and chicken 218, 222
  precipitation of acute attacks of porphyria
    by 230–232
3-Methylcholanthrene
  decrease in heme oxygenase activity 286
  increase in hepatic Y protein 293
  inducer of
    bilirubin GT 299
    cytochrome P-448 59, 178
    mixed function oxidase system 55, 56,
      58, 59, 61, 62, 66, 69, 178, 179
Methyl dopa
  precipitation of acute attaks of porphyria
    by 244
1-Methyl-3-isobutylxanthine
  and ALA-S induction in cell culture
    261
3-Methyl-4-monomethylaminoazobenzene
  N-demethylation of 82
Methyltesterone
  production of cholestasis by 304
Methyltestrenolone
  production of cholestasis by 304
4-Methylumbelliferone
  inhibition of bilirubin GT by 300
  substrate for UDP-glucuronyl transferase
    64, 295
Methyl mercury
  decrease in cytochrome P-450 caused by
    115, 116
  increase in liver heme turnover caused by
    116, 121
  inhibition of drug metabolism caused by
    352
Methyprylon
  inducer of ALA-S and porphyrin in chick
    embryo and chickens 224, 230, 232
  precipitation of acute attacks of porphyria
    by 230, 232
Methylvinylmaleimide
  product of bilirubin photodegradation
    307
Microsomal enzymes
  induction of 63, 64

Mitochondria
  changes induced by
    clofibrate 68
    lead 348
    nafenopin 68, 69
  deposition of iron in lead poisoning 348
Mitochondrial cytochromes 4, 50, 68–69
Mitomycin c
  effect on induction of ALA-S 264
Mixed-function oxidases (monooxygenases)
  53–55
  chemical inducers of 55–59
  induced by
    HCB and PCBs 177–179
    3-methylcholanthrene 59, 177–179
    phenobarbital 59, 178, 179
    TCDD 61, 177, 179
  inhibited by
    cadmium 88
    cobalt 85
    CS$_2$ 105
    lead 352
    methyl mercury 352
  levels in fetus and newborn 62, 355
  nutritional and hormonal factors 62, 63
  oxidative desulfuration reactions catalysed
    by 105
Monoamine oxidase inhibitors
  cause of cholestasis 304
Monooxygenase (see Mixed-function
  oxidase)
Morphine
  considered safe in hereditary hepatic por-
    phyria 230, 231, 251
  increased UDP-glucuronic acid supply due
    to 301
Morphine glucuronide
  effect of novobiocin on biliary excretion
    of 303
Myoglobin 3, 5

NAD Glycohydrolase 111
NADH
  cofactor for biliverdin reductase 25
  liver concentration in experimental por-
    phyria 32
  role in oxidative desulfuration 107
NADH-cytochrome c reductase 66, 67
NADPH
  cofactor for
    biliverdin reductase 25
    mixed-function oxidases 103,
      105–107, 113
  formation during drug oxidation 64
  possible role in glucose effect on ALA-S
    261
  role in lipid peroxidation 113

NADPH-cytochrome c reductase 23, 25,
  53, 55, 82, 89, 90, 113, 114
  conversion of heme to biliverdin by 276
  in liver biopsy specimens 58
  increased by
    cobalt 85
    inducing drugs 59
    thyroxine 62
  possible site of activation of CCl$_4$ 110
  requirement for heme degradation to bile
    pigments 275, 276
NADPH cytochrome P-450 reductase
  (see NADPH-cytochrome c reductase)
Nafenopin
  increase in
    liver Z protein caused by 293
    mitochondria caused by 68, 69
  proliferation of hepatic peroxisomes
    caused by 68
  stimulation of liver growth by 65
Naphthalene
  hemolysis in G6PD deficiency 282
β-Naphthoflavone
  inducer of cytochrome P-450 59–61
α-Naphthylisothiocyanate (ANIT)
  increased bilirubin production by 285
  induction of cholestasis by 285
  loss of cytochrome P-450 caused by
    107
Neonates
  albumin-binding capacity in 290
  bilirubin metabolism in 305
Neostigmine
  considered safe in hereditary hepatic por-
    phyria 230, 231, 251
Neuropsychiatric disorders
  in hereditary hepatic porphyrias
    239–243, 353
  in lead poisoning 353
Nialamide
  interference with glucuronidation 300
Nickel
  loss of cytochrome P-450 caused by 115
  stimulation of liver heme oxygenase 116
Nicotinic acid
  bilirubin displacement by 289
  increase in
    blood CO caused by 286
    serum bilirubin caused by 286
Nikethamide
  inducer of cytochrome P-450 56
Nitrazepam
  effect on ALA-S 219
p-Nitroanisole demethylation 58, 177
  impaired in lead-treated animals 247, 251
p-Nitrobenzoate
  nitro-reduction of 177

Nitrofurantoin
  hemolysis in G6PD deficiency 282
Nitrofurazone
  hemolysis in G6PD deficiency 282
p-Nitrophenol
  inhibition of bilirubin GT 300
Nonanamide 206
Norcodeine
  N-demethylation of 82
Norethanodrolone
  interference with glucuronidation 300
  production of cholestasis by 304
Norethindrone
  reduced bile flow caused by 304
Norethynodrel
  reduced bilirubin excretion caused by 304
Nortriptyline 61
Novobiocin
  bilirubin displacement by 289, 290
  effect on UDP-glucuronic acid supply
    301
  hyperbilirubinemia caused by 300
  reduction of bilirubin excretion 303
Nucleoside diphosphatase 63

Octachlorostyrene
  formula 158
  induction of porphyria by 157, 175, 176
Octanamide 206
n-Octylamine
  cytochrome P-450 spectral changes 55
Oleic acid
  effect on binding of bilirubin 289, 292
Oleyl-CoA
  formation in steroyl-CoA desaturase sy-
    stem 66
Oral contraceptives
  elevated ALA level in urine after 219
  production of cholestatic jaundice by 304
Oral contraceptive steroids
  effect on ALA-S in chick embryo 220
Ornithine decarboxylase
  effect of theophylline on 260
Ornithine-δ-transaminase
  induction repressed by carbohydrate
    feeding 256
Orotic acid
  treatment of hyperbilirubinemia with 301
Orphenadrine
  inducer of cytochrome P-450 56
Ouabain
  effect of phenobarbital on biliary excretion
    of 303
  reduction in bile flow caused by 302
Oxacillin
  bilirubin displacement by 289, 290
Oxazepam 219

α-Oxyheme 25
α-Oxymesohemin 25
Oxyphenbutazone
  bilirubin displacement by 289, 290

Pamaquine
  hemolysis in patients with G6PD defi-
    ciency caused by 282
Paracetamol
  considered safe in hereditary hepatic por-
    phyria 251
Paraldehyde
  inducer of ALA-S in chick embryo 219,
    221
Paraoxon 105, 107
Parathion
  covalent binding of sulphur to microso-
    mes 107
  loss of cytochrome P-450 during metabo-
    lism of 107
  oxidative desulfuration of 105, 107
Pembe yara
  skin condition of infants exposed to HCB
    164
Penicillins
  bilirubin displacement by 288, 290
  considered safe in hereditary hepatic por-
    phyria 230, 231, 251
  hemolysis caused by 283
Pentacarboxylate porphyrin
  excretion in HCB porphyria 183
Pentacarboxylate porphyrinogen III
  metabolism of 170, 181—185, 188, 189
Pentachlorobenzene 160
Pentachlorophenol
  accumulation of uroporphyrin in vitro
    caused by 190
  metabolite of HCB 161
Pentachlorothiophenol
  metabolite of HCB 161
  urinary excretion in HCB porphyria 190
Pentanamide 206
  hemolysis in patients with G6PD defi-
    ciency caused by 282
Pentobarbital
  hydroxylation of 177
  induction of
    ALA-S in chick embryo 219, 221
    porphyria in rodents 225
  precipitation of acute attacks of porphyria
    by 230
Perferryl ion 113
Perfluoro-n-hexane 67
Peroxidase 3
Peroxidase assay
  for measurement of bilirubin displace-
    ment 289—291

Peroxides
  in the erythrocyte 281
Peroxisomes
  catalase content of 50
  increase in enzymes caused by phenobarbital 65
  proliferation of caused by clofibrate and nafenopin 67—69
  urate oxidase content of 68
Phenacetin (Acetophenetidin)
  hemolysis in patients with G6PD deficiency caused by 281, 282
  reversed type I spectrum caused by 54
Phenelzine
  interference with glucuronidation by 300
Phenobarbital
  decrease of serum bilirubin in
    Dubin-Johnson syndrome 305
    Gunn rats 306
    neonatal jaundice 297
  decrease of serum bilirubin in
    type II Crigler-Najjar syndrome 296
  displacement of bilirubin by 289, 290
  effect on
    catalase 146
    early labelled bilirubin and CO production 284—286
  general changes in liver induced by 64, 65
  increase in
    bile flow caused by 302, 303
    bilirubin clearance after 295, 296, 306
    heme saturation of tryptophan pyrrolase by 53, 142
    liver mRNA by 145
    liver uptake of bilirubin and BSP caused by 292, 293
  inducer of
    ALA-S 89, 219, 221, 222, 225
      effect of theophylline 261
    bilirubin GT 295, 296
    cytochrome b₅ 67, 69
    cytochrome P-450 31, 55, 56, 59—61, 221
      effect reversed by
        acetate 90
        cobalt 84, 85
        PABA 89
    ferrochelatase 84
    ligandin 293
    mixed-function oxidases 55—59, 62, 65, 66, 69, 178, 179
    NADPH-cytochrome c reductase 89, 90
  inhibition of hepatic β-glucuronidase 305
  porphyrin accumulation caused by 222, 225
  potentiation of experimental porphyria in rats 143, 144
  precipitation of acute attacks of porphyria by 230
  proliferation of smooth endoplasmic reticulum by 63, 65
  stimulation of liver toxicity of
    AIA 97—99, 102
    CCl₄ 109
    CS₂ 105
    fluroxene 103
    phosphorothionate 107
  treatment of cholestasis with 305
Phenoclor 159, 173
Phenol 3,6-dibromophthalein
  biliary excretion of 303
Phenolphthalein
  inhibition of bilirubin GT by 300
Phenothiazines
  cholestasis caused by 304
  inhibition of Na/K ATPase activity by 304
Phenylbutazone
  bilirubin displacement by 289, 290
  increased heme saturation of tryptophan pyrrolase caused by 53
  inducer of cytochrome P-450 56, 60
  metabolism of in lead poisoning 352
  potentiation of ALA-S induction 247
  potentiation of DDC porphyria 143, 144
  use in neonatal hyperbilirubinemia 298
Phenylhydrazine
  hemolytic anemia induced by 351
Phenylthiourea 107
Phenylurea 107
Phosphate
  conjugation with bilirubin 279
Phosphatidylcholine
  binding of lead to 350
  in liver mixed-function oxidase reactions 54
Phosphodiesterase
  xanthine inhibitors of 260, 261
Phosphoenolpyruvate carboxykinase
  and glucose effect 257
  induction of 257
6-Phosphogluconate dehydrogenase 281
Phosphorothionates
  liver toxicity of 107, 108
Photosensitivity
  in porphyrias 240—242, 345
Phototherapy of jaundice
  in Crigler-Najjar syndrome 307
  in Gunn rats 303
  in newborn 306, 308
Pica
  in lead poisoning and iron-deficiency anemia 358

Piperazine
  bilirubin displacement by 289
Piperonyl butoxide
  inhibiton of
    hepatic β-glucuronidase by 305
    induced formation of uroporphyrin 190
    parathion-dependent loss of cytochrome
      P-450 107
Polychlorinated biphenyls (PCBs)
  effect on
    ALA-S 180
    drug-metabolising enzymes 177
    microsomal hemoproteins 177—179
  hepatomegaly produced by 177
  induction of
    cytochrome P-450 57
    glucuronyl transferases 299
  liver damage produced by 187, 188, 193
  metabolism of 161, 162
  poisoning in Japan by 157, 172
  porphyria produced by 173
  porphyrin accumulation in chickens
    caused by 157
Polyhalogenated biphenyls
  chemistry and nomenclature 159, 160
Polyvinylpyrrolidone
  effect on bilirubin metabolism in Gunn
    rats 305
Porphin
  formula 2
Porphobilin 353
Porphobilinogen (PBG)
  accumulation in liver in porphyrias 143,
    144, 243
  excretion of in
    HCB porphyria 167, 169—171
    human porphyria 240—242
    lead poisoning 336, 346
    PCB porphyria 173
  formula 7
Porphobilinogen deaminase
  (uroporphyrinogen I synthetase)
  activity in
    DDC porphyria 143
    HCB porphyria 185
    various tissues 16, 23
  assay of 15
  genetic defect in AIP 16, 241, 353
  inhibition by lead 334, 345
  mechanism of the enzyme reaction
    16—18
Porphobilinogen oxygenase
  (PBG oxygenase)
  activity in liver microsomes 35
Porphyria
  concept of 129
  glucose effect in experimental animals 255

heme catabolism in 287
induced by
  AIA in
    birds 222
    cell cultures 201, 203,
      205—207, 210—212
    chick embryo 217, 218, 226—229
    rodents 132, 138, 224
induced by
  chlorinated benzenes (other than
    HCB) 175, 176
  DDC
    in birds 222
    in chick embryo 203, 210, 211, 223
    in rodents 129, 130, 132, 137, 139
    drug interactions 143, 144
    reversal by Na benzoate or PABA
      89
  griseofulvin
    in chick embryo 203, 218, 223
    in rodents 129, 130, 132, 136, 137,
      139
  HCB in
    man 162—167
    rat 167—171, 224
    other species 171, 172, 222
  octachlorostyrene 175
  polyhalogenated biphenyls 157,
    161, 173
  TCDD 157, 174, 175
mechanism of induction by drugs
  132—150
role of drug metabolism in 146—148
Porphyria Cutanea Tarda (PCT)
  ALA-S activity in 158
  alcoholism and 158, 171
  body iron stores in 158, 171, 176, 190,
    264
  caused by HCB 157, 162, 167
  defect of UROG-D in 158, 184, 192, 193,
    242
  excretion of porphyrins in 165—167, 171,
    184, 189, 191, 240, 245
  insensitivity to enzyme-inducing drugs
    252
  isocoproporphyrin in feces in 19
  liver damage in 187, 189, 193
  liver cytochrome P-450 in 158
  role of
    estrogens in 158, 176, 193, 242
    iron in production of 190—193
  photosensitivity in 157, 242
  in herbicide factory workers 157, 173,
    174, 220
Porphyric patients
  drugs considered safe in 230—232,
    251

Porphyrin-inducing compounds (in chick
    embryo cell cultures)
  lipophilicity of 203—208
Porphyrins
  structure of 2, 3, 7
Porphyrin-metal chelatase (heme synthetase,
    ferrochelatase)
  assay of 22, 335, 336
  activity in different tissues 23
  inhibition by
    cobalt 86—88
    DDC 31, 135—137, 144
    griseofulvin 31, 135, 136, 138
    lead 87, 88, 333, 336, 341—345,
      360
    manganese 88
  location within cell 6, 21, 22, 149
  role of copper 86, 87
  substrate specificity of 22, 84, 335, 341
Porphyrinogens (hexahydroporphyrins) 3
Potassium
  loss from erythrocytes caused by lead and
    other metals 350, 360
Pregnandiol
  induction of ALA-S by 266
  inhibition of GT by 301
5β-Pregnan-3α-17α-diol-11,20-dione
  induction of ALA-S in chick embryo 220
Pregnandione
  induction of ALA-S by 220, 266
Pregnanolone
  induction of ALA-S by 265
Pregnantriol
  induction of ALA-S by 266
Pregnenolone
  effect on PBG oxygenase 35
Pregnenolone-16-α-carbonitrile (PCN)
  inducer of
    bilirubin GT 299, 303
    cytochrome P-450 56
    hepatic Y protein 293
  increase in bile flow caused by 302, 303
Primaquine
  hemolysis induced by 239, 282
Probenecid
  bilirubin displacement by 289
  binding to Y and Z proteins 291, 292
Propentdyopents
  products of bilirubin photodegradation
    307
Progestagens
  precipitation of acute attacks of porphyria
    by 244
Progesterone
  effect on ALA-S potentiated by lead 246
  effect on ALA-S and PBG oxygenase 35,
    220

induction of cytochrome P-450 by 249
prophyrin-inducing activity in cell culture
  265
Promazine
  interference with glucuronidation 300
Propanidid
  effect on ALA-S stimulated by BNPP
    221, 232
  formula 202
  uncertain whether safe for use in porphy-
    ric patients 230—232
Propranolol
  considered safe in hereditary hepatic por-
    phyria 231, 251
2-Propyl-2-isopropylacetamide (PIA)
  comparison with AIA in inducing por-
    phyria 138, 139, 226—229
  formula 131, 202
  increase in cytochrome P-450 caused by
    139, 222
  porphyrin-inducing activity of 205, 207,
    210, 211
Prostigmine
  considered safe in hereditary hepatic por-
    phyria 251
Protein
  dietary intake and
    AIA porphyria 255, 256
    human porphyria 256
Protein synthesis
  role of in stimulation of ALA-S by drugs
    146, 148, 149
Protoporphyrin
  isomers of 2, 7
Protoporphyrin IX
  accumulation in the liver in DDC and
    griseofulvin porphyria 137
  distribution 335
  excretion of in HCB porphyria 166, 170,
    172
  excretion of in human porphyrias 240,
    242
  formula 7
  formation of in chick embryo liver cells
    189, 190, 210, 211
  in erythrocytes
    chelation with zinc 344, 345
    correlation with blood lead levels
      342—344
    correlation with bone marrow lead 343
  in anemias 335, 342
  in erythropoietic porphyria 335, 342
  in lead poisoning 335, 336, 341, 343,
    344, 358—360
  in diagnosis of lead toxicity 357, 359,
    360
  methods of assay 342, 344

Protoporphyrin IX in skin in erythropoietic
  protoporphyria 345
  spectrum of 101
Protoporphyrinogen IX 20, 21, 240
  formula 7
Protoporphyrinogen oxidase 21
Pyrazinamide 223
Pyridoxal phosphate
  cofactor for ALA-S 8, 263
Pyrimidine 5′-nucleotidase
  inhibition by lead 348
Pyruvate-kinase 281

Quinacrine
  hemolysis in G6PD deficiency 282
Quinidine
  bilirubin displacement by 289, 290
  hemolysis caused by 283
Quinine
  hemolysis caused by 283
Quinocide
  hemolysis in G6PD deficiency 282

Rhodopseudomonas spheroides
  ALA-S from 8, 10, 11
  coproporphyrinogen oxidase in 20
Rifampicin
  hemolysis caused by 283
  effect on mixed-function oxidase system
    56, 58
Rifamycin
  effect on hepatocellular bilirubin trans-
    port 291
  hepatic clearance of 291
Rifamycin SV
  binding with Y and Z liver proteins 291,
    292
RNA
  increase of messenger type after lipid-solu-
    ble drugs 145, 147—149
Rose bengal
  excretion by hepatocyte 280
  hepatic clearance of 291
  interference with glucuronidation 300
  reduction in bile flow caused by 302

Safrole
  inducer of cytochrome P-450 57
Salicylates
  bilirubin displacement caused by
    288—290
  binding to ligandin 292
  effect on
    pyruvate-kinase deficient erythrocytes
      281
    serum bilirubin in Gunn rats 306
Salicylamide
  metabolism of in AIP 249, 251

Scleroderma 90
Secobarbital
  conversion to an epoxide 103
  formula 202
  inducer of ALA-S 221, 225, 232
  induction of porphyrins caused by 219,
    222, 224, 225
  loss of cytochrome P-450 caused by 103,
    287
  precipitation of acute attacks of porphyr-
    ia 230, 232
Secretin
  increase in bile flow caused by 302
Sedormid (allylisopropylacetylurea)
  effect on liver catalase 142
  formula 202
  hepatic porphyria caused by 201
  production of green pigments by 98
Serine dehydratase
  glucose effect on 257, 259
  induction by
    glucagon 259
    tryptophan 258
Serum
  effect on porphyrin formation in cell cul-
    ture 210, 211
Sex difference
  in response to halogenated compounds
    170, 179, 187
Sex hormones
  effect on heme synthesis 265
Sickle cell anemia
  lead toxicity in 357
  zinc deficiency in 357
SKF 525-A (2-Diethylaminoethyl-
    3,3-diphenylpropylacetate)
  effect on
    PIA metabolism in liver 223, 225
    hexobarbital metabolism in liver 223,
      225
  inhibition of
    AIA-dependant loss of cytochrome P-
      450 48, 102
    ALA-S induction 146, 147
    bilirubin GT 300
    induced uroprophyrin formation 190
Skin lesions
  in HCB porphyria 163, 164, 168, 169
  in PCT 157
Sodium benzoate
  bilirubin displacement by 288—290
  reversal of DDC porphyria by 89, 90
Sodium dehydrocholate
  inhibition of bilirubin excretion by
    303
Sodium meralluride
  bilirubin displacement by 289, 290

Spironolactone
  increase in
    bile flow   302, 303
    bilirubin GT   299, 303
    hepatic Y protein   293
  inducer of cytochrome P-450   56
Starvation
  effect on liver heme metabolism   111, 112,
    117—119
  induction of heme oxygenase by   117, 287
Stercobilin   5
Steroids
  binding by ligandin   292
  effect on bile flow and bilirubin excretion
    302
  excretion of in porphyria   266
  17-alkylated (anabolic)
    cholestasis produced by   304
5α-H Steroids
  prophyrin-inducing activity of   223
5β-H Steroids
  basic formula   202
  effect on ALA-S   35, 219, 224, 265
  prophyrin-inducing activity of   223
  production in AIP   266
  stimulation of hemoglobin synthesis by
    29, 30, 265
Steroyl-CoA desaturase system   66
Stibophen
  hemolysis caused by   283
Streptomycin
  considered safe in hereditary hepatic por-
    phyria   230, 231
  interference with glucuronidation   300
Succinate
  effect on induction of ALA-S   261
  reversal of acetate inhibition of ALA-S   90
Succinate dehydrogenase
  inhibition by metalloporphyrins   348
Succinate-glycine cycle   258
Succinimides
  precipitation of acute attacks of porphyria
    by   244
Succinyl-CoA
  availability for heme biosynthesis   32, 90,
    91
Succinyl CoA synthetase   11, 32
Sulfanilamide
  reversal of DDC porphyria by   90
Sulfapyridine
  hemolysis in G6PD deficiency by   282
Sulfate
  conjugation with bilirubin   279
Sulfhemoglobinemia
  caused by phenacetin   281
Sulfisoxazole
  hemolysis in G6PD deficiency   282

Sulfobromophthalein (see BSP)
Sulfonamides
  displacement of bilirubin caused by
    288—290
  hemolysis due to   282, 283
  kernicterus caused by   288
  precipitation of acute attacks of porphyria
    by   230, 231, 244
Sulfonic acid
  hemolysis due to   282
Sulfur
  reactive form produced from
    CS_2 106—109
    phosphorothionates   107, 108
Surmesan   162

Taurine
  conjugation with bilirubin   279
Taurocholate
  production of cholestasis by   304
Taurolithocholate
  production of cholestasis by   304
Terpene compounds
  porphyrin-inducing activity in cell cul-
    tures   202, 203, 208
Testosterone
  effect
    in HCB porphyria   170
    on erythropoietin   265
  increase in cytochrome P-450 caused by   62
  production of porphyrins in cell culture
    265
Tetrachlorocatechol
  metabolite of HCB   161
1,2,4,5-Tetrachlorobenzene   175
  formed from HCB in the gut   161
2,3,7,8-Tetrachlorodibenzo-p-dioxin
  (TCDD)
  acute toxicity of   162, 175
  analogues of
    induction of ALA-S in chick
      embryo by   220
  binding protein in mouse liver   61
  contaminant of 2,4,5-T   61, 157, 174, 220
  effect on mixed-function oxidase system
    57, 61, 66, 177, 179
  formula   158, 202
  increase in kidney Y protein caused by
    293
  induction of ALA-S in chick embryo   157,
    175, 220
  liver damage caused by   187, 188, 193
  porphyria cutanea tarda caused by   173, 220
  production of
    prophyria in mice   157, 175, 187,
      192
    uroporphyrin in cell cultures   189

Tetrachlorodibenzofuran 175
Tetrachlorophenol 190
Tetrachloroquinone
  metabolite of HCB 161
Tetracycline
  bilirubin displacement by 288, 290
Tetraethyl lead
  lymphoma produced in mice 355
  toxicity of 355
N,N,N′,N′-Tetramethyl-p-
  phenylenediamine 114
2,3,5,6-Tetramethylterephthalate
  (diethyl ester)
  porphyrin-inducing activity in cell cul-
    tures 204, 205
Thalidomide
  induction of ALA-S in chick embryo 219,
    221
Theophylline
  effect on ALA-S induction 260 – 262
  increase in bile flow caused by 302
  induction of ornithine decarboxylase 260
Thiazide diuretics
  production of cholestasis and hyperbiliru-
    binemia by 304
Thiazosulfone
  hemolysis in G6PD deficiency 282
Thiopental
  induction of ALA-S in different species
    221, 222, 225
  precipitation of acute attacks of porphyria
    by 230, 231, 244
Threonine dehydrase
  induction repressed by carbohydrate feed-
    ing 256
α-Thujone 203
β-Thujone 203
Thyroid
  effect of aminotriazole on 83
Thyroxine
  binding to Z protein 292
  increase in NADPH-cytochrome c-reduc-
    tase by 62
  mitochondrial changes induced by 69
α-Tocopherol 116
Tolbutamide
  bilirubin displacement by 288 – 290
  inducer of cytochrome P-450 56
  precipitation of acute attacks of porphyria
    by 230, 231, 244
2,4,5-Trichlorophenoxyacetic acid
  (2,4,5-T)
  porphyria in workers exposed to 157,
    173, 174
  commercial product contaminated with
    TCDD 61, 174, 220
Trihydrocoprostane

induction of ALA-S by 266
Triiodothyronine
  effect on AIA-mediated induction of
    ALA-S 264
Tryptophan
  induction of
    ALA-S 257
    tryptophan pyrrolase 52, 53
Tryptophan pyrrolase 4, 5
  after AIA treatment 135
  and regulatory heme 141, 146
  biological half-life 50, 51
  contribution to heme catabolic pool 283
  heme saturation of 142
  induction by cortisone, tryptophan and
    drugs 49, 51 – 53, 69, 259
  role in induction of ALA-S by trypto-
    phan 257
Tumors
  induced by lead 355
Tyrosine aminotransferase
  glucose effect on 257, 261
  induction by
    cortisone 51, 52
    cyclic AMP 259
    glucagon 259
    hydrocortisone 259
    tryptophan 258

UDP-Glucose 27
  treatment of hyperbilirubinemia with 301
UDP-Glucose dehydrogenase 301
UDP-Glucuronic acid
  effect of drugs on supply of 64, 301
  substrate for UDP-glucuronyl transferase
    27, 278
UDP-Glucuronyl transferase
  (see glucuronyl transferases, GT)
UDP-xylose 27
Urate oxidase 68
Urobilogens
  excretion of 280
  formation from bilirubin 280
Uroporphyrin
  accumulation and storage in hepatocytes
    189
  excretion in
    HCB porphyria 164 – 166, 168, 169,
      171, 176
    lead poisoning 336, 346
    PCB porphyria 173, 176
    PCT 189, 240, 242
  isomers of 2
  formation in cell culture 189, 190, 210, 211
Uroporphyrinogen I
  product of PBG deaminase 6, 14, 16
  substrate for UROG-D 19, 181

Uroporphyrinogen III 6, 15—19
  formula 7
  substrate for UROG-D 181, 182
Uroporphyrinogen decarboxylase (UROG-
  D)
  activity in
    PCT 184, 192, 193, 158, 242
    porphyria caused by polyhalogenated
      compounds 180—186, 188—190,
      192, 193, 210
  effect of iron on 191, 192
  inhibition by SH reagents 19
  mechanism of the enzyme reaction 18, 19
  properties 18, 19
  substrates for 181, 182
Uroporphyrinogen III cosynthetase 14—18
  activity in
    congenital erythropoietic porphyria 15
    human, mouse and squirrel tissues 15
    PCT 191
  assay 15
Uroporphyrinogen I synthetase
  (see porphobilinogen deaminase)

Valeramide 203
Valium
  used in neonates to lower serum bilirubin
    298
Variegate Porphyria (VP)
  glucose effect in 156
  induction of ALA-S in 252
  porphyrin excretion 240, 242
  photosensitivity in 242
Vitamin B
  safe in hereditary hepatic porphyria 251
Vitamin B$_{12}$

corrin ring of 2
  deficiency anemia
    decreased red cell protoporphyrin
      in 335
Vitamin C
  safe in hereditary hepatic porphyria 251
Vitamin E 112
  safe in hereditary hepatic porphyria 251
Vitamin K
  hemolysis in G6PD deficiency 282
  hyperbilirubinemia in neonates caused by
    300

Y Protein (see Ligandin)

Z Protein
  compounds which bind to 292
  diminished by DDT and dieldrin 293
  increased by clofibrate and nafenopin 68,
    293
  role in uptake and transport of bilirubin
    277, 278
Zinc
  chelation with protoporphyrin 344, 345
  deficiency in sickle cell anemia 357
  loss of cytochrome P-450 caused by 115,
    116
  role of in ALA dehydratase activity 334,
    338, 357, 360
  stimulation of heme oxygenase by 116
Zinc-protoporphyrin
  in erythrocytes 344
    in iron-deficiency anemia 344, 348
    in lead poisoning 345, 348, 357
Zoxazolamine
  hydroxylation of 177

Handbuch der experimentellen Pharmakologie/ Handbook of Experimental Pharmacology

Heffter-Heubner, New Series

Volume 4:

General Pharmacology

Volume 10:

Die Pharmakologie anorganischer Anionen

Volume 11:

Lobelin und Lobeliaalkaloide

Volume 12:

Morphin und morphin-ähnlich wirkende Verbindungen

Volume 14: Part 1

The Adrenocortical Hormones I

Part 2
The Adrenocortical Hormones II

Part 3
The Adrenocortical Hormones III

Volume 16:

Erzeugung von Krank-heitszuständen durch das Experiment/ Experimental Production of Diseases

Part 1
Blut (In Vorbereitung)

Part 2
Atemwege

Part 3
Heart and Circulation

Part 4
Niere, Nierenbecken, Blase

Part 5
Liver

Part 6
Schilddrüse
(In Vorbereitung)

Part 7
Zentralnervensystem

Part 8
Stütz- und Hartgewebe

Part 9
Infektionen I

Part 10
Infektionen II

Part 11A
Infektionen III

Part 11B
Infektionen IV

Part 12
Tumoren I

Part 13
Tumoren II

Part 14
Tumoren III
(In preparation)

Part 15
Kohlenhydratstoff-wechsel, Fieber/ Carbohydrate Metabolism, Fever

Volume 17: Part 1

Ions alcalino-terreux I

Part 2
Ions alcalino-terreux II

Volume 18: Part 1
Histamine

Part 2
Anti-Histaminics

Volume 19:

5-Hydroxytryptamine and Related Indolealkylamines

Volume 20: Part 1

Pharmacology of Fluorides I

Part 2
Pharmacology of Fluorides II

Volume 21:

Beryllium

Volume 22: Part 1

Die Gestagene I

Part 2
Die Gestagene II

Volume 23:

Neurohypophysial Hormones and Similar Polipeptides

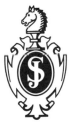

Springer-Verlag
Berlin
Heidelberg
New York

Handbuch der experimentellen Pharmakologie/ Handbook of Experimental Pharmacology

Heffter-Heubner, New Series

Volume 24:

Diuretica

Volume 25:

Bradykinin, Kallidin and Kallikrein

Volume 26:

Vergleichende Pharmakologie von Überträgersubstanzen in tiersystematischer Darstellung

Volume 27:

Anticoagulantien

Volume 28: Part 1

Concepts in Biochemical Pharmacology I
Part 3
Concepts in Biochemical Pharmacology III

Volume 29:

Oral wirksame Antidiabetika

Volume 30:

Modern Inhalation Anesthetics

Volume 32: Part 1

Insulin I
Part 2
Insulin II

Volume 34:

Secretin, Cholecystokinin, Pancreozymin and Gastrin

Volume 35: Part 1

Androgene I

Part 2
Androgens II and Antiandrogens/ Androgene II und Antiandrogene

Volume 36:

Uranium – Plutonium – Transplutonic Elements

Volume 37:

Angiotensin

Volume 38: Part 1

Antieoplastic and and Immunosuppressive Agents I

Part 2
Antineoplastic and Immunosuppressive Agents II

Volume 39:

Antihypertensive Agents

Volume 40:

Organic Nitrates

Volume 41:

Hypolipidemic Agents

Volume 42:

Neuromuscular Junction

Volume 43:

Anabolic-Androgenic Steroids

Volume 44:

Haem and Haemoproteins

Volume 45: Part 1
Drug Addiction I
Part 2
Drug Addiction II

Volume 46:

Fibrinolytics and Antifibrinolytics
(In Preparation)

Volume 47:

Kinetics of Drug Action

Volume 48:

Arthropod Venoms

Volume 49:

Gangliomic Transmission (In preparation)

Volume 50:

Inflammation and Antiinflammatory Drugs
(In preparation)

Volume 51:

Ergot Alkaloids and Related Compounds
(In preparation)

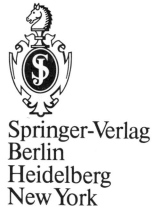

Springer-Verlag
Berlin
Heidelberg
New York